Stress and Immunity

Nicholas Plotnikoff
Anthony Murgo
Robert Faith
Joseph Wybran

CRC Press
Boca Raton Ann Arbor London

Library of Congress Cataloging-in-Publication Data

Stress and immunity / [editors] Nicholas P. Plotnikoff . . . [et al.].
    p.   cm.
    Includes bibliographical references and index.
    1. Stress (Physiology)   2. Stress (Psychology)   3. Psychoneuroimmunology.   I. Plotnikoff,
Nicholas P.
    [DNLM: 1. Adjuvants, Immunologic.   2. Endorphins—immunology.   3. Stress—
immunology.   4. Stress, Psychological—immunology.   QZ 160 S9143]
QP82.2.S8S863   1991
616.07'9—dc20
DNLM/DLC   91-10821
                                                                                     CIP

Developed by Telford Press

© 1991 by CRC Press, Inc.

International Standard Book Number 0-8493-8845-7

Library of Congress Card Number 91-10821
Printed in the United States of America   1 2 3 4 5 6 7 8 9 0

WE DEDICATE THIS BOOK TO THE MEMORY OF
PROFESSOR JOSEPH WYBRAN

MEMORIUM FOR JOSEPH WYBRAN

October 1989 will always stand in our memory as a time of loss. Joseph Wybran's death by an unknown assassin was a shock to the entire scientific community. We will miss him very much!

Dr. Joseph Wybran was the Director of the Department of Immunology, Hematology, Transfusion at Hospital Erasme, Universite Libre de Bruxelles. In his memory, it is fitting to reflect on his many achievements and contributions to the progress of medicine. The most widely quoted studies by Professor Wybran were "the human rosette forming cell as a marker of a population of thymus-derived cells," as well as "isolation of normal T cells in chronic lymphatic leukemia" and "thymus-derived rosette forming cells in human disease states: cancer, lymphomas, viral and bacterial infections and other diseases." His research included studies on transfer factor, thymosin, BCG, levamisole, lynestrenol, isoprisosine, imuthiol, corticosteroids, cyclosporine, interferons, tumor necrosis factor, interleukin 2, and methionine enkephalin. It can be said that he was one of the early pioneers of immunomodulation research. Perhaps one of his most outstanding contributions was the discovery of opioid peptide receptors on human T cells. This basic finding led to a series of *in vitro* studies demonstrating that the opioid peptides (methionine and leucine enkephalin) were potent immunomodulators, increasing T cells, B cells, macrophage activation, mitogen blastogenesis, chemotaxis, as well as natural killer (NK), killer (K), and lymphokine activated killer (LAK) cell functions. These basic immunological functions of the opioid peptides were focused in terms of stress responses. Clearly, the enkephalins were defined as stress hormones being released from the adrenal glands concomitantly with the steroid hormones and catecholamines.

The important finding in recent years that murine T helper cells contained the prohormone for methionine enkephalin, proenkephalin A, adds further significance to Joe Wybran's discovery of lymphocyte associated opioid receptors. In the presence of mitogen activation, post-translational processing of the prohormone occurred releasing methionine enkephalin peptides into the media. Like interleukin 2 and gamma interferon, it can now be said that methionine enkephalin is an interleukin, a potent lymphokine of the immune system. All of these exciting discoveries of the role of the enkephalins in the immune system can clearly be credited to the original discovery of enkephalin receptors on human T cells by Professor Wybran.

The clinical application of these basic developments are manifold and still very much in progress. Professor Wybran was always considered by his many friends a world-class scientist and a gentleman. He was always warmly received at scientific meetings and his presentations well attended. His patient attitude was particularly helpful in our collaborative studies which required frequent communication. In conclusion, we offer this present consortium of outstanding contributions to the field of stress and immunity as a lasting tribute to the memory of Professor Wybran, who, in reflection, helped set the stage for the clinical development of immunomodulators.

DISCLAIMER STATEMENT

This book was co-authored by Dr. Anthony J. Murgo in his private capacity. No official support or endorsement by the Food and Drug Administration is intended or should be inferred.

CONTENTS

Part I
Clinical Studies on Stress and Immunity

Stress-Associated Modulation of the Immune Response in Humans

Joel E. Hillhouse
Department of Medical Microbiology and Immunology,
The Ohio State University Medical Center,
Columbus, Ohio

Janice K. Kiecolt-Glaser
Department of Psychiatry,
The Ohio State University Medical Center,
Columbus, Ohio

Ronald Glaser
Department of Medical Microbiology and Immunology,
The Ohio State University Medical Center,
Columbus, Ohio

INTRODUCTION

The proposed relationships between emotional and disease states have a long and colorful history. As early as the second century A.D., Galen reported that melancholy women appeared more likely to develop cancer than sanguine women. Despite the lengthy history of such conjectures, it is only recently that the knowledge base and methodological skills have sufficiently developed to allow empirical testing of these ideas.

Psychoneuroimmunology (PNI), as the field has come to be known, has its roots in ancient ideas and practices (Lloyd, 1987). Scientific exploration of this topic has progressed slowly over several decades, only to explode in the 1980s following the publication of Ader and Cohen's landmark work (Ader and Cohen, 1975). The complexity of the fields subsumed by PNI (psychology, behavioral medicine, endocrinology, neuroscience, and immunology, to name a few) have provided a wealth of information. However, this very complexity poses problems for the researcher trying to integrate and study this area. In this chapter, we will attempt to overview the relevant human studies in this expanding field, in particular, highlighting major areas of human studies with respect to specific types of stressors, health implications, and effects.

DEPRESSION AND BEREAVEMENT

Among the earliest reported human work in this area was a study by Bartrop et al. (1977) that explored the effects of spousal death on mitogen-stimulated lymphocyte proliferation. These researchers examined immune function (T- and B-lymphocyte number and function) in 26 bereaved spouses 2 and 6 weeks after bereavement; 26 hospital staff members served as controls. Results indicated that average T-cell function as measured by mitogen-induced stimulation was reduced following bereavement.

In a later prospective study, Schleifer et al. (1983) examined 16 men whose wives were dying of breast cancer. Peripheral blood was collected before and after the wives' deaths. Blastogenic responses following the death of their spouse were significantly suppressed compared to both prebereavement values. Consistent with these results, Irwin et al. (1989) reported that women whose husbands had recently died of lung cancer evidenced greater depression in immune function than women whose husbands were undergoing treatment for metastatic lung cancer, or women with healthy husbands. In a related study, Linn et al. (1984) found that only bereaved subjects with high depressive symptom scores (measured by the Hopkins Symptom Check List) demonstrated reduced lymphocyte responsiveness.

One possible explanation for the change in the immune response seen in bereaved subjects involves the mediating role of depression. The Linn et al. (1984) study provides some support for this hypothesis since bereavement in the absence of moderate to severe depression was not sufficient to bring about immune change.

A number of studies have further examined the relationship between depression and immune function. Stein and colleagues have performed a series of studies looking at the depression-immune function relationship. In their initial study, they found that depressed subjects had lower total T- and B-lymphocyte numbers, as well as lower mitogen-induced lymphocyte stimulation (Schleifer et al., 1984). These results were not replicated in a follow-up study (Schleifer et al., 1985). However, in a more recent study (Schleifer et al., 1989), while they did not find differences between depressed patients and controls in lymphocyte stimulation, natural killer (NK) cell activity, or lymphocyte numbers, there were age- and severity-related differences (i.e., as age and severity increased, there appeared to be an increasing negative association between depression and immune function).

In contrast, some studies have failed to find a relationship between depression and the immune system. Albrecht and colleagues (1985) studied 27 depressed patients and did not find altered immune function relative to normal controls. Similarly, Sengers et al. (1982) reported normal T- and B-cell function and numbers in 25 manic-depressed patients. However, both research groups provide an interpretational caveat, i.e., their results may have been affected by the treatment (e.g., electroconvulsive therapy, lithium, and/or tricyclic antidepressants) that a majority of the patients were concurrently receiving.

Considering specific mechanisms, some researchers have conjectured that depression and immune function are linked through cortisol secretion. Several studies have found both suppressed immune function and increased cortisol secretion in depressed subjects (Schleifer et al., 1984, 1989; Kronfol and House, 1984; Denney et al., 1988). Stein and colleagues (1985) have further suggested that immune changes may be related to underlying biological processes associated with depression. However, it must be pointed out that in the Denney et al. (1988) study, cortisol levels were not related to any lymphocyte measure, nor was cortisol related to depression itself. Furthermore, it is apparent in the depression literature that only subsets of depressed patients exhibit the abnormal cortisol secretion patterns (Rubin et al., 1987). As these relationships are not unambiguous, such findings should be interpreted cautiously. Further work in this area should attempt to more clearly delineate the relationships among cortisol, depression, and immune function. Special emphasis might be given to those suppressed patients who do exhibit abnormal cortisol patterns. There is also a need to look carefully at cortisol measurement methods.

Other researchers have considered the depression-immune relationship from a different angle, positing a role for the effect of chronic stress associated with depression. The link between chronic and acute stressors in immune function will be explored in the following sections.

ACUTE OR COMMONPLACE STRESSORS

In contrast to chronic stress, there is a relatively large body of literature that has examined more commonplace, or "acute" stressors. Lazarus and Folkman (1984) have suggested that everyday hassles and stressors are better predictors of health and psychological problems. The study of acute stressors provides methodological advantages as well, allowing for better experimental manipulation, as well as more careful delineation of mechanisms and direct health consequences.

A favorite paradigm for examining immunological effects of acute stressors has involved the study of college or postgraduate students engaged in examinations. As early as 1950, several researchers had begun assessing the immunological effects of examination stress (Humphreys and Raab, 1950; Kerr, 1955). More recently, research in our own and several other laboratories has utilized this stress paradigm.

Dorian and colleagues (Dorian et al., 1981, 1982) explored the effects of oral examinations on psychiatry residents compared to age- and sex-matched physician controls. Results indicated higher levels of emotional distress, reduced mitogen-induced lymphocyte proliferation, and some evidence for higher T- and B-lymphocyte counts in the preexamination residents, when compared to either controls or their own postexamination values.

Halvorsen and Vassend (1987) measured the psychological and immunological status of 12 psychology undergraduates taking an examination and 11 control subjects. Preexamination students demonstrated higher anxiety, greater self-reported distress, increased numbers of circulating monocytes, reduced expression of interleukin-1 (IL-2) receptors, and a reduction in lymphocyte responsiveness to PHA.

We have conducted a series of studies in our laboratory examining the relationship of examination stressors to changes in psychological and immune functioning in first- and second-year medical students. Our basic design involves a battery of psychological assessments and quantitative and functional immunological assays administered during a relatively nonstressed period (usually the beginning of the quarter, or immediately following spring, Christmas, or summer break) as well as during the week of their mid-terms or final examinations. The medical school curriculum at Ohio State University is such that the entire medical student class cycles through several 3-d examination blocks over the academic year.

The results of the first study revealed that examination stress was associated with declines in NK activity (Kiecolt-Glaser et al., 1984). Evidence of a decrease in NK cell number was shown in a second study that utilized a different target cell (Glaser et al., 1986b). In subsequent studies, we have identified changes in total T-lymphocytes, T_4/T_8 ratios, mitogen responsiveness, γ-interferon production by mitogen-stimulated peripheral blood leukocytes (PBLs), and ability of the cellular immune response to control latent herpesviruses (Glaser et al., 1985a; Glaser et al., 1987).

This last finding is of particular interest, as it may have implications for health-related outcomes. Significant changes in antibody titers to herpesviruses are thought to reflect functional changes in cellular immunity systems

(Henle and Henle, 1982). For example, it has been noted that immunosuppressed patients (i.e.,those with immunosuppressive illnesses or receiving immunosuppressive therapy) characteristically have elevated herpesvirus antibody titers. Elevation in antibody titers is thought to reflect inability of the cellular immune response to control the reactivation of viral products and infectious virus. We have found increased antibody titers to three herpesviruses: EBV, the etiological agent for infectious mononucleosis (IM), HSV-1 responsible for cold sores, and CMV, which produces a mononucleosis syndrome.

Recent findings have indicated that the activity of a lymphokine-designated leukocyte migration inhibition factor (LIF) that is suppressed during recrudescence of HSV type 2 infections (Sheridan et al., 1982) was also suppressed during examination periods. Also associated with examination stress were alterations in plasma and intracellular levels of cyclic AMP. This last finding may point to a possible mechanism explaining the changes in PBLs in the cellular immune response. Lastly, more self-reported illnesses were associated with exam periods than with baseline (Glaser et al., 1987).

With regard to psychological variables, several studies from our laboratory have identified a relationship between loneliness and decreased immune function (Kiecolt-Glaser et al., 1984; Glaser et al., 1985a). Lonelier students had poorer immune function than their less lonely counterparts. This represents an interesting finding, as it implies a potential role for personal relationships and/or social relations in affecting or buffering immune system changes.

A number of studies have examined the influence of examination stress on endocrine function. Hellhammer et al. (1985) studied ten healthy males taking final examinations in medicine or psychology. These authors found a relationship between salivary cortisol levels and examination stress, in which inadequate coping attempts were positively correlated with cortisol elevations. However, as cortisol levels were abnormally high in control (non-exam) subjects, this suggests that students may in fact represent a chronically stressed sample. In a similar study, Hudgens et al. (1989) found elevated cortisol levels both before and after an examination in 18 third- and fourth-year medical students. Prolactin levels, however, were elevated only during preexamination. Luteinizing hormone levels were negatively correlated with anxiety levels both before and after the examination. The finding of elevated cortisol levels at both time points is suggestive of the experience of a more chronic stressor.

Extended space flight is yet another long-term mental and physical stressor in which immunological measures have been studied. Kimzey (1975) reported that sky lab astronauts had a depressed lymphocyte proliferative response to PHA post-flight as compared to pre-flight. He also reported a reduction in circulating T-lymphocytes. Taylor and Dardano (1983) reported lower post-flight lymphocyte stimulation to PHA in the space shuttle astronauts. They reported a relationship between crew member ranking in terms of in-flight difficulties and decreased blastogenic response. In contrast, Voss (1984) failed to find any postflight differences in serum IgG, IgA, and IgM levels in sky lab astronauts.

In examining the effects of stress on immune function, few studies have utilized laboratory stressors. In a series of experiments, Palmblad and colleagues (Palmblad et al., 1976, 1979) examined the effects of sleep deprivation on immunological responses. In the first study, 8 female subjects underwent a 77-h sleep deprivation stressor. Results indicated that interferon-producing capacity rose during and after the vigil. Decreases in phagocytic activity were also demonstrated during the sleep deprivation period. In the second study, 12 male students participated in a 48-h sleep deprivation paradigm. Phyto-hemagglutinin-induced lymphocyte stimulation was reduced following the stressor.

In an another example of an experimentally manipulated stressor, Landmann et al. (1984) subjected 15 normal individuals to a mental stress test (a variation of the Stroops Color-Word Conflict Test). This brief psychological stressor was found to produce higher cortisol levels, slight increases in lymphocyte and leukocyte numbers, and a significant increase in the number of circulating monocytes.

The greater ease of experimental manipulation in measurement of physiological response provided by laboratory-induced stressors makes them particularly attractive at this point in the field's development. Nevertheless, these manipulations must be carefully thought out, not only with regard to the psychological stressor itself, but in relation to the kinetics of the endocrine and immunological measures of interest as well. Such experimentally manipulated stressors could provide elegant methods with which to carefully map out the mechanisms and kinetics of these complex relationships.

As noted with chronic stress, the acute stress literature also demonstrates relatively robust and consistent findings of generally reduced immune function in response to stress. However, the mechanisms behind these effects remain unclear. To clarify these relationships, a careful examination of the interaction of psychological stress and endocrine and immunological systems is needed. Such a study is currently in progress in our laboratory.

Utilizing a paradigm of baseline nonstress and examination stress, we are currently assessing the subgroup of medical students with regard to psychological, endocrinolial, and immunological factors in collaboration with Dr. William Malarkey. One hundred male medical students (20 students per year over 5 years) will provide 24-h samplings of various "stress hormones" from blood taken at the following intervals: 1 month prior to, within 3 d of, and 2 weeks after a major examination. We will be assaying growth hormone, prolactin, adrenalcorticotropic hormone (ACTH), cortisol, and catecholamines along with immunological measures. Subjects will also complete a battery of psychological and health assessments. In this study, it is hoped that we will be better able to delineate the interactions and mechanisms involved in stress-endocrine-immune relationships.

CHRONIC STRESSORS

There are a variety of studies examining the effects of chronic stressors on immune function in humans. Among the stressors studied are divorce/separation, caregiving for Alzheimer's disease (AD) patients, the effects of extended space flight, and living near the Three-Mile Island (TMI) nuclear power plant.

Epidemiological data indicate that separated and divorced individuals are at a greater risk for mental and physical illness on an acturial basis than married, single, or widowed individuals (Bloom et al., 1978; Verbrugge, 1979). Divorce can be conceptualized as a chronic stressor for those experiencing it, since adjustment appears to occur over several years (Weiss, 1975). Furthermore, continued preoccupation with the (ex)spouse (attachment to the former spouse) has been hypothesized to lead to distress-related symptoms (Weiss, 1975).

We have examined the immunological effects of divorce as a chronic stressor in two studies (Kiecolt-Glaser et al., 1987a, 1988). In the first study, 38 separated/divorced women were compared to sociodemographically matched married controls. Immunological assays included mitogen-stimulated lymphocyte proliferation to Con A and PHA, antibody titers to a latent herpesvirus, Epstein-Barr virus (EBV), and T- and NK cell numbers. The separated/divorced group evidenced significantly higher EBV antibody titers, significantly lower percentages of NK cells, and significantly different blastogenic response to PHA. Furthermore, "attachment" to the former spouse was negatively associated with immune function in this group.

In a follow-up study examining the effects of marital discord in males, 32 separated/divorced men were compared with matched married controls. Separated/divorced men appeared more psychologically distressed, lonelier, and reported more recent illnesses than married men. These individuals also had significantly poorer immune function in terms of antibody titers to EBV and herpes simplex virus type 1 (HSV), and T-helper to suppressor ratios. Separated/divorced men who had both initiated the separation and were separated within the last year appeared less distressed and reported better health than the noninitiators.

Caring for a patient with AD also represents a chronic stressor. Research has indicated that AD caregivers are at high risk for depression (Crook and Miller, 1985). We have been studying the immunological effects of this long-term stressor in our laboratory (Kiecolt-Glaser et al., 1987b). Immunological and psychological data were collected from 34 caregivers and 34 matched comparison subjects. Caregivers demonstrated significantly greater emotional distress (as measured by the Beck Depression Inventory and other self-report assessments) and generally poorer immune functioning (e.g., higher EBV antibody titers and lower percentage of T-lymphocytes, and helper T-lymphocytes).

Living near the site of the nuclear disaster at TMI has also been examined as another potential chronic stressor (McKinnon et al., in press). There were persistent behavioral and endocrinological differences in TMI residents compared to matched controls living 80 miles from the power plant. These differences include elevated levels of urinary epinephrine and norepinephrine, as well as elevated cortisol levels. Immunological data revealed that the TMI residents have fewer B-lymphocytes, NK cells, and suppressor T-lymphocytes than comparison subjects. Differences have also been reported with regard to neutrophil numbers and antibody titers to cytomegalovirus (CMV), another latent herpesvirus. Thus, across a variety of subjects, situations, and immunological measures, chronic stressors appear to have deleterious effects on the immune system. However, the effects have not typically been either strong or consistent. Unfortunately, up to this time, little attempt has been made to delineate the kinetics, nor have the health implications been carefully examined. It would seem that one of the major problems facing this area is the absence of a strong conceptual base underlying the categorization of the psychological stressors or their individual effects. There is growing evidence that specific stressors can exert specific physiological reactions, and therefore may have specific immunological effects.

INFECTIOUS DISEASE

The influence of stress on the incidence and duration of infectious disease is one interesting area of study with particular relevance to health. In an early, often-cited study, Kasl et al. (1979) examined psychosocial risk factors in the development of IM in a class of 1400 West Point cadets. The cadets who became infected and developed clinical IM could be distinguished from the infected cadets not manifesting clinical symptoms of IM on the basis of three factors: (1) having fathers who were overachievers, (2) having higher levels of motivation for a military career, and (3) scoring poorly on indices of relative academic performance. These factors were also related to length of stay in the hospital and levels of EBV antibody titers.

In a laboratory-controlled experiment, Broadbent et al. (1984) reported that virus shedding in subjects experimentally exposed to rhinoviruses and influenza viruses was related to their personality status as either introverts or extroverts. Individuals who reported greater distress on a self-report inventory had more evidence of nasal secretion after infection. Other researchers (Clover et al., 1989) have found that infection with influenza B virus was associated with family cohesion and adaptability (measured by the Family Adaptability and Cohesion Scale), thus suggesting that family dysfunction may be related to altered immune response.

A series of studies have focused on the role of psychosocial factors in the recurrence of herpes labialis and the herpes viruses associated with cold sores (HSV-1 and HSV-2), or genital herpes. In their examination of the incidence of cold sore recurrence in a group of 61 nursing students, Katcher et al. (1973) found that psychosocial factors such as mood, social assets, and life change were able to account for 14% of their recurrence variance. In a follow-up study, Friedmann and colleagues (1977) found that mood was negatively associated with cold sore recurrence in 149 nurses.

Other studies have focused on the recurrence rates of genital herpes. Goldmeier and Johnson (1982) studied 58 patients with confirmed genital herpes. Patients evidencing higher distress demonstrated a much greater rate of recurrence than did less distressed patients. Schmidt et al. (1985) examined the role of stress in 35 genital herpes patients. The authors found that patients reported an increase in stressful life events, elevated anxiety, and increased daily hassles and frustrations prior to the appearance of a recurrent lesion, in contrast to the period after the lesion had disappeared. On a subgroup of 10 patients, these same authors collected immunological data 0 to 3 d after the appearance of a lesion, and found blunted T-lymphocyte blastogenesis at time of recurrence compared to nonrecurrent periods.

Silver et al. (1986) examined the relationship of psychological factors in recurrent HSV-induced lesions. HSV recurrences and pain were related to level of psychological distress. The most important variable in this study appeared to be coping strategies, as the greatest rates of recurrence were found in those subjects who took an emotional-focused, avoidant-coping approach. Vanderplate et al. (1988) examined the role of stress on HSV lesions as moderated by social support. Results indicated that both duration of disease and disease-specific social support were significant moderators of the relationship between HSV recurrence and stress in their 59 subjects. Specifically, when illness duration is short, stress and number of recurrences are positively associated. No relationship was noted with longer duration. At lower levels of social support, there was a positive relationship of stress to recurrence; however, with high support, no relationship was found.

Lastly, Kemeny and colleagues (1989) performed a prospective study that examined stress, life change, mood, HSV recurrence, and several immunological measures. While stress and mood scores were found to be uncorrelated with HSV recurrence, they were negatively associated with the proportion of helper and suppressor T-lymphocytes in the overall sample. Although helper T-lymphocyte proportions were not related to recurrence, suppressor T-cells were negatively correlated with this variable. An association between depressive mood and recurrence was found in those patients not experiencing other infections.

The potential value of this line of research cannot be overstated, as the herpes virus literature provides a linkage between psychosocial factors and health behaviors that is crucial to this field. However, a majority of the reported studies have been retrospective in nature, and must be interpreted with caution, particularly with regard to inferences of causality. Furthermore, few of the studies have attempted to assess immunological function as well as disease status, with the exception of Kemeny et al. (1989). Based on the results of our medical student studies with regard to herpesvirus antibody titers, it is interesting to conjecture direct links among stress, immune function, and disease recurrence. However, the mechanism underlying this relationship awaits more accurate delineation. It would be of great interest to prospectively examine the relationships among stress, endocrine measures, carefully chosen immunological measures, and health status, such as HSV recurrence.

CANCER

Another area of interest is the relationship of psychosocial variables to cancer. Considerable literature has developed over the years, and will not be fully reviewed here. Temoshok et al. (1985) have suggested that this rather prodigious literature could be divided into seven main categories. Of these, the categories of major interest to PNI include (1) studies examining psychosocial characteristics of noncancer patients vs. cancer patients, (2) studies in which patients with suspicious lumps or lesions are assessed prior to biopsy, with results compared to actual diagnosis post-biopsy, (3) studies taking a prospective or retrospective approach to pre-morbid stress, psychosocial characteristics, or health habits, (4) studies examining the relationship of psychosocial variables to disease progress and/or survival times, and (5) studies focusing on the association of immunological variables presumed to be related to cancer initiation or exacerbation and psychosocial factors. The interested reader is referred to reviews of the first four of these areas (Bahnson, 1980, 1981; Cox and MacKay, 1982; Fox, 1978; Greer, 1983; LeShan, 1959) that also detail the contradictory results and methodological inadequacies found throughout this literature.

Of specific interest to this chapter are those studies that examine the relationship of psychological factors, specific immunological functioning, and cancer, although these are unfortunately rare within the literature. In one such study, Pettingale et al. (1977) examined the relationship of emotional expression and serum IgA in 160 breast cancer patients. Several studies have reported rises in serum IgA levels in patients with breast cancer (Roberts et al., 1975). Serum IgA levels were found to be higher in all patients who tended to suppress their anger preoperatively. At the postoperative follow-ups, this pattern was demonstrated only by breast cancer patients.

In a follow-up to this study, Pettingale and colleagues (1981) examined serum immunoglobulin (IgG, IgA, and IgM), several hormones (progesterone, testosterone, estradiol, cortisol, prolactin, growth hormone, and thyroxine), and lymphocyte proliferation in response to PHA in 69 women with breast cancer. Patients were classified according to their psychological response to cancer diagnosis (i.e., denial, fighting spirit, stoic acceptance, or helpless/hopeless). At preoperative assessment, no relationship was found between psychological response style and the biological measures. However, at 3-month follow-up, patients in the denial group demonstrated increased levels of serum IgM compared to the other groups. There were no associations between psychological response styles and PHA-induced lymphocyte proliferation.

Levy et al. (1987) examined the associations among stress, NK cell activity, and predicted prognosis in 75 women with breast cancer. Using multiple regression analyses, these authors report that, in general, patients reporting depressive, fatigue-like symptoms and complaining of a lack of family support at baseline had a decrease in NK activity at 3 months follow-up.

Levy et al. (1987) have suggested that emotional, cognitive, and behavioral responses are "biological response modifiers" that have relevance for cancer risk and progression. While the authors admit that the biology of the tumor is the most important determinant of cancer outcome, they point out that numerous epidemiological risk factors for breast (and possibly other) cancers have possible endocrine pathways (i.e., sex, age at menarche, etc.). The possibility arises that response styles mediated through endocrine changes may be associated with cancer outcome.

Unfortunately, there have been few well-controlled, prospective human studies that have examined cancer-immunology-psychosocial associations in sufficient detail. While the work by Levy and others is encouraging, it is clear that further delineation of the relationships among cancer onset, progression, and endocrine and immune system function is needed. One avenue of future study might involve the examination of specific and well-defined populations across many data points. The use of treatment interventions as experimental manipulations may also prove fruitful in clarifying these associations.

Some interesting data from our laboratory may shed some light on the psychoimmunology-cancer relationship. In both human (Kiecolt-Glaser et al., 1985b) and animal studies (Glaser et al., 1985c), we have demonstrated that stress can affect DNA repair mechanisms. In the human study, DNA repair (recovery of nucleoid sedimentation following irradiation of PBLs with 100 rad of X-irradiation) was assessed in 28 newly admitted, nonmedicated, nonpsychotic, psychiatric inpatients. A significant difference in DNA repair was found between high- and low-distress subject groups (measured by scale 2 depression on the Minnesota Multiphasic Personality Inventory, MMPI), with the high-distress group evidencing poorer DNA repair. Such alterations in DNA repair might have a number of potentially important consequences, not the least of which could include increased risk for cancer. Most carcinogens appear to induce cancer by damaging the DNA in cells, resulting in abnormal cells. The body's ability to repair damaged cells is therefore critical, and there is evidence that faulty DNA repair is associated with an increased incidence of cancer (Takabe et al., 1983). In the next section, we will consider the application of psychological interventions to this field.

INTERVENTIONS

Few studies have examined the effects of psychosocial interventions on immune status and/or infectious disease status. This likely reflects the relative "youth" of the field and difficulties associated with the conduct of well-controlled treatment intervention research.

Among the earliest studies exploring the ability of an intervention to affect immunological reactivity were several experiments with hypnosis reported by Black and colleagues (Black, 1963a, 1963b; Black et al., 1963). These authors assessed the effects of hypnotic suggestion on the delayed hypersensitivity reaction to tuberculin, using four highly selected subjects. Skin biopsies revealed that these subjects exhibited normal cellular infiltration, but demonstrated a reduced amount of edema. As this work was not controlled, conclusions must remain very tentative.

In an attempt to follow-up this line of evidence, as well as the more recent conditioned immunosuppression animal work of Ader and Cohen (1975), Smith and McDaniels (1983) examined the effects of conditioning on the tuberculin reaction in 7 human subjects. Using the color of the skin test vial (red for saline, green for tuberculin) as the conditioned stimulus, subjects were assessed monthly over 6 months. When the vials were reversed (red for tuberculin, green for saline) at the sixth trial, results indicated that the tuberculin response at this trial was reduced in terms of erythema and induration.

Gould and Tissler (1984) reported on two case studies (32- and 26-year old females) that examined the effects of hypnotic suggestion on genital HSV recurrence. After three sessions of hypnosis, as well as audio tape-guided self-hypnosis, the older subject was able to go 3 months without a recurrence, while the 26 year old went 7 months without a recurrence. These results are particularly impressive in light of the fact that both women had been experiencing almost monthly recurrences prior to treatment. Unfortunately, this work lacked experimental controls.

Our laboratory has been involved in a number of studies examining the effects of psychosocial interventions on immunological parameters. In one study that examined the effects of relaxation training in a geriatric sample (Kiecolt-Glaser et al., 1985a), the relaxation group was able to significantly decrease distress at post-treatment (as measured by the Hopkins Symptom Checklist) relative to social contact or no contract controls. Immunologically, these subjects also demonstrated increased NK cell activity and decreased HSV-antibody titers, with the latter presumably reflecting some increase in the ability of the cellular immune response to control the latent virus.

In a second study examining the effects of relaxation, we studied 34 first-year medical students randomly divided into relaxation and control groups (Kiecolt-Glaser et al., 1986). Students were bled at the beginning of their school quarter and again during final examinations. The relaxation group received relaxation training preceding the second blood draw. At examination time, the relaxation group reported decreased anxiety and distress compared to controls. For both groups, there was a decrease in the percentage of T-helper cells, T-helper/T-suppressor ratio, and NK cell lysis at examination time, but no interaction was found. Interestingly, the frequency of relaxation practice was a significant predictor of the T-helper cell percentage during examinations.

In a collaborative study with Dr. James Pennebaker, we examined whether actively confronting upsetting experiences might have positive effects on immune function (Pennebaker et al., 1988). Twenty-five of 50 undergraduate subjects spent 4 d writing about personal traumatic experiences which they had not revealed to others. The remaining 25 students spent the same amount of time writing about trivial experiences. Following this writing experience, the "trauma subjects" were found to have a higher blastogenic response to PHA and a decreased number of health center visits for illnesses. These subjects also reported feeling happier than did controls at 3-month follow-up. When the trauma group was split into high- and low-disclosure groups, the high disclosures had an improved mitogen-induced lymphocyte response compared to low disclosures and controls.

Lastly, there is one recent study that failed to demonstrate positive immunological effects as a result of a psychosocial intervention. Coates and colleagues (1989) reported that stress reduction training (relaxation, stress management) did not change immunological measures of lymphocyte subsets, NK cell function, mitogen-induced lymphocyte response, or serum IgA levels in 64 men who were positive for HIV. The authors conjectured that the immune response may be difficult to modulate in a person who is debilitated due to HIV infection.

The body of work which has examined the effects of intervention on the immune system is exciting in several respects. Most obvious are its possible implications regarding the treatment and prevention of immunologically relevant disorders. However, there are several difficulties in this area which must be overcome before we will be able to demonstrate a significant affect. At this point, it should be pointed out that most of the effects found in the above studies are relatively small and are of unknown physiological significance. One of the problems which remains for this area is our lack of understanding of the relationship of immunological variables and health status. Further research is clearly needed.

In the future, theoretically grounded, basic research that explores the mechanisms of the immune response and the long-term kinetics of its various components is strongly encouraged. Another major difficulty concerns our lack of well-defined assessments of immune-related health. Most studies have relied on retrospective accounts or number of health center visits, which is clearly not adequate to delineate this complex relationship. The work with herpesvirus is exciting in this respect, as these studies provide a clearly defined health outcome, namely, lesion recurrence or release of infectious virus. The inclusion of relevant immunoloigcal measures is particularly important as well.

In our laboratory, a research project is currently underway that will attempt to address at least some of these issues. We will be examining the effects of a stress-management-based intervention on the immunological status of hospital nurses. Both immune parameters and health information will be assessed. It is hoped that nurses will represent a population that is able to provide accurate and relevant health data. Assesssments will include daily diary generated data as well as blood drawn on consecutive days to obtain a clearer picture of the kinetics of the immune response to such intervention.

Intervention-based studies are also noteworthy as an experimental manipulation of stress. While this paradigm has largely been overlooked to date, it has a potential to yield important and relevant data. The basic concept is as follows: if stress has the effect of modulating the immune system in some fashion, then the reduction of stress should serve to return the immune system to its prior state. Viewing stress intervention as an experimental manipulation allows us to provide more causal inferential information, as well as to map out the kinetics of the response. With interventions we can carefully time and quantify our manipulations with an eye toward enhanced understanding of the relationships.

OVERVIEW OF THE STRESS-IMMUNO RELATIONSHIP

In the past decade, researchers have begun to map out the cognitive, emotional, physiological, and behavioral aspects of stress. Of particular interest to PNI is how stress-related physiological changes impinge upon immune function. For the purposes of this chapter, we have focused primarily on the immunological effects of psychological stress. Psychological stress can be differentiated from physical stress in that it is subject to cognitive appraisal (Paterson and Neufeld, 1989).

Psychological stressors have been conceptualized as interactions among external threats, internal evaluations of threats, personal resources available to deal with the threat, and potential physical and psychological outcomes (Lazarus and Folkman, 1984). These interactions are thought to result in the cognitive, emotional, physiological, and behavioral manifestations of stress mentioned above.

The physiological effects of stress can generally be categorized under the rubric of arousal. Arousal would include such physical alterations as elevated heart rate, blood pressure, and respiration, as well as the endocrine changes associated with stress. Emotional presentations are typically interrelated with physiological arousal, and are often grouped under the heading of anxiety. Anxiety has more simply been described as a disagreeable emotion associated with fear, and involving short-term physiological responses (Lewis, 1970). Alternatively, others have characterized anxiety as a state of general arousal related to diverse emotions such as anger, fear, excitement, or depression (Paterson and Neufeld, 1989). This last definition would seem to have the greatest relevance for the present discussion.

Most researchers would agree that anxiety and/or stress has a necessary cognitive component. Stress can act to affect both the content and capacity of cognitive functioning (Paterson and Neufeld, 1989). With respect to content, stress tends to create worry or rumination. Stress also affects performance (capacity) in a well-defined manner. This effect is known as the Yerkes-Dodson law, which states that as arousal increases, performance improves, and with further increases, decays.

Lastly, stress may affect behavior generally by boosting activity level. In addition, it leads the individual to attempt to engage in coping behaviors. Of particular interest in this regard is the interaction and influence of this behavioral component of stress upon other domains, and the modifications which result. Thus, the stress response is not a static response. Rather, it fluctuates and changes as the person interacts with and responds to the stressor. It is this type of change and flux that should be kept in mind when attempting to understand or describe the endocrine and immune consequences of stress.

ENDOCRINE RESPONSE TO STRESS

The endocrine reaction to stress is very complex and only partially understood. The hypothalamus (HT) appears to play a central role in coordinating the endocrine, autonomic, and behavioral responses to stress. Select cell populations within the HT exert neural control over the two main axes (pituitary-adrenocortical and sympathetic-adrenomedullary). These axes are responsible for the glucocorticoid- and proopioimelanocorticortin (POMC)-derived peptides and the release of epinephrine and norepinephrine into circulation.

The HT neural regulation of these systems involve several neuropeptides, including corticotropin-releasing factor (CRF), vasopressin (VP), and oxytocin (OT) (Silverman et al., 1989). Specifically, CRF stimulation leads to co-secretion of ACTH and POMC-derived peptides (in particular β-endorphin) from the pituitary. The release of catecholamines (norepinephrine and epinephrine) constitutes an initial response to stressors, and is controlled via regional activation of sympathetic neurons and discharged from the adrenal medulla (Kopin et al. 1988). It appears that POMC-derived peptides act as a "brake" on the sympathetic and adrenomedullary systems whenever they are activated (Grossman, 1989). In this way, they probably serve to counterbalance stress-hormone release, possibly diminishing harmful consequences of frequent overstimulation by chronic stress. However, central opioids are also capable of eliciting catecholamine release.

Epinephrine, in yet another potential feedback loop, has been shown to be a potent releaser of ACTH and related POMC-derived peptides (Smelik et al., 1989). Lastly, glucocorticoids have been found to inhibit the release of ACTH from the pituitary through the action of a negative feedback loop (Dallman and Yates, 1969). Munck et al. (1984) propose that the physiological function of stress-induced increases in glucocorticoid levels is to protect, not against the stress itself, but against the normal defense reactions that are activated by stress. Glucocorticoids probably produce this effect by inhibiting defense reactions such as the release of insulin, lymphokines, and prostaglandins, thus preventing undesirable hypoglycemia, excessive lymphocyte activation, and uncontrolled inflammatory responses.

EFFECTS OF STRESS AND/OR COPING ON THE ENDOCRINE RESPONSE

Of special interest to PNI is the impact of chronic stress and/or coping responses on endocrine function, and the interaction of hormones with immune system function. The processes that control the blend and amount of neural hormone release (CRF, VP, and OT) depend on both the current physiological state of the organism and its prior exposure (Silverman et al., 1989). Silverman and colleagues found that in rats, exposure to complex, chronic stressors leads to physiological modifications of CRF cells in the paraventricular nucleus (the section of the HT containing the most numerous population of CRF-producing cells). The stress of prolonged immobilization leads to a reduction of CRF receptor number in the pituitary (Hauger et al., 1989).

While cortisol secretion is frequently elevated in response to a variety of stressors, it is the initial response that is most vigorous, with prolonged exposure leading to adaptation (Ursin et al., 1978). However, even in cortisol-adapted animals that are chronically stressed, exposure to novel stimuli results in an even more rapid endocrine response (Sakellaris and Vernikos-Danellis, 1975). It has also been reported that the adrenocortical response is dependent on the individual's perception of the stressor's impact (Bourne et al., 1968). Chronic stress may also reduce the sensitivity of the brain's pituitary unit to glucocorticoid negative feedback (Keller-Wood and Dallman, 1984).

Considering catecholamines, it is of interest that at least one study has demonstrated that relaxation practice was associated with higher norepinephrine concentration in response to a physical stressor (Hoffman et al., 1982). The authors interpreted these results as reflecting reduced norepinephrine endorgan responsivity (i.e., more norepinephrine was required to produce compensatory increases in heart rate and blood pressure). It appears that the quality and magnitude of both the ACTH and catecholamine response depends upon the stressor attributes, individual personality, and previous exposure and experience with the stressor.

Thus, the endocrine response to stress is a complex one and involves numerous feedback loops. This response is individualized with respect to stressors and may be modified by behavior, prior exposure, and coping responses. Because of its complexity and tendency to fluctuate, it is crucial that the endocrine-stress response not be conceptualized as a linear function. It is difficult to predict the kinetics of this response based on one or even several data points or hormonal measures. Thus, there is a critical need for further exploration of the kinetics of the endocrine response to stress in relation to psychological processes. Wiener (1989) has suggested that one of the most important issues in stress research is to "develop classification schema of stressors based on broad biological principles."

Goldstein and Halbreich (1987) offer another opinion, arguing that "stress should not be defined by hormonal response." These authors correctly point out that a situation can be quite stressful without concomitant increases in "stress hormones." Conversely, an increase in "stress hormones" does not always indicate the impact of the stressor. It would seem that much could be gained by assessing psychological responses and interpretations to ultimately define and quantify stress, while still utilizing hormone response profiles to assist in the categorization and specificity of stressors. It is clear that we must move away from unitary concepts of stress and begin to explore individual responses and patterns.

EFFECT OF ENDOCRINE RESPONSE AND IMMUNE FUNCTIONING

In general, stress appears to down-regulate the immune response in humans. More specifically, individual hormones have been shown to have distinctive effects on varying elements of the immune system. However, one should keep in mind that the majority of these studies involve *in vitro* assessments and/or administration of pharmacological doses of specific hormones.

Cortisol has been shown to inhibit (1) the proliferative response of T-cells to mitogens, (2) lymphokine production (IL-1, IL-2, T-cell growth factor), (3) monocyte function, (4) suppressor cells, (5) cytotoxic response, and (6) serum immunoglobulin production (Tsokos and Balow, 1986). It can also affect lymphocyte trafficking.

ACTH has been demonstrated to affect lymphocyte activation by enhancing intracellular Ca^{2+} increases in response to mitogens (Kavelaar et al., 1988) as well as *in vitro* antibody responses to T-cell-dependent and -independent antigens and the production of γ-interferon (Smith and Blalock, 1986).

POMC-derived peptides (i.e., β-endorphin) can (1) suppress NK cell activity, (2) modulate tumor growth, (3) inhibit T-lymphocyte chemotactic factor production, (4) augment interferon production, and (5) act as a potent inhibitor of PHA-induced lymphocyte proliferation (McCain et al., 1986).

Felten and Felten (1989) have presented evidence for noradrenergic innervation of lymphoid organs, thereby providing for the possibility of direct contact between these two systems. Epinephrine has been shown to increase the activity of NK cells (Kristoffer et al., 1985). Norepinephrine completely blocked the capacity of interferon to activate murine peritoneal macrophages to a tumoricidal state (Koff and Dunegan, 1985). Norepinephrine can also enhance (1) the primary antibody response, and (2) the ability of cytotoxic T-lymphocytes to lyse target cells.

Thus, "stress hormones" can have a variety of effects on immune function. It should be noted that many of these studies were performed *in vitro,* often using pharmacological doses and testing the hormone in isolation. *In vivo,* there exists an endocrine "milieu" of many hormones in varying amounts. In a study examining the *in vitro* effects of a "physiological" hormone mixture, little immunological effect was found (Deitch and Bridges, 1987). These authors conjectured that the hormones acted to "cancel out" their individual effects on immune function. It is not possible to interpret from this *in vitro* study how such a hormone balance may be affected by infection, chronic stress, or behavioral coping.

In addition, recent work by Blalock's laboratory suggests that the role of hormones may be more complicated than classic endocrinologists had conceded. They have shown that lymphocytes can produce ACTH and β-endorphin (Blalock and Smith, 1985). This lymphocyte-derived ACTH can be stimulated by CRF (Meyer et al., 1987) and the ACTH released may be responsible for stimulating adrenal corticosterone production in hypophysectomized mice (Smith et al., 1982).

PSYCHOLOGICAL STRESS: ENDOCRINE AND IMMUNE INTERACTIONS

The kinetics and interaction of psychological stress, endocrine response, and immune function are complex. In an attempt to clarify this complexity, we offer a greatly simplified example. We can imagine an individual experiencing a major life stressor, such as marital difficulties. As the problems mount, the individual's perceived stress level would be assumed to rise and eventually peak.

Based on the literature reviewed here, it would be expected that this individual's hormone response might also change concomitant with this rise in stress. "Stress hormones" might rise as the stress worsens, and then eventually there would be an adaptation in this response.

The immune system would probably be affected by these endocrine changes, with a down-regulation of the immune response, at least initially. However, by Jerne's network hypothesis (1974), the immune system has its own counterbalancing self-regulatory system. This could cause the immune system to "overshoot" and lead to transitory immune enhancement before eventually modulating "back and forth" until it reaches equilibrium (much like the physical action of a spring).

Therefore, depending on at what time one attempts to assess these systems, different results could be obtained. At one time, we may see the typically reported high stress, high "stress hormones," and suppressed immune response. At another time, it may be high stress and high "stress hormone," but enhanced immune function (a result that has also been reported in the literature). At still another time, there could even be high stress, low "stress hormones," and enhanced or suppressed immune function.

The point is that no single point measure provides the "true" picture of this complex interrelationship. Instead, longitudinal studies with many data points across the different systems are needed to understand these processes. It will not be possible to understand these systems until the time and effort is extended to carefully map out these interactions. As this model may vary across different categories of stressors, coping responses, and their interactions, such clarification will require a considerable expenditure of resources.

Returning again to the model, it should be noted that despite its complexity, this model does not consider (1) the effects of the introduction of infectious agents or (2) the possible health implications of these changes. The first question could be explored utilizing creative experimental models, while the latter question awaits more accurate immunological markers of health status.

REFERENCES

Ader R and Cohen N: Behaviorally conditioned immunosuppression. *Psychosom Med* 1975; 37:333.

Albrecht J, Helderman JH, Schlesser, MA, and Rush AJ: A controlled study of cellular immune function in affective disorders before and during somatic therapy. *Psychiatr Res* 1985; 15:185.

Bahnson CB: Stress and cancer: the state of the art, part 1. *Psychosomatics* 1980; 21:975.

Bahnson CB: Stress and cancer: the state of the art, part 2. *Psychosomatics* 1981; 22:207.

Bartrop RW, Luckhurst E, Lazarus L, Kiloh LG, and Penney R: Depressed lymphocyte function after bereavement. *Lancet* 1977; 1:834.

Black S, Humphrey JH, and Niven JS: Inhibition of Mantoux reaction by direct suggestion under hypnosis. *Br Med J* 1963; 1:1649.

Black S: Inhibition of immediate-type hypersensitivity response by direct suggestion under hypnosis. *Br Med J* 1963a; 1:925.

Black S: Shift in dose-response curve of Prausnitz-Kustner reaction by direct suggestion under hypnosis. *Br Med J* 1963b; 1:990.

Blalock JE and Smith EM: A complete regulatory loop between the immune and neuroendocrine systems. *Fed Proc* 1985; 44:108.

Bloom B, Asher S, and White S: Marital disruption as a stressor: a review and analysis. *Psychol Bull* 1978; 85:867.

Bourne PG, Rose RM, and Nason JW: 17-OHCS levels in combat-special forces "A" team under threat of attack. *Arch Gen Psychiat* 1968; 19:135.

Broadbent DE, Broadbent MHP, Phillpotts RJ, and Wallace J: Some further studies on the production of experimental colds in volunteers by psychological factors. *J Psychosom Res* 1984; 28:511.

Clover RD, Abell T, Becker LA, Crawford S, and Ramsey CN Jr: Family functioning and stress as predictors of influenza B infection. *J Fam Pract* 1989; 28:535.

Coates TJ, McKusick L, Kuno R, and Stites DP: Stress reduction training changed number of sexual partners but not immune function in men with HIV. *Am J Public Health* 1989; 79:885.

Cox T and MacKay C: Psychosocial factors and psychophysiological mechanisms in the aetiology and development of cancers. *Soc Sci Med* 1982; 16:381.

Crook TH and Miller NE: The challenge of Alzheimer's disease. *Am Psychol* 1985; 40:1245.

Dallman MF and Yates FE: Dynamic asymmetries in the corticosteroid feedback path and distribution-metabolism-binding elements of the adrenocortical system. *Ann NY Acad Sci* 1969; 156:696.

Deitch EA and Bridges RM: Stress hormones modulate neutrophil and lymphocyte activity in vitro. *J Trauma* 1987; 27:1146.

Denney DR, Stephenson LA, Penick EG, and Weller RA: Lymphocyte subclasses and depression. *J Abnorm Psychol* 1988; 97:499.

Dorian BJ, Garfinkel PE, Brown GM, Shore A, Gladman D, and Keystone E: Aberrations in lymphocyte subpopulations and function during psychological stress. *Clin Exp Immunol* 1982; 50:132.

Dorian BJ, Keystone E, Garfinkel PE, and Brown GM: Immune mechanisms in acute psychological stress (abstr.). *Psychosom Med* 1981; 43:84.

Felten SY and Felten DL: Are lymphocytes targets of noradrenergic innervation? In *Frontiers of Stress Research*. Weiner H, Florin I, Murison R, and Hellhammer D, Eds. Hans Huber, New York 1989, pp. 56–71.

Fox BH: Premorbid psychological factors as related to cancer incidence. *J Behav Med* 1978; 1:45.

Friedmann E, Katcher AH, and Brightman VJ: Incidence of recurrent herpes labialis and upper respiratory infection: a prospective study of the influence of biologic, social and psychologic predictors. *Oral Surg* 1977; 43:873.

Glaser R, Kiecolt-Glaser JK, Speicher CE, and Holliday JE: Stress, loneliness, and change in herpesvirus latency. *J Behav Med* 1985a; 8:249.

Glaser R, Kiecolt-Glaser JK, Stout JC, Tarr KL, Speicher DE, and Holliday JE: Stress-related impairments in cellular immunity. *Psychiat Res* 1985b; 16:233.

Glaser R, Mehl VS, Penn G, Speicher CE, and Kiecolt-Glaser JK: Stress-associated changes in plasma immunoglobulin levels. *Int J Psychosom* 1986a; 33:41.

Glaser R, Rice J, Sheridan J, et al: Stress-related immune suppression: health implications. *Brain Behav Immun* 1987; 1:7.

Glaser R, Rice J, Speicher CE, Stout JC, and Kiecolt-Glaser JK: Stress depresses interferon production by leukocytes concomitant with a decrease in NK cell activity. *Behav Neurosci* 1986b; 100:675.

Glaser R, Thorn BE, Tarr KL, Kiecolt-Glaser JK, and D'Ambrosio SM: Effects of stress on methyltransferase synthesis: an important DNA repair enzyme. *Health Psychol* 1985c; 4:403.

Goldmeier D and Johnson A: Does psychiatric illness affect the occurrence rate of genital herpes? *Br J Vener Dis* 1982; 54:40.

Goldstein S and Halbreith V: Hormones and stress. In *Handbook of Clinical Psychoneuroendocrinology* Nemeroff CB and Loosen PT, Guilford Press, New York, 1987, pp. 460–469.

Gould SS and Tissler DM: The use of hypnosis in the treatment of herpes simplex II. *Am J Clin Hypn* 1984; 26:171.

Greer S: Cancer and the mind. *Int J Psychiatry* 1983; 143:535.

Grossman A: Opioids and stress: The role of ACTH and epinephrine. In *Neuropeptides and Stress* Tache Y, Morley JE, and Brown MR, Eds. Springer-Verlag, New York, 1989, pp. 313–324.

Halvorsen R and Vassend O: Effect of examination stress on some cellular immunity functions. *J Psychosom Res* 1987; 31:693.

Hauger RL, Millan M, Harwood JP, Lorang M, Catt KJ, and Aguilera G: Receptors for corticotropin releasing factor in the pituitary and brain: regulatory effects of glucocorticoids, CRF and stress. in *Molecular Biology of Stress* Breznitz S and Zinder O, Eds. Alan R. Liss, New York, 1989, pp. 3–17.

Hellhammer DH, Heib C, Hubert W, and Rolf L: Relationship between salivary cortisol release and behavioral coping under examination stress. *IRCS Med Sci* 1985; 13:1179.

Henle W. and Henle G: Epstein-Barr virus and infectious mononucleosis. In *Human Herpesvirus Infectious: Clinical Aspects*. Glaser R. and Gotleib-Stematsky T, Eds. Dekker, New York 1982, pp. 151–162.

Hoffman JW, Benson H, Arns PA, et al: Reduced sympathetic nervous system responsivitiy associated with relaxation response. *Science* 1982; 215:190.

Hudgens GA, Chatterton RJ, Torre J, et al: Hormonal and psychological profiles in response to a written examination. in *Molecular Biology of Stress* Breznitz S and Zinder O, Eds. Alan R. Liss, New York, 1989, pp. 265–275.

Humphreys RJ and Raab W: Response of circulating eosinophils to nor-epinephrine, epinephrine and emotional stress in humans. *Proc Soc Exp Biol Med* 1950; 74:302.

Irwin M, Daniels M, Smith TL, Bloom E, and Weiner H: Impaired natural killer cell activity during bereavement. *Brain Behav Immunol* 1989; 1:98.

Jerne NK: Toward a network theory of the immune system. *Ann Immunol* 1974; 125:373.

Kasl SV, Evans AS, and Niederman JC: Psychosocial risk factors in the development of infectious mononucleosis. *Psychosom Med* 1979; 41:445.

Katcher AH, Brightman V, Luborsky L, and Ship I: Prediction of incidence of recurrent herpes labialis and systemic illness from psychological measurements. *J Dent Res* 1973; 52:49.

Kavelaars A, Ballieux RE, and Heijnen CJ: The role of IL-1 in the corticotropin-releasing factor and arginine-vasopressin-induced secretion of immunoreactive beta-endorphin by human peripheral blood mononuclear cells. *J Immunol* 1988; 142:2338.

Keller-Wood M and Dallman M: Corticosteroid inhibition of ACTH secretion. *Endocrinol Rev* 1984; 5:1.

Kemeny ME, Cohen F, Zegans LS, and Conant MA: Psychological and immunological predictors of genital herpes recurrence. *Psychosom Med* 1989; 51:195.

Kerr AC: The effect of mental stress on the eosinophil leucocyte count in man. *Q J Exp Physiol* 1955; 41:18.

Kiecolt-Glaser JK, Kennedy S, Malkoff S, Fisher L, Speicher CE, and Glaser R: Marital discord and immunity in males. *Psychosom Med* 1988; 50:213.

Kiecolt-Glaser JK, Fisher L, Ogrocki P, Stout JC, Speicher CE, and Glaser R: Marital quality, marital disruption, and immune function. *Psychosom Med* 1987a; 49:13.

Kiecolt-Glaser JK, Garner W, Speicher CE, Penn GM, Holliday J, and Glaser R: Psychosocial modifiers of immunocompetence in medical students. *Psychosom Med* 1984; 46:7.

Kiecolt-Glaser JK, Glaser R, Dyer C, Shuttleworth E, Ogrocki P, and Speicher CE: Chronic stress and immunity in family caregivers of Alzheimer's disease victims. *Psychosom Med* 1987b; 49:523.

Kiecolt-Glaser JK, Glaser R, Williger D, et al: Psychosocial enhancement of immunocompetence in a geriatric population. *Health Psychol* 1985a; 4:25.

Kiecolt-Glaser JK, Glaser R, Strain EC, et al: Modulation of cellular immunity in medical students. *J Behav Med* 1986; 9:5.

Kiecolt-Glaser JK, Stephens R, Lipetz P, Speicher CE, and Glaser R: Distress and DNA repair in human lymphocytes. *J Behav Med* 1985b; 8:311.

Kimzey SL: The effects of extended spaceflight on hematologic and immunological systems. *J Am Med Women's Assoc* 1975; 30:218.

Koff WC and Dunegan MA: Modulation of macrophage-mediated tumoricidal activity by neuropeptides and neurohormones. *J Immunol* 1985; 125:350.

Kopin IJ, Eisenhofer G, and Goldstein D: Sympathoadrenal medullary system and stress. In *Mechanisms of Physical and Emotional Stress* Chrousos GP, Loriaux DL, and Gold PW, Eds. Plenum Press, New York, 1988, pp. 11–24.

Kristoffer H, Svante H, and Orjan S: Evidence for a beta-adrenoceptor-mediated regulation of human natural killer cells. *J Immunol* 1985; 134:4095.

Kronfol Z and House JD: Depression, cortisol, and immune function. *Lancet* 1984; 1:1026.

Landman RMA, Muller FB, Perini CH, Wesp M, Erne P, and Buhler FR: Changes of immuno-regulatory cells induced by psychological and physical stress: relationship to plasma catecholamines. *Clin Exp Immunol* 1984; 58:127.

Lazarus RS and Folkman S: *Stress, Appraisal and Coping* Springer-Verlag, New York, 1984.

LeShan L: Personality states as factors in the development of malignant disease: a critical review. *J Natl Cancer Inst* 1959; 22:1.

Levy SM, Heberman R, Lippman M, and D'Angelo T: Correlation of stress factors with sustained depression of natural killer cell activity and predicted prognosis in patients with breast cancer. *J Clin Oncol* 1987; 5:348.

Levy SM: Behavior as a biological response modifier: psychological variables and cancer prognosis. In *Women with Cancer* Andersen BL, Ed. Springer-Verlag, New York 1986, pp. 289–306.

Lewis A: The ambiguous word "anxiety." *Int J Psychiatry* 1970; 9:62.

Linn MW, Linn BS, and Jensen J: Stressful events, dysphoric mood, and immune responsiveness. *Psychol Rep* 1984; 54:219.

Lloyd R: *Explorations in Psychoneuroimmunology* Grune and Stratton, New York, 1987.

McCain HW, Lamster IB, and Bilotta J: Immunosuppressive effects of the opiopeptins. In *Enkephalins and Endorphins* Plotnikoff NP, Faith RE, Murgo AJ, and Good RA, Eds. Plenum Press, New York, 1986, pp. 159.

McKinnon W, Weisse, CS, Reynolds CP, Bowles CA, and Baum A: Chronic stress, leukocyte subpopulations, and humoral response to latent viruses. *Health Psychol.* In press.

Meyer WJ II, Smith EM, Richards GE, Cavallo A, Morrill AC, and Blalock JE: In vivo immunoreactive adrenocorticotropin (ACTH) production by human mononuclear leukocytes from normal and ACTH-deficient individuals. *J Clin Endocrinol Metab* 1987; 64:98.

Munck A, Guyre PM, and Holbrook NJ: Physiological functions of glucocorticoids in stress and their relation to pharmacological actions. *Endocr Rev* 1984; 5:25.

Palmblad J, Cantell K, Strander H, et al: Stressor exposure and immunological response in man: interferon-producing capacity and phagocytosis. *J Psychosom Res* 1976; 20:193.

Palmblad J, Petrini B, Wasserman J, and Akerstedt T: Lymphocyte and granulocyte reactions during sleep deprivation. *Psychosom Med* 1979; 41:273.

Paterson RJ and Neufeld RWJ: The stress response and parameters of stressful situations. In *Advances in the Investigation of Psychological Stress* Neufeld RWJ, Ed. John Wiley & Sons, New York, 1989, pp. 7–42.

Pennebaker JW, Kiecolt-Glaser JK, and Glaser R: Disclosure of traumas and immune function: health implications for psychotherapy. *J Consul Clin Psychol* 1988; 56:239.

Pettingale KW, Greer S, and Tee DEH: Serum IgA and emotional expression in breast cancer patients. *J Psychosom Res* 1977; 21:395.

Pettingale KW, Philalithis A, Tee, DEH, and Greer S: The biological correlates of psychological responses to breast cancer. *J Psychosom Res* 1981; 25:453.

Roberts MM, Bathgate EM, and Stevenson A: Serum immunoglobulin levels in patients with breast cancer. *Cancer* 1975; 36:221.

Rubin RT, Poland RE, Lesser IM, Winston RA, and Blodgett ACN: Neuroendocrine aspects of primary endogenous depression. *Arch Gen Psychiatry* 1987; 44:328.

Sakellaris PC and Vernikos-Danellis J: Increased rate of response of the pituitary-adrenal system in rats adapted to chronic stress. *Endocrinology* 1975; 97:597.

Schleifer SJ, Keller SE, Bond RN, Cohen J, and Stein M: Major depressive disorder and immunity. *Arch Gen Psychiatry* 1989; 46:81.

Schleifer SJ, Keller SE, Camerino M, Thornton JC, and Stein M: Suppression of lymphocyte stimulation following bereavement. *JAMA* 1983; 250:374.

Schleifer SJ, Keller SE, Meyerson AT, Reskin MJ, Davis KC, and Stein M: Lymphocyte function in major depression. *Arch Gen Psychiatry* 1984; 41:484.

Schleifer SJ, Keller SE, Siris SG, Davis KC, and Stein M: Depression and immunity. *Arch Gen Psychiatry* 1985; 42:129.

Schmidt DD, Zyzanski S, Ellner J, Kumar ML, and Arno J: Stress as a precipitating factor in subjects with recurrent herpes labialis. *J Fam Pract* 1985; 20:359.

Sengars DPS, Waters BGH, Dunne JV, and Bover IM: Lymphocyte subpopulations and mitogenic responses of lymphocytes in manic-depressive disorders. *Biol Psychiatry* 1982; 17:1017.

Sheridan JG, Donnerberg AD, Aurelian L, and Elpern DJ: Immunity to herpes simplex virus type 2. IV. Impaired lymphokine production during recrudescence correlates with an imbalance in T-lymphocyte subsets. *J Immunol* 1982; 129:326.

Silver PS, Auerbach SM, Vishniavsky N, and Kaplowitz LG: Psychological factors in recurrent genital herpes infection: stress, coping style, social support, emotional dysfunction, and symptom recurrence. *J Psychosom Res* 1986; 30:163.

Silverman AJ, Hou-Yu A, and Kelly DD: Modification of hypothalamic neurons by behavioral stress. In *Neuropeptides and Stress* Tache Y, Morley JE, and Brown MR, Eds. Springer-Verlag, New York, 1989, pp. 23–38.

Smelik PG, Tilders FJH, and Berkenbosch F: Participation of adrenaline and vasopressin in the stress response. In *Frontiers of Stress Research* Weiner H, Florin I, Murison R, and Hellhammer D, Eds. Hans Huber, New York 1989, pp. 94–99.

Smith EM and Blalock JE: A complete regulatory loop between the immune and endocrine systems operates through common signal molecules (hormones) and receptors. In *Enkephalins and Endorphins: Stress and the Immune System* Plotnikoff NP, Faith RE, Murgo AJ, and Good RA, Eds. Plenum Press, New York, 1986, pp. 119–128.

Smith EM, Meyer WJ, and Blalock JE: Virus-induced corticosterone in hypophysectomized mice: a possible lymphoid adrenal axis. *Science* 1982; 218:1311.

Smith GR and McDaniel SM: Psychologically mediated effect on the delayed hypersensitivity reaction to tuberculin in humans. *Psychosom Med* 1983; 45:65.

Stein M, Keller SE, and Schleifer SJ: Stress and immunomodulation: the role of depression and neuroendocrine function. *J Immunol* 1985; 135:827s.

Takabe H, Yagi T, and Satoh Y: Cancer-prone hereditary diseases in relation to DNA repair. In *International Cancer Congress, Part B, Biology of Cancer* Mirand EA, Hutchinson WB, and Mihich E, Eds. Alan R. Liss, New York 1983.

Taylor GR and Dardano JR: Human cellular immune responsiveness following space flight. *Aviat Space Environ Med* 1983; 555.

Temoshok L, Heller BW, Sagebiel RW, et al: The relationship of psychosocial factors to prognostic indicators in cutaneous malignant melanoma. *J Psychosom Res* 1985; 29:139.

Tsokos GC and Balow JE: Regulation of human cellular immune responses by glucocorticoids. In *Enkephalins and Endorphins: Stress and the Immune System* Plotnikoff NP, Faith RE, Murgo AJ, and Good RA, Eds. Plenum Press, New York 1986, pp. 159–172.

Ursin H, Baade E, and Levine S: *Psychobiology of Stress* Academic Press, New York, 1978.

Vanderplate C, Aral SO, and Magder L: The relationship among genital herpes simplex virus, stress, and social support. *Health Psychol* 1988; 7:159.

Verbrugge LM: Marital status and health. *J Marriage Fam* 1979; 41:267.

Voss EW: Prolonged weightlessness and humoral immunity. *Science* 1984; 225:214.

Weiner H: Overview. In *Frontiers of Stress Research* Weiner H, Florin I, Murison R, and Hellhammer D, Eds. Huber, New York, 1989, pp. 405–418.

Weiss RS: *Marital Separation* Basic Books, New York, 1975.

Behavior as A Biological Response Modifier

Lynda A. Heiden
Department of Psychology
San Jose State University
San Jose, California

Sandra M. Levy
Pittsburgh Cancer Institute
University of Pittsburgh School of Medicine
Pittsburgh, Pennsylvania

INTRODUCTION

A number of behavioral and psychological variables have been associated with immune modulation and immunologically mediated diseases. The initial focus of this chapter will be on psychological modifiers of cancer progression and, to a much lesser extent, cancer etiology. Although a variety of psychological variables have been studied, we will focus on those examined most extensively: social support, helplessness and hopelessness, emotional expression/suppression, and depression. A discussion of psychosocial variables specifically associated with natural immunity in cancer patients will follow, including studies at the Pittsburgh Cancer Institute.

CANCER

Social Support

While most would agree that adequate psychosocial support can improve a cancer patient's quality of life (Stoll, 1979), the role of social support in disease progression is much less clear. Funch and Marshall (1983) studied predictors of survival in women with breast cancer. After 20 years of observation, it was found that survival in the youngest and oldest groups was clearly longer among those who reported better social support than among those with poorer social support, but this was not as strongly so in the middle age group. In a large population study, Reynolds and Kaplan (1987) reported that male cancer patients who were most socially isolated, and reported more feelings of isolation, were at significantly poorer risk of survival.

In a study by Cassileth et al. (1985), social support was unrelated either to survival in a metastatic group of mixed cancers or to relapse in a stage I and II group of melanoma and breast patients. At follow-up, 7% of the metastatic group were still alive, and 59% of the second group were still in remission. Comparing psychosocial indices, including social support, of the living vs. deceased patients, and relapsed patients with those in remission, no significant differences were found. It is important to note that one issue raised about these studies is that the measure of social support used by Cassileth and colleagues (1985, 1987) (items from Berkman and Syme's Social Network Index) is quite limited in terms of measuring perceived emotional or qualitative support. It has been suggested by Cohen (1988) that perceived availability of support may provide a "buffer" between life stress and host response.

Social support interventions have been utilized in attempts to increase the survival time of cancer patients. Morgenstern and colleagues (1984) found no significant relationship between attendance at psychosocial group sessions and survival in breast cancer patients after corrections were made for duration of disease upon entering the treatment program. However, more recently, Spiegel and colleagues (1989) reported a significant increase in survival time for metastatic breast cancer patients who were randomized to a support group condition compared to controls. The latter finding was consistent with a recent review concerning the survival value of social support (House, 1989) and underscores the likely value of such support related to positive health outcome.

Only a few investigators have examined the possible mediating mechanisms linking social support to host vulnerability (Levy et al., 1985; Kiecolt-Glaser et al., 1985). Perceived social support from family members proved to be a significant variable in one of our (SML's) studies of early stage breast cancer patients. Those women reporting a lack of social support in their environment, with decreased spousal communication, poor quality of spousal relationship, and general inadequacy of the family support system, tended also to have unfavorable biological predictors of risk, e.g., lower natural killer (NK) cell activity. More recently, we have found this same social variable to predict time to recurrent disease in this same sample of patients followed longitudinally (Levy et al., 1989).

The association between increased social support and decreased distress has not been consistently demonstrated. Further, it is not absolutely clear at this point whether the social support/health outcome relationship may extend to cancer. The evidence from several studies, including animal (Heisel, 1985; Laudenslager et al., 1985), clinical (Funch and Marshall, 1983), and epidemiological studies (Reynolds and Kaplan, 1987), suggests that it might. While the complex nature of this type of research is reflected in other studies and reviews (Cassileth et al., 1985, 1987; Kiecolt-Glaser et al., 1985; Morgenstern, et al., 1984), the weight of the evidence (for example, as summarized by House, 1989) suggests that support from significant others may indeed enhance physical as well as mental health in a variety of populations.

Helplessness and Hopelessness

The theory of learned helplessness has frequently been tested for its relevance to health, and has been linked to poor cancer outcome (Greer et al., 1985). Helplessness is defined as "the psychological state that frequently results when events are uncontrollable" (Seligman, 1975, p. 9). Originating in laboratory work, animals subjected to uncontrollable shock learned that, regardless of which behavior they engaged in, they were unable to escape the aversive stimuli. "Helpless" behavior was conditioned with repeated exposure to uncontrollable shock; the animals gave up attempts to cope behaviorally, passively cowering in their cages. This passive behavior persisted into subsequent trials, even when they could control and avoid shock.

Numerous animal studies have been conducted examining the effects of helplessness on experimental tumor growth (Laudenslager et al., 1983; Shavit et al., 1984; Greenberg et al., 1984; Justice, 1985); however, results have been inconsistent. In a study by Visintainer et al. (1982), tumors were implanted in three groups of rats: one group received escapable shock, one inescapable shock, and one served as an unstressed control group. Tumor rejection was comparable in the escapable shock and unstressed control groups (53 and 50%, respectively), but only 27% of the inescapable shock group rejected the implanted tumors. This and other animal studies (Shavit et al., 1984; Greenberg et al., 1984) have demonstrated not only plausible biological mediating mechanisms linking helplessness and tumor outcome, but some of them have also demonstrated causation, that is, lack of control or predictability is one source of the differential tumor response. However, in other studies (Justice, 1985; Burchfield et al., 1978), mice exposed to uncontrollable stress showed no differences in tumor development when compared to unstressed mice. As Justice (1985) and Newberry (1981) point out, such inconsistencies may in fact be explained by the use of different tumor systems, different stress and tumor exposure schedules, and different strains and species studied.

In human studies, hopelessness is a term or concept often used interchangeably with helplessness, and describes a feeling or belief that a situation or problem is without solution. Hopelessness-helplessness has often been associated with early relapse and mortality in human cancer studies. Examining the relationship between biological outcome and psychological response post-surgery, Greer et al. (1985) assessed survival among stage I and II breast cancer patients 10 years after a psychological interview. Those displaying a giving-up or helpless attitude and those showing stoic acceptance of their disease had recurrent disease or died earlier than those responding to their disease either with "denial" or a "fighting spirit". These findings have continued to hold on 13 years of follow-up. Similar results were found in studies by Jensen (1984) and DeClemente and Temoshok (1985). Achte and Vauhkonen (1980) also found helplessness to be a predictor of earlier mortality in a group of males, although the relationship was a relatively weak one.

Using a standard measure of hopelessness, Cassileth and colleagues (1985, 1987) did not find a relationship between hopelessness and survival duration. These results applied to both a metastatic cancer group and a group with stage I and II breast cancer or melanoma. In a study of metastatic breast cancer patients, Jamison et al. (1987) also found no relationship of hopelessness to survival.

The predictive properties of hopelessness, as well as other psychological variables, was examined in a study of cervical cancer severity (Goodkin et al., 1986). Scores on a scale of future despair and hopelessness were related to disease severity along a continuum from early precancer to established stage I invasive cancer. While hopelessness intensified the predictive power of important life events, hopelessness showed only marginal significance in predicting severity of disease.

Depression

Clinical depression has been related to cancer incidence in a number of studies, although no studies exist on clinical depression and survival. In a 4-year follow-up of patients with diagnosed affective disorders, Kerr et al. (1969) found a higher than expected mortality rate among men treated for first-episode endogenous or reactive depression. Attempting to replicate this study, Whitlock and Siskind (1979) followed 39 male and 90 female patients with a primary diagnosis of depression for 2 years 4 months to 4 years. All patients were 40 years of age or older, with ages ranging from 40 to 82 years of age. Using the exact Poisson probabilities test, results indicated that male cancer deaths were significantly higher than expected, while female deaths were no greater than expected.

Nonpathological depression has also been associated with poor cancer prognosis (Jensen, 1984; Achte and Vauhkonen, 1980; Temoshok, 1985; Levy and Schain, 1987). However, several investigators reported no such trends (Jamison et al., 1987; Schonfield, 1981; Stavraky et al., 1968), or even reverse trends (Derogatis et al., 1979).

The phenomenon of happiness or joy could be conceptualized as being the opposite side of the depression ''coin''. In a study by Levy and colleagues (1988), advanced breast cancer patients who reported more joy, optimism, and enthusiasm at the time of recurrence lived significantly longer than others in the sample. In fact, of the predictor variables significant for survival — the disease-free interval, joy, physician's prognosis, and measures of metastatic sites — the ''joy factor'' was the second most potent predictor of survival time.

Evidence suggests that it is possible, under some conditions, and for some kinds of tumor events, for patients with nonpathological depression to have a poorer prognosis than those without such depression. Considering the inconsistent nature of study results, however, it is inadvisable to designate any specific subpopulation, and certainly not the population at large (Zonderman et al., 1989), as being subject to increased risk of poor prognosis in the presence of nonpathological depression.

Emotional Expression/Suppression

In spite of the fact that researchers have hypothesized a relationship between failure to express emotion and cancer occurrence (Cox and MacKay, 1982; Weinberger et al., 1979), there are few well-designed studies in which expression of emotion has been a specific predictor variable for relapse or survival. In studies where little emotional expression is reported, it is unclear which respondents were suppressing emotional expression or actually *felt* little emotion.

The issues in this type of research are further complicated by the difficulty in assessing whether emotional reactivity experienced at any given time is repressed (in the psychodynamic sense), or is suppressed consciously. Investigators have specifically tested for these differences (Temoshok, 1985; Jensen, 1984; Weinberger et al., 1979; Kneier and Temoshok, 1984), and in one of these studies (Jensen, 1984), this issue was directly related to cancer survival. Using multivariate analyses, Jensen (1984) found a repressive-defensive coping style, helplessness-hopelessness, chronic stress, and comforting, future-oriented daydreaming to be associated with malignant spread and deterioration.

Some investigators have attempted to place the response to disease described as ''stoic acceptance'' under the rubric of ''inability to express emotion''. Greer et al. (1985) found that stage I and II breast cancer patients described as having stoic acceptance tended to survive a shorter time than those having what they called ''fighting spirit''. It should be noted, however, that Greer and colleagues do not relate the term stoic acceptance to that of inability to express emotion, and we also believe that the two terms should remain distinct.

NATURAL IMMUNITY

Again, with respect to mechanisms, a pilot study of stress, coping, and biological vulnerability in advanced melanoma patients was conducted by Levy and colleagues (1987) at the National Cancer Institute. Although the sample was quite small (n = 13), significant relationships emerged between NK cell activity and self-reported distress symptoms. Interestingly, positive correlations were found between NK activity and vigor (r = 0.70), state and trait curiosity (r = 0.55, 0.74), and state anger (r = 0.60), and negative associations were found between NK activity and vigor (r = −0.87), depression (r = −0.61), fatigue (r = −0.85), total Profile of Mood States score (r = −0.64), and state anxiety (r = −0.69). Generally, these findings make clinical sense and are in the expected direction.

Through studies conducted at the National Cancer Institute and the Pittsburgh Cancer Institute, Levy and colleagues (1987) have investigated immunological and behavioral factors predicting cancer prognosis in both early and late disease. Although some of this work has been published, new data are only now emerging on prospective follow-up.

As indicated earlier, in a study of prognosis in early-stage breast cancer patients (Levy et al., 1985), it was found that baseline NK activity was significantly associated with the spread of cancer to the axillary region. Patients who had higher levels of NK activity tended to have fewer lymph nodes positive for cancer. Additionally, 51% of the NK activity variance could be accounted for by three factors: the patient's "adjustment to illness", perception of family support, and report of fatigue-depressive symptoms. Those who appeared "adjusted", who complained about a lack of social support in their faimilies, and who responded to their disease in a listless, apathetic manner tended to have lower levels of NK activity, and potentially had the greatest risk for recurrence. It should be recognized that while potentially disease or treatment related, the fatigue reported could have resulted in part from underlying physiological causes, and that adjustment, depression, and perception of support could all have partial origins in the fatigue or other biological causes.

A 3-month follow-up study produced the same findings (Levy et al., 1987). Nodal status was found to be more strongly related to NK activity levels than interim chemotherapy and/or radiotherapy. That is, there were no apparent chronic effects on NK function as a result of interim adjuvant treatment, but patients who had greater disease burden had lower NK activity — both at baseline and on follow-up. In addition, NK activity could also be predicted at 3 months based on the same three psychological factors that we had identified as important at baseline. We are just now examining predictors of recurrent disease in our sample and, along with other biological predictors, both baseline and follow-up NK activity, and the reports of perceived social support and overall distress, are being tested. The data suggest that higher NK activity and lower distress predicted a longer disease-free interval.

DEPRESSION, BEREAVEMENT, AND IMMUNITY

Depression, according to a number of psychosocial researchers (Dohren-wend and Dohrenwend, 1981; Brown and Harris, 1986), can be initiated by a combination of life events, chronic stresses, and lack of appropriate social support. Biological explanations include arguments that depression represents a disease state produced by alterations in neuropeptide concentrations, neu-rotransmitter, neurophysiologic, and/or neuroendocrine abnormalities (Thase et al., 1985; Post et al., 1984). It is a psychological disorder affecting millions of people each year and, in addition to its many psychosocial ramifications, can have deleterious effects on physical health as well.

As previously discussed, clinical depression has been related to cancer incidence in at least one well-conducted epidemiological study which followed a cohort of originally healthy individuals over a period of 2 decades. Depres-sion has also been associated with altered immunity in physically healthy individuals, although results in this area have been inconsistent.

A critical review of studies of depression and immunity will first be provided. Studies examining the effects of bereavement on immunity will be incorporated into this review, since severity of depressive symptoms is com-monly included for study. It is acknowledged, however, that depression and bereavement, while overlapping in symptomatology, are different clinical entities, both in etiology and course. An analysis of these studies will then follow, including discussion of methodological issues inherent in this type of research. Bringing together this review and analysis, current work at the Pittsburgh Cancer Institute and Western Psychiatric Institute and Clinic will subsequently be described, and future research directions will be considered.

OVERVIEW OF STUDIES

Depression

In a study comparing clinically depressed patients with nondepressed psychiatric patients and normal controls, Kronfol and co-workers (1982) found blunted responses to phytohemagglutinin (PHA), concanavalin A (ConA), and pokeweed mitogen (PWM) stimulation. All patients were drug free for at least 2 weeks prior to immunological evaluation. Support for these findings was provided in a pilot study by Darko et al. (1986); however, a study of 32 moderately depressed patients (Albrecht et al., 1985) failed to replicate the results of the Kronfol et al. (1982) study.

Schleifer and colleagues have completed several studies of immunity and depression. In their first study (1984), 18 psychiatric inpatients meeting Research Diagnostic Criteria (RDC) for major depressive disorder, and with a Hamilton Depression Rating Scale Score of 18 or greater, were matched with nondepressed controls on the basis of age, sex, and race. Blood samples of both groups were obtrained during morning hours. The total number of lymphocytes, and numbers of T- and B-cells, were lower in the depressed group, although there were no significant differences in the percentage of T- and B-cells. Proliferative responses to PHA, ConA, and PWM were all consistently lower in depressed patients, as compared to controls.

To evaluate whether these observed alterations in immunity may be associated specifically with depression or may be attributable to either hospitalization effects or to other psychiatric disorders, Schleifer and colleagues (1985) conducted a study of ambulatory depressed patients, schizophrenic inpatients, and patients hospitalized for herniorrhaphy. Immunological assessment included numbers of lymphocytes, T-cells, and B-cells, percentage of T- and B-cells, and proliferative response to PHA, PWM, and ConA mitogens. Separate controls were established for each group, matching for age, sex, and race. Schizophrenic inpatients and the herniorrhaphy patients did not differ significantly from their controls on any immunological parameter. PHA, PWM, and ConA responses of the ambulatory depressed patients were similar to controls; however, the number of T-cells was significantly lower in the depressed group. Differences in total lymphocytes, percentage of T-cells, and number and percentage of B-cells were not significant. According to the authors, these results suggest that the lower proliferative responses observed in the 1984 study of hospitalized depressed patients were more likely related to the severity of depression rather than to hospitalization effects.

In their most recent study, Schleifer and colleagues (1989) evaluated immunological differences between 91 patients with major depressive disorder and concurrently studied controls matched for age and sex. Using an extensive immune system assessment, no mean differences were found between depressives and matched controls in mitogen-induced lymphocyte proliferation, enumeration of lymphocyte subsets, or NK cell activity. Summarizing their work to date, they concluded that the observed discrepancies may be attributed to population differences in age, severity of depressive illness, and hospitalization status.

Examining a different set of immune parameters, a retrospective comparison was made of leukocyte counts in 177 untreated depressive patients and 178 untreated schizophrenic controls (Kronfol et al., 1984). Significant increases in the absolute and relative number of neutrophils and significant decreases in the absolute and relative number of lymphocytes were found in depressed patients. Additionally, when compared to normative values, the depressed group showed higher frequencies of both neutrophilia and lymphocytopenia than did those in the schizophrenic group. The authors suggest that these results are in the expected direction considering that elevated concentrations of cortisol are frequently associated with depression and with an increase in neutrophils and decrease in lymphocytes. However, in a later study, Kronfol and colleagues (1986) examined the role of urinary free cortisol (UFC) excretion in lymphocyte response to mitogen stimulation and did not find elevated UFC to be signficantly related to immune response in depressed patients.

One possible mechanism for the immune changes noted among depressed individuals is that a chronic activation of the HPAC system produces persistent cortisol elevations, which, in turn, has an immunosuppressive effect. To examine the role of baseline and post-dexamethasone cortisol levels in proliferative response to mitogens, Cosyns et al. (1989) conducted a prospective study of 30 hospitalized depressed women. Using DSM-III diagnostic criteria, patients with major depression showed a significantly lower mitogenic response to PHA, ConA, and PWM than those with minor depression, although differences between groups were not affected by severity of distress as measured by the Hamilton Depression Rating Scale. DST suppressors and nonsuppressors did not differ on immunological measures, nor could differences be attributed to age, body weight, weight loss, total number of leukocytes, menopausal status, sleep disturbances, concomitant use of low-dosage benzodiazepines, or length of drug-free period before testing.

Unipolar and bipolar patients in a depressed phase are frequently grouped together in studies of depression and immunity. Recognizing the need for a unipolar/bipolar distinction, Murphy et al. (1987) retrospectively examined lymphocyte numbers in 50 unipolar patients and 30 bipolar patients with major depression. Reduced numbers of circulating lymphocytes were evident in many of the patients, with abnormalities more common in the unipolar group (52%) than in the bipolar group (27%). Although no functional evaluation of immunity was done in this study, these differences do suggest a need to more clearly distinguish between these two clinical diagnostic groups.

Bereavement

Bereavement, a single, presumably catastrophic, and inherently stressful event, has been correlated with immunosuppression in several studies. Bartrop et al. (1977) compared the immunocompetence of 26 bereaved spouses with that of a matched control group. Mitogenic response to PHA and ConA was significantly more depressed in bereaved subjects than controls at 6 weeks post-bereavement, but not at 2 weeks. No significant differences were observed in other measures of immunity. Stress-related hormone concentrations (e.g., cortisol, thyrosine) were also measured, with no significant changes in concentration demonstrated for either group at either 2 or 6 weeks, suggesting that these hormones did not serve as mediators in the mitogenic responses. That hormone concentrations remained constant while T-cell function declined substantiates the evidence for multiple biological pathways affecting immune response.

Linn et al. (1982) studied the degree of depression following a family death or serious illness, and its effect on the immune system. Divided by their median depression scores on the Hopkins Symptom Checklist, immunological tests were run on 60 males who had experienced family death or illness in the 6 months prior to study. *In vivo* cellular responses were measured by three delayed hypersensitivity skin tests, with significantly less responsiveness in the high depression group. IgG and IgM levels were also significantly lower in the high-depression group, although values remained in the normal range.

In a prospective study of 15 spouses of women with cancer (Schleifer et al., 1983), significant suppression of lymphocytic proliferative response was found during the first 2 months following death of a spouse when compared with the pre-loss period. Some persistence in these alterations was suggested by the intermediate mitogenic responsiveness observed in the 4- to 14-month period following loss. The total number of lymphocytes, and B- and T-cell counts did not change significantly either pre- or post-loss.

Hypothesizing that changes in NK activity in the bereaved might be related to the severity of the depressed mood, Irwin and colleagues (1987) studied NK activity and depressive symptoms in six women prior to and following the death of their husbands. Increases in depressive symptoms from pre-loss to post-loss, as measured by the Hamilton Depression Rating Scale, were strongly correlated with decreases in NK activity. In another component of this study, Irwin et al. (1987) examined NK cell function in ten women whose husbands had died of cancer 1 to 4 months previous to blood sampling with immune function, as compared to eight female controls. Lymphocyte numbers did not differ between the two groups; however, NK lytic activity was significantly lower and depression scores were significantly higher in the bereaved group when compared to controls.

SUMMARY AND ANALYSIS

In summary, observations from these studies suggest that some, but not all, patients with major depressive disorder or depressed mood show immune system changes (Krueger et al., 1984). Evidence certainly supports variables such as age and severity of depressive symptoms as important factors accounting for some of the discrepancies observed in immune outcome measures. However, some of the differences demonstrated across studies may be due to differing, and sometimes flawed, methodologies.

Many of the methodological issues in behavioral immunology research have been addressed in a paper by Kiecolt-Glaser and Glaser (1988). As pointed out by the authors, when studying stress and immunity, there is considerable need to identify and control for behavioral concomitants of emotional distress (e.g., increased alcohol intake, tobacco use, and changes in appetite, sleep, and exercise) which may alter immune parameters. Of those studies reviewed above, only a few investigators controlled well for alcohol use (Irwin et al., 1987). Prescribed psychotropic drug use, as well as other drug use, is highly variable across depression studies; in some studies, controls for medication were entirely excluded, particularly in earlier work (Linn et al., 1982; Bartrop et al., 1977). In those studies in which patients are drug free, they may be so for time periods ranging from 2 weeks (e.g., Darko et al., 1986) to 3 months or more (e.g., Schleifer et al., 1984). More recently, investigators have noted the need for evaluation of nutritional status (Cosyns et al., 1989), although its importance has not always been recognized (Schleifer et al., 1984, 1985, 1989; Kronfol et al., 1985, 1986, 1987). While modifications in sleep quality are frequently seen in both depressed patients and the bereaved, and sleep deprivation has demonstrated immunologic effects (Palmblad et al., 1979), no attempts have been made to control for changes in either sleep quantity or quality in studies of depression and immunity. Comparability of data is also restricted by differing laboratory procedures, although thorough discussion of this issue lies beyond the scope of this chapter.

In addition to these methodological difficulties, some issues remain which are unique to the depression-immune system research area. For example, some studies have been performed without the benefit of standardized psychiatric diagnostic procedures (Kronfol et al., 1984). When standardized assessments have been made, a variety of psychometric measures and procedures have been utilized, severely restricting the comparability of studies. The DSM-III, the Schedule of Affective Disorders Schedule, the Research Diagnostic Criteria for depression, the Hamilton Depression Rating Scale, and the Hopkins Symptom Checklist have all been utilized to diagnose and assess the severity of depression. Correlations among these measures can be expected to be high; however, some are specifically designed to assess symptoms through a written self-report of the patient, while others are designed to diagnose depression by structured clinical interview. Additionally, each measure targets at least a slightly different set of depressive symptoms.

Probably the most conspicuous and serious shortcoming evident in the research is the assumption that depressed individuals are a homogenous group. Those with bipolar illness in a depressed cycle frequently are not differentiated from those suffering a single episode of depression, nor are single-episode depressed patients well differentiated from those experiencing recurrent episodes of depression. Biological as well as psychological profiles are likely to differ among these and other subgroups of depressives; thus, collapsing them into a single group only serves to "muddy the waters".

THE PITTSBURGH CANCER INSTITUTE AND WESTERN PSYCHIATRIC INSTITUTE AND CLINIC STUDY

Although investigators have found age, severity of depression, and hospitalization status to consistently correlate with immune response in depressed patients (Schleifer et al., 1989; Monjan, 1987), only minimal attempts have been made to identify other, possibly more potent, vulnerability factors. As distinct circadian patterns have been demonstrated in the immune system, it is possible that depression-linked alterations in the "biological clock" may increase vulnerability to immunological changes.

Circadian rhythm disturbances, such as in the sleep/wake cycle and in patterns of hormonal release, have been well documented in depressed patients (Monjan, 1987), although the causal direction of the depression-circadian dysfunction link is not known at present (Monk et al., in press). To integrate the concept of biological clock disruption in depression with what is known about environmental factors most commonly associated with depression, a "social zeitgeber" theory of depression has been proposed (Ehlers et al., 1988). In biological research, a "zeitgeber" (or "time giver") refers to certain external forces (e.g., light) with the capacity to synchronize body rhythms. It has been found, however, that in addition to physical forces, social contacts and environment ("social zeitgebers") also serve as powerful entraining and maintaining agents of the circadian system (Bernton et al., 1987; Monk et al., in press). Of interest in the study of immunity and depression is whether some of the variability in the effect of depression on immune response may be explained by alterations in social rhythms. To our knowledge, this relationship has not been studied. Additionally, while there is some evidence that prolonged sleep deprivation can alter immune function (Palmblad et al., 1979), it is not yet known whether those changes in sleep associated with depression are related to immunological change.

In hopes of extending knowledge in this area, as well as providing a clearer picture of the relationship between depression and immune function, a study is presently underway in Pittsburgh prospectively examining the direct association of social rhythms, sleep patterns, and severity of distress to immune function and infectious disease incidence in recurrently depressed patients. In addition to the usual demographic information (e.g., age), data are being collected on menstrual cycle phase, nutritional status, tobacco and alcohol use, and exercise, while controlling for circadian variations in immune response. The immunological evaluation is quite extensive, including functional and quantitative measures of cellular, humoral, and natural immunity.

While most studies to date have evaluated patients either at a single point in time or over only brief follow-up periods, this study focuses on recurrently depressed patients. Thus, understanding of the association between depression and immunity may also be increased by determining if altered immunity is specific for the state of depression, or persists into remission. Recurrent depression may be particularly relevant to health outcome because it represents a psychological and biological response *pattern* occurring over time, as opposed to being a relatively isolated psychological response state.

BEHAVIORAL INTERVENTIONS AND IMMUNE RESPONSE

When considering behavior as a biological response modifier, it is important to examine specific behavioral coping strategies with demonstrated immune-altering properties. Several behavioral interventions and behavioral coping patterns have been hypothesized to influence the immune system. As suggested by the Irwin study of immunity in bereaved individuals, response to the stressor (death of spouse) is equally, if not more important than the stressor itself. Thus, most researchers have focused on modulation of the immune response by either decreasing the distress or enhancing the well-being of the individual. The primary distress-reducing interventions associated with immunological alterations have included relaxation training (Kiecolt-Glaser et al., 1985) and writing about personal, traumatic life events (Pennebaker et al., 1988). A psychosocial intervention providing health information, relaxation and stress management training, and an imagery technique was effective in reducing the frequency of recurrent HSV infection episodes, as well as facilitating adjustment to the disease (Longo et al., 1988). In a single-case protocol, a meditation was used to significantly reduce both induration of delayed hypersensitivity skin test reactions and *in vitro* lymphocyte stimulation to varicella zoster (Smith et al., 1985). Aerobic exercise training, with demonstrated psychological benefits (Griest et al., 1979), has also been shown to have potentially beneficial increases in T-lymphocyte subsets among HIV-1 seropositive individuals (Laperriere et al., 1988) and to have immunomodulatory effects in healthy males (Watson et al., 1986).

While evidence supporting intentional modulation of immune response continues to grow, less is known about the relevance of these immunological changes to health outcome. Longitudinal studies will be needed to determine what, if any, impact specific behavioral interventions may have.

BEHAVIOR AS A BIOLOGICAL MODIFIER

In this chapter, we have provided (1) a review and analysis of behavioral and psychosocial variables which may influence natural immunity and the progression of immunologically mediated disease, (2) evidence suggesting that a specific psychopathological state may diminish immunological defenses, and (3) an examination of specific behavioral coping strategies with immune-altering properties. Although the pathways linking the central nervous system, the endocrine and the immune system, and host vulnerability are multiple and complex — and as yet poorly understood — that such pathways exist is, we believe, indisputable. This biological plausibility has provided the base upon which our research program has been founded.

REFERENCES

Achte K and Vauhkonen ML: Psychic factors in cancer. I., *Cancer and Psyche* Monogr. 1, Psychiatric Clinic of Helsinki University Central Hospital 1980.

Albrecht J, Helderman J, Schlesser M, and Rush JA: A controlled study of cellular immune function in affective disorders before and during somatic therapy. *Psychiatr Res* 1985; 15:185–193.

Bartrop RW, Lazarus R, Luckhurst E, Kiloh LG, and Penney R: Depressed lymphocyte function after bereavement. *Lancet* 1977; 1:834–836.

Brown GW and Harris T: Stressor, vulnerability and depression: a question of replication. *Psychol Med* 1986; 16:739–744.

Burchfield S, Woods S, and Elich M: Effects of cold stress on tumor growth. *Psychol Behav* 1978; 21:537–540.

Cassileth BR, Lusk EJ, Miller DS, Brown LL, and Miller C: Psychosocial correlates of survival in advanced malignant disease? *N Engl J Med* 1985; 312:1551–1555.

Cassileth B, Lusk EJ, Walsh W, Altman H, and Pisano M: Psychosocial correlates of unusually good outcome three years after cancer diagnosis. *Proc Am Soc Clin Oncol* 1987; 6:253 (Abstr).

Cohen S: Psychosocial models of the role of social support in the etiology of physical disease. *Health Psychol* 1988; 7:269–297.

Cosyns P, Maes M, Vandewoude M, Stevens WJ, DeClerck LS and Schotte C: Impaired mitogen-induced lymphocyte responses and the hypothalamic-pituitary-adrenal axis in depressive disorders. *J Affect Disord* 1989; 16:41–48.

Cox T and MacKay C: Psychosocial factors and psychophysiological mechanisms in the etiology and development of cancers. *Soc Sci Med* 1982; 16:381–396.

Darko DF, Lucas AH, and Gillin JC: Replication of lower lymphocyte blastogenesis in depression. *Am J Psychiatry* 1986; 143:1492.

Derogatis L, Abeloff M, and Melisaratos N: Psychological coping mechanisms and survival time in metastatic breast cancer. *JAMA* 1979; 242:1504.

DiClemente RJ and Temoshok, L: Psychological adjustment to having cutaneous malignant melanoma as a predictor of follow-up clinical status. *Psychosom Med* 1985; 47:81 (Abst).

Dohrenwend BS and Dohrenwend BP: Eds. *Stressful Life Events and Their Contexts* Neal Watson, New York, 1981.

Ehlers EL, Frank E, and Kupfer SJ: Social zeitgebers and biological rhythms. *Arch Gen Psychiatry* 1988; 45:948.

Funch D and Marshall J: The role of support in relation to recovery from breast surgery. *Soc Sci Med* 1983; 16:91.

Goodkin K, Antoni MH, and Blaney PH: Stress and hopelessness in the promotion of cervical intraepithelial neoplasia to invasive squamous cell carcinoma of the cervix. *J Psychosom Res* 1986; 30:67.

Greenberg A, Dyck D, and Sandler L: Opponent processes, neuro-hormones, and natural resistance. In *Psychoneuroendocrine Systems in Cancer and Immunity* Fox B and Newberry B, Eds. Hogrefe, Toronto 1984.

Greer S, Pettingale K, Morris T, and Haybittle J: Mental attitudes to cancer: an additional prognostic factor. *Lancet* March 1985; 30:750.

Greist JH, Klein MH, Eischens RR, Faris J, Gurman AS and Morgan WP: Running as treatment for depression. *Comp Psychiatry* 1979; 20:41–53.

Heisel S: Immigration induces a rise in natural killer cell activity in male vervet monkeys. *Am J Primatol* 1985; 8:342 (Abstr).

House JS, Landis KR and Umberson D: Social relationships and health. *Science* 1989; 241:540–545.

Irwin M, Daniels M, Smith TL, Bloom E, and Weiner H: Impaired natural killer cell activity during bereavement. *Brain Behav Immun* 1987; 1:98–104.

Jamieson RN, Burish TG, and Wallston KA: Psychogenic factors in predicting survival of breast cancer patients. *J Clin Oncol* 1987; 5:768.

Jensen M: Psychobiological factors in the prognosis and treatment of neoplastic disorders. Ph.D. thesis. Department of Psychology, Yale University 1984.

Justice A: Review of the effects of stress on cancer in laboratory animals: importance of time of stress application and type of tumor. *Psychol Bull* 1985; 98:108.

Kerr TA, Schapira K, and Roth M: The relationship between premature death and affective disorder. *Br J Psychiatry* 1969; 115:1277.

Kiecolt-Glaser J and Glaser R: Methodological issues in behavioral immunology research with humans. *Brain Behav Immun* 1988; 2:67–78.

Kiecolt-Glaser JK, Glaser R, Williger D, Stout J, Messick G, Shepard S, Ricker D, Romisher SC, Briner W, Bonnell G, and Donnerburg R: Psychosocial enhancement of immunocompetence in a geriatric population. *Health Psychol* 1985; 4:25.

Kneier R and Temoshok L: Repressive coping reactions in patients with malignant melanoma as compared to cardiovascular patients. *J Psychosom Res* 1984; 28:145.

Kronfol A, Nasrallah HA, Chapman S, and House JD: Depression, cortisol metabolism, and lymphocytopenia. *J Affect Disord* 1985; 9:169–173.

Kronfol A, Silva J, Greden J, Dembinski S, and Carroll BJ: Cell-mediated immunity in melancholia. *Psychosom Med.* 1982; 44 (Abstr.).

Kronfol Z, Turner R, Nasrallah H, and Winokur, G: Leukocyte reguation in depression and schizophrenia. *Psychiatry Res* 1984; 13:13.

Kronfol Z, House JD, Silva J, Greden J, and Carroll BJ: Depression, urinary free cortisol excretion and lymphocyte function. *Br J Psychiatry* 1986; 148:71.

Kronfol Z, Quinn J, House D, and Nasrallah HA: Immunologic abnormalities in depressive illness. In *Viruses, Immunity, and Mental Disorders* Kurstak E, Lipowski ZJ, and Morozov PV, Eds. Plenus, New York, 1987, pp. 363–367.

Krueger R, Levy E, and Cathcart E: Lymphocyte subsets in patients with major depression: preliminary findings. *Advances* 1984; 1:5.

Laperriere R, Schneiderman N, Antoni MH, and Fletcher MA: Aerobic exercise training and psychoneuroimmunology in AIDS research. In *Psychological Aspects of AIDS* Temoshok L and Baum A, Eds. Lawrence Erlbaum Associates, Hillsdale, NJ 1988.

Laudenslager M, Capitanio JP, and Reite M: Possible effects of early separation experiences on subsequent immune function in adult macaque monkeys. *Am J Psychiatry* 1985; 142:862.

Laudenslager ML, Ryan SM, Drugan SM, Hyson RL, and Maier SF: Coping and immunosuppression: inescapable but not escapable shock suppresses lymphocyte proliferation. *Science* 1983; 221:568.

Levy S, Herberman R, Maluish A, Schlien B, and Lippman M: Prognostic risk assessment in primary breast cancer by behavioral and immunological parameters. *Health Psychol.* 1985; 4:99.

Levy S and Schain W: Psychological response and breast cancer: direct and indirect contributions to treatment outcome. In *Diagnosis and Treatment of Breast Cancer* Lippman M, Lichter A, and Danforth D, Eds. W.B. Saunders, New York, 1987.

Levy SM, Herberman R, d'Angelo T, and Lippman M: Mastectomy versus excisional biopsy: distress sequelae as a function of choice. *J Clin Oncol* 1989; 7:367–375.

Levy SM, Herberman R, and Lippman M: Correlation of stress cofactors with sustained depression of natural killer cell activity and predicted prognosis in patients with breast cancer. *J Clin Oncol* 1987; 3:348–353.

Levy SM, Herberman R, Whiteside T, Sanzo K, Lee J, and Kirkwood, J: Perceived social support and tumor estrogen/progesterone receptor status as predictors of natural killer cell cytotoxicity in breast cancer patients. *Psychosom Med* Provisionally accepted 1989.

Levy S, Lee J, Bagley C, and Lippman M: Survival hazards analysis in first recurrent breast cancer patients: seven-year follow-up. *Psychosom Med* 1988; 50:520–528.

Linn BS, Linn MW, and Jensen J: Degree of depression and immune responsiveness. *Psychosom Med* 1982; 44:128–129.

Longo DJ, Clum GA, and Yaeger NJ: Psychosocial treatment for recurrent genital herpes. *J Consult Clin Psychol* 1988; 56:61–66.

Monjan A: *Behavioral Modulation of Immune Functioning* Paper presented at The Society of Behavioral Medicine. 1987.

Morgenstern H, Gellert G, Walter S, Ostfeld A, and Siegel B: The impact of a psychosocial support program on survival with breast cancer: the importance of selection bias in program evaluation. *J Chron Dis* 1984; 37:273–282.

Murphy D, Gardner R, Greden JF, and Carroll BJ: Lymphocyte numbers in endogenous depression. *Psychol Med* 1987; 17:381–385.

Newberry BH: Effects of presumably stressful stimuli (PSS) on the development of animal tumors: some issues. In *Perspectives in Behavioral Medicine* Weiss SM, Herd JA, and Fox, BH, Eds. 1981, pp. 329–350.

Palmblad J, Petrini B, Wasserman J, and Adkerstedt T: Lymphocyte and granulocyte reactions during sleep deprivation. *Psychosom Med.* 1979; 41:273–278.

Pennebaker JW, Kiecolt-Glaser JK, and Glaser R: Disclosure of traumas and immune function health implications for psychotherapy. *J Consult Clin Psychol* 1988; 56:239–245.

Post RM, Jimerson DC, Ballenger, JC, Lee, CR, Uhde TW, and Goodwin FK: Cerebrospinal fluid norepinephrine and its metabolites in manic-depressive illness. In *Neurobiology of Mood Disorders* Vol. 1. *Frontiers of Clinical Neuroscience* Post RM and Ballenger JC, Eds., Williams & Wilkins, Baltimore.

Reynolds R and Kaplan G: Social connections and risk for cancer: prospective evidence from the Alameda County Study. Submitted 1987.

Shavit J, Lewis J, Terman G, Gale R, and Liebeskind J: Opioid peptides mediate the suppressive effect of stress on natural killer cytotoxicity. *Science* 1984; 223:188–190.

Schleifer SJ, Keller SE, Camerino M, Thornton JC, and Stein M: Suppression of lymphocyte stimulation following bereavement. *JAMA* 1983; 250:374–377.

Schleifer SJ, Keller SE, Siris SG, Davis KL, and Stein M: Depression and immunity: lymphocyte function in ambulatory depressed patients, hospitalized schizophrenic patients, and patients for herniorraphy. *Arch Gen Psychiatry* 1985; 42:129–133.

Schleifer SJ, Keller SE, Meyerson AT, Raskin MJ, Davis KL, and Stein M: Lymphocyte function in major depressive disorder. *Arch Gen Psychiatry* 1984; 41:484–486.

Schleifer SJ, Keller SE, Bond RN, Cohen J, and Stein M: Major depressive disorder and immunity: role of age, sex, severity, and hospitalization. *Arch Gen Psychiatry* 1989; 46:81–87.

Schonfield J: Psychologic factors in the recovery from and recurrence of early breast cancer. In *Living and Dying with Cancer* Attmed P, Ed. Elsevier, New York, 1981.

Seligman M: *Helplessness: On Depression, Development and Death* W.H. Freeman, San Francisco 1975.

Spiegel D, Bloom JR, Kraemer HC, and Gottheil E: Effect of psychosocial treatment on survival of patients with metastatic breast cancer. *Lancet* October 14 1989.

Smith RG, McKenzie JM, Marner DJ, and Steele RW: Psychologic modulation of the human immune response to varicella zoster. *Arch Intern Med* 1985; 145:2110–2112.

Stavraky KM, Buck CW, Lott SS, and Wanklin JM: Psychological factors in the outcome of human cancer. *J Psychosom Res* 1968; 12:251–259.

Stoll B: *Mind and Cancer Prognosis* John Wiley & Sons, Chicester 1979.

Temoshok L: Biopsychosocial studies on cutaneous malignant melanoma: psychosocial factors associated with prognostic indicators, progression, psychophysiology, and tumor-host response. *Soc Sci Med* 1985; 20:833–840.

Thase ME, Frank E, and Kupfer DJ: Biological processes in major depression. In *Handbook of Depression: Treatment, Assessment, and Research* Beckham EE and Leber WR, Eds. Dorsey Press, Homewood, IL 1985.

Visintainer MA, Volpicelli JR, and Seligman M: Tumor rejection in rats after inescapable or escapable shock. *Science* 1982; 216:437–439.

Watson RR, Moriguchi S, Werner L, Wilmore JH, and Freund BJ: Modification of cellular immune functions in humans by endurance exercise training. *Med Sci Sports Exercise* 1986; 18:95–100.

Weinberger DA, Schwartz GW and Davidson RJ: Low-anxious, high-anxious, and repressive coping styles: psychometric patterns and behavioral and physiological responses to stress. *J Abnormal Psychol* 1979; 88:369–380.

Whitlock FA and Siskind M: Depression and cancer: a follow-up study. *Psychol Med* 1979; 9:747–752.

Zonderman AB, Costa PT, and McCrae RR: Depression as a risk for cancer morbidity and mortality in a nationally representative sample. *JAMA* 1989; 262:1191–1198.

The Effects of Psychological and Physical Stress in Humans

Alan Breier
Outpatient Research Program
Maryland Psychiatric Research Center
Department of Psychiatry
University of Maryland School of Medicine
Baltimore, Maryland

Margot Albus
Mental State Hospital Haar
Vokestraße 72
Haar, Germany

Owen M. Wolkowitz
Department of Psychiatry
University of California at San Francisco School of Medicine
San Francisco, California

Theodore P. Zahn
Laboratories of Psychology and Psychopathology
National Institutes of Mental Health
Bethesda, Maryland

Stephen M. Paul
Director, Intramural Research Program
National Institutes of Mental Health
Bethesda, Maryland

David Pickar
Experimental Therapeutics Branch
National Institutes of Mental Health
Bethesda, Maryland

INTRODUCTION

Stress is a pervasive factor of everyday life that contributes to the pathophysiology of nearly all psychiatric illnesses and a range of medical illness. Immense strides have been made in the preclinical laboratory in elucidating the neurobiological processes involved in the stress response. However, progress in the transfer of information from preclinical studies to clinical application has been impeded, in part, because of the lack of sufficient strategies to examine stress in humans. Our work has focused on the development of strategies to examine the behavioral and neurobiologic processes of human stress in healthy volunteers and patients with severe psychiatric illnesses (Breier et al., 1988, 1987a, 1987b, 1986a, 1986b; Breier and Paul, 1988; Breier, 1989; Charney et al., 1984, 1986; Roy et al., 1985; Wolkowitz et al., 1986, 1987).

In this paper, we present data from two different laboratory-based paradigms developed to assess human stress. One paradigm was designed to assess the effects of psychological stress and the second paradigm was developed to assess the effects of physical stress. The first study involves examining the behavioral and neuroendocrine effects of uncontrollable and controllable stress in healthy volunteers and depressed patients with a paradigm based on the so-called "learned helplessness" studies in animals (Seligman and Maier, 1967). The second study assesses the immunologic effects of metabolic stress through 2-deoxy-D-glucose (2DG) infusion.

CONTROLLABLE AND UNCONTROLLABLE STRESS IN VOLUNTEERS AND AFFECTIVELY ILL PATIENTS

The rationale for studying the effects of controllable and uncontrollable stress comes from a large body of preclinical and clinical literature. Preclinical studies demonstrate that exposure to uncontrollable stress in comparison to identical amounts of controllable stress results in a range of deficits. These deficits include impaired immunologic function (Laudenslager et al., 1983), increased catecholaminergic release leading to central norepinephrine depletion (Weiss et al., 1981; Anisman et al., 1980), altered hypothalamic-pituitary-adrenal axis (HPA) function (Swenson and Vogel, 1983; Davis et al., 1977; Hanson et al., 1976; Nealis and Bowman, 1972), and specific neurovegetative behavioral effects (Anisman, 1984; Weiss and Simson, 1985; Seligman and Maier, 1967). All of these deficits have parallels to data found in clinical studies of affective illness such that exposure to uncontrollable stress has been proposed as an animal model of human depression. Clinical studies have shown that stress is associated with the onset of depressive illness (Brown et al., 1973; Paykel et al., 1969; Leff et al., 1970; Thompson and Hendric,

1972; Goodwin and Bunney, 1973; Lloyd, 1980). Moreover, the types of stressful events most frequently associated with the onset of depression are events termed "exit" events that are generally outside the individual's control and therefore contribute to feelings of powerlessness. Examples of these events are death of a relative, serious physical illness, and loss or change in occupational status. We first examined the effects of controllable and uncontrollable noise stress on behavior and HPA axis function in healthy volunteers (Breier et al., 1987a). Our second experiment utilized the noise stress paradigm to compare stress effects in depressed patients and controls to address the hypothesis that affective illness is associated with altered behavioral and neuroendocrine sensitivity to uncontrollable stress (Breier, 1989).

Methods

In the first experiment, 10 healthy volunteers (6 males, 4 females; mean ± SD age: 33 ± 9 years) participated in two alternately assigned test days, a controllable test day and an uncontrollable test day. The noise stress apparatus was modified from other studies that have examined uncontrollable stress in humans (Hiroto, 1974; Gatchel and Proctor, 1976) and has been described in depth previously (Breier et al., 1987a, 1989). Briefly, on the controllable stress test day, aversive loud noise (60 trials of 100 dB pure tones delivered through headphones) was administered and could be terminated, providing a simple button push sequence was learned. On the uncontrollable stress test day, the button responses did not affect noise termination and the subjects were unable to stop the noise. Following the noise stress, subjects were presented a mental task consisting of solving 20 five-letter, single-solution anagrams (Tresselt and Mayzner, 1966). A mental task was incorporated into the paradigm because animal studies have shown that deficits resulting from uncontrollable stress can be manifested subsequent to the stress when the animal is challenged by a performance test. The degree of "success", "helplessness", and "control" which subjects experienced during the noise stress was determined using a visual analog, self-rating scale administered at the end of the noise condition. Serial blood samples for adrenocorticotropic hormone (ACTH) and cortisol were collected throughout the test procedure.

In the second experiment, seven patients (4 females, 3 males; mean ± SD age: 41 ± 11 years) who met DSM III criteria for major depression and were hospitalized for assessment of their affective illness participated in the uncontrollable-controllable noise stress study. Patients were drug free for a minimum of 3 weeks prior to participation and had moderate levels of depressive symptoms the week of the study (McNair and Lorr, 1971; depression-dejection score: 25 ± 8). The seven patients participated in an uncontrollable test day and six of the seven participated in a controllable test day using the

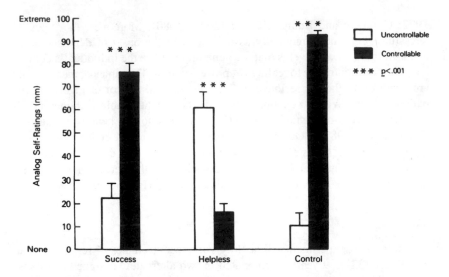

Figure 3-1. Comparison of the effects of uncontrollable and controllable noise stress on behavioral ratings (mean ± S.E.M.) in healthy volunteers (n = 10). (From Breier 1989. With permission.)

noise stress apparatus and following the procedure described above. The effects of uncontrollable and controllable noise stress on behavioral ratings and plasma cortisol levels were compared between depressed patients and the healthy volunteers described above.

Results

In healthy volunteers, uncontrollable, in comparison to controllable, noise stress produced greater ratings of lack of success ($p < 0.001$), helplessness ($p < 0.001$), and lack of control ($p < 0.0001$) (Figure 1). The behavioral changes resulting from exposure to uncontrollable stress were accompanied by alterations in ACTH and cortisol secretion. There were significant differences (condition × time) between uncontrollable and controllable stress on secretion of ACTH (F = 5.6, p = 0.006) (Figure 2) and a trend toward differences for cortisol (F = 2.2, p = 0.07). Although the magnitude of the ACTH rise was relatively modest, ACTH levels were significantly elevated in the uncontrollable stress condition when compared to controllable stress at 15 min (during the mental task, $p < 0.05$) and 45 min (at the end of the study, $p < 0.05$) following cessation of the noise stress.

The depressed patients had stronger behavioral and neuroendocrine responses to uncontrollable stress than the volunteers. The depressives, in comparison to the volunteers, had significantly lower ratings of feelings of success following uncontrollable noise stress exposure (Figure 3). In contrast, there

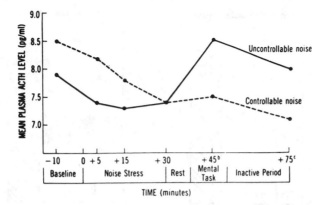

Figure 3-2. Plasma ACTH levels during exposure to controllable and uncontrollable stress. *$p < 0.05$, comparison between uncontrollable and controllable levels during the mental task and at the end of the inactive period. (From Breier et al., 1979. With permission.)

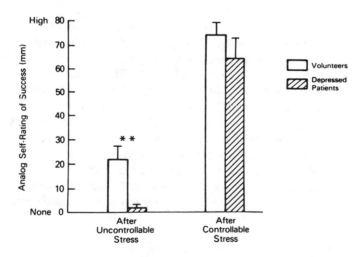

Figure 3-3. Comparison of ratings of success (mean ± S.E.M.) following uncontrollable and controllable stress. **$p = 0.02$, comparison of depressed patients and volunteers after uncontrollable stress. (From Breier, 1989. With permission.)

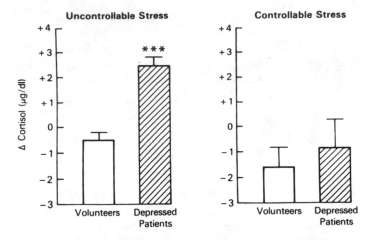

Figure 3-4. Comparison of change in plasma cortisol (end of noise stress value–baseline value; mean ± S.E.M.) during uncontrollable and controllable noise stress. *** $p = 0.001$, comparison between depressed and volunteer values. (From Breier, 1989. With permission.)

were no significant differences between the two groups in success ratings following controllable noise stress. Moreover, the depressed patients, in comparison to volunteers, had a significantly greater peak change in cortisol levels during uncontrollable stress exposure (Figure 4). The uncontrollable cortisol baseline values (mean ± S.D.) for depressives (10 ± 5) and volunteers (7.1 ± 3) were not significantly different. Uncontrollalble peak cortisol levels were significantly correlated with uncontrollable ratings of helplessness (r = 0.80, $p = 0.02$). There were no significant differences between depressive and volunteer change in cortisol levels during controllable stress exposure (Figure 4). Both groups effectively terminated the controllable noise stress. There were no differences between depressive and volunteer ratings of helplessness and control following uncontrollable and controllable noise exposure.

Discussion

The results of the normal volunteer study demonstrate that exposure to brief, uncontrollable aversive stimuli produces greater alterations in behavioral responses and HPA axis function than exposure to identical amounts of controllable aversive stimuli. Uncontrollable stress administration, in comparison to controllable stress, resulted in increased ratings of helplessness, lack of control and success, and greater plasma ACTH levels. In addition, we have previously reported that uncontrollable noise stress exposure in healthy volunteers results in elevated skin conductance activity and increased plasma epinephrine levels (Breier et al., 1987a).

These data are similar to those reported from various "learned helplessness" paradigms in animals, although there are also important differences between the human uncontrollable stress paradigm reported here and uncontrollable stress experiments in animals. In many animal studies (Weiss et al., 1981; Anisman et al., 1980), both the magnitude and duration of stress exposure are greater than that used in this and other human studies. The latter may account for the more profound neurobiological and behavioral changes in animals exposed to uncontrollable stress. Nevertheless, the determination of behavioral changes such as "helplessness" following uncontrollable stress in animals can only be indirectly inferred from behavioral observation and performance tasks, whereas direct assessment of mood state changes is possible in humans. There are, however, several parallels between the results of this study and studies of uncontrollable stress in animals. In the rhesus monkey, increases in plasma cortisol and decreases in social activity were observed following exposure to aversive uncontrollable noise (100 dB) stress when compared to either pre-stress baseline values or to animals exposed to identical amounts of controllable noise stress (Hanson et al., 1976; Nealis and Bowman, 1972). Similar results have also been observed in rodents, where significantly higher plasma levels of corticosterone have been observed following exposure to uncontrollable stress when compared to controllable stress (Swenson and Vogel, 1983).

The data indicating that uncontrollable stress resulted in greater behavioral and neuroendocrine effects in the depressed patients than the volunteers suggests that affectively ill patients may have altered HPA axis function and behavioral responsivity to uncontrollable stress. Furthermore, the significant correlation between uncontrollable stress-induced ratings of helplessness and cortisol secretion suggests that there may be an important relationship between the well-described cognitive deficits of depression (Beck et al., 1981) and increased HPA axis activation observed in many depressed patients (Carroll et al., 1976, 1981; Pfohl et al., 1985). The uncontrollable effects in depressed patients do not appear to be related to nonspecific stress effects because there were no significant behavioral and neuroendocrine differences between depressed and volunteer subjects when exposed to identical amounts of controllable stress. The data are in agreement with previous studies that have demonstrated that depressed subjects have increased behavioral and neurobiologic responses to uncontrollable stress (Gatchel et al., 1977). We conclude from this study that depressed patients may have increased sensitivity to uncontrollable stress and that their altered stress response may contribute to the pathophysiology of the behavioral and neuroendocrine deficits of depression.

2DG-INDUCED GLUCOPRIVIC STRESS

2-Deoxy-D-glucose (2DG) is a glucose analog that competitively inhibits intracellular glucose metabolism. Because neurons are critically dependent on glucose for metabolic activity, the central nervous system is especially sensitive to the effects of 2DG-induced glucoprivation. 2DG-induced glucoprivic effects include strong activation of the HPA axis (Woolf et al., 1977; Brodows et al., 1973) and adrenomedullary (Welle et al., 1980) activity, and stimulation of appetite centers (Muller et al., 1972; Miselis and Epstein, 1970; Yamamoto et al., 1984). Thus, 2DG administration is an attractive stress paradigm to address a wide variety of research questions.

We have developed a stress paradigm that involves 2DG infusion (50 mg/kg) for human studies and examined a range of questions. In a study of healthy volunteers, we examined the interrelationship among HPA axis, adrenomedullary, and sympathoneural function during 2DG-induced glucoprivic stress (Breier et al., 1987c; Breier, 1989). We found that 2DG produced robust elevations in plasma levels of ACTH, cortisol, and epinephrine; modest increases in plasma norepinephrine; and significant decreases in plasma dihydroxyphenylglycol (DHPG), the intraneuronal metabolite of norepinephrine (Eisenhofer et al., 1987). Plasma increases in ACTH and cortisol were not correlated with increases in plasma epinephrine levels, suggesting that one central modulator alone, such as corticotropin-releasing factor (CRF), is probably insufficient to explain glucoprivic stress-induced activation of the HPA axis and adrenomedullary system. Moreover, the decrease in DHPG suggests that glucoprivation may result in suppression of sympathoneural activity. We also found that the epinephrine and norepinephrine elevations were significantly correlated, which, together with the finding of decreased DHPG levels, suggests that the modest 2DG-induced increases in plasma norepinephrine may originate from adrenomedullary sources. This contention is supported by data indicating that significant amounts of stress-induced peripheral norepinephrine originate from adrenomedullary stores (Goldstein et al., 1983).

In another study using the 2DG-stress paradigm, we examined the effects of stress on dopamine function in neuroleptic-treated schizophrenic patients and healthy volunteers by comparing post-2DG infusion plasma levels of the dopamine metabolite homovanillic acid (HVA) (Breier, 1989). We found that 2DG-induced stress produced significantly greater elevations in HVA in schizophrenic patients as compared to the healthy volunteers. This study suggests that schizophrenic patients may have altered stress-induced dopamine activity. To further clarify the effects of stress in schizophrenic patients, we are currently examining the effects of 2DG in drug-free and matched, neuroleptic-treated schizophrenic patients.

We present data here from a third study that examined the effects of glucoprivic stress on mitogen T-cell proliferation (Breier et al., 1987b).

Methods

Four healthy female volunteers (age range, 21 to 33 years) participated in an active 2DG (50 mg/kg) infusion test day and a placebo (normal saline) infusion test day. Blood samples were obtained at two points on each test day: at baseline prior to infusion and 150 min after infusion. The procedure for assessing T-cell proliferation was described in detail previously (Breier et al., 1987b; Arora et al., 1987). Briefly, cells were cultured in the presence of mitogen for 72 h (concanavalin A [ConA] was added in a concentration of 0.5 μg per culture and phytohemagglutinins [PHAs] at a concentration of 2.5 μg per culture) and pulsed with tritiated thymidine (sp act, 6.7 Ci/mmol) for the final 18 to 20 h. The data were expressed as cpm and each value represents the mean of six individual wells.

Results

2-Deoxy-D-glucose caused rapid suppression of T-cell proliferation to both ConA and PHA mitogens (Figure 5). The average percent suppression 2 h following 2DG administration for ConA and PHA was 68 and 46%, respectively, with significant reductions in cell counts following 2DG administration, compared with baseline counts for ConA ($p < 0.02$) and PHA ($p < 0.025$). There were no significant changes in T-cell proliferation following placebo. There were significant increases in plasma cortisol levels following 2DG administration.

Discussion

The data from the immune study demonstrated that 2DG-induced stress results in rapid and robust suppression of mitogen stimulated T-cell proliferation. The mechanism of 2DG-induced immunosuppression is under investigation. *In vitro* incubation of 2DG and human lymphocytes for 2 h does not suppress T-cell function (Arora, 1987, unpublished data), suggesting that the effects of 2DG administration on T-cell activity observed in this study were not because of the direct effects of 2DG on the T-cells themselves. 2DG administration at the doses used in this study results in robust activation of the HPA axis (Breier, 1989). Glucocorticoids, which are known to suppress mitogen-stimulated T-cell activity, may have had an effect on the T-cell proliferation in the present study. However, we did not find a relationship between the degree of cortisol secretion and T-cell suppression in individual subjects. Moreover, the extent of suppression observed in this study is probably greater than would be expected by glucocorticoids alone, suggesting that additional processes may have contributed to the T-cell suppression observed in this study.

There is a growing body of literature indicating that altered immune func-

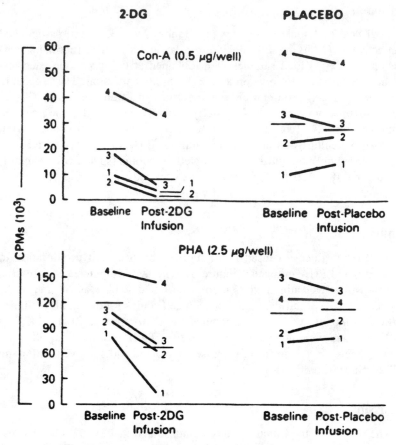

Figure 3-5. Effects of 2-deoxy-*D*-glucose (2-DG)-induced stress on mitogen T-cell proliferation. Each value represents a mean of six wells. Each subject is represented by the same numeral (N = 4). ConA indicates concanavalin A; PHA, phytohem-agglutinin; and cpm, counts per minute. (From Breier et al., 1987b. With permission.)

tion may play an important role in the pathophysiology of severe psychiatric illnesses such as depression (Schleifer et al., 1983, 1984) and schizophrenia (DeLisi and Crow, 1986). Thus, the 2DG paradigm may be a useful approach to examine immune function in these and other illnesses.

CONCLUSION

In summary, we have presented data from two different laboratory-based stress paradigms designed to examine the effects of psychological and physical stress in humans. The psychological stressor assessed the effects of controllable and uncontrollable noise stress in healthy volunteers and depressed patients. In healthy volunteers, we found that uncontrollable stress produces robust behavioral responses and significant, although relatively modest, neuroendocrine responses. Moreover, depressed patients, in comparison to normal controls, have increased sensitivity to both the behavioral and neuroendocrine effects of uncontrollable stress, whereas depressed patients and controls have similar responses to controllable stress. In the 2DG study, we reported that 2DG-induced glucoprivic stress produces robust elevations in plasma levels of epinephrine, cortisol, and ACTH, and that the levels of activation of the adrenomedullary system and HPA axis were not correlated. We presented data here from a study that demonstrated that 2DG-related stress causes rapid suppression of T-cell activity and suggest that the 2DG paradigm may be a useful tool to study stress effects on immune function.

We have reported previously that the effects of psychological and physical stress on neurobiological function and behavior are qualitatively and quantitatively quite different (Breier, 1989), indicating that the choice of stress paradigm is a crucial issue for human studies. Future studies using a range of stress paradigms will be needed to further elucidate the neurobiology of the human stress response.

REFERENCES

Anisman H, Pizzino A, and Sklar LS: Coping with stress, norepinephrine and escape performance. *Brain Res* 1980; 191:583–588.

Anisman H: Vulnerability to depression: contribution of stress. In *Neurobiology of Mood Disorders* Vol 1. Post RM and Ballenger JC, Eds. Williams & Wilkins, Baltimore 1984.

Arora PK, Hanna EE, Paul SM, and Skolnick P: Suppression of the immune response by benzodiazepine receptor inverse agonists. *J Neuroimmunol* 1987; 15:1–9.

Arora PK: Unpublished data, 1984.

Beck AT, Rush AJ, Shaw BF, and Emery G: *Cognitive Therapy of Depression* Guilford Press, New York, 1981.

Breier A, Charney DS, and Heninger GR: Agoraphobia with panic attacks: development, diagnostic stability and course of illness. *Arch Gen Psychiatry* 1986; 43:1029–1036.

Breier A, Charney DS, and Heninger GR: Intravenous diazepam fails to effect growth hormone and cortisol secretion in humans. *Psychiatry Res* 1986b; 18:293–299.

Breier A, Albus M, Pickar D, Zahn TP, Wolkowitz OM and Paul SM: Controllable and uncontrollable stress in humans: alterations in mood, neuroendocrine and psychophysiologic function. *Am J Psychiatry* 1987a; 144:1419–1425.

Breier A, Arora PK, Wolkowitz OM, Pickar D, and Paul SM: Metabolic stress produces rapid immunosuppression in humans. *Arch Gen Psychiatry* 1987b; 44:1108–1109.

Breier A, Goldstein D, Rappaport M, Paul SM, and Pickar D: Metabolic stress effects in normal volunteers and schizophrenic patients. *Proc ACNP*, 1987c.

Breier A and Paul SM: The neurobiological substrates of anxiety. In *Handbook of Anxiety* Roth M, Burrows GD, and Noyes R, Eds. Elsevier, Cambridge 1988.

Breier A, Kelsoe JR, Kirwin PD, Bellar SA, Wolkowitz OM, and Pickar D: Early parental loss and the development of adult psychopathology, *Arch Gen Psychiatry* 1988; 45:987–993.

Breier A: Experimental approaches to human stress research: assessment of neurobiological mechanisms of stress in volunteers and psychiatric patients. *Biol Psychiatry* 1989; 26:438–462.

Brodows RG, Pi Sunyer FX, and Campbell RG: Neural control of counter-regulatory events during glucopenia in man. *J Clin Invest* 1973; 52:1841–1845.

Brodows RG, Pi Sunyer FX, and Campbell RG: Sympathetic control of hepatic glycogenolysis during glucopenia in man. *Metabolism* 1975; 24:617–624.

Brown GW, Harris TO, and Peto J: Life events and psychiatric disorders. II. Nature of causal links. *Psychol Med* 1973; 3:159–176.

Carroll BJ, Curtis GC and Mendels J: Neuroendocrine regulation in depression. II. Discrimination of depressed from nondepressed patients. *Arch Gen Psychiatry* 1976; 33:1051–1058.

Carroll BJ, Feinberg M, Greden JF, et al: A specific laboratory test for the diagnosis of melancholia: standardization, validation and clinical utility. *Arch Gen Psychiatry* 1981; 38:15–22.

Charney DS, Heninger GR, and Breier A: Noradrenergic function in panic anxiety: effects of yohimbine in healthy subjects and patients with agoraphobia and panic disorder. *Arch Gen Psychiatry* 1984; 41:751–763.

Charney DS, Breier A, Jatlow PI, and Heninger GR: Behavioral, biochemical and blood pressure responses to alprazolam in healthy subjects: interaction with yohimbine. *Psychopharmacology* 1986; 88:133–140.

Davis H, Porter JW, Livingstone J, et al: Pituitary-adrenal activity and lever press shock escape behavior. *Physiol Psychol* 1977; 5:280–284.

DeLisi LE and Crow TJ: Is schizophrenia a viral or immunological disorder? *Psychiatr Clin N Am* 1986; 9(1):115–132.

Eisenhofer G, Goldstein DS, Stull R, Keiser HR, Sunderland T, Murphy DL, and Kopin IJ: Simultaneous liquid chromatographic determination of 3,4-dihydroxyphenylglycol, catecholamines, and 3,4-dihydroxyphenylalanine and their responses to inhibition of monamine oxidase. *Clin Chem* 1986; 32:2030–2033.

Eisenhofer G, Ropchak TG, Stull RW, Goldstein DS, Keiser HR, and Kopin IJ: Dihydroxyphenylglycol and intraneuronal metabolism of endogenous and exogenous norepinephrine in the rat vas deferens. *J Pharm Exp Ther* 1987; 241:547–553.

Forrest AD, Fraser RH, and Priest RG: Environmental factors in depressive illness. *Br J Psychiatry* 1965; 111:243–253.

Gatchel RJ and Proctor DJ: Physiologic correlates of learned helplessness in man. *J Abnorm Psychol* 1976; 85:27–34.

Gatchel RJ, McKinney ME, and Koebernick LF: Learned helplessness, depression, and physiological response. *Psychophysiology* 1977; 14:25–31.

Goldstein DS, McCarty R, Polinsky RJ, and Kopin IJ: Relationship between plasma norepinephrine and sympathetic neural activity. *Hypertension* 1983; 5:552–559.

Goodwin FK and Bunney WE: Psychobiological aspects of stress and affective illness. In *Separation and Aggression: Clinical and Research Aspects* Scott JP and Senay EC, Eds. AAAS, Washington, D.C. 1973.

Hanson JD, Larson ME, and Snowdon CT: The effects of control over high intensity noise on plasma cortisol levels in rhesus monkeys. *Behav Biol* 1976; 16:333–340.

Hiroto DS: Locus of control and learned helplessness. *J Exp Psychol* 1974; 102:187–193.

Laudenslager ML, Ryan SM, Drugan RC, Hyson RL, and Maier SF: Coping and immunosuppression: inescapable but not escapable shock suppresses lymphocyte proliferation. *Science* 1983; 221:568–570.

Leff MJ, Roatch JF, and Bunney WE: Environmental factors preceding the onset of severe depression. *Psychiatry* 1970; 33:298–311.

Lloyd C: Life events and depressive disorder reviewed. II. Events as precipitating factors. *Arch Gen Psychiatry* 1980; 37:541–548.

McNair DM, Lorr M, and Droppleman LF: *Profile of Mood States (POMS)* Educational Testing Service, San Diego 1971.

Miselis R and Epstein AN: Feeding induced by 2DG injection into the lateral ventricle of the rat. *Physiologist* 1970; 73:3.

Muller EE, Cocchi D, and Mantegazza P: Brain adrenergic system in the feeding response induced by 2DG. *Am J Physiol* 1972; 223:945–950.

Nealis PM and Bowman RE: The effects of man-made noise on social behaviors and plasma cortisol levels of rhesus monkeys. In *National Science Foundation Final Report* 1972; Grant 64–9634.

Paykel ES, Myers JK, Dienelt MN, et al: Life events and depression: a controlled study. *Arch Gen Psychiatry* 1969; 21:753–760.

Pfohl B, Herman B, Schlechte J, et al: Pituitary-adrenal axis rhythm disturbances in psychiatric depression. *Arch Gen Psychiatry* 1985; 42:897–903.

Schleifer SJ, Keller SE, Camerino M, Thornton JC, and Stein M: Suppression of lymphocytes stimulation following bereavement. *JAMA* 1983; 250:374–377.

Schleifer SJ, Keller SE, Meyerson AJ, and Stein M: Lymphocyte function in major depressive disorder. *Arch Gen Psychiatry* 1984; 41:484–486.

Seligman MEP and Maier SF: Failure to escape traumatic shock *J Exp Psychol* 1967; 74:1–9.

Seligman MEP, Klein DC, and Miller WR: Depression. In *Handbook of Behavior Modification and Behavior Therapy* Leitenberg H, Ed. Prentice-Hall, Englewood Cliffs, NJ 1976.

Swenson RM and Vogel WH: Plasma catecholamine and corticosterone as well as brain catecholamine changes during coping in rats exposed to stressful foot shock. *Pharmacol Biochem Behav* 1983; 18:689–693.

Thompson K and Hendric H: Environmental stress in primary depressive illness. *Arch Gen Psychiatry* 1972; 26:130–132.

Tresselt ME and Mayzner MS: Normative solution times for a sample of 134 solution words and 378 associated anagrams. *Psychon Monogr Suppl.* 1966; 1:293–299.

Weiss JM, Goodman PA, Losito BG, et al: Behavioral depression produced by an uncontrollable stressor: relationship to norepinephrine, dopamine and serotonin levels in various brain regions. *Brain Res Rev* 1981; 3:167–205.

Weiss JM and Simson PG: Neurochemical basis of stress-induced depression. *Psychopharm Bull* 1985; 21:447–457.

Welle SL, Thompson DA, Campbell RG, and Lilavivathana U: Increased hunger and thirst during glucoprivation in humans. *Physiol Behav* 1980; 25:397–403.

Wolkowitz OM, Doran AR, Breier A, Cohen MR and Pickar D: Endogenous opioid regulation of hypothalamo-pituitary-adrenal axis activity in schizophrenia. *Biol Psychiatry* 1986; 21:366–373.

Wolkowitz OM, Doran AR, Breier A, Roy A, Jimerson DC, Sutton ME, Golden RN, Paul SM, and Pickar D: The effects of dexamethasone on plasma homovanillic acid and 3-methoxy-4-hydroxyphenylglycol: evidence for abnormal corticosteroid-catecholamine interactions in major depression. *Arch Gen Psychiatry* 1987; 44:782–789.

Woolf PD, Lee LA, Leebaw W, Thompson D, Lilavivathana U, Brodows R, and Campbell R: Intracellular glucopenia causes prolactin release in man. *J Clin Endocrinol Metab* 1977; 45:377–383.

Yamamoto H, Nagai K, and Nakagawa H: Bilateral lesions of the SCN abolish lipolytic and hyperphagic responses to 2DG. *Biol Behav* 1984; 32:1017–1020.

Psychosocial Stress and Disease: A Historical Sketch*

Robert Kellner
Department of Psychiatry, School of Medicine
The University of New Mexico
Albuquerque, New Mexico

INTRODUCTION

The scientific study on the effects of social stress and disease had slow beginnings. Poets had written about broken hearts long before epidemiologists became aware of the risks of bereavement. Sir Henry Wooten wrote, "He first deceased/ She tried/ To live without him/ She liked it not/ And died." In the short story, *Camille,* by Alexander Dumas, which later became the libretto for *La Traviata,* the beautiful heroine dies of tuberculosis after she had been abandoned by her highborn lover, long before the relationship of a broken love link and a susceptibility to tuberculosis was known to scientists. The relationship between stress and disease remained the domain of folklore and speculations by physicians and was not a topic of scientific pursuit until the second half of this century.

The earliest data on the relationship of psychosocial stress and disease were serendipitous; they did not stir interest in the scientific community at the time, were often not emphasized by the authors of the study, and some were dismissed as unexplained or as statistical flukes. Downes and Simons (1953) carried out a family study in Baltimore, MD, during World War II.

*This chapter is based on the C. Charles Burlingame, M.D. award lecture at the Institute of Living, Hartford, CT, April, 1988.

The authors compared families of patients with psychoneurosis to other families. They found a higher incidence of physical illness and psychosomatic illness in the families of psychoneurotics than in other families. The nature of the study does not allow conclusions about causation. Chronic and severe physical illness in the family can act as a stressor and could be a precipitant or an aggravating factor in neurosis (Kellner, 1963); conversely, having a psychoneurotic family member could be a stressor that predisposes to disease. There was, however, a finding in this study which did not make sense: rheumatic fever, a disease caused by streptococcal infections, was more common in the families of the psychoneurotics. To my knowledge, this result was not pursued at the time and an explanation for this finding had to wait for 2 decades.

Two pediatricians, Meyer and Haggerty (1962), decided to examine children's susceptibility to streptococcal infection, and in particular, whether the children developed infections at time of stress. In a prospective study, the authors counted the number of stressful events in each family, took throat swabs in children, and measured the number of antistreptolysin-o responses at regular intervals. They found that the complaints of sore throat, acquisition of infection, and antistreptolysin-o responses were higher 2 weeks after a stressful event in the family than in the 2 weeks before. When the relationship of these measures of infection and the scores of a psychological test measuring chronic family stress were compared, there was a significant positive correlation of chronic family stress and the acquisition of streptococcal infections. Dr. John Appley, a pioneer of research in the psychosomatic diseases of children, commented on this study in a lecture, "stress means streps".

A series of studies on the relationship of psychosocial stress and disease were carried out by Kissen (1982), a Scottish chest physician. Several of his studies showed clear associations between psychosocial stress and tuberculosis. In a retrospective study, the author found more deprivation of affection in childhood among patients with tuberculosis than other patients with chest disease who did not have tuberculosis. In a prospective study, he found that the Mantoux convertors who progressed to clinical TB had more recent psychosocial stressors than patients who did not develop a clinical illness, suggesting that emotional stress made the patient more vulnerable to the disease. The most important factor associated with clinical disease was a break in a love link such as abandonment, divorce, and bereavement.

Since then there have been numerous reports on the relationship of stress and impaired immunity. Several authors have reviewed this topic, for example, Kiecolt-Glaser and Glaser (1986), and the present volume attests to the progress in the field.

SOCIAL RELATIONSHIPS AND HEALTH

Social relationships and health have been recently reviewed by House et al. (1988). The survey of prospective studies and experimental research clearly shows that close social relationships and social integration have a protective value. They summarized studies that show that the unmarried and more socially isolated have higher rates of tuberculosis (Holmes, 1956). Other studies have since shown that social isolation, at least in the elderly, impairs immune competence and increases known risk factors (Thomas et al., 1985). The authors conclude that poor social relationships or social isolation constitute a major risk factor for health — rivaling the effects of well-established health risk factors such as cigarette smoking, elevated blood pressure, elevated blood lipids, obesity, and lack of physical activity. The evidence on social relationships and health increasingly approximates that available at the time of the U.S. Surgeon General's 1964 report on smoking and health, with similar implications for future research and public policy. Kennedy et al. (1988), in a review on the effects of stressors on immunity, concluded that the quality of interpersonal relationships may serve to attenuate the adverse immunological changes associated with psychological distress.

SOCIAL STRESS, MENTAL ILLNESS, AND PHYSICAL ILLNESS

In a series of studies, Holmes and Rahe (1968) showed a relationship between events and changes on one hand and distress such as anxiety and depression on the other; their studies show also a small but statistically significant association with physical illness. Later studies focusing on depression found that the changes have to be of a certain kind: the events are beyond the individual's control and have an "objective negative impact", in other words, they would be regarded by an outside observer as distressing (Fava et al., 1981). Depression, in turn, has been found to be associated with decreased immune competency on one hand (Editorial, 1987) and a substantially increased mortality (Avery and Winokur, 1976).

LONELINESS

The effects of loneliness have been reviewed by West et al. (1986). Loneliness is a subjective feeling, and is only weakly correlated with lack of contact with other people. Simple, self-rating scales of loneliness have been found to be associated with decreased immune competency (Kiecolt-Glaser et al., 1984b, 1984c) and poor health. Lynch, in his monograph *The Broken*

Heart (1979), surveyed the studies that evaluated the effects of loneliness and social isolation on health, and consistent trends emerged: the lonely and socially isolated were at higher risk. West and his colleagues conclude that studies of loneliness are linked with reported feelings of ill health, somatic distress, and visits to physicians. There is some link for a subjective feeling of loneliness and physical disease, but, to date, the feeling of loneliness is more closely associated with decreased immune competency (Kiecolt-Glaser et al., 1984a, 1984b, 1984c; Locke et al., 1981). In most studies, the effects of feeling lonely on the one hand and lack of social integration on the other have not been separately evaluated. A few findings suggest the relationship of loneliness to the development of cancer and cardiovascular disease, but the studies are too few to warrant conclusions.

MARRIAGE

The most thoroughly researched phenomenon and its effect on health is marriage, its dissolution, or absence. Marriage can be decidedly stressful, and studies have shown that stresses within marriage or poor marital adjustment are associated with depression. Although marital maladjustment could be a consequence of depression, there are other studies to show that a close relationship with another person at times of crisis has a protective effect and prevents depression (Brown et al., 1986; Kennedy et al., 1988). It would truly be hard to find a magazine that contained cartoons that did not also contain at least one pertaining to the hassles of married life. For example, a recent cartoon shows a man at a table. His wife in curlers, unattractive and slovenly dressed, is bringing him a cup of coffee; the caption is, "I don't know what I'd do without you Doris. But I'd like to give it a six months try." Another cartoon shows the inside of an empty house without any furniture, carpeting, or pictures; a man is coming through the door and is asking, "Honey, I'm home. Still mad?" In George Orwell's novel, *Coming Up For Air,* the hero says to himself after a quarrel with his wife that when someone is murdered, the first person the police cross-examine is the spouse; which goes to show what our society really thinks about marriage.

So while discord in marriage can cause anguish and pain and may have serious effects on mental and probably physical health, the overwhelming evidence points to the protective value of marriage. Since the sexual revolution, Western society has apparently decided that chastity is less important than charity, to my mind a gratifying change from the attitudes prevailing in the previous century. It is too soon to tell whether living with a person of the opposite sex has the same protective effects as having a legal contract of marriage and solemnization by religious vows.

People who are married tend to be healthier and live longer than those who are not. Mortality is increased after bereavement (Kaprio et al., 1987; Parkes 1972); the causes for this are probably multiple; there is a documented increase in drinking, smoking, depression, and, perhaps, a neglect of adequate nutrition. The mortality from virtually all diseases is higher in the widowed than in the married (Kraus and Lilienfeld, 1959).

Living alone in an unmarried state even if not bereaved also carries an increased risk (Lynch, 1979). Morowitz (1975) shows the well-known and robust association of smoking and increased mortality. However, married men smoking more than one pack a day had almost the same mortality as single nonsmoking men. The study again demonstrates the protective value of marriage; I am not sure, however, of the other practical implications of this finding. To paraphrase the author of this study, one of the implications is as follows: if a counselor or a health professional has a patient who is male, smokes more than one pack a week, and claims that he does so only because his wife is driving him to distraction, and that if he was not married to her, he could stop smoking; if longevity was his only consideration, one could safely counsel him that he may just as well stay put. One might also quote similar statistics to those who are thinking of marriage but are undecided; the chances are that they are going to live longer.

CAUSES FOR THE ASSOCIATION

Impaired immune competency mediated by psychosocial stressors and depression is probably only one of the many factors and probably not even the most important one. In a study of treated and untreated depressives, one of the causes of high mortality in the untreated was an increased rate of myocardial infarction (Avery and Winokur, 1976), so the cardiovascular consequences of stress are probably one of the important contributing factors. Similarly, in the study of bereavement, mortality was highest in the first week after bereavement and the risk was higher for ischemic heart disease.

The relationship of stress within marriage and families is even more complex and the effects of stress are difficult to isolate from other factors. Families differ in health. Diseases tend to cluster in some families, whereas other families are fortunate and stay healthy. Genetics, assortative mating, shared socioeconomic factors, the spread of infection within the family, stresses that affect the whole family, and interaction within the family all may be playing a role. The causes are probably multiple, arriving at different times in people's and families' lives. Illness in the family, even if noninfectious, poses at least a slightly increased risk for the other members (Kellner, 1963).

WHAT CAN BE DONE?

The differences in morbidity and mortality among social classes in Western countries and the striking differences in life expectancy between developed and underdeveloped countries show a strong link between poverty and poor education on the one hand and disease on the other. Determined action by a society can improve health. In several Western democracies, deliberate policies aimed at combating poverty have eventually decreased it. Organized public health measures to prevent disease and the availability of medical care clearly affect longevity as well as health. A description of the numerous ways by which the delivery of medical care saves lives and prevents disease from becoming chronic is beyond the scope of this chapter.

The axiom of antiquity that a healthy mind resides in a healthy body has been confirmed by research (Kellner, 1987). There is evidence that disease impairs mental health and, conversely, mental disorders impair health in many ways and increase mortality. Eysenk (1987, 1988) reviewed the relationship of personality, stress, and death from cancer and heart disease and found that stress was a potent cause of death, and stressed individuals had a 40% higher death rate than nonstressed ones. Energetic treatment of mental illness with drugs or ECT has been shown to be associated with decreased mortality and depression (Avery and Winokur, 1976). Appropriate treatment of mental illness probably improves the health of the family members as well. Recent controlled studies of psychotherapy have also shown evidence that it leads to improvement in mental health and others have shown beneficial effects on the prognosis in physical disease. For example, there are two controlled studies in the literature in which psychotherapy has helped the healing rate of peptic ulcer (Chappell and Stevenson, 1936; Sjödin, 1986). Grossarth-Maticek et al. (1984) carried out a controlled study of psychotherapy in patients with disseminated cancer. The psychotherapy was devised by the author and addressed specifically the problems which he believed were important in cancer patients. Psychotherapy had the same effect on survival time as chemotherapy and the survival time with the combination of psychotherapy and chemotherapy was significantly longer than with chemotherapy alone.

A PREDICTION

Predictions are the most cost-effective activities of scientists. If the predictor is correct, he or she can proudly claim to have been right all along; conversely, when the prediction is wrong, the writer will not draw attention to the previous forecasts, and the predictor is seldom blamed for it. Prediction involves only little work, and offers a quick way for self-aggrandizement. The trouble is, as one cartoon character recently said, ''Prediction is difficult, particularly if it pertains to the future.''

The present volume shows that research in psychoimmunology is expanding, and a survey of the literature of recent years suggests that research on the relationship of psychosocial stress and disease will continue to increase. There is also evidence to suggest that a substantial benefit of physical health can come from the use of psychotropic drugs from psychotherapy and probably in the future from the application of knowledge from psychoimmunology. In years to come, healers will aim at a healthy mind when they treat an ill body.

REFERENCES

Avery D, and Winokur G: Mortality in depressed patients treated with electroconvulsive therapy and antidepressants. *Arch Gen Psychiatry* 1976; 33:1029.

Brown GW, Andrews B, Harris T, Adler Z, and Bridge L: Social Support, self-esteem and depression. *Psychol Med* 1986; 16:813.

Calabrese JR, Kling MA, and Gold PW: Alterations in immunocompetence during stress, bereavement, and depression: focus on neuroendocrine regulation. *Am J Psychiatry* 1987; 144:1123.

Downes J and Simon K: Characteristics of psychoneurotic patients and their families as revealed in a general morbidity study. *Psychosom Med* 1953; 15(5):463.

Editorial: depression, stress, and immunity. *Lancet* June 1987.

Eysenck HJ: Personality as a predictor of cancer and cardiovascular disease, and the application of behaviour therapy in prophylaxis. *Eur J Psychiatry* 1987; 1(1):29.

Eysenck HJ: Personality, stress and cancer: prediction and prophylaxis. *Br J Med Psychol* 1988; 61:57.

Fava GA, Munari F, Pavan L, and Kellner R: Life events and depression, a replication. *J Affect Disord* 1981; 3:159.

Grossarth-Maticek R, Schmidt P, Vetter H, and Arndt S: Psychotherapy research in oncology. In *Health Care and Human Behaviour* Steptoe A and Matthews AM, Eds. Academic Press, London 1984, pp. 325–341.

Holmes TH and Rahe RH: The Social Readjustment Rating Scale. *J Psychosom Res* 1968; 11:213.

Holmes TH: *Personality, Stress and Tuberculosis* Sparer PJ, Ed. International Universities Press, New York, 1956.

House JS, Landis KR, and Umberson D: Social realtionships and health. *Science* 1988; 241:6640.

Kaprio J, Koskenvuo M, and Rita H: Mortality after bereavement: a prospective study of 95,647 widowed persons. *Am J Publ Health* 1987; 77:283.

Kellner R: *Family Ill Health, An Investigation in General Practice* Tavistock Publications and Charles C Thomas, London 1963.

Kellner R: Physical health, mental health and exercise. In *Sports Medicine* Appenzeller O, Ed. Urban & Schwarzenberg, Baltimore 1987, pp. 73–81.

Kennedy S, Kiecolt-Glaser JK, and Glaser R: Immunological consequences of acute and chronic stressors: mediating role of interpersonal relationships. *Br J Med Psychol* 1988; 61:77.

Kiecolt-Glaser JK, Ricker D, George J, et al: Urinary cortisol levels, cellular im-munocompetency, and loneliness in psychiatric inpatients. *Psychosom Med* 1984a; 46:15.

Kiecolt-Glaser JK, Garner W, Speicher C, et al: Psychosocial modifiers of immu-nocompetency in medical students. *Psychosom Med* 1984b; 46:7.

Kiecolt-Glaser JK, Speicher CE, Holliday JE, et al: Stress and the transformation of lymphocytes by Epstein-Barr virus. *J Behav Med* 1984c; 7:1.

Kiecolt-Glaser JK and Glaser R: Psychological influences on immunity. *Immunity* 1986; 27:621.

Kissen DM: *Emotional Factors in Pulmonary Tuberculosis* Tavistock, London 1982.

Kraus AS and Lilienfeld AM: Some epidemiological aspects of the high mortality rate in the young widowed group. *J Chron Dis* 1959; 10:207.

Locke SE, Hurst MW, Heisel JS, et al: The influence of stress and other social factors on human immunity. Paper presented at American Psychosomatic Meeting. Cited in *Psychoneuroimmunology* Academic Press, Orlando 1981, pp. 129–138.

Lynch JJ: *The Broken Heart. The Medical Consequences of Loneliness* Basic Books, New York, 1977.

Meyer RJ and Haggerty RJ: Streptococcal infections in families. *Pediatrics* 1962; 29:539.

Morowitz HJ: Hiding in the Hammond Report. *Hosp Pract,* 1975; August:35.

Parkes CM: *Bereavement. Of Grief in Adult Life* International Universities Press, New York, 1972.

Pennebaker JW, Kiecolt-Glaser JK, and Glaser R: Disclosure of traumas and immune function: health implications for psychotherapy. *J Consult Clin Psychol* 1988; 56:239.

Sjödin I, Svedlund J, Ottoson JO, and Dotevall G: Controlled study of psychotherapy in chronic peptic ulcer disease. *Psychosomatics* 1986; 27(3):187.

Thomas PD, Goodwin JM, and Goodwin JS: Effect of social support on stress-related changes in cholesterol level, uric acid level, and immune function in an elderly sample. *Am J Psychiatry* 1985; 142:735.

West DA, Moore-West M, and Kellner R: The effects of loneliness: a review of the literature. *Compr Psychiatry* 1986; 27(4):351.

Widmer RB and Cadoret RJ: Depression in primary care: changes in pattern of patient visits and complaints during a developing depression. *J Fam Pract* 1978; 7:293.

Chapter

5

Stress and Immunity: A Behavioral Medicine Perspective

Edward A. Workman
Department of Psychiatry
University of Virginia
Roanoke/Salem Program
Salem, Virginia

Mariano F. La Via
Department of Pathology and Laboratory Medicine
Medical University of South Carolina,
Charleston, South Carolina.

THE IMMUNE SYSTEM: A BASIC OVERVIEW

The immune system has been defined classically as comprising two distinct arms: humoral and cellular. The humoral immune system effector cells are B-lymphocytes which can (1) differentiate into antibody-secreting plasma cells or (2) remain in a nondividing resting state as memory B-cells which, on second contact with an antigen, differentiate into antigen-specific plasma cells. Antibodies are circulating protein molecules which confer protection against certain bacteria, neutralize bacterial toxins, prevent reinfection with viruses, and mediate allergic reactions.

The cellular immune system, unlike the humoral system, confers immunity by cell-to-antigen contact rather than indirectly through antibodies. This system comprises T-lymphocytes, mononuclear phagocytes (macrophages), and polymorphonuclear (PMN) phagocytes. T-lymphocytes include T-helper (CD4 +) and T-suppressor cells (CD8 +). CD4 + lymphocytes help

69

other cells recognize antigens — specifically, macrophages and other T- and B-lymphocytes. CD4+ cells, after contacting an antigen presented by a macrophage, produce interleukin-2, a lymphokine which is capable of stimulating other T-helper cells, natural killer (NK) cells, cytotoxic CD8+ lymphocytes, and CD8+ T-suppressor cells. NK and cytotoxic T-cells both serve antiviral, antitumor, and antifungal functions. The difference between these cell types lies in the NK cells' unique ability to attack and destroy infected cells without prior interaction with these cells. CD8+ T-suppressor cells function to modulate antibody-producing plasma cells, thus supplying a "governing system" which keeps the immune system from cycling out of control.

PMN phagocytes or granulocytes are circulating "white cells" which have the ability to engulf antigens and digest them via complex enzyme systems contained in granules. PMNs include neutrophils, eosinophils, and basophils, and are involved in the early defense response to bacteria, parasites, and various allergens. Mononuclear phagocytes (monocytes in peripheral blood and macrophages in tissue) have multiple functions, including (1) direct killing by ingestion of pathogenic invaders, (2) the processing of antigens to be presented to helper T-cells, and (3) the direct stimulation of T-helpers via production and secretion of a lymphokine, interleukin-1, which activates T-helpers (Roitt et al., 1989).

THE IMMUNOLOGICAL EFFECTS OF STRESS

The interrelationships of the central nervous and immune systems have been the subject of ever increasing attention on the part of several investigators who have directed their efforts to elucidating various aspects of these interactions (Ader, 1981; Ader et al., 1991). In particular, numerous investigators have examined the immunomodulation induced by stress and have attempted to uncover its mechanisms and its relationship to morbidity.

A number of recent reviews have summarized studies of the effects of various psychological stressors on the immune system (Workman and La Via, 1987a; Calabrese et al., 1987; Dantzer et al., 1989; Khansari, 1990). The majority of studies have focused on the effects of three types of stressors, including examinations, bereavement, and marital discord. Almost without exception, these studies have found that psychological stress affects principally the cellular immune system, having little, if any, impact on plasma cell antibody production.

EXAMINATION STRESS

Dorian et al. (1982) compared eight psychiatric residents who were under high levels of stress (prior to Board Exams) to 16 similar-aged psychiatrists on multiple measures of immune system functioning. Two weeks prior to exams, the highest stress group exhibited significantly decreased responsiveness to the T-cell mitogens phytohemagglutinin (PHA) and concanavalin A (ConA). Also, NK cell activities were significantly depressed and total white counts and total lymphocytes were significantly elevated. Two weeks after the Board Exams, PHA response (in the high-stress group) had increased significantly compared to controls, and all other variables were nonsignificant.

Kiecolt-Glaser et al. (1984a) evaluated the immunological effects of stress in 75 medical students taking major examinations. As a group, the students exhibited a significant drop in NK cell activity during exams, as compared to baseline levels. Plasma IgA levels were increased, but no other variables were significantly altered. Interestingly, the most severe depression of NK activity was observed in medical students with the highest levels of overall life stress, as measured by the Holmes-Rahe Social Readjustment Rating Scale (SRRS).

BEREAVEMENT STRESS

Schleifer et al. (1983) used a multiple baseline design to evaluate the effects of stress on 15 male volunteers whose spouses were in a breast cancer treatment program. The subjects' immune responses were measured three times during treatment, on two occasions after the spouses' death, and during a 4- to 14-month follow-up period. During the period following their spouses' death, subjects exhibited significant reduction of responses to PHA, ConA, and pokeweed mitogen (PWM). The response to mitogens returned to baseline levels during the follow-up period.

Bartrop et al. (1977) compared the immune responses of 28 subjects whose spouses had died within 3 weeks (of accidents or illnesses) to 26 age-, sex-, and race-matched controls. At 1 to 3 weeks following the spouses' death, there was no significant difference between the two groups on mitogen responses (PHA, ConA) or numbers of T- or B-lymphocytes. However, at 6 weeks post-bereavement, bereaved subjects exhibited significantly lower PHA and ConA responses, indicating defects in the CD4+ lymphocyte system.

MARITAL DISCORD

Kiecolt-Glaser et al. (1988) compared 32 separated or divorced men to 32 married men, matched on age, number of children, and duration of marriage. Immunological dependent variables included antibody titers to Epstein-Barr virus (EBV) and herpes simplex virus type I (HSV-1), and relative percentages of helper (CD4+) and suppressor (CD8+) T-lymphocytes. Separated/divorced men exhibited significantly increased depression and distress (measured by the Brief Symptom Inventory) and loneliness (measured by the UCLA Loneliness Scale) when compared to matched controls. Furthermore, the separated/divorced group exhibited significantly more medical illnesses in the past 2 months, and significantly higher EBV and HSV-1 antibody titers as compared to controls. The latter finding suggests decreased cellular immune control of latent viruses, consistent with prior studies showing that stress depresses the function of the cell mediated responses. Interestingly, there were no significant differences in CD4 + and CD8 + lymphocyte percentages between the two groups. Also, no changes were observed in body weight, sleep pattern, or caffeine and alcohol intake.

Kiecolt-Glaser et al. (1987) compared 32 separated/divorced (S/D) women to 32 matched married women. Lymphocytes from S/D women exhibited significantly reduced responses to the mitogens PHA and ConA. Women who had been separated within the past year exhibited the most extreme reduction in mitogen response, and also exhibited significantly reduced NK and CD4 + cell percentages, as well as increased EBV antibody titers.

An interesting finding in both of the above studies was obtained when the married groups were analyzed in terms of marital quality (measured by the Dyadic Adjustment Scale). Poorer marital quality among males (Kiecolt-Glaser et al., 1988) was significantly associated with increased distress and depression, increased loneliness, and, most importantly, increased EBV antibody titers and decreased CD4/CD8 ratios. Poorer marital quality among females (Kiecolt-Glaser et al., 1987) was associated with decreased response to PHA and ConA, and increased EBV antibody titers. These subgroup findings strengthen the conclusion that stress from marital discord results in decreased cellular immune competence. Furthermore, subgroup differences in apparent responsiveness to stress lead to the concept of behavioral subtypes in stress-induced immunomodulation.

Having established that stress of various types will induce a reduction in the ability of T lymphocytes to respond to mitogen stimulation, attention has been turned to uncovering mechanisms which mediate their immunomodulatory effect.

Of particular interest in this respect are the recent observations of Glaser et al. (1990). These authors examined the expression of interleukin 2 receptors (IL2R) and the synthesis of mRNA in lymphocytes of students under stress. Their results showed a decrease of IL2R positive lymphocytes and of IL2R mRNA during the stress period as compared to baseline, non stress values. Moreover, they demonstrated that an increase of interleukin 2 could not overcome the stress-induced depression of IL2R positive cells and IL2R mRNA by up regulating IL2R. These observations are of great interest in that they suggest a possible mechanism for stress induced immunodepression and also indicate that stress may be acting at the level of gene expression. The search for pathogenetic mechanism of stress induced immunomodulation is of paramount importance in order to plan intervention strategies to reverse the depressive effects of stress on immune functions.

BEHAVIORAL SUBTYPES IN STRESS RESPONSES

The concept of behavioral subtypes involves the observation that different subgroups of individuals respond differentially to the same stressor. Although this concept is relatively new in the human stress literature, several early animal stress studies strongly suggested the existence of behavioral subtypes in stress response (Ingram and Corfman, 1980; Wahlsten, 1975). More recently, Irwin and Livnat (1987) compared shock stress modulation of NK activity in two distinct strains of mice. These researchers found that one strain (C57Bl/6J) exhibited significantly depressed NK activity with chronic shock administration. Interestingly, the comparison strain (DBA/2J) exhibited no significant changes during any shock conditions, suggesting that the former strain was more vulnerable to stress through some undetermined mechanism.

In the human stress literature, several studies have isolated behavioral subtypes of individuals who exhibit increased sensitivity to the immunological effects of stress. Workman and La Via (1987b) examined the effects of examination stress on 15 medical students matched, on age and sex, to 15 low-stress controls. Examination stress resulted in a significant (72%) reduction in the T-lymphocyte response to PHA. Most importantly, stressed subjects who were characterized by high scores on "stress intrusion" using the Impact of Events Scale (Horowitz et al., 1979) exhibited a significantly greater reduction of the response to PHA than did other stressed subjects. In fact, subjects with a high stress-intrusion response style exhibited a 34% greater reduction in the mitogen response than subjects characterized as "stress avoiders". Furthermore, stress intrusion subjects experienced an increased incidence of viral upper respiratory infections following stress as compared to stress avoidance subjects.

High stress-intrusion subjects are individuals who are hyperresponsive to stress. They are characterized by a tendency to ruminate about stressful events — they daydream about them, are unable to put stressors "out of mind", and sometimes tend to have nightmares about specific stressors. Proposed criteria (based on our clinical experience) for the stress-intrusion subtype are shown in Table 1. It seems possible that high stress-intrusion subjects represent individuals who are not only particularly susceptible to the immunosuppressive effects of stress, but may well be at enhanced risk for developing diseases that are secondary to this immunosuppression (e.g., viral syndromes, neoplastic processes). Recently Workman and Short (1991) have investigated the hypothesis that stress intrusion subjects may suffer from an anxiety disorder.

TABLE I.
Proposed Clinical Criteria for Identification of the Stress Intruder
Subtype

During the past week, the patient has been exposed to at least one stressful event which (1) generates recurrent ruminative thoughts at least five times per day on a daily basis, (2) keeps the patient from falling asleep within 30 min of usual bedtime at least three of the past five nights, and (3) prompts the patient to discuss with friends the stressful event at least three times per day on four of the past five days.

Following exposure to a stressful event, the patient either
(1) finds his/her appetite drastically reduced, or
(2) increases food intake significantly.

Following vivid thoughts of the stressful event, in 1 above, the patient either
(1) experiences waves of tension/anxiety or
(2) develops feelings of nausea, with or without vomiting.

Approximately 50% of a group of females volunteering for a study of the biochemistry of stress exhibited a high degree of stress intrusion. Over 85% of these subjects met the DMSIII-R criteria for panic disorder or generalized anxiety disorder. These preliminary results suggest that high stress intrusion subjects may suffer from an anxiety disorder. Extensive research is needed to address this possibility.

An interesting question regarding the concept of the stress-intrusion response style involves its possible relationship to Kobasa's (1979) concept of "hardiness". Hardiness, according to Kobasa, involves three components: commitment, control, and challenge. "Hardy" individuals are high on all three of these dimensions, exhibiting, respectively, feelings of meaningfulness in their work and relationships, a sense of being in control of events around them, and a tendency to interpret stressors as challenges that will be overcome. Hardy individuals have been shown by Kobasa to exhibit significantly less susceptibility to stress-induced illness than non-hardy individuals. The question arises as to whether high stress-intrusion persons are low on hardiness. Future research should clarify this interesting possibility.

Another subtype which may be particularly susceptible to the effects of stress is the individual characterized by loneliness or a poor social support network. Kiecolt-Glaser et al. (1984b) examined the lymphocyte response to PHA among psychiatric patients with hypercortisolism (which may be suggestive of high stress). These researchers found that PHA response was substantially reduced in a subset of patients with high scores on the UCLA Loneliness Scale.

Also, Kiecolt-Glaser et al. (1984a) examined the effect of examination stress on NK activity. Although stress itself, as would be expected, reduced NK activity, this reduction was highly correlated with the subjects' loneliness scores on the UCLA Loneliness Scale. Although of a correlational nature, these data are strongly suggestive that loneliness modifies the immunological response to psychological stress.

In a similar investigation, Kiecolt-Glaser et al. (1984c) evaluated the effects of examination stress and loneliness on the activation of lymphocytes by Epstein-Barr virus. Medical students were median split on the UCLA Loneliness Scale, and high vs. low loneliness students were compared. The results rather clearly indicated that viral transformation of lymphocytes was significantly reduced in the high-loneliness group.

It appears that, like a "stress-intruder" response style, loneliness enhances the immunosuppressive effects of psychological stress. Information about such modifier variables could be extremely useful in detecting persons who are at particular risk for stress-induced illnesses, and, perhaps, taking preventive measures to moderate these risks. Clearly, much future research is needed to refine our methods of measuring these modifier variables and articulating their mechanisms and the extent of their effect on stress-induced immunomodulation.

STRESS, IMMUNITY, AND DISEASE

Ultimately, the clinical significance of stress-induced immunosuppression lies in the extent to which the dampened cellular immunity results in medical illness. In other words, stressed subjects may exhibit *statistically significant* reductions in specified immunological measures, but do they concomitantly, or subsequently, exhibit *medically significant* alterations in their health status? Only a very small number of investigations have evaluated this issue.

Rahe and Arthur (1978) reviewed a long history of investigations examining the effects of stress exposure on medical illnesses. Clearly, extensive prior research had shown that significant stress exposure reliably precedes the onset or exacerbation of a variety of medical conditions, including allergic, autoimmune, neoplastic, and infectious processes. However, it should be noted that none of these myriad investigations attempted to link causally specific stress-induced immunological processes to specific pathological processes. The data presented show only gross, correlative relationships between stress and medical illness.

Since the Rahe and Arthur review, there have been numerous "correlational" studies examining further the relationship between various forms of "distress" and illness, but none have prospectively and systematically examined the effect of specific stress-induced immune system alterations on the onset or exacerbation of specific, well-defined, *measurable* diseases. Interestingly, a rather well-controlled, 17-year prospective investigation demonstrated significantly increased cancer incidence among subjects with high Minnesota Multiphasic Personality Inventory (MMPI) depression scores

(Shekelle et al., 1981). Although there exist some limited factorial and extensive immunological similarities between stress and depression (Calabrese et al., 1987), we cannot draw valid, meaningful conclusions from this study in relation to stress and cancer. Furthermore, this investigation did not assess immunological mediating variables to allow for an assessment of immune system alterations secondary to depression. Nevertheless, the study by Shekelle et al. (1981), if extensive immunological monitoring were added, should serve as the model for the type of investigation that could answer important clinical questions regarding the effects of stress-induced immune changes on human diseases.

At this point in time, we agree with Stein et al. (1991) that the full clinical significance of stress induced immune alterations remains to be determined. However, it seems clear that the clinical significance of stress-induced immunomodulation will vary across subsets (i.e., subtypes) of patients. It is thus crucial that future research focus on interactions between clinically relevant dependent variables and reliable and valid subtype measures.

STRESS, IMMUNITY, AND HIV INFECTION

Much attention has been directed toward psychoimmunological aspects of HIV infection (Stein et al., 1991; Rabkin et al., 1991). Despite some inconsistent findings in this area, it seems important to address this aspect of CNS-immune system interactions.

The psychiatric impact of human immunodeficiency virus (HIV) infection is well documented in the literature. Specifically, HIV patients have been found to exhibit significant post-diagnosis stress responses, comparable to those seen in terminal cancer patients (Faulstich, 1987; Morin et al., 1984).

The medical community has responded affirmatively to the psychiatric sequelae of HIV infection. For example, Hausman (1983) suggested the use of anxiolytic medications (e.g., benzodiazepines) to manage excessive anxiety and stress reactions. Faulstich (1987) recommended that clinicians consider the use of antidepressive medications to manage HIV-related depressive reactions. Morin et al. (1984) advocated the use of behavioral stress management procedures.

While the management of psychiatric sequelae of HIV infection appears both humane and medically rational at this time, little is actually known about the direct interrelationships between stress, immune competence, and the progression of HIV-induced disease. Depending on the nature and direction of these interrelationships, the systematic alteration of stress levels could have a significant (and perhaps surprising) impact on HIV infection.

Given the demonstrated effects of stress on T lymphocyte proliferation, it becomes extremely interesting to examine the possibility of interactions between these psychological processes and HIV-induced disease processes. On the surface one could be tempted to hypothesize that since HIV infection involves a progressive deterioration of the CD4+ lymphocyte system (Gottlieb et al., 1981) with resulting increased susceptibility to viral, fungal, and parasitic infections, stress would likely exacerbate this immunological deterioration (via decreased T-lymphocyte function), with possible contributory effects on the patient's susceptibility to opportunistic infections. If this hypothesis were to prove correct, efforts aimed at reducing stress in HIV patients might be expected to contribute positively to the management of infection sequelae, in addition to facilitating the patient's emotional comfort.

On the other hand, a hypothesis radically different from the above can be generated from an analysis of the HIV reproduction cycle. Briefly, HIV retroviruses integrate into the target-cell (e.g., CD4+ lymphocyte) genome. When the HIV-infected cell replicates and divides, the viral genome is copied and carried with each daughter cell, perpetuating the viral infection (Folks et al., 1986). Furthermore, antigen stimulation is currently believed to represent a particularly important event in continuation of the HIV replication cycle (Zagury et al., 1986). Stimulation by an antigen results in CD4+ lymphocyte activation, which, in turn, results in (1) transcription of the viral genome into RNA, (2) the subsequent synthesis of viral proteins, and (3) their assembly with genomic viral RNA into new, mature, and infective viral particles which can infect additional CD4+ lymphocytes or other cells (e.g., glial cells) with the CD4 receptor. Thus, CD4+ lymphocyte polyclonal proliferation in the face of antigenic stimulating facilitates the proliferation of HIV and possibly its spread from one target cell to another, chronically increasing the patient's overall HIV load.

Since stress decreases lymphocyte activation (as measured by polyclonal proliferation in responses to mitogen), one could hypothesize that this psychological process might *decrease* the transmission of HIV from one target cell to another via dampening of the major mechanism of viral proliferation. In other words, stress could have a *protective effect* against the proliferation and subsequent cytopathological consequences of HIV. Furthermore, if this, perhaps oversimplistic, hypothesis is correct, a reduction in stress among HIV patients could conceivably result in increasing antigen-induced CD4+ lymphocyte activation and, thus, the proliferation and cell-to-cell spread of HIV.

Recent data presented by Patterson et al. (1991) support this hypothesis. These authors found that HIV+ patients with high levels of stress maintain better health status at follow up than patients with low stress. These findings, if confirmed by further study, may suggest new rationales for therapeutic intervention in HIV+ patients.

From the standpoint of our current knowledge of stress and immunity, it may be concluded that the psychiatric sequelae of HIV infection could have a complex relationship to the ongoing immunopathology. For example, the attempt to make patients more comfortable by decreasing stress could have a multitude of effects, which may be highly desirable or undesirable from a purely medical standpoint. Further rigorous research is obviously needed to evaluate the role of stress and its treatment in the clinical course of HIV infections. This research needs to take into account the importance of subtypes (intruders vs. avoiders, etc.) in evaluating results.

CONCLUSION

It should be clear from this brief review that psychological stress downregulates the cellular immune system, by depressing the mitogen response of T-lymphocytes and the activity of NK cells. Certainly, future research will isolate other stress-induced effects of which we are currently unaware.

The major clinical questions at this point no longer involve *whether* stress impacts immunity and health. The important questions now are how much, how, and for whom? One set of questions to be addressed in the 1990s and beyond involves *what diseases* result from or are exacerbated by what specific immunological effects of stress. Also, what are the effects of stress reduction on specific diseases? Another set of questions has to do with the concept that certain potentially identifiable individuals are clearly more susceptible to the immunological effects of stress than others. We need to further assess which additional characteristics predispose individuals to stress-induced immunosuppression, and, perhaps most importantly, we must learn to better measure these characteristics so as to reliably identify and provide prophylaxis to high-risk individuals.

The 1970s represented the period when behavioral immunology began to identify specific immunological effects of stress. This work was continued into the 1980s with much success. Also during the 1980s, researchers began to identify subtypes of individuals who are hyperresponsive to stress effects on the immune response. Surely this work will continue and expand. But we think that one of the most exciting aspects of behavioral immunology in the 1990s and beyond is that researchers will begin to seriously translate findings into clinically significant technologies of assessment and treatment of specific medical diseases — diseases that are modulated or, in some cases, caused by stress-immunity interactions.

REFERENCES

Ader R: Psychoneuroimmunology. Academic Press, New York; 1981.
Ader R et al: Depressed lymphocyte function after bereavement. *Lancet* 1977; 1:834–836.

Bartrop R et al: Depressed lymphocyte function after bereavement. *Lancet* 1977; 1:834–836.

Calabrese J et al: Alteration in immunocompetence during stress bereavement, and depression. *Am J Psychiatry* 1987; 144:1123–1134.

Dantzer R and Kelley KW: Stress and immunity: an integrated view of relationships between the brain and the immune system. *Life Sciences* 1989; 44:1995–2008.

Dorian B et al: Aberration in lymphocyte subpopulations and function during psychological stress. *Clin Exp Immunol* 1982; 50:132–138.

Faulstich M: Psychiatric Aspects of AIDS. *Am J Psychiatry* 1987; 144:551–556.

Folks T et al: Induction of HTLV-III/LAV from a non-virus producing T cell line: implications for latency. *Science* 1986; 231:600–602.

Glaser R et al: Psychological stress-induced modulation of Interleukin 2 receptor gene expression and Interleukin 2 production in peripheral blood leukocytes. *Arch Gen Psych* 1990; 47:707–712.

Gottlieb M et al: Pneumocystis pneumonia and mucosal candidiasis in previously healthy homosexual men: evidence of a new acquired cellular immunodeficiency. *N Engl J Med* 1981; 305:1425–1431.

Hausman K: Treating victims of AIDS poses challenges to psychiatrists. *Psychiatr News* 1983, August 5.

Horowitz M, Willner N, and Alvarez W: The impact of events scale. *Psychosom Med* 1979; 41:209–215.

Ingram DK and Corfman TP: An overview of neurobiological comparisons in mouse strains. *Neurosci Biobehav Rev* 1980; 4:421–435.

Irwin J and Livnat S: Behavioral influences on the immune system: stress and conditioning. *Progr Neuropsychopharmacol Biol Psych* 1987; 11:137–143.

Khansary DN et al: Effects of stress on the immune system. *Immunol Today* 1990; 11:170–175.

Kiecolt-Glaser J et al: Psychosocial modifiers of immunocompetence in medical students. *Psychosom Med* 1984a; 46:7–14.

Kiecolt-Glaser J, Ricker D, and George J: Urinary cortisol levels, cellular immunocompetence, and loneliness in psychiatric inpatients. *Psychosom Med* 1984b; 46:15–23.

Kiecolt-Glaser J et al: Stress and the transformation of lymphocytes by Epstein-Barr Virus. *J Behav Med* 1984c; 7:1–12.

Kiecolt-Glaser JK et al: Marital quality, marital disruption and immune function. *Psychosom Med* 1987; 49:13–34.

Kiecolt-Glaser JK et al: Marital discord and immunity in males. *Psychosom Med* 1988; 50:213–229.

Kobasa S: Stressful life events, personality and health. *J Pers Soc Psychol* 1979; 37:1–11.

Morin S, Charles K, and Malyon A: The psychological impact of AIDS on gay men. *Am Psychol* 1984; 49:1288–1293.

Patterson TL, Grant I, Atkinson JH, McCutchan A, Smith K and Day J: Psychosocial variables may moderate progress in HIV. *Psychosom Med* 1991: 2:211.

Rabkin JG, Williams JB, Remien RH, Goetz R, Kertzner R, and Gorman JM: Depression, distress, lymphocyte subsets, and human immunodeficiency virus symptoms on two occasions in HIV-positive homosexual men. *Arch Gen Psych* 1991; 48:111–119.

Rahe R and Arthur R: Life change and illness studies: past history and future directions. *J Hum Stress* 1978; 4:3–15.

Roitt I et al: *Immunology* 1989; Gower Medical Publishing.

Schleifer S et al: Suppression of lymphocyte stimulation following bereavement. *JAMA* 1983; 205:374–377.

Shekelle R, Raynor W, Ostfeld A, et al: Psychological depression and the 17 year risk of cancer. *Psychosom Med* 1981; 43:117–125.

Stein M, Miller A, and Trestman R: Depression, the immune system, and health and illness. *Arch Gen Psych* 1991; 48:171–177.

Wahlsten D: Genetic variation in the development of mouse brain and behavior: evidence from the middle postnatal period. *Devel Psychobiol* 1975; 8:371–380.

Workman EA and La Via MF: Immunologic effects of psychological stressors: a review of the literature. *Int J Psychosomatics* 1987a; 34:35–40.

Workman E and La Via M: T lymphocyte polyclonal proliferation: effects of stress and stress response style on medical students taking national board examinations. *Clin Immunol Immunopathol* 1987; 43:303–313.

Workman E and Short D: Stress response style in panic disorder and generalized anxiety disorder. In preparation.

Zagury D et al: Long term culture of HTLV-III infected cells: a model of cytopathology of T-cell depletion in AIDS. *Science* 1986; 231:850–853.

Chapter 6

Alterations in Immunocompetence During Stress: A Medical Perspective

Joseph R. Calabrese
Director, Mood Disorders Program
University Hospitals of Cleveland
Case Western Reserve University
School of Medicine
Cleveland, Ohio

Catherine Wilde
Biofeedback Therapist
Section of Biofeedback
Department of Psychiatry and Psychology
Cleveland Clinic Foundation
Cleveland, Ohio

INTRODUCTION

The last decade has produced a series of studies which indicate that psychological stress and psychiatric illness can compromise immunologic function. These studies suggest that psychological state may influence susceptibility to illness and/or course and prognosis. This overview is provided in an attempt to place into medical context the growing body of data that link psychological function and immunologic reactivity. The vast majority of the literature documenting the immunomodulating properties of stress have yielded data that suggest the cellular arm of the immunologic apparatus is principally affected by the experience of stress. Whether the abnormalities of cellular compromise that accompany the experience of stress are adequate to engender clinically significant changes of immune function in the healthy individual is quite controversial. At present, the data are more likely to suggest that these immunomodulating properties have significance in the already immunocompromised, the patient with a disorder that already affects the immune system. If the immunomodulating properties of stress are clinically significant, they are likely to be of particular importance in immunodeficient populations, i.e., healthy carriers of human immunodeficiency virus.

At present, there are few studies that have systematically assessed the immunomodulating properties of stress in an otherwise healthy individual. It may be that stress in this setting produces nothing more than an increased incidence of minor infections (Meyer and Haggerty, 1962). It is not the intent of this paper to review in detail the already vast literature documenting the specific immunomodulating properties of stress, as this has been done elsewhere (Calabrese et al., 1987; Kiecolt-Glaser and Glaser, 1986) and the reports are now too numerous to mention. The objective of this paper is to review a cross section of the literature and then attempt to comment on the clinical significance of these findings in humans. Do the immunomodulating properties of physical and psychosocial stressors have a relevance to the general medical health of both the well and medically ill population?

AUTONOMIC CONTRIBUTIONS TO STRESS AND IMMUNOREGULATION

Any discussion of the immunomodulating properties of stress must first begin with a brief historical review of what has now become known as the "generalized stress response". It was the nineteenth century physiologist Claude Bernard who first recognized the importance of homeostasis and adaptation and stated, "The constancy of the 'milieu interieur' is the condition of a free and independent existence" (Bernard, 1878). Later, the pioneering work of Cannon and Selye greatly advanced awareness of the role that emotion plays in homeostasis and adaptation. Cannon provided observations that he believed important to his "emergency theory of emotion" and in 1914 coined the term "fight-or-flight" response (Cannon, 1914). He argued that whereas the parasympathetic branch of the autonomic nervous system regulates such vegetative functions as digestion, the sympathetic branch prepares the body for defense against stress.

The work of Selye greatly clarified the coordinated roles of the autonomic nervous system, endocrine system, and immune system in the response to stress. He suggested that there were three distinct stages in the body's response to stress. The first stage was accompanied by activation of both the hypothalamic pituitary adrenal cortical and sympathoadrenal medullary axes and was called the "alarm reaction". The second was the "stage of resistance", during which the most appropriate local defense against stress was organized. The third stage occurred if the stress was too strong or too prolonged. In this "stage of exhaustion", the body's resistance declined and death usually followed (Selye, 1936, 1956). During the first stage of the stress response, neuroendocrine changes are initially seen and believed to be important in the orchestration of a multisystem stress response involving the autonomic nervous system. During the stress response, there is an outpouring of cortisol and catecholamines that results in truly profound physiologic changes. These changes are mediated by a secondary cascade of neuroendocrine changes that include altered levels of renin, calcitonin, thyroxine, parathyroid hormone, glucagon, erythropoietin, gastrin, and insulin (Borsyenko, 1987). The changes in epinephrine and norepinephrine cause a variety of cardiovascular changes resulting in increased cardiac output, stroke volume, and systolic blood pressure. Blood flow, strength, and glucose content to skeletal muscles also increases. The circulatory changes that are seen include increased blood coagulation and increased blood glucose due to hepatic glycogenolysis. In addition to these changes, there is a generalized decrease in the activity of the digestive apparatus. Palmar sweating is a well-known concomitant of the stress response and is routinely used to study the relationship between the autonomic nervous system and stress (Asterita, 1985). During the second stage of the stress response, the neuroendocrine changes are believed to counterregulate the immune response. This has recently been reviewed by Munck et al. (1984), who have proposed that the most important physiologic effect of glucocorticoid secretion is to suppress immunity, thereby punctuating the immune response. If the stress response is chronic, exhaustion occurs. The counterregulatory immunomodulating properties of the neuroendocrine changes persist unnecessarily and then lead to what is now recognized as stress-related immunocompromise.

Of additional interest is the observation that the body is wonderfully unbiased in its appreciation of the immunomodulating properties of stress. It would appear that our bodies are unable to distinguish the immunomodulating properties of a physical stressor from those of a psychological or social stressor. When one reviews the literature regarding the stress responses that are seen during acute paradigms, one observes that the neuroendocrine changes that follow are similar regardless of the modality of the stressor. Within the category of psychological stressors, however, the qualitative features of the stressor do appear to have importance, as uncontrollable, unpredictable stressors have more potent effects on immunity than those which are controllable and predictable (Breier et al., 1987; Kubitz et al., 1986; Maier et al., 1982; Sklar and Anisman, 1981).

STRESS AND PSYCHOSOMATIC ILLNESS

A small number of illnesses traditionally were labeled "psychosomatic" disorders because of the observation that they were strongly influenced by intrapsychic conflict and psychosocial stress (Alexander, 1948) or personality type (Mirsky, 1958). These included headaches, asthma, dermatitis, ulcers, arthritis, colitis, coronary heart disease, diabetes, and hypertension. In the past 15 years, the interdisciplinary field of behavioral medicine has focused attention on the interactive effects of psychological, behavioral, and biomedical phenomena and has expanded our awareness of the many ways in which psychosocial stressors can influence illness. For example, symptom expression in the traditional psychosomatic illnesses is often mediated by the same neuroendocrine changes that occur during periods of stress. Most of these illnesses, however, have multiple pathways by which symptoms may occur, and stress may act as a predisposing, precipitating, and/or sustaining factor in the illness (Weiner, 1972). Not surprisingly, many of these disorders are associated with immune alterations, though it is often not clear how immunity interacts with these illnesses. This section discusses interactive mechanisms involved in some of these disorders.

Friedman and Booth-Kewley (1987) recently conducted a meta-analysis of personality variables associated with five psychosomatic disorders—asthma, headaches, ulcers, arthritis, and heart disease. This technique combined data from studies done between 1945 and 1984 and identified a probably "disease-prone" personality involving depression, anger/hostility, and anxiety. Interestingly, increased levels of sympatho-medullary and pituitary-cortical hormones have been demonstrated during all of these states, and evidence of psychobiologic suppression of immunity is most closely associated with depression (discussed below). Hostility is a significant factor associated with greater risk of coronary heart disease (CHD) in the type A individual (Dembroski et al., 1978). Type As have increased cortisol levels which may interfere in the metabolism of lipids and cholesterol and contribute to formation of fatty plaques in the arteries. In both hypertension and coronary heart disease, there is an abnormally high sympathetic stimulus to the heart and blood vessels and a combination of borderline hypertension, and type A behavior may predispose an individual for coronary heart disease later in life (Julius, 1987). Suppressed hostility and poor frustration tolerance also have been associated with essential hypertension and with elevated catecholamine levels (Henry et al., 1986). While hypertension is not generally identified as an immune disorder, there is evidence suggesting that both autonomic and immune factors may have a role in its etiology. In a series of studies, Norman and Dzielak (1986) demonstrated that development and maintenance of hypertension in rats is dependent on the combined role of overactivity of the sympathetic nervous system and immunologic dysfunction involving the T-lymphocyte system. A number of risk factors associated with hypertension also are associated with immunocompromise. These include age, obesity, smoking, dietary factors (e.g., sodium, caffeine, and alcohol), and life stress and are discussed further in the next section.

Recently, McClelland and associates identified a construct called "inhibited power motivation" which is similar to suppressed hostility and has been related to psychosomatic illness (reviewed in Jemmott and Locke, 1984). Three criteria identify people with high inhibited power motivation: (1) a strong need for power, (2) a need for power that is stronger than the need for affiliation, and (3) a high degree of activity inhibition. A longitudinal study found that men who showed the inhibited power motivation syndrome in their 30s had higher blood pressures in their 50s than other men (McClelland, 1979). People high in inhibited power motivation have high resting levels of epinephrine and norepinephrine (Steele, 1973) and are more susceptible to severe upper respiratory illnesses during periods of power-related life stress (McClelland and Jemmott, 1980). Excessive alcohol consumption was found in men displaying strong power motivation but low activity inhibition (McClelland, 1980).

The airways of asthma patients are hyperresponsive to airway constricting stimuli, including chemical substances, allergens, physical stimuli, and emotional stressors. Clear allergen-precipitated asthma occurs in 10 to 20% of the adult asthmatic population and is known to be IgE mediated. Secondary hypersensitivity of bronchial airways to environmental agents is a complex pheonomenon and may be acquired through prolonged exposure, infection, or the process of classical conditioning (Bouhays, 1974; Khan, 1974). Stress, through modulation of catecholamine secretion, can influence airway responses in asthmatics. Airway muscle contraction occurs via efferent cholinergic pathways and dilation results from the relaxant action of β-adrenergic stimuli (MacFadden et al., 1969). Panic-fear is a frequently cited personality dimension associated with this disorder (e.g., Dirks et al., 1977).

Diabetes is not a disease with a specific etiology, but, rather, describes a heterogenous group of disorders having elevated plasma glucose as a common denominator (Rosenbaum, 1983). Autoimmunity may be involved in insulin resistance. It has long been accepted that emotional factors are related to fluctuations in the course of diabetes mellitus (Treutman, 1962). Glucogen, catecholamines, cortisol, and growth hormone are always elevated during diabetic ketoacidosis, but it has been shown that a combination of insulin deficiency and stress hormone excess is required to produce the metabolic decompensation (Eaton and Schade, 1979). High-anxiety diabetics have been found to have elevated glucohemoglobin scores compared to moderate and no-anxiety cases. Under experimental conditions, stress states have reported to induce insulin deficiency and glucagon excess (Gerich and Lorenzi, 1978).

It can be seen that all of the above disorders are susceptible to mediation at some level by psychosocial stressors. The influence of stress, however, may be complex and quite indirect. For example, Weiner (1977), in his study of gout, found that exacerbations of this inflammatory disorder were mediated by dietary habits. Flare-ups occurred during stress if patients ate more and had less dietary control, consumed greater amounts of alcohol, took medication less reliably, and got less sleep. Friedman (1987) noted that the experience of the psychosomatic disorder is in itself stressful and that psychological factors are likely to influence progression of the illness in immune-related, slow-developing psychosomatic diseases such as arthritis. Interestingly, obesity, diabetes, atherosclerosis, hypertension, mental depression, metabolic immunodepression, autoimmune disturbances, and cancer have been identified as diseases of compensation associated with the homeostatic weakness inherent in normal aging (Dilman, 1971).

Finally, there is increasing evidence that stress management interventions can make a significant contribution to the treatment of these diseases. For example, biofeedback-assisted relaxation has been effective in reducing hypoglycemic episodes and reducing insulin intake in diabetic patients (Turkat, 1982) and has been used alone and in combination with medication to lower and control blood pressure in patients with essential hypertension (see Shellenberger and Green, 1986, for a review). Desensitization has proved effective in the treatment of asthma (Khan, 1977). The possibility of a role for stress management in resisting the immune-compromising effects of stress is currently a major area of interest and has been addressed elsewhere in this volume.

PHYSICAL STRESSORS IN HUMANS AND IMMUNITY

It is a well-recognized fact that a variety of physical stressors are known to alter immunity in reproducible and clinically meaningful ways; of particular note is the effect of normal aging. It has been demonstrated that advanced age is normally accompanied by both quantitative and qualitative changes in immune function. Shifts in lymphocyte subsets such as T- and perhaps B-cell lymphocytopenias have been documented. Functional measures of lymphocyte activity have, in addition, been noted to be negatively affected by normal aging as assessed by lymphocyte transformation testing. Lymphocyte responses to T-cell mitogenic challenges with phytohemagglutinin (PHA), concanavalin A (ConA), and allogeneic cells have been noted to be impaired in old age. Interestingly, lymphocyte responses to the B-cell pokeweed mitogen were not significantly different (Clot et al., 1972; Kishimoto et al., 1978). Malnutrition distinguishes itself as a particularly potent stressor in that it leads to not only abnormalities of cellular immunity, but also humoral immunity. Single-nutrient deficiencies involving vitamins, minerals, and amino acids have been noted to decrease lymphocyte responses to mitogen stimulation as well as cause T-cell lymphocytopenias. Decreased antibody responses to antigenic challenge as well as B-cell lymphocytopenias have also been documented (Beisel et al., 1981). Protein calorie malnutrition has been reported to cause anergy with delayed hypersensitivity skin testing and generalized lymphocytopenias (Bistrian et al., 1975). This kind of malnutrition has also been noted to decrease lymphocyte responses to allogeneic cells in mixed lymphocyte cultures, cause T-cell lymphocytopenias, and decrease helper cells and serum thymic hormone (Chandra, 1983).

There is an extensive literature regarding the immunomodulating properties of a number of drugs that are frequently abused, i.e., alcohol, nicotine, opiates, etc. The ability of alcohol to alter immunity *in vivo* and *in vitro* has been most extensively studied and is now well recognized to cause such clinically significant changes as anergy with delayed hypersensitivity skin testing as well as the more subtle changes involving decreased lymphocyte responses to PHA and ConA. This drug may also have such differential effects on T-cell subsets as increased numbers of helper cells and decreased numbers of suppressor cells (Watson et al., 1984). Heavy cigarette smoking has been demonstrated to cause leukocytosis in the presence of a generalized lymphocytopenia. Suppressor cells increase and as a result of this, the helper-to-suppressor cell ratio decreases (Miller et al., 1982). Opiate addiction causes anergy with delayed hypersensitivity skin testing and increased IgG and IgM (Lazzarin et al., 1984).

Such diverse stressors as auditory stimulation, sleep deprivation, and marathon running have all been documented as having the ability to impair various aspects of the cellular arm of the immunologic apparatus. Auditory stimulation during sleep has increased lymphocyte synthesis of interferon and decreased neutrophil and monocyte phagocytosis (Palmblad et al., 1976). Sleep deprivation decreases lymphocyte responses to PHA (Palmblad et al., 1979). Marathon running decreases lymphocyte responses to PHA, ConA, and purified protein derivative (PPD). White blood counts as well as neutrophil counts were increased and all in the presence of hypercortisolism (Eskola et al., 1978). These findings are systematically tabulated in Table I (Calabrese et al., 1978).

PSYCHOSOCIAL STRESS IN HUMANS AND IMMUNITY

In their landmark paper in 1977, Bartrop et al. first reported a relationship between psychological state and immunologic function. The subjects who participated in that study were 26 men and women whose spouses were seriously ill. Each subject provided a blood sample 1 to 3 weeks and 6 weeks after the death of his or her spouse; a group of 25 age- and sex-matched control subjects provided similarly spaced blood samples. Bartrop was the

TABLE I.
Common Immunologic Findings During Physical Stress

Study	Stressor	Cellular Immunity	Humoral Immunity
Clot et al., 1972	Advanced age	Decreased number of T-lymphocytes; decreased number of monocytes	Decreased number of B lymphocytes
Kishimoto et al., 1978	Advanced age	Decreased lymphocyte responses to PHA and ConA; decreased lymphocyte responses to allogeneic cells (missed lymphocyte cultures)	Normal lymphocyte responses to pokeweed mitogen
Palmblad et al., 1979	Auditory stimulation during sleep deprivation	Increased lymphocyte synthesis of interferon; decreased neutrophil and monocyte phagocytosis during sleep deprivation, but increased afterward	
Palmblad et al., 1979	Sleep deprivation	Decreased lymphocyte responses to PHA	
Eskola et al., 1978	Marathon running	Decreased lymphocyte responses to PHA, ConA, and purified protein derivative; incresed WBC and neutrophil count; increased plasma cortisol	
Bistrian et al., 1975	Protein calorie malnutrition	Anergy with delayed hypersensitivity skin testing; decreased number of lymphocytes	
Chandra, 1983	Protein calorie malnutrition	Decreased lymphocyte responses to allogeneic cells; increased plasma cortisol; decreased number of T-lymphocytes and helper cells; decreased serum thymic hormone	
Beisel et al., 1981	Single nutrient deficiencies (vitamins, minerals, amino acids)	Decreased lymphocyte responses to mitogen stimulation; decreased number of T-lymphocytes	Decreased antibody response to antigenic challenge; decreased number of lymphocytes

Miller et al., 1982	Heavy cigarette smoking	Increased WBC and number of suppressor cells; decreased number of total lymphocytes; decreased helper-to-suppressor cell ratio
Watson et al., 1984	Heavy alcohol use	Anergy with delayed hypersensitivity skin testing; decreased lymphocyte responses to PHA and ConA; increased number of helper cells; decreased number of suppressor cells
Lazzarin et al., 1984	Opiate addiction	Anergy with delayed hypersensitivity skin testing; Increased IgG and IgM

From Calabrese et al. (1978). With permission.

TABLE II.
Common Immunologic Findings in Stress, Bereavement, and Depression

Study	Stressor	Cellular Immunity	Humoral Immunity
Bartrop et al., 1977	Bereavement	Decreased lymphocyte responses to PHA and ConA	
Schleifer et al.	Bereavement	Decreased lymphocyte responses to PHA and ConA	Decreased lymphocyte responses to PWM
Linn et al.	Bereavement	Decreased lymphocyte responses to allogeneic lymphocytes (mixed lymphocyte cultures)	
Kronfol et al.	Depression	Decreased lymphocyte responses to PHA and ConA	Decreased lymphocyte responses to PWM
Kronfol et al.	Depression	Neutrophilia and lymphocytopenia in nonsuppressors	
Schleifer et al.	Depression	Decreased lymphocyte responses to PHA and ConA	Decreased lymphocyte responses to PWM
		Decreased number of T-lymphocytes	Decreased number of B-lymphocytes
Schleifer et al.	Depression	Normal lymphocyte responses to PHAS and ConA	Normal lymphocyte responses to PWM
		Decreased number of T-lymphocytes	
Calabrese et al., 1987	Depression	Decreased lymphocyte responses to PHA and ConA	Decreased lymphocyte responses to PWM
		Elevated plasma levels of prostaglandin E_1 and E_2	
Albrecht et al.	Depression	Normal lymphocyte responses to PHA and ConA	Normal lymphocyte responses to PWM
Kiecolt-Glaser et al.	Loneliness	Decreased lymphocyte responses to PHA	Normal lymphocyte responses to PWM
		Increased natural killer cell activity	
Kiecolt-Glaser et al.	Examination stress	Decreased natural killer cell activity	Increased plasma IgA

Study	Stressor	Findings	Findings (humoral/B-cell)
Kasl et al., 1979	Examination stress	Increased incidence of infectious mononucleosis in students with poor academic performance, overachieving fathers, and high needs for achievement	
Dorian et al.	Examination stress	Decreased lymphocyte responses to PHA and ConA	
Baker et al.	Examination stress	Increased number of T-lymphocytes; Increased serum cortisol; increased number of helper cells; no change in number of lymphocytes, helper cells, or suppressor cells	Decreased number of B-lymphocytes
Locke and Heisel	Stressful life events		No change in antibody responses to influenza vaccine
Greene et al.	Stressful life events	Normal lymphocyte responses to PHA and ConA	Normal lymphocyte responses to PWM; No change in antibody responses to influence vaccine
Cohen-Cole et al.	Stressful life events	Decreased lymphocyte responses to ConA; decreased neutrophil chemotaxis; Decreased phagocytosis; Decreased natural killer cell activity; Increased WBC; increased neutrophils	
Locke et al.	Stressful life events		
Mora et al.	Elective hospitalization		
Linn et al.	Nonelective hospitalization	Decreased lymphocyte responses to PHA; Anergy with delayed hypersensitivity skin testing	Normal lymphocyte responses to PWM
Linn and Jensen	Elective hospitalization	Normal lymphocyte responses to PHA, ConA, and allogeneic cells; Normal delayed hypersensitivity skin testing	No quantitative changes in immunoglobulins
Schleifer et al.	Elective hospitalization	Normal lymphocyte responses to PHA and ConA	Normal lymphocyte responses to PWM

first to study the immunomodulating properties of the stress and bereavement with mitogen stimulation, one of the most widely applied *in vitro* probes of immunologic function in subsequent studies. Bartrop isolated lymphocytes from the blood of each subject and cultured them with mitogens, substances known to stimulate lymphocyte proliferation. At higher doses of PHA and ConA, lymphocyte responses in bereaved subjects were significantly lower at 6 weeks than at the first sampling, suggesting a cumulative, time-dependent effect of stress. In addition to *in vitro* stimulation with potent nonspecific T-cell mitogens, Bartrop assessed *in vivo* T-cell lymphocyte function by challenging this system with several specific antigens known to produce a characteristic delayed hypersensitivity reaction apparent on routine skin testing. In contrast to the abnormal responses to mitogen stimulation, the bereaved subjects responded normally at all times to the skin testing procedures, suggesting that the wide variety of cellular interactions required for delayed hypersensitivity were largely intact. Subsequently, these findings have been replicated by Schleifer et al. (1983) and Linn et al. (1984). Table II summarizes a cross section of the available studies which have documented significant changes in immunity during a variety of psychosocial stressors.

At the present time, there have been only either epidemiologic or retrospective studies of bereaved and chronically stressed individuals to assess their vulnerability to disease. There can be no firm conclusion concerning the clinical implications of blunted lymphocyte responses to mitogenic or allogeneic stimulation. These responses merely suggest that in an artificial, *in vitro* situation, lymphocytes are less capable of undergoing mitoses, a finding that need not translate into clinically relevant immunocompromise. Studies that have assessed vulnerability to disease have been epidemiologic and convey a sense, though not definitive, that psychological factors can influence an individual's capacity to fend off disease. For example, Meyer and Haggerty (1962) showed that chronic stress was related to increases in streptococcal infection in 16 families. Kasl et al. (1979) showed that military cadets who experienced greater academic pressure were more likely than others to contract infectious mononucleosis. Baker and Brewerton (1981) reported an increased incidence of stressful life events in the months preceding the onset of acute rheumatoid arthritis. On the other hand, the prospective findings of Shekelle et al. (1981), who studied depression with the Minnesota Multiphasic Personality Inventory, reported a twofold increase in the odds of death from cancer during a 17-year follow-up of middle-aged employed men with baseline evidence of mood disturbance.

CLINICAL SIGNIFICANCE

The vast majority of studies evaluating the immunomodulating properties of stress have repeatedly reported impaired lymphocyte responses to a variety

COMPLEX INTERACTIONS OF THE IMMUNE RESPONSE

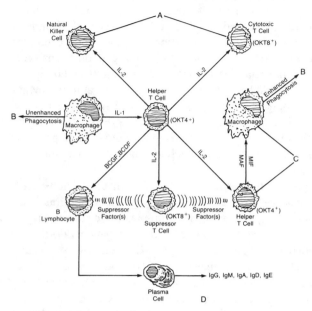

Figure 1. (A) Immunity against tumor cells and allograft transplants, and viruses (both extracellular and intracellular). (B) Immunity against nonspecific exogenous antigens such as dead self-components. (C) Delayed hypersensitivity — fungal infections, mycobacterium tuberculosis, and other granuloma-producing agents. (D) Immunity against bacteria, toxins, and allergens (immediate hypersensitivity), and viruses (only extracellular).

of antigenic challenges, including PHA, ConA, pokeweed mitogen, and allogeneic cells. A review of Figure 1 shows that many factors could account for the abnormalities of cellular immunity that have been seen in the variety of stressors reviewed in the last section. Functionally, defects in T-cell activity have been described that could compromise immune mechanisms important in resistance to viral and fungal agents and in the impairment of the integrity of tumor cell surveillance. In addition, since T-cells also contribute to B-cell proliferation by secreting B-cell differentiation factors, functional defects in T-cell activity could also affect humoral-mediated immunity.

Figure 1 diagramatically outlines the different cellular and humoral components of the immune response. One notes that abnormalities impairing the number or function of either the natural killer cell or the cytotoxic T-cell result in an impairment of the body's ability to fend off foreign tissues (see Figure 1A). The list of foreign tissues these two cells fight includes tumor cells and allograft transplants, as well as viruses (both intracellular and extracellular). If stress is able to alter macrophage or neutrophil activity, it could do so by altering either unenhanced phagocytosis or enhanced phagocytosis (see Figure 1B). This would impair the body's ability to nonspecifically fight exogenous antigens as well as dead self-components. The anergy on skin testing, which is only seen in this literature on rare occasion, suggests delayed hypersensitivity is impaired (see Figure 1C). This kind of immune response is important in fighting fungal infections, mycobacterium tuberculosis, and other granuloma-producing agents. If plasma cell functions were impaired during stress, abnormalities involving the function and/or quantity of immunoglobulins would be present. This would result in impairment on the part of the body to fight bacteria, toxins, allergens (immediate hypersensitivity), and viruses (only extracellular). As mentioned previously, however, the great majority of the evidence regarding the immunomodulating properties of stress suggests that this arm of the immunologic apparatus, the humoral arm, is left largely intact.

At the present time, there can be no firm conclusions concerning the clinical implications of data suggesting immunocompromise during stress, bereavement, and depression. *In vitro* immunologic studies suggest that lymphocytes taken from stressed and/or depressed patients do not reproduce as well when challenged by foreign antigens. Of note, however, is little evidence of anergy on skin testing, suggesting the gross intactness of the cellular arm of the immunologic apparatus. Only retrospective studies have been conducted in these reports to assess vulnerability to disease. There exists a need for prospectively designed studies to assess quantitative and qualitative evidence of immunocompromise. The complex interdependence and redundance of the different components of the immunologic apparatus suggests that stimuli like psychosocial stressors that lead to only subtle changes in immunocompetence are not likely to result in clinically significant changes in study populations which are otherwise healthy. Although not yet definitively demonstrated, on the other hand, it is likely that already-immunocompromised patient populations will have their baseline vulnerability enhanced.

REFERENCES

Alexander F: *Psychosomatic Medicine*. W.W. Norton, New York, 1948.

Asterita MF: *The Physiology of Stress with Special Reference to the Neuroendocrine System*. Human Sciences Press, New York, 1985.

Baker GHB and Brewerton DA: Rheumatoid arthritis: a psychiatric assessment. *Br. Med. J.* 1981; 282:2014.

Bartrop RW, Luckhurst E, Lazaraus L, et al.: Depressed lymphocyte function after bereavement. *Lancet* 1977; 1:834–836.

Beisel WR, Edelman R, Nauss K, et al.: Single nutrient effects on immunologic functions. *JAMA* 1981; 245:53–58.

Bernard C: *Les Phenomenes de la Vie*, Vol. 1. J-B Bailliere et Fils, Paris, 1878, p. 879.

Bistrian BR, Blackburn GL, Schrimshar NS, et al.: Cellular immunity in semistarved states in hospitalized adults. *Am. J. Clin. Nutr.* 1975; 28:1148–1155.

Borsyenko M: The immune system. An overview. *Ann. Behav. Med.* 1987; 9:3–10.

Bouhuys A: *Breathing: Physiology, Environment and Lung Disease.* Grune Å Stratton, New York, 1974.

Breier A, Albus M, Pickar D, Zahn TP, Wolkowitz, and Paul ST: Controllable and uncontrollable stress in humans: alterations in mood and neuroendocrine and psychophysiological function. *Am. J. Psychiatry* 1987; 144:1419–1425.

Calabrese JR, Kling A, and Gold PW: Alterations in immunocompetence during stress, bereavement, and depression: focus on neuroendocrine regulation. *Am. J. Psychiatry* 1987; 144:1123–1134.

Cannon WB: The emergency function of the adrenal medulla in pain and the major emotions. *Am. J. Physiol.* 1914; 33:356–372.

Chandra RK: Numerical and functional deficiency in T helper cells in protein energy malnutrition. *Clin. Exp. Immunol.* 1983; 51:126–132.

Clot J, Charmasson E, and Brochier J: Age-dependent changes of human blood lymphocyte subpopulations. *Clin. Exp. Immunol.* 1972; 32:346–351.

Delman VM: Age-associated elevation of hypothalamic threshold to feedback control and its role in development, aging, and disease. *Lancet* 1971; 1:1211–1219.

Dembroski TM, Weiss SM, Shields JL, Haynes SG, and Feinlieb M., Eds.: *Coronary-Prone Behavior.* Springer, New York, 1978.

Dirks JF, Jones F, and Kinsman RA: Panic-fear: a personality dimension related to intractability in asthma. *Psychosom. Med.* 1977; 39:120–126.

Eaton RP and Schade DS: Stress hormones and metabolic decompensation in man, in *Diabetes, 1979. Proceedings of the 10th Congress of the International Diabetes Foundation,* Wasdhausl WK, Ed., Excerpta Medica, Princeton, 1979, pp. 700–703.

Eskola J, Rauskanen O, Soppi E, et al.: Effect of sport stress on lymphocyte transformation and antibody formation. *Clin. Exp. Immunol.* 1978; 32:339–345.

Friedman HS and Booth-Kewley SB: The "disease-prone" personality. *Am. Psychol.* 1987; 42:539–555.

Gerich JE and Lorenzi M: The role of the autonomic nervous system and somatostatin in the control of insulin and glucagon secretion, in *Frontiers in Neuroendocrinology,* Vol. 5, Ganong WR and Martini L, Eds., Raven Press, New York, 1978, pp. 265–288.

Henry JP, Stephens P, and Ely DL: Psychosocial hypertension and the defense and defeat reactions. *J. Hypertens.* 1986; 4:687–697.

Jemmott JB III and Locke SE: Psychosocial factors, immunological mediation, and human susceptibility to infectious diseases: how much do we know? *Psychol. Bull.* 1984; 95:78–108.

Julius S: Role of the sympathetic nervous system in the pathophysiology of cardiovascular disease. *Am. Heart J.* 1987; 114:232–234.

Kasl SV, Evans AS, and Niederman JC: Psychosocial risk factors in the development of infectious mononucleosis. *Psychosom. Med.* 1979; 41:445–466.

Khan AU: Acquired bronchial hypersensitivity in asthma. *Psychosomatics* 1974; 15:188–189.

Kiecolt-Glaser JK and Glaser R: Psychological influences on immunity. *Psychosomatics* 1986; 27:621–624.

Kishimoto S, Tomino S, Inomata K, et al.: Age-related changes in the subsets and functions of human T lymphocytes. *J. Immunol.* 1978; 121:1773–1780.

Kubitz KA, Peavey BS, and Moore BS: *Biofeedback Self-Regul.* 1986; 11:115–123.

Lazzarin A, Mella L, Trombini M, et al.: Immunologic status in heroin addicts: effects of methadone maintenance treatment. *Drug Alcohol Depend.* 1984; 13:117–123.

MacFadden ER Jr, Luparello T, Lyons MA, and Blucker ER: The mechanism of action of suggestion in the induction of acute asthma attacks. *Psychosom. Med.* 1969; 31:134–141.

Maier SF, Drugan RC, and Grau JW: Controllability, coping behavior, and stress induced analgesia in the rat. *Pain* 1982; 12:47–56.

McClelland DC: Inhibited power motivation and high blood pressure in men. *J. Abnorm. Psychol.* 1979; 88:132–190.

McClelland DC and Jemmott JB III: Power motivation, stress, and physical illness. *J. Hum. Stress* 1980; 6(4):6–15.

Meyer RJ and Haggerty R: Streptococcal infections in families: factors altering individual susceptibility. *Pediatrics* 1962; 29:539–549.

Miller LG, Goldstein G, Murphy M, et al.: Reversible alterations in immunoregulatory T cells in smoking. *Chest* 1982; 82:526–529.

Mirsky IA: Physiologic, psychologic, and social determinants in the etiology of duodenal ulcer. *Am. J. Dig. Dis.* 1958; 3:285–315.

Munck A, Guyre PM, and Holbrook NJ: Physiological functions of glucocorticoids in stress and their relation to pharmacological actions. *Endocr. Rev.* 1984; 5:25–44.

Norman RA and Dzielak DJ: Immunological dysfunction and enhanced sympathetic activity contribute to the pathogenesis of spontaneous hypertension. *J. Hypertens.* 1986; 4:S437–S439.

Palmblad J, Cantell K, Strander H, et al.: Stressor exposure and immunologic response in man: interferon-producing capacity and phagocytosis. *J. Psychosom. Res.* 1976; 20:193–199.

Palmblad J, Petrini B, Wasserman J, et al.: Lymphocyte and granulocyte reactions during sleep deprivation. *Psychosom. Med.* 1979; 41:273–278.

Patel CH: Yoga and biofeedback in the management of "stress" in hypertensive patients. *Clin. Sci. Mol. Med.* 1975; 48:171S–174S.

Rosenbaum L: Biofeedback-assisted stress management for insulin-treated diabetes mellitus. *Biofeedback Self-Regul.* 1983; 8(4):518–532.

Selye H: A syndrome produced by diverse nocuous agents. *Nature* 1936; 138:32.

Selye H: *The Stress of Life.* McGraw-Hill, New York, 1956.

Shekelle RB, Raynor WJ, Ostfeld AM, et al.: Psychological depression and 17 year risk of death from cancer. *Psychosom. Med.* 1981; 43:117–125.

Shellenberger R and Green JA: *From the Ghost in the Box to Successful Biofeedback Training.* Health Psychology Publications, Greeley, CO, 1986.

Sklar LS and Anisman H: Stress and cancer. *Psychol. Bull.* 1981; 89:369–406.

Turkat D: The use of EMG biofeedback with insulin-dependent diabetic patients. *Biofeedback Self-Regul.* 1982; 7(3):301–304.

Watson RR, Eskelson C, and Hartman BR: Severe alcohol abuse and cellular immune function. *Ariz. Med.* 1984; 41:665–668.

Weiner H: *Psychobiology and Human Disease.* Elsevier, New York, 1977.

Weiner H: Presidential address: some comments on the transduction of experience by the brain: implications for our understanding of the relationship of mind to body. *Psychosom. Med.* 1972; 34:355–380.

Chapter 7

Behavioral Effects of Natural Stress Hormones

Charles D. Kimball
Virginia Mason Research Center
Seattle, Washington

The natural stress of childbirth provides an ideal opportunity to study the effects of stress-induced hormones and observe their influence on survival behavior.

The profound changes observed in the mood and attitude of maternity patients following the birth of the baby aroused wonder and amazement when I began an obstetrical internship on the University of Chicago Lying-In Hospital home delivery service during the great depression. After exhausting hours of painful stress in labor with no analgesic drugs, the moment the baby was born, effort was rewarded and a vast majority of these mothers suddenly manifested joyful elation, happy contentment, and an affectional attitude that was pervasive, heartwarming, and contagious. This abrupt mood change is reminiscent of the elated sense of accomplishment and happy satisfaction evidenced by Bruce Jenner, Mary Lou Retton, and other Olympic champions upon winning gold medals. It also calls to mind the prompt improvement in mood and demeanor of confirmed narcotic addicts suffering withdrawal symptoms, upon receiving an injection of morphine.

New concepts of what motivates moods, attitudes, and behavior began to take shape when I read of the discovery that peptide molecules secreted by endocrine cells bind the same receptors as morphine. News reports in 1976 and 1977 that peptide residues of β-lipotropin hormone bind brain cell opiate receptors, are antagonized by naloxone, and mimic the effects of opiate drugs in laboratory animals renewed long-standing interest in maternal attitudes and behavior and provoked questions. Do endorphins and other endogenous opiate receptor ligands transmit information to the brain centers where visceral contentment and pleasurable moods induced by opiate drugs are experienced? Are maternal moods and behavior influenced by endorphins reported to be essential to stimulate the release of prolactin hormone and secretion of breast milk (Meites et al., 1979)? Prolactin has long been alleged to stimulate maternal behavior and will induce typical nurturing behavior of virgin female rats toward pups placed with them in the cage (Bridges et al., 1984). Are endorphins another hormone species similar to the adrenalamines that influence both vital organ functions and survival behaviors (Cannon, 1911)? Do endorphin hormones become addictive, and reward and reinforce maternal performance and nurturing behavior? These questions prompted investigation of the placenta, a well-known hormone factory, as a possible source of endorphin hormone.

First by radioreceptor assay (RRA) (Kimball, 1979) and later by radioimmuno assay (RIA) (Houck et al., 1980), we found significant amounts of immunoreactive (ir) β-endorphin-like peptide hormone in homogenized extracts of human term placentas.

Subsequently, RIAs of human maternal and infant umbilical cord blood samples taken at the time of birth showed significant increase of both ir β-endorphin-like and prolactin hormone. At birth, term infants have nearly double the mothers' blood prolactin ($p = 0.001$) (Kimball et al., 1981).

Women who produced below average blood levels of ir β-endorphin-like peptide during the stress of labor were found to have significantly increased risk ($p = 0.05$) of suffering postpartum depression requiring psychiatric intervention, as shown in Figure 1 (Kimball et al., 1984).

The mood-elevating antidepressant effects of stress evoked by running, and referred to as "runners' high" in a surge of popular books on the subject, coincided in time with our studies of mother and infant blood. This facilitated RIAs on runners' blood for ir β-endorphin-like and prolactin hormones.

Blood samples taken from recreational (fun) and endurance (marathon) runners before and after running showed marked elevation of both hormones. The elevation was greater in fun than in endurance runners, who appeared to secrete decreasing amounts of prolactin in proportion to the increased distance they ran per week, which suggests tolerance (Figure 2).

RIAs of a number of other tissue extracts were done as controls for the placenta study. This led to the serendipitous discovery of significant amounts of ir β-endorphin-like peptide in acid acetone extracts of pork pancreas (Houck et al., 1980; Kimball et al., 1991).

Investigation of some biological characteristics of the pancreatic extract by the mouse tail-flick test (Figure 3) showed that intravenous injections of the ir β-endorphin-like peptide purified by high-performance liquid chro-

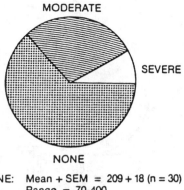

NONE: Mean + SEM = 209 + 18 (n = 30)
           Range = 70-400

MODERATE: Mean + SEM = 188 + 15 (n = 13)
           Range = 130-300

SEVERE: Mean + SEM = 125 + 13.5 (n = 4)
           Range = 90-160

P < 0.05

Figure 1. Significantly lower immunoreactive β-endorphin mean values in patients who reported severe postpartum blues.

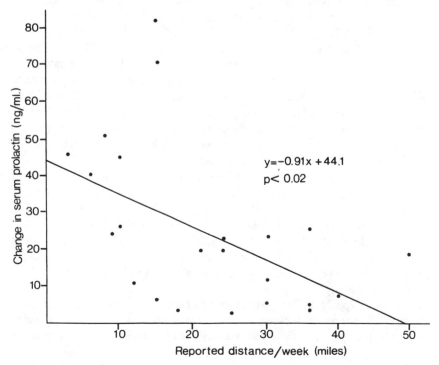

$$y = -0.91x + 44.1$$
$$p < 0.02$$

Figure 2. Regression line showing prolactin secretion decreases as habitual running distance increases.

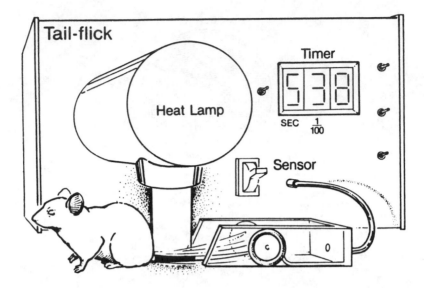

Figure 3. Mouse tail-flick test method of measuring tolerance to radiant heat.

matography produced analgesia to radiant heat stimulation (comparable to morphine) that was reversed by the opiate antagonist naloxone (Figure 4).

The purified pancreatic extract also inhibited the *in vitro* electrostimulation of guinea pig ileal muscle strip that was blocked by naloxone (Figure 5) (Kimball, 1987).

Our finding that pancreas is a source of ir β-endorphin-like hormone is supported by reports of other investigators as well as by interpretations of clinical data. For example, the presence of ir β-endorphin in D_2 pancreatic islet cells was demonstrated by immunohistochemical stains and by RIA of extracts of human, rat, and guinea pig pancreas (Bruni et al., 1979; Watkins et al., 1980). In addition to our findings in porcine pancreas, β-endorphin-like immunoreactivity was reported in extracts of bovine pancreas (Tung and Cockburn, 1984). Conflicting data indicate that the opioid peptide in guinea pig pancreatic extracts is enkephalin and not β-endorphin (Stern et al., 1982).

A number of clinical reports involve β-endorphin hormone in the regulation of insulin, glucagon, and blood sugar (Reid and Yen, 1981), and in diabetes mellitus (Feldman et al., 1983; Awoke et al., 1984; Reid et al., 1984; Giugliano, 1984; Curry et al., 1987; Giugliano et al., 1987). These reports show that pancreatic endorphin exerts regulatory influence on insulin secretion and imply deficiency of pancreatic endorphin secretion in obese (type 2) diabetes.

Obese (type 2) diabetics are known to have fluctuating insulin secretion and excessive appetites for sweets. Sugar stimulates islet cell secretions, which suggests that appetite satiety and the feelings of contentment and well being

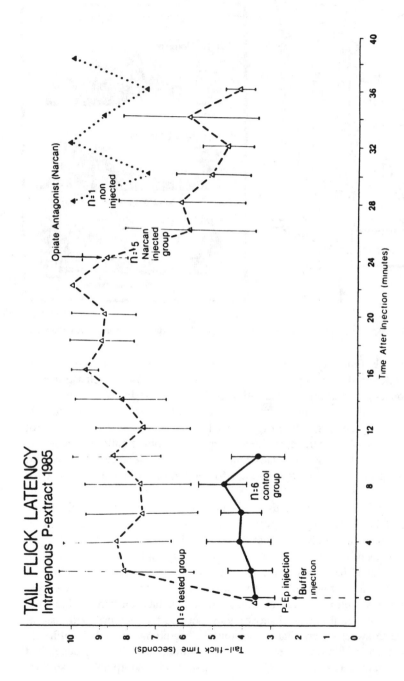

Figure 4. Tail-flick response to intravenous pancreatic endorphin peptide *(P-EP)* in test group (n = 6), control group (n = 6), and response to antagonist (n = 1).

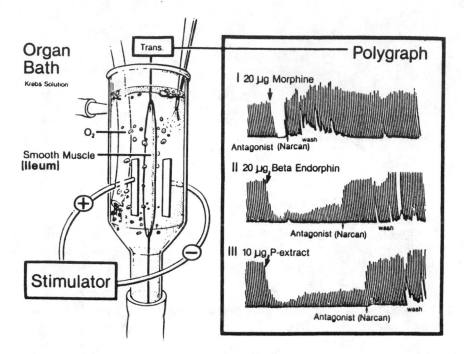

Figure 5. Response of bowel muscle strip to morphine, β-endorphin, and pancreatic endorphin.

that normally follow ingestion of a good meal may be due to pancreatic islet D_2 cell release of β-endorphin-like peptide when islet B-cells release insulin in response to increasing concentration of blood sugar. In fact, some investigators insist that the primary function of endorphin hormone in evolution is appetite satiety and regulation of feeding habits (Morley and Levine, 1980; Giugliano, 1984). Hyperendorphinemia reported in obese children and adults (Genazzani et al., 1986) indicates abnormally high tolerance to endorphin. Thus, it appears obese people overeat for endorphin hormones and not for calories.

The epidemic of drug abuse in America may be a latent result of the custom of bottle feeding newborn infants milk formulas containing sweet sugar that became widely prevalent during World War II. Eating habits, food preferences, and the set points for appetite satiety and visceral contentment are programmed in early infancy. Bottle feeding newborn infants milk formulas containing fermentable sugars (sucrose, glucose) that stimulate excessive insulin secretion instead of breast milk that has nonfermentable low-insulin-evoking milk sugar (lactose) may set food preference patterns for fermentable sweet sugars that overstimulate secretions of both insulin and pancreatic endorphin hormones. As a result, infants may become dependent on and tolerant to abnormally high levels of pancreatic endorphin-like peptides that bind opiate receptors on nerve cells in brain centers where pleasurable feelings of contentment and well-being are experienced.

Despite elevated blood endorphin at birth, infants have low tolerance to β-endorphin and morphine (Panksepp, 1986). Sucrose ingestion produced naloxone-reversible analgesia to heat pain and separation distress in infant rats (Blass, 1987). Sucrose ingestion was commonly used for analgesia in infants undergoing circumcision or laparotomy for pyloric stenosis. Cross tolerance between β-endorphin hormone and morphine has been clearly demonstrated. Intravenous injections of synthetic β-endorphin will relieve and prevent withdrawal symptoms of high-dose heroin addicts (Su et al., 1980; Catlin et al., 1981).

The assumption that pancreatic endorphin-like peptide may activate the same receptors and neuron circuits as opiate drugs to induce pleasurable rewards and set habitual patterns of appetite satisfaction is sustained by impressive laboratory data (Koob and Bloom, 1988), as well as by clinical studies and observations. Koob and Bloom postulate that drugs "have specific endogenous ligands on which they act at specific places to produce distinct patterns of behavior relevant to dependence . . . patterns of behavior emerge because drugs are able to usurp the crucial reinforcement systems and the small finite number of transmitters and response sites that operate normally to shape survival of the organism." The point is, early exposure to excessively high levels of sugar-induced pancreatic β-endorphin-like hormone at the critical imprinting period appears to produce tolerance and sets appetite satiety limits for opiate ligands of both obese and addiction-prone people at abnormally high levels.

The importance of hormone and drug mechanisms that dominate moods, attitudes, thoughts, and behavior cannot be overstated. Both endorphins and opiate drugs evoke prolactin hormone thought to be held in tonic inhibition by dopamine, which is an aggression hormone. Endorphins suppress dopamine, reward the mother, release prolactin, and initiate secretion of breast milk. Prolactin, as noted earlier, stimulates nurturing behavior in virgin female rats, ostensibly engenders tender maternal feelings of affection, compassion, and altruism in most women, and protective, food sharing, paternal attitudes in most men.

The intangible flow of pleasurable emotions between mother and infant during breast feeding is the crucial imprinting experience that conditions affectional trust and basic security subserving the infant's personality, character development, and sense of self-esteem (Kimball, 1967). Affectional security during early childhood (in T.S. Eliot's terms, feeling lovable and loved) is the basis of self-image and self-protective immunity that insulates people against chemical dependency (as well as obesity) during the identity-criss turmoil of adolescence. In other words, appetite satiety depends on self-esteem and feelings of being lovable and loved, presumably engendered by pancreatic endorphins, as it does on calories. Sugar is a poor substitute for TLC.

The symbiotic effects of stress-evoked endorphin and prolactin on the reproductive physiology and behavior of both sexes may be the *sine qua non* of species survival as well as the pursuit of happiness and evolution of domestic tranquility in civilized cultures. The ultimate purpose of this dual hormone mechanism must be to motivate and sustain species-specific feeding, nurturing, and protective behavior patterns essential to infant survival and parental happiness. Thus, it appears the struggle for survival is rewarded and reinforced by a stress-induced happiness-hormone linkage that initiates and sustains mother-infant, husband-wife interdependency.

REFERENCES

Awoke S, Voyles NR, et al.: Alterations of plasma opioid activity in human diabetics. *Life Sci.* 1984; 34:1999.

Blass EM, Fitzgerald E, and Kehoe P: Interactions between sucrose, pain and isolation distress. *Pharmacol. Biochem. Behav.* 1987; 26:483.

Bridges RS, DiBaise R, et al.: Prolactin stimulation of maternal behavior in female rats. *Science* 1984; 227:782.

Bruni JF, Watkins WB, and Yen SSC: Beta endorphin in human pancreas. *J. Clin. Endocrinol. Metab.* 1979; 49:649.

Cannon WB: The stimulation of adrenal secretions by emotional excitement. *JAMA* 1911; 56:226.

Catlin DH, Gorelick DA, and Gerner RH: Studies of β-endorphin in patients with pain and drug addiction, in *Hormonal Proteins and Peptides,* Vol. 10, Li CH, Ed., Academic Press, New York, 1981, pp. 312–336.

Curry DL, Bennett LL, and Li CH: Stimulation of insulin secretion by beta endorphin 1–27 and 1–31. *Life Sci.* 1987; 40:2055.

Feldman M, Kisner RS, Unger RH, and Li CH: Beta endorphin and the endocrine pancreas. *N. Engl. J. Med.* 1983; 308:349.

Genazzani AR, Facchinetti F, et al.: Hyperendorphinemia in obese children and adolescence. *J. Clin. Endocrinol. Metab.* 1986; 62:36.

Giugliano D: Morphine, opioid peptides and pancreatic islet function. *Diabetes Care.* 1984; 7:92.

Giugliano D, Ceriello T, et al.: B-endorphin infusion restores acute insulin response to glucose in type-2 diabetes. *J. Clin. Endocrinol. Metab.* 1987; 64:944.

Houck JC, Chang CM, Kimball CD, et al.: Placental β-endorphin-like peptide. *Science* 1980; 207:78.

Houck JC, Chang CM, and Kimball CD: Pancreatic beta endorphin-like polypeptides. *Pharmacology* 1981; 23:14.

Kimball CD: Ethology in clinical obstetrics. *Am. J. Obstet. Gynecol.* 1967; 98:616.

Kimball CD: Do endorphin residues of beta lipotropin hormone reinforce reproductive functions? *Am. J. Obstet. Gynecol.* 1979; 134:127.

Kimball CD: Do opioid peptides mediate appetites and love bonds? *Am. J. Obstet. Gynecol.* 1987; 156:1463.

Kimball CD, Chang CM, et al.: Immunoreactive endorphin peptides and prolactin in umbilical vein and maternal blood. *Am. J. Obstet. Gynecol.* 1981; 140:157.

Kimball CD, Chang CM, and Chapman MB: Endogenous opioid peptides in intrapartum uterine blood. *Am. J. Obstet. Gynecol.* 1984; 149:79.

Kimball CD, Iqbal M, Huang JT, and Sutton D: An opioid pancreatic peptide produces ileal muscle inhibition and haloxone reversible analgesia. *Pharmacol. Biochem. Behav.* 1991; 38:909–912.

Koob GF and Bloom EE: Cellular and molecular mechanisms of drug dependence. *Science* 1988; 242:715.

Meites J, Bruni JF, et al.: Relations of opioid peptides and morphine to neuroendocrine functions. *Life Sci.* 1979; 24:1325.

Morley JF and Levine AS: Stress induced eating is mediated through endogenous opiates. *Science* 1980; 209:1259.

Morley JF and Levine AS: The role of endogenous opiates as regulators of appetite. *Am. J. Clin. Nutr.* 1982; 35:757.

Panksepp J: The psychobiology of prosocial behaviors: separation distress, play, and altruism, in *Altruism and Aggression: Biological and Social Origins,* Zahn-Waxler, Cummings, and Iannotti, Eds., Cambridge University Press, London, 1986, pp. 19–57.

Reid RL and Yen SSC: Endorphin stimulates the secretion of glucagon and endorphin in humans. *J. Clin. Endocrinol. Metab.* 1981; 33:197.

Reid RL, Sandler JA, and Yen SSC: Beta endorphin stimulates the secretion of insulin and glucagon in diabetes mellitus. *Metabolism* 1984; 33:196.

Stern AS, Wurzburger RJ, et al.: Opioid peptides in guinea pig pancreas. *Neurobiology* 1982; 79:6703.

Su CY, Lin CS, et al.: Suppression of morphine abstinence in heroin addicts by β-endorphin, in *Neural Peptides and Neuronal Communications,* Costa E and Trabucci M, Eds., Raven Press, New York, 1980, pp. 503–509.

Tung AK and Cockburn E: β-endorphin-like immunoreactivity in extracts of the fetal bovine pancreas. *Diabetes* 1984; 33:235.

Watkins WB, Bruni JF, and Yen SSC: β-endorphin and somatostatin in the pancreas D-cell localization by immunocytochemistry. *J. Histochem. Cytochem.* 1980; 28:1170.

Life Stress, Depression, and Reduced Natural Cytotoxicity: Clinical Findings and Putative Mechanisms

Michael Irwin
Associate Director, Clinical Center for Research on Alcoholism
San Diego Veterans Administration Medical Center (VAMC)
San Diego, California

Lee Jones
Research Fellow, Department of Psychiatry
University of California San Diego School of Medicine
La Jolla, California

OVERVIEW

This chapter will provide a review of recent evidence that describes an association between severe life stress, psychological depression, and alterations in natural killer (NK) cell activity. In addition, we will discuss an animal model that addresses the potential role of the neuroendocrine and the autonomic nervous systems in mediating changes in natural cytotoxicity during stress and depression. To help in the organization of data supporting the association between stress, depression, and alterations in NK cell activity, the following idealized model is briefly discussed and then used to illustrate relevant conclusions in each of the following sections.

MODEL OF STRESS-INDUCED IMMUNE ALTERATIONS

Figure 1 illustrates a hypothesized model that can be used to understand how social, psychological, and biological domains might theoretically be related to immune dysfunction following adverse life events, recognizing that the paths among these psychosocial and psychological domains are certainly more complex than what is shown. In addition, the causal pathways between these domains which result in immune changes or potential development of disease during adverse life events are not yet characterized and have been only tentatively constructed using cross-sectional data. Longitudinal studies are necessary if we are to test these proposed causal paths.

This model hypothesizes that adverse life events and buffers in the social environment, such as social support and coping, act through individual adaptation to produce changes in the endocrine and immune systems. Alterations in psychological adaptation, as measured by symptoms of insomnia, anxiety, and/or depression, mediate changes in neuroendocrine and autonomic efferent pathways from the brain to alter immune function. Decrements in immune function are then assumed to be related to increased disease susceptibility and changes in health outcome, although data have not yet demonstrated that stress-related changes of *in vitro* measures of immunity such as NK cell activity are associated with poor health outcome in either stressed or depressed persons.

The following sections will review the clinical findings that link stressful events, depression, and immune function and further document the proposed paths shown in Figure 1. To place these relationships between stress and immunity into a broader context, the relevance of life change to health status will first be discussed.

ADVERSE LIFE EVENTS, DEPRESSION, AND HEALTH OUTCOME

Adverse life events, psychological distress, and depressive symptoms have been linked to the development and course of many human diseases. For example, one of the most stressful life experiences, the death of a spouse, is associated with an elevated mortality rate among bereaved spouses that varies with age, sex, and time elapsed after the loss (Rees and Lutkins, 1967; Kraus and Lilienfeld, 1959; Helsing and Szklo, 1981; Parkes et al., 1969; Bowling and Benjamin, 1985; Mellstrom, 1932; Clayton, 1974). While the results are heterogeneous, there appears to be an excess mortality during the early periods after the loss that is especially found among widowers up to the age of 75. It is important to note, however, that one well-conducted study

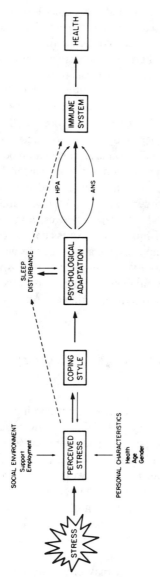

Figure 1. Hypothetical model to explain the association between stress and immune alterations in man.

failed to show this effect (Helsing and Szklo, 1981), and another recent study showed no association between bereavement and mortality due to cancer (Jones et al., 1984).

Other studies have hypothesized that it is object loss and depression that are the settings in which diseases occur. For example, within 1 week of a significant loss, there is an increased likelihood for the onset of an illness (Schmale and Iker, 1966a). Furthermore, an association between depressive profiles and the diagnosis of cervical cancer has been described (Schmale and Iker, 1966b), and epidemiologic evidence suggests that depressive profiles and symptoms are correlated with an increased incidence of cancer. Two studies, one which evaluated 1353 persons for a total of 10 years (Grossarth-Maticek, et al., 1985) and another study which conducted a 20-year follow-up of 2018 men (Persky et al., 1987), found an association between depressive profiles and an increased incidence of mortality from cancer. Likewise, several prospective studies have demonstrated an increased cancer morbidity and mortality among affective disorder patients (Whitlock and Siskind, 1979; Varsamis et al., 1972; Kerr et al., 1969). However, a more comprehensive review of studies on the relationship between stress and cancer does not yield consistent findings, and future approaches are needed in which experimental sophistication is adopted that involves well-controlled prospective and prognostic evaluations in which the analyses are based on types of tumors and include social, cultural, and demographic variables (Anisman and Zacharko, 1983).

NATURAL KILLER CELLS AND IMMUNE SURVEILLANCE

Our studies on the relationship between stress and immune function have primarily focused on the lytic activity of NK cells. NK cells are found in the peripheral blood of all normal persons and represent a distinct functional population of lymphocytes in addition to T- and B-cells. Capable of spontaneous cytotoxic activity against a wide variety of both autologous and allogeneic target cells, NK cells lyse these targets without any apparent previous sensitization and without involvement of major histocompatibility antigens. While a number of observations argue that NK cells play an important role in immune surveillance, it is important to emphasize that disturbances of NK cell activity as well as other cell-mediated immune parameters in depressed patients or stressed persons may either not be of sufficient magnitude to affect disease susceptibility or may be completely offset by increased function or numbers of other cell types.

NK cells are thought to have a role in surveillance against primary tumor development. For example, inhibition of an effective NK response results in a growth of primary metastatic carcinoma (Reid et al., 1981); selective depletion of NK cells renders mice unable to regulate the growth of an NK-susceptible lymphoma (Kawase et al., 1982); and mice congenitally deficient in NK cells have a marked increase in metastases following tumor transplantations (Talmadge et al., 1980). In man, a series of clinical trials has demonstrated that enhancement of NK cell activity by administration of interleukin-2 either alone or in conjunction with lymphokine-activated killer cells promotes the regression of metastatic tumors; both renal cell carcinomas and melanoma show regression in some patients who are treated with lymphokine-activated killer cells or interleukin-2 (Rosenberg et al., 1987).

Substantial experimental evidence also supports a role of NK cells in the control of herpes virus and cytomegalovirus infections. An enhanced susceptibility to herpes simplex virus type 1 (HSV-1) has been found in mice who are selectively depleted of NK activity and receive HSV-1 simultaneously, but not in mice in which NK cell depletion is postponed 5 d after the virus inoculation (Habu et al., 1984). Likewise, sensitivity to murine cytomegalovirus (CMV) infection increases in the absence of NK cells; whereas, resistance to CMV can occur if cells characteristic of NK cells are transferred (Bukowski et al., 1985; Bancroft et al., 1981). In humans, positive correlations have been made between sensitivity to viral infections in a number of disorders (Litzova and Herberman, 1986), although it is important to emphasize that these relationships may be merely coincidental with the underlying disease processes in which other immune abnormalities are also present. However, a recent report by Biron et al. (1989) has found that extreme susceptibility to herpes virus infections is found in association with specific loss of NK cells, killer cell function, and inducible killer cell activity. Overall, these data support the hypothesis that NK cells are important in the defense against herpes viruses, but not against other viruses (Ritz, 1989).

IMMUNE ALTERATIONS IN BEREAVEMENT

Clinical studies of immune function in bereavement have demonstrated altered immunity, including suppression of lymphocyte responses to mitogenic stimulation, reduced NK cell activity, and changes in T-cell subpopulations in bereaved men and women. The first study on the effects of bereavement on immune function demonstrated that T-cell responses to the mitogens phytohemagglutinin (PHA) and concanavalin A (ConA) were reduced at both 3 and 6 weeks after the death of the spouse as compared to the lymphocyte responses in age- and sex-matched control subjects (Bartrop et al., 1977). Schleifer and colleagues confirmed the findings of Bartrop et al. and found suppressed mitogen responses in 15 men during the first 2 months following the death of a spouse as compared to responses in the pre-bereavement period (Schleifer et al., 1983).

While these two studies document an association between adverse life events such as bereavement and suppressed responses to mitogenic stimulation, it might be that immunologic responses to loss would be found only in those subjects who demonstrate depressive symptoms. As proposed by the illustrated model (Figure 1), the psychological response to the loss, not merely the event, might mediate alterations in immune function. Consistent with the role of depressive symptoms in mediating immune changes during bereavement, Linn et al. (1984) found that reduced lymphocyte responses to the mitogen PHA were found in bereaved subjects who had high depression scores, but not in those with few signs of depression. However, responses of lymphocytes to the mitogen ConA and pokeweed mitogen did not differ between those with and without depressive symptoms. Irwin and colleagues (1987a) further clarified the role of psychological processes to modulate immune function in bereavement, assessing the relationship between depressive symptoms and alterations in both T-cell subpopulations and NK cell activity in bereaved women. In the first study, measures of total lymphocyte counts, T-helper and T-suppressor cell numbers, and NK cytotoxicity were compared among three groups of women: those whose husbands were dying of lung cancer, those whose husbands recently died, and women whose husbands were in good health. Using the Social Readjustment Scale (SRS) (Holmes and Rahe, 1967), concurrent changes in the spousal relationship as well as other life experiences were assessed; women whose husbands were healthy were more likely to be classified in the low SRS group, whereas women who either were anticipating or had experienced the death of their husbands were likely to be in the middle or high SRS groups, respectively. Age was similar between the three groups.

Depressive symptoms as measured by the Hamilton Depression Rating Scale (HDRS) were significantly ($p < 0.001$) more severe in the moderate and high SRS groups as compared to that found in the low SRS group. NK activity expressed in lytic units was significantly ($p < 0.001$) different between the three groups: the groups with moderate and high SRS scores were found to have reduced NK activity as compared to that found in the low SRS control subjects (Figure 2). However, the two groups did not differ in either absolute number of lymphocytes or T-cell subpopulations, including number of T-helper cells, T-suppressor/cytotoxic cells, or the ratio of T-helper to T-suppressor/cytotoxic cells.

Consistent with the work of Linn and colleagues (1984) in which the psychological response appeared to be an important correlate of immunologic changes in bereavement, we found that NK activity was negatively correlated with Hamilton Depression total score ($r - 0.28$, $p < 0.05$) as well as the Hamilton Depression subscales, depressed mood ($r - 0.39$, $p < 0.01$), and insomnia ($r - 0.28$, $p < 0.04$). Furthermore, the severity of depressive symptoms as measured by the total HDRS score was correlated with the loss of

T-suppressor/cytotoxic cells ($r - 0.42$, $p < 0.01$) as well as an increase in the ratio of T-helper to T-suppressor cells ($r + 0.54$, $p < 0.002$). A loss of T-suppressor cells has also been found in aged women as compared to younger women (Makinodan and Kay, 1980) and in depressed patients as compared to controls (Syvalahti et al., 1985). While the association between these immune changes and health outcome was not evaluated in these studies of bereaved women, lower T-suppressor cells might be associated with the emergence of autoantibodies (Mackinodan and Kay, 1980; Smith and Stein-

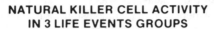

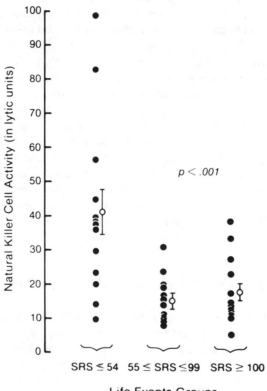

Figure 2. NK cell activity in women with low, moderate, and high scores. Each point represents the mean of multiple measures for individual subjects. NK activity was significantly different between the groups. (F = 8.3, df = 2,34; $p < 0.001$). Post hoc tests demonstrated that the groups with moderate and high SRS scores had significantly ($p < 0.05$) lower NK activity than did the group with low SRS scores.

berg, 1983), and it has been reported that autoantibodies occur more often in depressed patients than in control subjects (Shopsin et al., 1973; Deberbt et al., 1976; Johnstone and Whaley, 1975; Nemeroff et al., 1985).

To characterize further the contribution of depressive symptoms to changes in natural cytotoxicity during bereavement, a second study was conducted in which bereaved women were followed in a longitudinal design with concurrent measures of depressive symptoms and NK activity before and after the death of the spouse (Irwin et al., 1987). While neither mean NK activity nor Hamilton Depression scores differed from anticipatory to the actual bereavement, variance in both of these measures was significantly greater after bereavement as compared to pre-bereavement values, suggesting that individual differences are more likely in response to the death of the husband as compared to basal values. Importantly, change in severity of depressive symptoms from anticipatory bereavement to bereavement was strongly correlated ($r-0.89$, $p < 0.01$) with changes in NK activity during this interval; as depressive symptoms increased in individual subjects, NK activity was likely to decrease.

Together, these studies of immunity in bereavement have demonstrated that measures of cell-mediated immunity, including lymphocyte responses to mitogenic stimulation, NK activity, and T-cell subpopulations, are altered in persons undergoing major life stress such as bereavement. An important determinant of the magnitude of change in these cellular immune responses appears to be the severity of depressive symptoms in response to the loss. Thus, consistent with the model previously illustrated, it is changes in depressive symptoms, not merely the death of the spouse, that might predict and potentially determine the reduction in cell-mediated immunity. The important role of psychological processes in mediating a reduction in natural cytotoxicity will be discussed in the following sections.

DEPRESSION AND IMMUNE DYSFUNCTION

Major depression might also be associated with immune changes since bereaved subjects and distressed persons often manifest depressed mood and symptom patterns similar to those of patients with major depressive disorder (Clayton et al., 1972). Studies of depressed patients have found significant alterations of T-cell subpopulations as well as measures of cell-mediated immune function. Consistent with the findings of Irwin et al. (1987a) in which the severity of depressive symptoms was correlated with an increase in the ratio of T-helper to T-suppressor/cytotoxic cells in bereaved women, Syvalahti et al. (1985) found that depressed patients show a lower percentage of T-suppressor/cytotoxic cells and a higher ratio of T-helper to T-suppressor/cytotoxic cells than that found in control subjects. However, differences in quantitative measures of lymphocytes have not been found in all studies (Darko et al., 1988; Schleifer et al., 1989).

To examine the role of depression to reduce immune *function*, as well as *number* of immune cells, lymphocyte responses to mitogenic stimulation have been compared between depressed patients and control subjects. In psychotically depressed patients during the first days of illness, Cappell et al. (1978) found that PHA responses were significantly lower than those found at the time of clinical remission. Kronfol and colleagues observed a similar reduction in lymphocyte mitogenic stimulation with either ConA, PHA or pokeweed mitogens in 26 drug-free depressed patients as compared to controls (Kronfol et al., 1983). Finally, a series of studies conducted by Schleifer and colleagues has found that severity of depressive symptoms is a correlate of suppressed lymphocyte reactivity in depressed patients. In severely depressed inpatients (Schleifer et al., 1984), but not in more mildly depressed outpatients (Schleifer et al., 1985), reduced lymphocyte responses have been demonstrated. Furthermore, in a large study comprised of 91 age- and sex-matched pairs of depressed patients and control subjects, severity of depressive symptoms was correlated with reduced lymphocyte proliferative activity within the depressives even though no significant reduction of mitogen responses was found between the depressed patients and the control subjects (Schleifer et al., 1989).

These observations of altered lymphocyte responses in depressed patients have been extended to include the measurement of the cytolytic activity of peripheral lymphocytes. Irwin et al. (1987c) initially compared the values of natural cytotoxicity between a group of 19 hospitalized, depressed patients and age- and sex-matched control subjects. NK cell activity was significantly lower in these 19 hospitalized, male patients who were free of medication and met criteria for major depressive disorder than that found in the matched control subjects (Figure 3). Furthermore, total scores on the HDRS were negatively correlated with NK activity ($r - 0.44$, $p < 0.005$). This reduction of NK activity, which was demonstrated in a select group of depressives restricted to middle-aged men who were hospitalized for major depression, has now been replicated by two independent investigations (Urich et al., 1988; Mohl et al., 1987), although another large study found no significant difference in natural cytotoxicity in depressed patients as compared to controls (Schleifer et al., 1989).

These data, from studies of depressed patients and bereaved persons, have supported the hypothesis that both depression and depressive symptoms associated with threatening life events can lead to changes in immune function. However, in addition to the separate effects of either depression or adverse life events on immunity, it is also possible that depression and severe stress might *interact* to contribute together to a further additional decrease of cellular immune measures. For example, depressed patients are likely to experience severe life events during their depressive episodes, and such depressed patients who are undergoing severe stress might exhibit *more* immunologic distur-

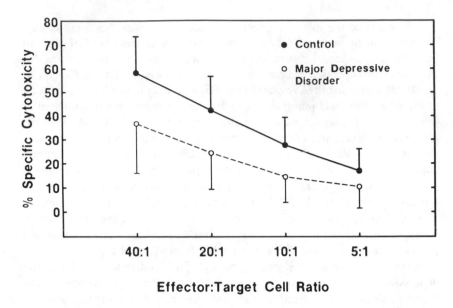

Figure 3. NK cytotoxicity in depressed patients and controls. Each point represents the mean of the percent specific cytotoxicity for each group (n = 19) across the four effector-to-target cell ratios. A repeated measures analysis of variance demonstrated a significant group effect (F = 13.2, df = 1,36; $p < 0.001$).

bances than equally depressed persons free of marked life stress. Conversely, immune changes that are found in persons who suffer adverse life events might be present only if such persons show depressive symptoms or have clinical depressions. Thus, to evaluate the individual and joint contribution of depression and severe, threatening life events (Brown and Harris, 1978) to alter immune function, both depressed patients and persons with and without high stress were evaluated simultaneously (Irwin et al., 1989).

Two groups of men were studied in a matched-pair design: 36 hospitalized, unmedicated depressed patients and 36 nonpatient control subjects. Life events and difficulties were assessed using an interview guided by the Psychiatric Epidemiologic Research Interview (Hirshfeld et al., 1977) and rated as *severe* using the criteria of Brown and Harris (1978). The presence of marked life stress was identified in 61% of the depressed group and in 22% of the controls.

Consistent with our earlier observations, a reduction of NK activity was found in the depressed patients as compared to the controls ($p < 0.05$) (Figure 4). Second, in persons undergoing severe, threatening life events (Brown and Harris, 1978) who are without signs of clinical depression, NK activity was also significantly ($p < 0.05$) reduced to a level comparable to that found in depressed patients. Finally, while lytic activity was lower in the high-stressed controls as compared to the low-stressed control subjects, the two groups of depressed patients who differed in their severity of life stress had similar values of NK activity. These data demonstrate that both depression and severe events or difficulties were associated with a reduction of NK cytotoxicity in an *independent* manner. However, the presence of severe life stress in depressed patients did not appear to produce a further reduction of NK activity.

Thus, an association between markedly threatening life events and a reduction of NK activity independent of depression and depressive symptoms

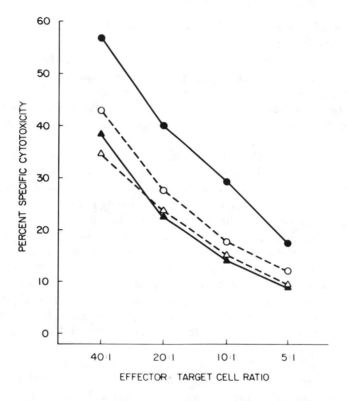

Figure 4. NK activity across the four effector-to-target cell ratios in control subjects with low (n = 28, ●———●) and high stress (n = 8, ▲———▲), and in the depressed patients with low (n = 14, ○---○) and high stress (n = 22, △---△). Using lytic unit values, a 2 (group: depressed, control) × 2 (condition stress: high, low) analysis of variance (ANOVA) demonstrated significant main effects for depression (F = 4.8, p <0.03) and stress (F = 4.1, p < 0.04). The group × stress interaction was not significant (F = 3.4, P = 0.06). Planned comparisons demonstrated that the mean value of lytic activity was significantly lower in the high-stress controls as compared to the low-stress controls (t = 2.6, p < 0.01). Lytic activity was similar in the two groups of depressed patients who differed in the severity of life stress (t = 1.6, p = 0.12).

has emerged from this study of stressed persons and depressed patients. Biological responses to threatening life change have been hypothesized to be similar to the physiologic changes of depression (Gold, 1988), and it appears that clinical depression and life distress share a common neuroimmunologic alteration of natural cytotoxicity. Central mechanisms which are common to depression and states of sustained high stress might mediate this immunologic change under both circumstances and will be discussed in the following sections.

CENTRAL NERVOUS SYSTEM MODULATION OF IMMUNITY

An animal model to understand how depression and/or severe life stress might produce changes in immune function involves the central administration of corticotropin-releasing factor (CRF) as a neuropeptide probe to determine the paths by which the brain communicates with the immune system. CRF is hypothesized to act in the brain to initiate biological responses to stress (Taylor and Fishman, 1988). If CRF is a physiological central nervous system regulator with integrative properties as has been proposed (Axelrod and Resine, 1984), this neuropeptide is to be expected to alter not only endocrine, but also autonomic and visceral functions, including immune function.

Neuroanatomic studies have demonstrated that the greatest density of CRF immunoreactive cells and fibers in the brain is found in the paraventricular nucleus of the hypothalamus and the median eminence (Paull et al., 1982). However, a wide distribution of CRF is also found throughout the brain (Olschowka et al., 1982; Swanson et al., 1983; Bloom et al., 1982), and CRF receptors which are relatively absent in the hypothalamus are mapped to a number of extrahypothalamic structures related to the limbic system and control the autonomic nervous system (DeSouza et al., 1984; Wynn et al., 1984).

Correspondingly, CRF may also act in the central nervous system at extrahypothalamic sites in addition to its well-established role as the hypothalamic regulator of pituitary secretion of ACTH and β-endorphin (Vale et al., 1981; Kalin et al., 1983). Studies have, in fact, demonstrated that CRF alters a variety of brain functions. For example, central administration of CRF increases the firing rate of the locus coeruleus (Valentino et al., 1983), produces EEG changes suggestive of increased arousal (Ehlers et al., 1983), and activates the autonomic nervous system as reflected by increased plasma concentrations of norepinephrine and epinephrine (Fisher et al., 1982; Brown et al., 1981). Furthermore, a pattern of behavioral responses such as decreased feeding and increased locomotor activity are produced in animals who are given central CRF (Sutton et al., 1982; Britton et al., 1982).

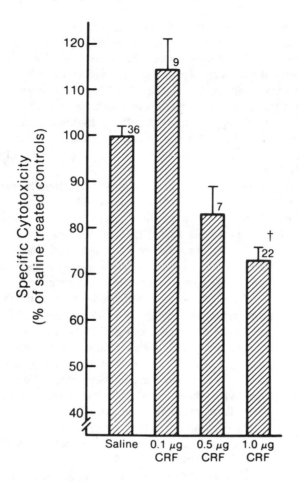

Figure 5. Effect of central administration of CRF (1.0 μg) on splenic NK cytotoxicity (expressed as mean percentage ± SEM of saline-treated controls to produce a dose-dependent reduction of NK activity (F = 11.4, df = 3.74; $p < 0.001$). (+): significantly ($p < 0.05$) different from saline group. The number of rats in each group is indicated next to the standard error bars.

Since increased concentrations of CRF have been found in the cerebro-spinal fluid of depressed patients (Nemeroff et al., 1984), it is tempting to speculate that CRF might coordinate the reduction of NK activity found in these patients. To explore this putative action of CRF to alter immunity, intraventricular CRF has been administered to rats and found to produce a significant decrement of NK activity (Figure 5) (Irwin et al., 1987d). Thus, CRF was capable of modulating immune function *in vivo* using the doses of CRF that are similar to those used to produce behavioral, pituitary, and autonomic activation.

CRF appears to act within the brain to induce changes in immune function. Neither administration of CRF subcutaneously nor incubation of CRF with NK cells *in vitro* produced a significant decrement in NK activity. Furthermore, the effects of CRF were significantly blocked by the central co-administration of the CRF antagonist, α-helical CRF (9–41). However, when the CRF antagonist was given peripherally, intracerebroventricular CRF was still able to significantly ($p < 0.05$) reduce NK activity. In summary, these findings support the hypothesis that CRF is a receptor-mediated phenomenon in the brain and not due to the nonspecific effects of exogenously administered intraventricular CRF.

The action of CRF to reduce splenic NK activity might be mediated by efferent outflow from the brain via either the neuroendocrine or the autonomic nervous systems. The autonomic nervous system is one pathway that can communicate changes in the brain to cells in the immune system. Primary, as well as secondary, lymphoid tissues are extensively innervated by nervous fibers localized in the vasculature as well as the parenchyma (Bulloch and Moore, 1981; Livnat, 1985). For example, fluorescence histochemical techniques have revealed abundant linear and varicose fibers that branch into areas of lymphocytes in the mouse spleen (Livnat et al., 1985). As visualized in recent electromicrographs, these noradrenergic fibers terminate on T-cells (Felten and Olschowka, 1987). Additional studies have demonstrated that lymphocytes are capable of receiving signals from these sympathetic nervous fibers. Monoamines such as norepinephrine, epinephrine, and dopamine bind to receptors on lymphocytes (Hadden et al., 1970; Hall and Goldstein, 1981) and are capable of regulating immune responses such as NK lytic activity. For example, direct *in vitro* application of norepinephrine or epinephrine reduces NK activity, an effect that is antagonized by preincubation with the β-antagonist propranolol (Hellstrand et al., 1985).

Autonomic activation appears to have a direct role in mediating CRF-induced suppression of NK activity (Irwin et al., 1988). Preadministration of the peripheral ganglionic blocker, chlorisondamine, antagonized CRF-induced elevations of norepinephrine and epinephrine (Lenz et al., 1987) and completely abolished the immuno-suppressive action of CRF (Figure 6) (Irwin et al., 1988). These results demonstrated that ganglionic blockade is capable of antagonizing the action of central CRF and that autonomic activation is one pathway which can communicate the action of CRF within the brain to NK cells.

CRF might also act through the pituitary adrenal axis to suppress NK activity. However, several studies now suggest that acute suppression of NK activity by CRF is dissociated from activation of the adrenal axis. For example, when the CRF antagonist α-helical (9–41) was administered at doses sufficient to inhibit CRF-induced release of ACTH and β-endorphin, a significant suppression of NK activity was still demonstrated (Irwin et al., 1987). Likewise, in experiments involving the co-administration of chlorisondamine and CRF, activation of the pituitary-adrenal axis with increased plasma levels of ACTH and corticosterone were found in animals who were administered CRF with and without chlorisondamine, whereas a reduction of NK activity was found only in those animals who received CRF alone (Irwin et al., 1988). Together, these experiments suggest that CRF-induced immune suppression is independent of the activation of the pituitary-adrenal axis. The action of CRF to reduce NK activity is found even when activation of the pituitary-adrenal axis is significantly antagonized. Furthermore, CRF-induced increases in plasma levels of these neurohormones can occur acutely without producing a significant reduction of NK activity.

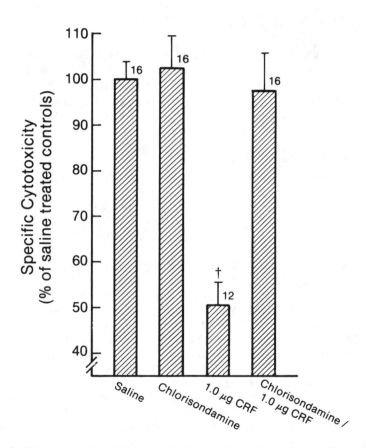

Figure 6. Effect of ganglionic blockade with chlorisondamine (3 mg/kg, i.p. 60 min before ICV injection) on CRF (1.0 µg/ICV)-induced suppression of NK cytotoxicity (expressed as mean percent ± SEM of saline-treated controls). (+): significantly ($p < 0.001$) different from saline group. The number of rats in each group is indicated next to the SE bars.

SUMMARY

Depressive states and distressing experiences are associated with reduced NK activity. Since both pituitary-adrenal and autonomic nervous mechanisms are capable of modulating cytotoxicity, the role of psychologic or central nervous processes in coordinating these efficients to produce changes in immune function is being examined. In a preclinical model, CRF is hypothesized to act as a central integrator of behavioral and biological responses to stress. Furthermore, central CRF has been found to activate the autonomic nervous system and to reduce natural cytotoxicity, providing a physiologic mechanism relevant to the interaction between the brain and NK cells.

ACKNOWLEDGMENTS

This work was supported by Grants from VA Merit Review, the Clinical Research Center on Alcoholism, and NIMH #R29-MH44275-01. Lee Jones was a UCSD Fellow in Clinical Psychopharmacology and Psychobiology (#MH18399) at the Mental Health Clinical Research Center (#MH 30914). Parts of this chapter have been previously published.

REFERENCES

Anisman H and Zacharko RM: Stress and neoplasia: speculations and caveats. *Behav. Med. Update* 1983; 5:27–35.

Axelrod J and Reisine TD: Stress hormones: their interaction and regulation. *Science* 1984; 224:452.

Bancroft GJ, Shellam GR, and Chalmer JE: Genetic influences on the augmentation of natural killer cells (NK) during murine cytomegalovirus infection: correlation with patterns of resistance. *J. Immunol.* 1981; 124:988–994.

Bartrop RW, Lazarus L, Luckherst E, and Kiloh LG: Depressed lymphocyte function after bereavement. *Lancet* 1977; 1:834–836.

Biron CA, Byron KS, and Sullivan JL: Severe herpes virus infections in an adolescent without natural killer cells. *N. Engl. J. Med.* 1989; 320:1732–1735.

Bloom FE, Battenberg EL, Rivier J, et al.: CRF: immunoreactive neurons and fibers in the rat hypothalamus. *Regul. Peptides* 1982; 4:43–48.

Bowling A and Benjamin B: Mortality after bereavement: a follow-up study of a sample of elderly widowed people. *Biol. Soc.* 1985; 2:197–203.

Britton KT, Koob GF, and Rivier J: ICV-CRF enhanced behavioral effects of novelty. *Life Sci.* 1982; 31:363–367.

Brown GW and Harris T: *Social Origins of Depression.* Tavistock, London, 1978.

Brown MR, Fisher LA, Rivier J, Spiess J, Rivier C, and Vale W: CRF: effects on the sympathetic nervous system and oxygen consumption. *Life Sci.* 1981; 30:207–210.

Bukowski JF, Warner JF, Dennert G, and Welsh RM: Adoptive transfer studies demonstrating the antiviral effect of natural killer cells in vivo. *J. Exp. Med.* 1985; 131:1531–1538.

Bulloch K and Moore RY: Innervation of the thymus gland by brainstem and spinal cord in the mouse and rat. *Am. J. Anat.* 1981; 162:157–166.

Cappell R, Gregoire F, Thiry L, and Sprecher S: Antibody and cell mediated immunity to herpes simplex virus in psychotic depression. *J. Clin. Psychiatry* 1978; 39:266–268.

Clayton PJ, Halikes JA, and Maurice WL: The depression of widowhood. *Br. J. Psychiatry* 1972; 120:71–78.

Clayton PJ: Mortality and morbidity in the first year of widowhood. *Arch. Gen. Psychiatry* 1974; 30:747–750.

Darko DF, Gillin JC, Bulloch SC, Golshan S, Tasevska Z, and Hamburger RN: Immune cells and the hypothalamic-pituitary axis in major depression. *Psychiatry Res.* 1988; 25:173–179.

Deberbt R, Hooren JV, Biesbrouck M, and Amery W: Antinuclear factor-positive mental depression: a single disease entity? *Biol. Psychiatry* 1976; 11:69–74.

DeSouza EB, Perrin MH, Insel TR, Rivier F, Vale W, and Kuhar M: CRF receptors in rat forebrain: autoradiographic identification. *Science* 1984; 224:1449–1451.

Ehlers CL, Henriksen SJ, Wang M, Rivier J, Vale W, and Bloom FE: CRF produces increases in brain excitability and convulsive seizures in rats. *Brain Res.* 1983; 332:336.

Felten SY and Olschowka J: Noradrenergic sympathetic innervation of the spleen. II. Tyrosine hydroxylase (TH)-positive nerve terminals form synaptic like contacts on lymphocytes in the splenic white pulp. *J. Neurosci. Res.* 1987; 18:37–48.

Fisher LA, Rivier J, Rivier C, Spiess J, Vale W, and Brown MR: CRF: central effects on mean arterial pressure and heart rate in rats. *Endocrinology* 1982; 11:2222–2224.

Gold PW: Stress-responsive neuromodulators. *Biol. Psychiatry* 1988; 24:371–374.

Grossarth-Maticek R, Bastinans J, Kanazir DT, Vetter H, and Schmidt P: Psychosocial factors as strong predictors of mortality from cancer, ischemic heart disease, and stroke. *J. Psychosom. Rev.* 1985; 33:129–138.

Habu S, Akamatsu K, Tamaoki N, and Okumura K: In vivo significance of NK cells on resistance against virus (HSV-1) infections in mice. *J. Immunol.* 1984; 133:2743–2747.

Hadden JW, Hadden EM, and Middleton E: Lymphocyte host transformation. I. Demonstration of adrenergic receptors in human peripheral lymphocytes. *J. Cell. Immunol.* 1970; 1:583–595.

Hall NR and Goldstein AL: Neurotransmitters and the immune system, in *Psychoneuroimmunology*, Ader R, Ed., Academic Press, New York, 1981, pp. 521–543.

Hellstrand K, Hermodsson S, and Strannegard O: Evidence for a beta-adrenoceptor mediated regulation of human natural killer cells. *J. Immunol.* 1985; 134:4095–4099.

Helsing KJ, Szklo M, and Comstock EW: Mortality after bereavement. *Am. J. Publ. Health* 1981; 71:802–809.

Hirschfeld RMA, Kleeman GL, and Schless AP: Modified Life Events section of the Psychiatric Epidemiology Research Interview (PERI), for use in the Clinical Studies of the NIMH Clinical Research Branch Collaborative Program on the Psychology of Depression, 1977.

Holmes TH and Rahe RH: The social readjustment rating scale. *J. Psychosom. Rev.* 1967; 11:213–218.

Irwin M, Daniels M, Bloom E, Smith TL, and Weiner H: Life events, depressive symptoms and immune function. *Am. J. Psychiatry* 1987a; 144:437–441.

Irwin MR, Daniels M, Smith TL, Bloom E, and Weiner H: Impaired natural killer cell activity during bereavement. *Brain Behav. Immun.* 1987b; 1:81–87.

Irwin M, Smith TL, and Gillin JC: Reduced natural killer cytotoxicity in depressed patients. *Life Sci.* 1987c; 41:2127–2133.

Irwin MR, Britton KT, and Vale W: Central corticotropin releasing factor suppresses natural killer cell activity. *Brain Behav. Immun.* 1987d; 1:98–104.

Irwin MR, Hauger RL, Brown MR, and Britton KT: Corticotropin-releasing factor activates the autonomic nervous system and reduces natural cytotoxicity. *Am. J. Physiol.* 1988; 255:R744–R747.

Irwin MR, Patterson T, Smith TL, Caldwell C, Brown SA, and Grant I: Suppression of immune function by life stress and depression. *Biol. Psychiatry* 1989 (in press).

Johnstone EC and Whaley K: Antinuclear antibodies in psychiatric illness: their relationship to diagnosis and drug treatment. *Br. Med. J.* 1975; 28:724–725.

Jones DR, Goldblatt PO, and Leon DA: Bereavement and cancer: some data on deaths of spouses from the longitudinal study of Office of Population Censuses and Surveys. *Br. Med. J.* 1984; 289:461–464.

Kalin NH, Shelton SE, Kraemer GW, and McKinney WT: CRF administered intraventricularly to rhesus monkeys. *Peptides* 1983; 4:217–220.

Kawase I, Urdol DL, and Brooks CG: Selective depletion of NK cell activity in vivo and its effect on the growth of NK sensitive and NK resistant tumor cell variants. *Int. J. Cancer* 1982; 29:507.

Kerr TA, Schapiro K, and Roth M: Relationship between premature death and affective disorders. *Br. J. Psychiatry* 1969; 115:1277–1282.

Kraus AS and Lilienfeld AM: Some epidemiologic aspects of the high mortality rate in the young widowed group. *J. Chron. Dis.* 1959; 9:207–217.

Kronfol Z, Silva J, Greden J, Dembinski S, Gardner R, and Carroll B: Impaired lymphocyte function in depressive illness. *Life Sci.* 1983; 33:241–247.

Lenz HJ, Raedler A, Greten H, and Brown MR: CRF initiates biological actions within the brain that are observed in response to stress. *Am. J. Physiol.* 1987; 252:R34–R39.

Linn MW, Linn BS, and Jensen J: Stressful events, dysphoric mood, and immune responsiveness. *Psychol. Rep.* 1984; 54:219–222.

Livnat S, Felten SJ, Carlton SL, Bellinger DL, and Felten DL: Involvement of peripheral and central catecholamine systems in neural-immune interactions. *Neuroimmunology* 1985; 10:5–30.

Lotzova E and Herberman RB: *Immunobiology of NK Cells.* CRC Press, Boca Raton, FL, 1986.

Makinodan R and Kay MMB: Age influence on the immune system. *Adv. Immunol.* 1980; 29:307.

Mellstrom D, Nilsson A, Oden A, Rundgren A, and Svanborg A: Mortality among the widowed in Sweden. *Scand. J. Soc. Med.* 1982; 10:33–41.

Mohl PC, Huang L, Bowden C, Fischbach M, Vogtsberer K, and Talal N: Natural killer cell activity in major depression (lett.). *Am. J. Psychiatry* 1987; 144:1619.

Nemeroff CB, Widerlov E, Bissette G, et al.: Elevated concentrations of CSF corticotropin-releasing-factor-like immunoreactivity in depressed patients. *Science* 1984; 226:1342–1344.

Nemeroff CB, Simon JS, Haggerty JJ, and Evans DL: Antithyroid antibodies in depressed patients. *Am. J. Psychiatry* 1985; 142:840–843.

Olschowka JA, O'Donohue TL, Mueller GP, and Jacobowitz DM: The distribution of corticotropin releasing factor-like immunoreactivity neurons in rat brain. *Peptides* 1982; 3:995–1015.

Parkes CM, Benjamin B, and Fitzgerald RG: Broken heart: a statistical study of increased mortality among widows. *Br. Med. J.* 1969; 1:740–743.

Persky VS, Kempthorne-Rawson J, and Shekelle RB: Personality and risk of cancer: 20-year follow-up of the Western Electric study. *Psychosom. Med.* 1987; 49:435–449.

Paull WK, Scholer J, Arimura A, Meyers CA, Chang JK, and Chong D: *Peptides* 1982; 18:3–191.

Rees WD and Lutkins SG: Mortality of bereavement. *Br. Med. J.* 1967; 4:13–6.

Reid LM, Minato N, Gresser I, et al.: Influence of anti-mouse interferon serum on the growth and metastasis of tumor cells persistently injected with virus and human prostatic tumor in athymic mice. *Proc. Natl. Acad. Sci. U.S.A.* 1981; 78:1171.

Ritz J: The role of natural killer cells in immune surveillance. *N. Engl. J. Med.* 1989; 320:1748–1749.

Rosenberg SA, Lotze MT, Muul LM, et al.: A progress report on the treatment of 157 patients with advanced cancer using lymphokine activated killer cells and interleukin-2 or high-dose interleukin-2 alone. *N. Engl. J. Med.* 1987; 316:899–906.

Schleifer SJ, Keller SE, Camerino M, Thornton JC, and Stein MM: Suppression of lymphocyte stimulation following bereavement. *JAMA* 1983; 250:374–377.

Schleifer S, Keller SE, Meyerson AT, Raskin MD, Davis KL, and Stein M: Lymphocyte function in major depressive disorder. *Arch. Gen. Psychiatry* 1984; 41:484–486.

Schleifer SJ, Keller SE, Siris SG, Davis KL, and Stein M: Lymphocyte function in ambulatory depressed patients, hospitalized schizophrenic patients, and patients hospitalized for herniorrhaphy. *Arch. Gen. Psychiatry* 1985; 42:129–134.

Schleifer SJ, Keller SE, Bond RN, Cohen J, and Stein M: Major depressive disorder and immunity. *Arch. Gen. Psychiatry* 1989; 46:81–87.

Schmale AH and Iker HP: The effect of hopelessness and the development of cancer. I. Identification of uterine cervical cancer in women with atypical cytology. *Psychosom. Med.* 1966a; 28:714–721.

Schmale AH and Iker H: Hopelessness as a predictor of cervical cancer. *Soc. Sci. Med.* 1966b; 5:95–100.

Shopsin B, Sathananthan GL, Chan TL, Kravitz H, and Gershon S: Antinuclear factor in psychiatric patients. *Biol. Psychiatry* 1973; 7:81–87.

Smith HR and Steinberg AD: Autoimmunity: a perspective. *Annu. Rev. Immunol.* 1983; 1:197–205.

Sutton RE, Koob GF, LeMoal M, et al.: Corticotropin releasing factor produces behavioral activation in rats. *Nature* 1982; 297:331–333.

Swanson LW, Sawchenko PE, Rivier J, et al.: The organization of ovine corticotropin releasing factor (CRF). *Neuroendocrinology* 1983; 36:165–186.

Syvalahti E, Eskola J, Ruuskanen O, and Laine T: Nonsuppression of cortisol in depression and immune function. *Prog. Neuropsychopharmacol. Biol. Psychiatry* 1985; 9(4):413–422.

Talmadge JD, Meyrs KM, Prien DJ, et al.: Role of NK cells in tumor growth and metastases in beige mice. *Nature* 1980; 284:622.

Taylor AI and Fishman LM: Corticotropin releasing hormone. *N. Engl. J. Med.* 1988; 319:213–222.

Urich A, Muller C, Aschauer H, Resch F, and Zilinski CC: Lytic effector cell function in schizophrenia and depression. *J. Neuroimmunol.* 1988; 18:291–301.

Vale W, Spiess J, Rivier C, and Rivier J: Characterization of a 41-residue ovine hypothalamic peptide that stimulates secretion of corticotropin and beta-endorphin. *Science* 1981; 213:1394–1397.

Valentino RJ, Foote SL, and Aston-Jones G: CRF activates noradrenergic neurons of the locus coeruleus. *Brain Res.* 1983; 270:363–367.

Varsamis J, Zuchowski T, and Main KK: Survival rate and causes of death in geriatric psychiatric patients. *Can. Psychiatr. Assoc. J.* 1972; 17:17–21.

Whitlock FA and Siskind M: Depression and cancer: a follow-up study. *Psychol. Med.* 1979; 9:747–752.

Wynn PC, Hauger RL, Holmes MC, Millan MA, Catt KJ, and Aguilera G: Brain and pituitary receptors for corticotropin releasing factor's localization and differential regulation after adrenalectomy. *Peptides* 1984; 5:1077–1084.

Bereavement: Effects on Immunity and Risk of Disease

Georgia D. Andrianopoulos
Departments of Surgery and Psychiatry
University of Illinois, College of Medicine
Chicago, Illinois

Joseph A. Flaherty
Department of Psychiatry
University of Illinois, College of Medicine
Chicago, Illinois

OVERVIEW

The notion that emotions can alter the risk of occurrence of certain diseases can be traced back to as early as the 2nd century A.D., when the Greek physician Galen noted a greater tendency for development of breast cancer among melancholic women than those with more sanguine traits. A correlation between single marital status and increased mortality was noted in France by Deparcieux over 2 centuries ago. Absence or loss of a spouse has been related to the "broken heart" syndrome that is frequently described in poetry and prose.

While numerous investigations have examined the association between bereavement and susceptibility to illness or mortality, specific high-risk patterns in bereavement that may be predictive of physical and psychological morbidity remain largely unknown. This may be due in part to wide variations in results reflecting geographical and cultural variations of bereavement, experimental design (retrospective vs. prospective), and sampling techniques. The absence of a clear definition of bereavement may have also contributed to the wide variation in results.

129

Bereavement has been defined as both a state and a reaction to the death or loss of someone to whom the individual had been attached (Raphael et al., 1987). Evidence based on data from animals, children separated from parents, and bereaved individuals suggest a similar temporal sequence in bereavement: separation anxiety, protest, sadness, and depression followed by reorganization (Bowlby, 1980). The adaptive value of bereavement and its relationship with other parallel states involving loss, life events, psychological trauma, and depression has not been clearly defined. Most investigators agree that a coherent model of bereavement is needed from which testable theoretical hypotheses may be generated to predict high-risk responses for physical and psychological morbidity related to bereavement. The absence of criteria that define the underlying normal course and constituents of bereavement make it difficult to determine abnormal or delayed bereavement.

As currently defined, bereavement may be too heterogeneous a concept for experimental investigation since it appears to be inclusive of numerous interactive psychological, social, and physical factors. Factors that are known or suspected to complicate bereavement include depression, adverse impact from chronic stress, sleep and nutritional disturbances, age, changes in physical activity, use of alcohol and tobacco, and duration of the illness of the deceased spouse. The relative contribution of individual components such as depression or distress on physical and psychological morbidity in bereavement has not been assessed. Thus, the task of accurate prediction, screening, and intervention of bereaved individuals at high risk for physical and psychological morbidity remains incomplete.

A possible explanation for the lack of separation of the aforementioned factors in clinical and experimental research of bereavement may have originated in the initial epidemiologic studies where bereavement was defined as the immediate period preceding and following the death of a spouse. However, while this all-encompassing definition of bereavement may have been useful for epidemiologic studies, examination of some of the major components of bereavement may be more heuristic in clinical and experimental research. The concept of bereavement as a multicomponent process inclusive of somatic disturbances, preoccupation with images of the deceased, guilt, anger, and disorganized behavior was recognized by Lindemann as early as 1944.

Presently, there appears to be sufficient homogeneity in epidemiologic and experimental data to support the notion that bereavement can increase the rate or the likelihood of occurrence of certain psychological and physical illnesses.

This chapter will provide a summary of epidemiologic studies that have investigated the association between the state of bereavement or commonly noted constituents of bereavement such as depression and the risk for physical and psychological morbidity. Since depression seems to relate to bereavement-related immunosuppression, and possibly to the increased risk of physical and psychological morbidity in bereavement, studies on depression, immune function, and illness will also be briefly reviewed.

Since animal models are frequently used to examine epidemiologic associations between various risk factors and susceptibility to illness, results from animal studies that have examined epidemiologic associations of depression and illness will be discussed.

Lastly, future areas of investigation that may further our understanding of the mechanisms that may potentially link bereavement and other behavioral factors to disease risk will be outlined.

HEALTH CONSEQUENCES OF BEREAVEMENT

During the impending or actual loss of a spouse, the surviving spouse is faced with a variety of short-term and long-term issues and demands that occur irrespective of their degree of ability to handle these demands or their level of preparedness. Short-term issues facing the surviving spouse may include concern and empathy toward the ill spouse, anxiety and sadness about the impending loss, helping with treatment decisions, communciation about the medical status of spouse to other family members or friends, adjustments in work schedule or daily responsibilities, adjustment of role within the family, and alterations in the preexisting balance between personal, private, and professional aspects of his (her) life. Some of the long-term concerns facing the surviving spouse as a result of impending or actual loss of a spouse include loneliness or isolation, financial issues, adjustment in altered marital status, and changes in future plans.

The impact of these issues on the spouse is expected to vary according to past coping style, the number of past crises and the successful resolution of past crises, the duration of the spouse's illness, confidence and degree of effectiveness in financial issues, family and social integration, and overall physical and psychological health. This section will provide a review of studies that have investigated the association between bereavement and risk of physical and psychological illness.

Epidemiologic studies show an association between bereavement and increased risk of morbidity for medical (Jacobs and Ostfeld, 1977; Maddison and Viola, 1968; Mor et al., 1986; Clayton, 1979; Klerman and Izen, 1977; Parks and Brown, 1982) and psychological disorders (Parkes, 1984), as well as increases in mortality from all causes (Rees and Lutkins, 1967; Bowling and Benjamin, 1985; Bowling, 1987; Helsing et al., 1981).

In the so-called broken-heart study, Parks et al. (1969) described the increased mortality rates of widowers during the 6 months following the death of their spouse, primarily from coronary heart disease. The rate of death in individuals during the first week after the death of their spouse was twice the expected rate in a sample of 95,647 widowed individuals (Kaprio et al., 1987). In this group, ischemic heart disease accounted for the majority of the death cases.

Results of a prospective study of 4000 widowers (Helsing et al., 1981) showed increased rates of mortality during the first 10 years following the death of a spouse, but not during the first year. Additionally, among males, the rates of death from infectious diseases, accidents, and suicide were higher than expected, while among females, the rates of cirrhosis of the liver were significantly greater than expected. In a review of epidemiologic studies on bereavement and mortality, Jacobs and Ostfeld (1977) concluded that of the 35,000 deaths that occur annually among the recently widowed, an estimated 7000 can be attributed to the death of the spouse. Overall, about 67% of widowers noted a deterioration of health status within the first year after the death of their spouse (Jacobs and Ostfeld, 1977).

Results also suggest that the highest rate of morbidity among the bereaved may occur within 6 months after the death of a spouse. In a study of 4486 widowers at least 55 years old or older, 213 died within the first 6 months after the death of their spouse, or at a rate 40% above the expected level for age-matched, married controls (Young et al., 1963).

The majority of studies investigating the association between bereavement and mortality have shown an increased risk of mortality, particularly among bereaved males (Osterweiss et al., 1984).

Similar to morbidity, the increased mortality among males seems highest during the first 6 months following the death of their spouse (Bowling, 1987). The increase in mortality seems to be due to a variety of illnesses, particularly cardiovascular disorders. The rate of suicide has also been shown to increase in bereavement (Hesling et al., 1981). Evidence suggests an association between bereavement and increased rates of hyperthyroidism, diabetes, cancer, and cardiovascular disorders (Raphael and Middleton, 1987).

The mediating mechanisms for the increased rates in the aforementioned illness or disorders have not been delineated; however, there is some evidence to suggest that the risk of occurrence of certain illnesses may vary in a temporal fashion, with early and late effects of bereavement. Evidence suggests that the risk of cardiovascular disease may be highest shortly after the loss of a spouse and may be precipitated by ventricular arrythmias (Solomon et al., 1982). Parasympathetic rebound following intense stress or fear has been related to sudden death apparently due to severe cardiac arrythmia and is the hypothetical mechanism of the so-called "voodoo death" phenomenon. The increased risk of developing other illnesses such as diabetes or cancer is associated with the late effects of bereavement. The mechanisms by which the late effects of bereavement are mediated have been related to alterations in the immune system (Schleifer et al., 1983, 1985).

The most common initial reaction to the death of a spouse or close relative is characterized by increased, erratic, and at times violent motor movements and an overall state of agitation and arousal. These responses generally dissipate over a period of minutes or hours and a state of hypoactivity and hypoarousal ensues. It may be of value to relate these behavioral factors that occur in the course of bereavement to neuroendocrine activation and the risk of occurrence of illness. Specifically, more information is needed to determine whether cardiovascular disorders are early phenomena in bereavement and mediated by hypothalamic-pituitary-adrenal (HPA) neuroendocrine activation, while cancer and other illnesses are late phenomena and mediated by the immune system.

The age at which an individual becomes widowed seems to be a factor in the risk of mortality. Although studies have shown that individuals under the age of 35 who become widowed have a greater risk of fatality than married controls of comparable age (Kraus and Lilienfeld, 1959), it appears that widowers between the ages of 55 and 74 run the greatest risk of morbidity after loss of their spouse.

Bereavement has also been related to an increased rate of utilization of various medical services, although it is difficult to separate treatment-seeking behaviors from physical morbidity in the majority of these studies (Klerman and Izan, 1977). Data from the National Hospice Study showed an increase in physician visits during the first 4 months after the death of a relative, compared to national norms (Mor et al., 1986). However, rather than bereavement per se, increases in the utilization of medical services by the bereaved may be a manifestation of psychological distress, which is also prevelant in bereavement (Clayton, 1979).

A number of studies have shown increased use of tranquilizers, sedatives, and alcohol among the recently bereaved (Mor et al., 1986; Maddison and Viola, 1968; Osterweiss et al., 1984). Evidence suggests that alcohol, sedatives, and tranquilizers have an immunosuppressive influence and may therefore be contributing factors in the immune alterations commonly described in bereavement. Experimental results have not consistently supported the finding of excess mortality in bereavement. Notably, bereavement was not related to excess mortality from cancer (Jones et al., 1984).

Bereavement has also been associated with an increased risk of psychological morbidity. Patients who were admitted to a psychiatric hospital were significantly more likely than expected demographically (i.e., age, social group) to have sustained loss of a spouse (Parkes, 1965, 1974). Previous results show the frequency of depression at about 45% during the first postbereavement year (Clayton et al., 1972, 1974). The nature of depressive symptoms or depression in bereavement and its relationship to affective disorders needs to be better defined. For example, the characteristic finding of dexamethasone nonsuppression in patients with depression has been related to anxiety and not depression in bereavement (Schuchter et al., 1986). The rate of mania, anxiety, phobia, and other disorders may also be increased among the recently bereaved (Shackleton, 1984).

Results from the aforementioned studies suggest that men may be more vulnerable to bereavement-related physical and psychological morbidity, possibly due to greater changes among men in daily routines and roles and less availability of social support systems (Raphael and Middleton, 1987). Stress, depression, loneliness, anxiety, alienation (dysphoria), and the impoverishment of social support networks may occur more commonly in men, and they are also factors frequently associated with bereavement and poor health, including the etiology or course of infectious diseases, autoimmune diseases, and cancer (Solomon, 1987). Deficiency in social support has been more consistently related to increased mortality (Berkman, 1988) than physical illness. Reduced social support has been related to an increase in physical symptoms (Gore, 1978); however, no association between physical symptoms and social support was noted in another study (Schaefer et al., 1981). Thus, social support seems to be a more consistent factor in mortality and psychological illness rather than physical symptoms (Grant et al., 1988). Results have also shown that the quality of support rather than overall levels of support may be more important in predicting health outcomes (Grant et al., 1988).

There are sociocultural, ethnic, and social class differences in bereavement that define who is the bereaved, legitimate sources of support, their appropriate timing of involvement in bereavement, and acceptable methods of expressing distress (Eisenbruch, 1984a, 1984b). Generally, cultures that encourage public processing and expression of grief fare better than Western cultures which emphasize a private, deritualized system of handling loss with an aim to return to "normal" as quickly as possible.

Since normal and pathologic bereavement have not been operationally defined, the concepts of "delayed" or "disturbed" grief have not been clearly defined. A potentially useful tool for assessing the presence of bereavement-related symptoms and behaviors is the Texas Grief Inventory (Zisook et al., 1982). This instrument is made up of 34 items relating to present feelings and 24 items relating to feelings at the time of the person's death. This and other instruments may be used to elucidate the stages that follow major loss and help define normal and pathologic patterns of response to loss.

Bereavement-related therapeutic interventions may be offered to individuals with high-risk profiles with the aim of reducing symptomatology that has been previously linked to a complicated bereavement process. A variety of therapeutic approaches and models have been successfully applied to the bereaved, including psychotherapy (Osterweiss et al., 1984; Krupnick and Horowitz, 1985) and behavioral therapy (Mawson et al., 1981). Other therapies particularly suited to the bereaved include guiding the patient through the processes of "reliving, revisiting and reviewing" (Melges and DeMaso, 1980). Psychotherapeutic interventions have been shown to reduce the increased morbidity of the bereaved (Parkes, 1980); however, it is unclear whether mortality is similarly reduced with psychotherapeutic intervention (Parkes, 1980).

In summary, bereavement can be defined as a response to impending or actual loss of a person with whom there is attachment or love. The time period that precedes and follows the loss of a spouse is associated with increased risk of physical and psychological morbidity. This risk appears to be greater for males than females and during the first year following the death of a spouse; however, males remain at a higher risk for longer periods. The causes of mortality vary; however, cardiovascular disorders account for the majority of the death cases among bereaved people. Some components of the bereavement process seem to be present universally (i.e., phases of grief, postures and behaviors during the various phases), while other components appear to be more variable. The heterogeneity of the bereavement process may reflect the differences of individuals, sociocultural variations, social class, and overall physical and psychological health.

BEREAVEMENT: EFFECTS ON THE IMMUNE SYSTEM

As with other behavioral factors, the most widely investigated hypothetical mechanism by which bereavement increases the risk of disease and fatality is immunity. According to this hypothesis, bereavement or its constituents (i.e., depression, distress, chronic stress etc.) also suppress immune function by as yet undefined mechanisms, resulting in increased rates in certain types of illness. There are at least two pathways by which bereavement and its constituents can alter the risk of occurrence in certain diseases.

First, bereavement-associated neuroendocrine/neurohormonal activation may alter immune function in a manner that influences the risk of occurrence in certain diseases. Both depression and chronic stress, two commonly identified factors in bereavement, have been shown in animal (Monjan and Collector, 1977; Murison et al., 1989) and human (Dorian et al., 1980, 1982; Keller et al., 1981; Albrecht et al., 1985) studies to suppress some parameters of immune function or alter the structure of the immune organs (in the case of stress), perhaps by activation of the HPA axis. In addition to immunity, other studies have examined the effects of bereavement on cardiovascular and neuroendocrine systems.

A second pathway by which bereavement or its main constituents can alter the likelihood of occurrence in certain diseases is by increasing or decreasing the likelihood and frequency of occurrence in other health behaviors that in turn, either by way of the immune system or mechanisms independent of immunity, alter the risk of disease. For example, in addition to bereavement, individuals facing impending or actual loss of their spouse may also have a greater likelihood of altered levels of nutritional intake, sleep, physical activity, and tobacco and alcohol use, which have been shown to influence immune function.

The following section provides a summary of results describing the association between bereavement and immune function.

The relationship between bereavement and immunity was first examined by Bartrop et al. (1977) in a study of men and women whose spouses were seriously ill. Blood samples were collected from these subjects at two time points, first at approximately 1 to 3 weeks and again 6 weeks following the death of the spouse. Isolated lymphocytes were challenged by known mitogens (agents that increase the rate of mitosis) such as phytohemagglutinin (PHA) and concanavalin A (ConA). Results showed that T-cell responses to PHA and ConA were significantly lower in bereaved subjects, compared to non-bereaved controls at 6 weeks, but not at 1 month following the loss of a spouse. Comparing T-cell responses to stimulation of both mitogens between the two time-point samplings, results showed higher suppression in T-cell mitogenesis at the 6-week post-bereavement sampling. However, no differences were found in the number of T- and B-cells, immunoglobulins, delayed hypersensitivity responses, cortisol, prolactin, or the presence of autoantibodies between bereaved and control subjects. These results suggested that a time lag may exist in the suppression of mitogen-induced lymphocyte proliferation in bereavement. In contrast, mitogen-induced suppression of lymphocyte proliferation with other stressors such as 48-h sleep deprivation (Palmblad et al., 1979) and running a marathon (Escola et al., 1978) seems to persist for several days after the event. Since Bartrop et al. (1977) did not perform standardized psychiatric evaluations, the differences in mitogenesis between bereaved and control subjects could not be related specifically to bereavement.

In a prospective study, Schleifer et al. (1983) assessed lymphocyte proliferation in response to PHA, ConA and pokeweed mitogen (PWM). Responses of lymphocytes to the three mitogens were compared for samples taken before and during the first 2 months after the death of the spouse. Results showed suppression of mitogen-induced lymphocyte stimulation with each mitogen during the two post-bereavement months, compared to pre-bereavement. The results of this study also show that lymphocyte stimulation was suppressed in association with the actual loss of the spouse rather than the preexisting stress associated with the spouse's illness. Similar to the Bartrop et al. study, the number of peripheral blood lymphocytes and the number of T- and B-cells did not differ during the pre-bereavement and the 2-month post-bereavement time periods (Schleifer et al., 1983). However, in contrast to the Bartrop et al. study, Schleifer et al., noted alterations in immune reactivity to mitogenic stimulation as early as 1 month post-bereavement.

These differences in lymphocyte reactivity may be due to other factors such as age or sex, which have been shown to alter lymphocyte reactivity (Calabrese et al., 1989; Irwin et al., 1987c). As in the Bartrop et al. study, Schleifer et al. (1983) also omitted data on the standardized psychiatric assessment of their subjects. Thus, once again, the separate effects of bereavement and other factors associated with bereavement could not be examined separately.

Linn et al. (1984) also examined the effect of bereavement on cell-mediated and humoral immunity. However, in this study, subjects were evaluated with the Hopkins Symptoms Checklist (HSC). Results showed that PHA-induced lymphocyte stimulation was suppressed in the bereaved only when the depression scores on the depression subset of the HSC were elevated. Results on immune function by the "mixed lymphocyte culture procedure" in which lymphocytes are combined from two different donors also showed reduced cell-mediated immunity among the bereaved group. ConA and PWM-induced lymphocyte stimulation did not differ in the depressed and the non-depressed subjects. Results also showed no differences between bereaved subjects and controls to delayed hypersensitivity skin tests.

Results of later studies tend to support the hypothesis that depression is a frequent concomitant of bereavement and may indeed be the mediating mechanism by which bereavement can alter immunity (Parkes, 1984).

The weight of the aforementioned experimental evidence points to an association between bereavement and immune function as measured by mitogen-induced lymphocyte proliferation. In a series of well-conducted investigations of the relationship between additional parameters of immune function and bereavement or depression in bereavement, Irwin et al. (1986a, 1986b, 1987a, 1987b) have shown that T-cell subpopulations and the activity of natural killer cells (NKC) are altered when bereavement is inclusive of increased exposure to life events or depressive disorders.

Specifically, Irwin et al. (1986a, 1986b, 1987a) studied two groups of women whose husbands were either receiving medical treatment for metastatic lung cancer or whose husbands had died of lung cancer in the previous 1 to 6 months and a control group of women whose husbands were healthy. Women in all three groups completed the Hamilton Rating Scale for Depression (HRSD) and the Social Readjustment Rating Scale (SRS). NKC activity, the number of T-cells, and the ratio of T-cell subpopulations (T-helper and T-suppressor) were studied as parameters of immune function. Results showed first, that control women experienced fewer levels of life change events than women with husbands with advanced lung cancer or women within the first 6 months post-bereavement. Additionally, HDRS and NKC activity in women with moderate to high SRS scores was lower than in the low-SRS group, compared to the moderate- and high-SRS groups. No significant differences in either NK activity or HDRS scores were noted between moderate and high SRS scores. However, the level of SRS was not related to the absolute number of lymphocytes, percent of T-cells, and T-cell ratio of helper to suppressor.

However, the total mean HDRS score was significantly related to suppressed NKC activity. An examination of the association between several HDRS subscales and NKC activity showed that the depressed mood and insomnia subscales were also related to reduced NKC activity; however, the anxiety and somatic symptoms subscales were not related to NKC activity.

The total HDRS score and the subscales of depressed mood, insomnia, and anxiety were related to an enhanced ratio of T-helper to T-suppressor cells. Additionally, the total HDRS score was related to a reduction of T-suppressor cells. In this study, some known confounders of immune function such as nutritional status and physical activity were controlled.

These results demonstrate that women faced with the impending loss of their spouse or who have recently experienced an actual loss of a spouse experience more stress and depression than women whose husbands are healthy. Suppressed NKC activity, the ratio of T-helper to T-suppressor cells, and the number of T-suppressor cells was related to the severity of depression. In this study, SRS scores correlated highly with depression and bereavement status (pre- and post-bereavement), and the relative contribution of these factors on immune alterations was difficult to determine.

In order to delineate the effect of depression on immune function in bereavement, Irwin et al. (1987b) examined depression and concomitant changes in NKC activity in a prospective study of women 1 month before and 1 month after the death of their spouse. Results showed that the mean values of HDRS and NKC activity were not different between the anticipatory period and the period after the actual loss.

Interestingly, the variability in HDRS scores was greater after actual loss than during the anticipatory period, and this change was significantly related to suppression of NKC activity. This finding supports the hypothesis of heterogeneity of response among the bereaved group, especially after the experience of the loss.

In the preceding discussion of experimental results, it becomes apparent that frequently, rather than bereavement status per se, alterations in immunity and perhaps health are associated with the absence or presence of specific reactions to the loss of a spouse. Specifically, the presence of depression and life events-related distress more than bereavement status per se seem to relate to immune function.

Presently, it is unclear whether depression and stress are more detrimental to immune function in bereavement than in other settings or populations in which they occur. However, studies have shown that immune function may be altered under several bereavement-related behaviors, including sleep (Palmblad, 1979), caloric (Bistrian et al., 1975) or specific nutrient intake (Chandra, 1983; Beisel et al., 1981), smoking (Miller et al., 1982), age (Linn and Jensen, 1983), physical activity (Escola et al., 1978), alcohol intake (Watson et al., 1984), and use of certain drugs (Lazzarin et al., 1984). The presence of depression or stress occurring in this milieu may have a greater impact on immune function by way of interaction and perhaps facilitation by some of the aforementioned variables. However, previous results suggest that unlike depression in different settings, in bereavement, hypercortisolism relates to anxiety to a higher degree than to depression (Schuchter et al., 1986).

More information is required in order to further understand the unique qualities of depression and stress in bereavement vs. other settings and their respective influence on immune function.

It is also important to note that the triad in the equation, bereavement → immune function → risk of disease and death, has not been adequately examined in its entirety in a single study in humans, but, rather, in combinations of two variables at a time. The following list of variables known or suspected to be associated with response to death of a spouse and (or) immunity need to be considered: First, demographic factors known or suspected to influence immunity are age, sex, and level of income and education. Second, psychological factors potentially modifying both immunity and bereavement include coping style, adequacy of social support systems, "hardiness" (Kobussa, 1983), depressive disorders, exposure and impact of life events, acute or chronic stress (Kiecolt-Glazer et al., 1984), adequacy of social or marital support systems (Kiecolt-Glazer et al., 1987), length of illness of the spouse, and attribution of responsibility for maintaining health (Solomon, 1981).

The weight of the aforementioned evidence generally supports the notion that the impact of stressful events, including bereavement, more than the face value of the stressor per se may be the most significant predictor for the occurrence of immune alterations and depressive disorders. Thus, as with stress, Selye's concept that "it is not what happens to you but how you take it" appears to also hold in the area of bereavement.

Stressful life events, including bereavement, have been associated with changes in CNS activity that resemble depression (Schleifer et al., 1987). Additionally, similar to depression in other settings, bereavement has been related to alterations in sleep, appetite, physical activity, and socialization (Clayton et al., 1972; Clayton, 1979; Parkes, 1972). As depression is a frequent complicating factor in bereavement and may be a factor in the immunosuppressive properties of bereavement, some of the conceptual issues that may uniquely relate to depression, immunity, and risk of illness will be briefly reviewed.

DEPRESSION, IMMUNITY, AND ILLNESS

Disturbances in some parameters of immune function have been associated with depression. The most commonly supported hypothetical-mediating mechanism for depression-related immunosuppression is depression-related hypercortisolism.

Previous results have shown that PHA-induced activation of lymphocytes was suppressed among patients in an acute state of depression, compared to states of remission (Cappel et al., 1978). Similarly, lymphocyte function was altered in depressed individuals, compared to controls (Kronfol et al., 1984, 1985). Mitogen-induced lymphocyte stimulation in drug-free ambulatory patients with major depressive disorder were lower than hospitalized age- and sex-matched controls (Schleifer et al., 1985). In addition, severity of depressive disorder rather than hospitalization per se was related to suppressed mitogenesis. Decreased mitogen responses were also related to unipolar major depressive disorder, compared with age- and sex-matched controls (Schleifer et al., 1985). Age was either inversely related or unrelated to mitogenesis in patients with depressive disorder. In contrast, control subjects showed age-related increases in mitogenesis. Previous findings have shown that among patients with depression, the presence of dexamethasone nonsuppression may be a marker for immunosuppression in these patients (Kronfol et al., 1985).

Calabrese et al. (1986) provided additional support for depression-associated suppression of mitogen-induced lymphocyte activity. However, it is unclear whether the finding of increased levels of prostaglandins (PGE1, PGE2) in plasma of depressed individuals is sufficient to account for depression-related immunosuppression (Goodwin and Webb, 1980). It is likely that the elevated levels of these PGs in depressed individuals reflect local or systemic inflammatory processes. Essential fatty acids (nutritional status) have been shown to alter cell-mediated and humoral immunity (Hwang, 1989). Cyclooxygenase inhibitors that reduce PG synthesis have been shown to be immunoenhancing (Goodwin et al., 1978). Thus, the finding of increased serum levels of PGs in patients with depression may relate to nutritional status and mediate immunosuppression.

Previous findings offer extensive support that the immune system is altered in bereavement (Irwin et al., 1987; Schleifer et al., 1983; Locke et al., 1984; Calabrese et al., 1987), life stress (Irwin et al., 1987; Schindler, 1985), and depressive symptoms (Schleifer et al., 1989; Schindler, 1985). However, it is not clear whether these immune alterations alter the risk of occurrence of illness. Previous findings suggest that life stress, loss, and depression can alter susceptibility to certain illnesses, including infectious disease (Jemmott and Locke, 1984), autoimmune disorders (Solomon, 1981), allergies (Stein, 1981), and cancer (Fox, 1981).

Among psychosocial factors, the relationship between depression and cancer has been investigated most frequently in epidemiologic studies.

Schmale and Iker (1966b) found that the degree of helplessness, as measured by interview, and depression, as measured by the Minnesota Multiphasic Personality Inventory (MMPI), were significantly predictive of cancer in women who were hospitalized with class III Papanicolaou (pap) smears. In a 10-year follow-up prospective study of 1353 individuals, Grossarth-Maticek et al. (1983) noted that depression, low emotionality, and helplessness were the most powerful predictors of subsequent cancer development. However, in this study, the effects of age, smoking, weight, and alcohol intake were not adequately controlled and may have confounded the association between depression and risk of death due to cancer. An increased risk of death due to cancer was also related to depression in a 17-year follow-up study with appropriate controls for factors known to relate to cancer risk (Shekelle et al., 1981). In a 20-year follow-up prospective study of 2018 middle-age males, Persky et al. (1987) noted a positive association between depression, as measured by the MMPI, and the incidence of and mortality from cancer. The positive association between depression and cancer morbidity and mortality remained after adjustment for smoking history, alcohol intake, age, occupational status, body mass index, and serum cholesterol levels. Frequently, depression can be characterized by helplessness. Results by Schmale and Iker (1966a, 1966b) showed that hopelessness was predictive of the diagnosis of cervical carcinoma.

A number of investigations have reported no difference in cancer morbidity or mortality between depressed and nondepressed individuals as assessed by various standardized instruments for depression (Fox, 1978). In a prospective study by Zonderman et al. (1989), depression at the time of interview was not significantly related to cancer morbidity or mortality in a 7-year follow-up.

In reviewing investigations of the effect of depression on the immune system or on the development of medical and psychological illness, it may be important to consider that most investigations have not differentiated among the two major subtypes of depression, melancholic and atypical depression. Gold et al. (1988) have summarized the important differences in neuroendocrine activation between the two subtypes, hyperarousal and hypoarousal, respectively, for melancholic and atypical depression. These differences in neuroendocrine activation suggest that the impact on the immune system or other immune parameters differs between the two subtypes. Therefore, the risk of developing certain illnesses can also be expected to vary among individuals with melancholic and atypical depression. For instance, the characteristic feature of overfeeding in atypical depression may increase the likelihood of occurrence in obesity-related illnesses, including diabetes and cancer. In contrast, underfeeding or reduced body weight has been related to suppression of cancer development (Tannenbaum, 1942). Previous results also show that dexamethasone nonsuppression of cortisol is uncommon among patients with atypical depression, characterized by hyperarousal and increased sleeping and feeding (Casper et al., 1988).

Thus, epidemiologic studies that have examined the relationship between depression and cancer risk or cancer fatality (Shekelle et al., 1981; Persky et al., 1987; Zonderman et al., 1989) without differentiating among the two depression subtypes may have obscured the true nature of the association between depression and cancer, if indeed such a relationship exists.

Furthermore, a review of the literature in which depression has been related to cancer risk or fatality suggests that immune factors are considered as more likely mediators between depression and cancer than other factors like "health" behaviors (i.e., diet and exercise), which may also be altered in depression (Krauchi and Wirt-Justice, 1988; Farmer et al., 1988). Given that immunity is the most popular hypothetical mediating mechanism between depression and cancer, it would be of interest to examine the relationship between depression and the risk of occurrence of cancers which have been shown to be most sensitive to immune factors (Andrianopoulos, 1989a). Previous results have shown an increased incidence of only certain neoplasms in chronically immunodeficient patients (Penn, 1978, 1982). The incidence of lymphomas, carcinomas of the lip and skin, carcinomas of the vulva, *in situ* carcinomas of the uterine cervix, and leukemias is greater in organ transplant recipients and other chronically immunosuppressed individuals than in the general population (Penn, 1978). In contrast, the most frequently occurring cancers in the general population (colon, lung, and breast) are not increased in immunosuppressed patients. Although behavioral factors and depression may not be considered as immunosuppressive as pharmacotherapy, with a sufficent number of cases, a trend of effect between depression and some cancers may emerge, if indeed such a relationship exists.

Evidence also suggests that depression in bereavement may differ from depressive illness in other settings in a variety of ways. First, cortisol levels have not been as predictive of depression in bereavement as in depression in other settings. Second, it appears that the immunosuppressive effects of depression could be facilitated in bereavement possibly via other bereavement-related constituents such as alterations in sleep, feeding, socialization, physical activity, and alcohol consumption. In addition, the risk of recurrence of long-standing depression is increased in bereavement.

It is also possible to consider that immune changes during bereavement are the result of the separation experience itself. Studies of the infant's psychologic response to separation from its mother have shown disturbances in heart rate, body temperature, and sleep patterns in nonhuman primates (Reite et al., 1981). Using Bowlby's two-phased framework of separation, the initial protest phase has been linked to changes in activity (Lewis et al., 1976), vocalization (Reite et al., 1974), and food intake (Butler, 1978) as well as changes in cortisol (Smotherman et al., 1979), catecholamines (Breese et al., 1977), growth hormone (Kuhn et al., 1978), and T-cell activity (Keeler et al., 1983), and increase in hemolytic complement activity (Coe et al., 1988) and specific antibody activity (Coe et al., 1988b). Significant, though somewhat reduced immunological changes have been shown in peer separated nonhuman primates (Boccia et al., 1989). Maternal separation has a continued effect on immune function when imposed upon an early weaning condition in several animal studies (Kelley, 1980; Lunderslager and Perti, 1985).

Hofer (1984) and colleagues have provided extensive research into the "hidden regulators" in the mother-infant relationship that control physiological functioning. For example, activity level in the infant is partially controlled by maternal warmth (Hofer, 1975a) and tactile sensation from contact with the mother (Hofer, 1975b). The developing rhythmicity of REM cycles seems to be largely controlled by the periodicity of maternal milk and tactile sensation (Hofer and Shair, 1982). Hofer proposed a psychobiology of bereavement that suggests that psychologic and physiologic reactions are due to the abrupt withdrawal of the spouse who has acted as a zeitgeber (timekeeper) for entraining the biological functions to a circadian rhythm. Support for this hypothesis comes from various experiments showing that social interactions do serve as zeitgebers in regulating circadian rhythms and that withdrawal of these cues results in at least transient deregulation of circadian rhythms (Wever, 1974). Ehlers et al. (1988) have extended Hofer's argument into the social zeitgeber hypothesis of depression. These authors suggest that life events, such as death of a spouse, have a depressogenic effect through the alteration in daily social rhythms, resulting in altered biological rhythms, which lead to a common state of deregulation which, in vulnerable individuals, may lead to a clinical depression.

In the first test on the social zeitgeber hypothesis, we followed 147 widows and widowers during the first year of bereavement (Flaherty et al., 1987). Using a preliminary form of the daily rhythm metric (Monk et al., in press), we found that changes in the surviving spouse's daily rhythms (e.g., times for getting up, eating breakfast, lunch, and dinner, going to bed, etc.) were associated with higher depression scores and higher rates of depressive illness. Social rhythm changes were also associated with an increase in gastrointestinal and cardiovascular symptoms. Changes in the timing of these daily activities had a significant "predictive" effect of depression at 1 month and 1 year, using multiple regression analyses. A similar association was found for changes in daily rhythms and increased cardiovascular symptoms. As might be expected, bereavement caused by sudden death vs. after a prolonged illness resulted in greater social rhythms disruption and higher depression scores.

Given the repeated finding of a circadian rhythmicity to immune functioning (Levi et al., 1985, 1988; Knapp and Parnell, 1984; Ritchie et al., 1983) we find it plausible to suggest that bereavement-induced circadian changes may account for some of the variance in immune function in the course of bereavement.

Consideration of the aforementioned issues may improve the positioning of future studies in a manner that is consistent with the theoretical conceptualization of the etiology and mediation of psychosocial variables in physical illness.

ANIMAL STUDIES

Investigations of the association between psychosocial factors and physical illness in animals have been limited because of difficulties in creating in the laboratory conditions that simulate the human condition as well as difficulties in creating in animals the physical aspects of human diseases. However, animal models have contributed to the understanding of the conditions under which psychosocial variables may become risk factors in the development of illness and have been particularly useful in the identification of potential mechanisms by which psychosocial variables may modulate the risk of disease. Unlike human studies, the entire triad in the equation of psychosocial variables → immune alterations → development of disease has been examined in one combination in animal studies.

The current conceptualization of psychosocial factors in research is based largely upon Selye's view of stress as a consistent, specific response of the organism to phenomenologically different, nonspecific stimulation (Selye, 1950). Thus, stressors are defined in terms of their ability to evoke commonly recognized neuroendocrine responses, particularly the HPA system. While this definition of stress may constitute a tautologic error, it has proven to be most heuristic in terms of understanding somatic reactions to psychosocial factors.

Animal models have been particularly useful in investigating epidemiologically derived associations between illness and given risk factors, as well as in examining possible etiologic and mediating mechanisms for these associations. Most known risk factors in the development of illness, including cancer, have been identified in a two-step process: epidemiologic association between certain risk factors and an illness, followed by confirmation of these relationships under controlled conditions in animal models. A third step, that of examining possible mediating mechanisms, may require observations of the effects of a given factor on the cellular or biochemical level and may be accomplished in *in vivo* or *ex vivo* studies in humans or animals. For instance, epidemiologic findings of increased risk of cancer with high consumption of dietary fat have been further examined in animal studies.

Occasionally, results from animal studies fail to support epidemiologic associations, prompting reevaluation and reexamination of the original hypotheses. For instance, the epidemiologic finding of increased cancer risk with high consumption of dietary fat is becoming increasingly questionable because results from animal studies have pointed to inconsistencies, limitations, or qualifications of these associations.

Results from animal investigations have shown that psychosocial factors such as stress alter the structure and function of various somatic systems and the risk of occurrence of certain illnesses (Ader, 1964; Weiss, 1968, 1970, 1984). In animal research, stress is the most commonly investigated psychosocial risk factor in the development of illness. Previous studies have shown that the qualities of a given stressor and the choice of the disease model may modulate the nature and the direction of the somatic response. These interactions between disease and stress models have been difficult to predict and account to a large degree for the conflicting results in this area of research.

A hypothetical mediating mechanism for the adverse effects of stress on immunity and somatic function is via activation of the HPA axis and elevated levels of corticosterone (Murison et al., 1989). Psychological factors such as predictability and controllability of the stressor can reduce the adverse impact of physical stressors like electric shock and restraint on the gastrointestinal tract (Weiss, 1968, 1984) and the immune system (Mormede et al., 1988; Laudenslager et al., 1983).

Since stress has demonstrable adverse effects on the gastrointestinal tract (Weiss, 1970; Pare, 1976), we conducted a series of studies to examine the effect of chronic stress on the structure and morphology of the colon. Previous studies in humans have shown alterations in colonic morphology and function with stress and emotional states of hostility, anger, or dejection (Latimer, 1983). Stress is also considered to be a factor in the development and maintenance of disorders of colonic function such as irritable bowel syndrome (Whitehead et al., 1985), as well as colonic disorders of function and structure such as ulcerative colitis (Almy, 1980).

We examined the effects of a well-known stress model, "activity-stress" (A-S), that was previously shown to result in gastric ulcerations in rats on the morphology and structure of the colon and rectum. These results showed histopathologic and morphologic alterations in the colon with A-S treatment (Andrianopoulos and Wilcott, 1982; Andrianopoulos et al., 1987).

The A-S procedure is different from other stressors because it appears to be self-selected rather than imposed. In A-S, animals are housed individually in activity wheel cages (Wahman), and allowed to run spontaneously. Food is partially restricted, and made available for 1 h/d (Pare, 1976). Within 7 to 16 d of this regimen of spontaneous activity and partial food restriction, animals enter a disease phase characterized by increasing levels of physical activity, decreasing amounts of food consumption and body weight, gastrointestinal ulceration, and immunodeficiency (Pare et al., 1976; Hara and Ogawa, 1983). The disease phase appears to be a result of the unexplained increase in physical activity; thus, A-S is also known as "paradoxical stress".

In our studies, A-S treatment was related to decreased overall cellularity of the colonic mucosa, reduced number and altered architecture of mucos-secreting goblet cells, thinning of the mucosal layer, and chronic inflammation and infiltration of lymphocytes. These results showed that A-S treatment results in alterations of cellular activity and structure in the colonic mucosal layer. In addition, the A-S-related histopathologic alterations resembled those commonly found in the mucosae of patients with ulcerative colitis. Ulcerative colitis is an idiopathic, autoimmune, inflammatory disease of the colorectum of unknown etiology (Rachmilewitz, 1980). Psychosocial factors may exert an influence in the course of ulcerative colitis (Almy, 1980). In addition, the risk of occurrence of colorectal carcinoma is greater among patients with chronic ulcerative colitis than in the general population (Ballantyne, 1987).

Since A-S was shown to alter colonic structure and morphology and emotional factors have been related to increased cancer risk in epidemiologic studies (Persky et al., 1987; Shekelle et al., 1981), we also examined the effect of A-S on the development of colorectal carcinoma in rats.

We used the 1,2-dimethylhydrazine (DMH), colon carcinogenesis model to produce colorectal carcinoma. The DMH model is used most frequently in colorectal cancer research because it is specific to the colon and results in tumor formation that resembles the development as well as the anatomic distribution of human colorectal carcinoma, i.e., the formation of tumors is highest in the left colon, followed by the rectum and right colon (Rogers et al., 1985). We selected chemical carcinogenesis rather than innoculation or viral tumor systems because chemical carcinogenesis parallels more closely the development of human cancers (Justice, 1985). Over 63% of human cancers have been attributed to exposure to environmental pollutants and toxins. An additional reason for selecting the DMH model to investigate chronic stress as a risk factor in the development of colorectal carcinoma is the extensive use of this model in the identification of dietary and other risk factors in colorectal carcinogenesis (Nelson et al., 1987, 1988).

Since in the DMH model colorectal tumors develop approximately 4 months after a series of weekly injections with DMH and animals succumb to A-S treatment in 1 to 2 weeks, in the following experiment, A-S was adapted to an intermittent schedule (3.5 d of A-S alternating with 3.5 d of standard housing). These results showed that intermittent A-S was related to reduced DMH tumor induction in the rat colorectum (Andrianopoulos et al., 1988). Since the majority of animal studies have shown stress-related enhancement of tumorigenesis (Riley, 1981), our results of A-S-related suppression of colorectal carcinogenesis were examined further in a separate experiment. Additionally, since the properties of intermittent A-S as a stressor had not been previously described, it became questionable whether intermittent A-S was indeed stressful. Therefore, the effects of A-S treatment (non-intermittent) on the DMH-treated colon were further investigated in a separate short-term study.

In this study, rather than adapting the A-S procedure to the carcinogenesis model as done previously, the carcinogenesis model was adapted to the A-S procedure (Andrianopoulos et al., 1988). Animals were treated with A-S until they reached the disease phase, then given a single injection of DMH and sacrificed 24 h after injection. In this study, rather than carcinogenesis, the effect of A-S on DMH-induced nuclear damage and mucosal proliferation in the colorectum was assessed. Results showed that A-S treatment reduced DMH-induced nuclear damage and cellular aberrations in the colonic mucosa. These data supported the previous findings of suppressed DMH-induced carcinogenesis with intermittent A-S.

A-S treatment was also related to reduced cellular proliferation (cell multiplication) in the colon, as measured by the number of metaphases (Andrianopoulos et al., 1988). Rubio et al. (1989) have also demonstrated stress-related reduction of colonic mucosal cell proliferation. The finding of reduced colonic mucosal cell proliferation with A-S is consistent with the finding of A-S-related suppression of carcinogenesis. Colonic mucosal proliferation can be effected by substances or conditions that are known to exert an influence in the development of colorectal carcinoma. Substances known to suppress carcinogenesis (such as retinoids) also act on normal mucosa and invasive neoplastic cells by suppressing their proliferation (DiFronzo et al., 1987). Conversely, bile salts and certain kinds of fats that increase mucosal cell proliferation have also been found to promote DMH tumor induction (Newmark et al., 1984).

In order to identify the protective component of A-S in colorectal carcinogenesis, we examined the effect of spontaneous activity without food restriction on DMH tumor induction. Consistent with epidemiologic associations between physical activity and reduced colon cancer risk (Vena et al., 1985), results from this study reduced DMH-induced colorectal carcinogenesis in animals that were allowed spontaneous physical activity (Andrianopoulos et al., 1987). Therefore, the physical activity component of A-S per se was protective against carcinogenesis in this animal model. Thus, the effect of chronic stress separate from physical activity could not be ascertained from the aforementioned results.

The majority of previous stress and carcinogenesis studies have used viral or inoculation tumor systems, with the exception of dimethylbenzoanthracene (DMBA)-induced mammary tumorigenesis (Justice, 1985). Previous results have shown that frequently stress and carcinogenesis studies have utilized stressors that cause tissue damage or interfere with the nutritional status or body weight of the animal (Justice, 1985). As caloric restriction per se is consistently related to suppressed carcinogenesis (Tannenbaum, 1942; Kritchevsky and Klurfeld, 1987), the effect of stress independent from physical activity or caloric restriction had not been examined in a chemical carcinogenesis model.

In the following study, we examined the effects of three intermittent chronic stressors on the development of DMH-induced colorectal carcinoma. Animals were treated with oscillation stress (4 min, twice weekly), injection stress (2 i.m. injections of 0.2 ml isotonic saline twice weekly), and open-field stress (free exploration in children's wading pool, 4 min, twice weekly). Stress treatments were applied during DMH injections and were maintained throughout the experiment. Results showed mild enhancement of colorectal carcinogenesis in association with each of the three stressors that approached significance (Andrianopoulos et al., 1990). Colorectal carcinogenesis was significantly increased in the combined stress groups compared to controls. Final body weights did not differ between stress-treated and control groups. In order to assure that these three mild stressors evoked commonly recognized stress markers, plasma levels of epinephrine, norepinephrine, and dopamine and serum levels of corticosterone were also examined during the course of the experiment. Results showed significant increases in the levels of norepinephrine and dopamine in stressed groups compared to controls. These findings show that carcinogen-induced colorectal carcinogenesis is mildly enhanced when stress treatments are mild, intermittent, and exclusive of physical exercise and caloric restriction. However, DMH-induced colorectal carcinogenesis is suppressed when stressors result in alterations of physical activity, caloric restriction, and tissue damage.

To summarize, results from animal studies have shown that stress has an adverse impact on the cardiovascular, gastrointestinal, reproductive, and immune systems. Stress-activated central and peripheral mechanisms of immunomodulation are the hypothetical mediating mechanisms. Psychological factors modulate the impact of physical stressors on somatic function and structure and the immune system.

As depression is most consistently related to cancer risk in epidemiologic studies, the effect of various chronic stress treatments on the development of colorectal carcinoma was investigated in a series of studies. Chronic stress was related to structural and morphologic abnormalities in the rat colon. Chronic stress was also related to reduced colonic mucosal cell proliferation. When stress was inclusive of physical activity, colorectal carcinogenesis was suppressed. However, when stress was mild, intermittent, and exclusive of physical activity, it resulted in activation of commonly recognized neuroendocrine stress markers and increased DMH-induced colorectal carcinoma. These studies also show that the effects of chronic stress on colonic structure and morphology and on DMH-induced colorectal carcinogenesis are mediated at least in part by alterations in colonic mucosal cell proliferation. The proliferative rate may be another mechanism by which stress and other psychosocial factors can alter the risk of disease. Stress-activated increases in catecholamines may mediate the effects of stress on proliferative activity. Exogenously supplied catecholamines and centrally activated biogenic amines have been shown to modulate colonic mucosal cell proliferation by Tutton and Barkla (1987).

Therefore, the effects of stress on DMH-induced colorectal carcinogenesis are mediated at least in part by alterations in colonic mucosal cell proliferation. Further investigations are needed to examine the hypothetical equation: stress → catecholamines/biogenic amines → altered colonic mucosal proliferation → modulation of DMH-induced carcinogenesis.

CONCLUSIONS

The lack of a comprehensive definition of bereavement as normal process in reaction to loss of a valued and (or) loved object has made the definition of abnormal or delayed bereavement difficult.

1. There are sociocultural, religious, and ethnic differences in bereavement; however, societies that encourage open expression of grief through religion or rituals seem to enhance successful resolution of loss.
2. There are clusters of behavioral, emotional, and perhaps neuroendocrine features accompanying the major phases of bereavement from the early to late effects.
3. Susceptibility for illness may be specific to the given bereavement phase: increased risk for cardiovascular disorder associated with the early (acute) phases of bereavement and increased susceptibility to cancer or diabetes associated with the late effects of bereavement.
4. There is strong evidence of immunosuppression in bereavement-related depression; however, it is unclear whether the increased risk for illness in bereavement relates to immunosuppression.
5. Bereavement-related depression may be immunosuppressive per se. Bereavement-related depression may also alter the likelihood or frequency of occurrence of health behaviors like alcohol consumption, physical activity, sleep, and dietary factors which may in turn facilitate immunosuppression.
6. Although depression-related immunosuppression is a consistent finding in human studies, the notion of depression as a risk factor in the development of illness is not as widely supported. Nonetheless, there is sufficient homogeneity in epidemiologic studies to suggest an increased risk for physical and psychological morbidity in bereavement.
7. Psychotherapeutic intervention may be recommended to individuals with high-risk profiles for a complicated bereavement process. The high-risk profile may include: male gender, 55 years of age or older, 1 year or less post loss of spouse, previous history of depression or currently in depression, adverse impact of life stress (distress), and weak social and family support systems.
8. Medical screening, particularly for cardiovascular disorders, especially in the acute phases of bereavement, may also be recommended. Bereaved individuals should be particularly encouraged to follow national (ACS) guidelines for cancer screening.

REFERENCES

Albrecht J, Helderman JH, Schlesser MA, et al.: A controlled study of cellular immune function in affective disorders before and during somatic therapy. *Psychiatry Res.* 1985; 13:13–18.

Almy TP: Psychosocial aspects of chronic ulcerative colitis, in *Inflammatory Bowel Disease,* Kirsner JB and Shorter RG, Eds., Lea & Febiger, Philadelphia, 1980, pp. 44–54.

Andrianopoulos GD and Wilcott RC: Activity-stress induced pathology in the colon and rectum of the rat. *Physiol. Behav.* 1982; 28:191–193.

Andrianopoulos GD, Bombeck CT, and Nyhus LM: Influence of maturation of activity-stress related pathology in the rat colon. *Physiol. Behav.* 1986; 36:1105–1110.

Andrianopoulos GD, Nelson RL, Misumi A, et al.: Effect of activity stress on experimental rat colon carcinogenesis: early histopathologic changes and colon tumor induction. *Cancer Det. Prev.* 1988; 13:31–39.

Andrianopoulos GD, Nelson RL, Bombeck CT, et al.: The influence of physical activity in 1,2 dimethylhydrazine induced colon carcinogenesis in the rat. *Anticancer Res.* 1987; 7:49–52.

Andrianopoulos GD, Nelson RL, Barch DH, et al.: The effect of mild stress on DHM-induced colorectal cancer. *Cancer Det. Prev.* 1990; 14:577–581.

Andrianopoulos GD: Conceptual issues on the association between depression and cancer. *JAMA* 1990; 263:513.

Ballantyne G: Risk of colorectal cancer in patients with ulcerative colitis and Crohn's disease, in *Problems in Current Surgery. Controversies of Colon Cancer,* Nelson RL, Ed., Lippincott, Philadelphia, 1987, pp. 154–167.

Bartrop RW, Luckhurst E, Lazarus L, et al.: Depressed lymphocyte function after bereavement. *Lancet* 1977; 1:834–836.

Baker GHB and Brewerton DA: Rheumatoid arthritis: a psychiatric assessment. *Br. Med. J.* 1981; 282:2014.

Boccia MA, Reite M, Kaeningh K., et al.: Behavioral and autonomic responses to peer separation in Macaque monkey infants. *Dev. Biol.* 1988; 22(5):447–461.

Bowling A: Mortality after bereavement: a review of the literature on survival periods and factors affecting survival. *Soc. Sci. Med.* 1987; 24:117–124.

Bowling A and Benjamin B: Mortality after bereavement: a follow-up study of a sample of elderly widowed people. *Biol. Soc.* 1985; 2:197–203.

Bowlby J: Loss, sadness and depression, in *Attachment and Loss,* Hogarth Press, London, 1980.

Bistrian BR, Blackburn GL, Schrimshaw NS, et al.: Cellular immunity in semistarved states in hospitalized adults. *Am. J. Clin. Nutr.* 1975; 28:1145–1155.

Biesel WR, Elderman R, Nauss K, et al.: Single nutrient effects on immunologic functions. *JAMA* 1981; 245:53–58.

Berkman L: The relationship of social networks and social support to morbidity and mortality, in *Social Support and Health,* Cohen S and Syme SL, Eds., Academic Press, New York, 1988.

Calabrese JR, Kling MA, and Gold PW: Alterations in immunocompetence during stress, bereavement and depression: focus on neuroendocrine regulation. *Am. J. Psychiatry,* 1987; 144:1123–1134.

Calabrese JR, Skewrer RG, and Barna B: Depression, immunocompetence and prostaglandins of the E. series. *Psychiatr. Res.* 1986; 17:41–47.

Cappel R, Gregoire F, Thiry L, et al.: Antibody and cell mediated immunity to herpes simplex virus in psychotic depression. *J. Clin. Psychiatry* 1978; 39:266–268.

Chandra RK: Numerical and functional deficiency in T helper cells in protein energy malnutrition. *Clin. Exp. Immunol.* 1983; 51:126–132.

Clayton PJ, Hirjanic M, and Murphy GE: Mourning and depression: their similarities and differences. *Can. J. Psychiatry* 1974; 19:309–312.

Clayton PJ, Halikes JA, and Maurice WL: The depression of widowhood. *Br. J. Psychiatry* 1972; 120:71–78.

Clayton PJ: The sequelae and nonsequelae of conjugal bereavement. *Am. J. Psychiatry* 1979; 136:1530–1534.

Coe CL, Rosenberg LT, and Levine S: Effects of maternal separation on the complete system and antibody response in infant primates. *Int. J. Neurosci.* 1988; (40):289–302.

Cox, PR and Ford JR: The mortality of widows shortly after widowhood. *Lancet* 1964; 1:163–164.

DiFronzo G, Capelletti V, Miodini P, et al.: Role of cellular retinoic acid binding protein in patients with large bowel cancer. *Cancer Det. Prov.* 1987; 10:325–337.

Dorian BJ, Garfinkel PE, Brown G, et al.: Aberrations in lymphocyte subpopulations and functions during psychological stress. *Clin. Exp. Immunol.* 1980; 50:132–138.

Elhers CL, Track E, and Kupfer DJ: Social zeitgebers and biological rhythms: a unified approach to understanding the etiology of depression. *Arch. Gen. Psychiatry* 1988; 45:948–952.

Eisenbruch M: Cross cultural aspects of bereavement. I. A conceptual framework for comparative analysis. *Cult. Med. Psychiatry* 1984a; 8:283–309.

Eisenbruch MA: Cross cultural aspects of bereavement. II. Ethnic and cultural variation in the development of bereavement practices. *Cult. Med. Psychiatry* 1984b; 8:315–347.

Elliott GR and Eisdorfer C, Eds.: *Stress and Human Health: Analysis and Implications for Research*. Springer, New York, 1982.

Farmer ME, Locke BZ, Moscicki EK, et al.: Physical activity and depressive symptoms: the NHANES I epidemiologic follow up study. *Am. J. Epidemiol.* 1988; 128:1340–1351.

Flaherty JA, Frank E, Kupfer DJ, et al.: Social zeitgebers and bereavement, in New Research Abstract, Annu. Meet. American Psychiatric Association, Chicago, 1987.

Fox BH: Premorbid psychological factors as related to cancer incidence. *J. Behav. Med.* 1978; 1:45–133.

Fox BH: Psychosocial factors in the immune system and human cancer, in *Psychoneuroimmunology*, Ader R, Ed., Academic Press, New York, 1981, pp. 103–158.

Gold PW, Goodwin FK, and Chrousos GP: Clinical and biochemical manifestations of depression: relationship to neurobiology of stress. *N. Engl. J. Med.* 1988; 319:348–353.

Goodwin JS and Webb DR: Review: regulation of the immune response by prostaglandins. *Clin. Immunol. Immunopathol.* 1980; 15:106–122.

Goodwin JJ, Selinger DJ, Nessner RP, et al.: Effect of indomethacin in vivo on humoral and cell mediated immunity in humans. *Infect. Immunol.* 1978; 19:430–433.

Gore S: The effect of social support in moderating the health consequences of unemployment. *J. Health Soc. Behav.* 1983; 19:157–165.

Grant I, Patterson LT, and Yager J: Social supports in relation to physical health and symptoms in the elderly. *Am. J. Psychiatry* 1988; 145:1254–1258.

Grossarth-Maticek R, Bastiaans J, and Kanazin DT: Psychosocial factors as strong predictors of mortality from cancer, ischemic heart disease and stress: the Yugoslav prospective study. *J. Psychosom. Res.* 1983; 29:167–176.

Hara C and Ogawa N: Influence of maturation of ulcer development and immunodeficiency induced by activity—stress in rats. *Physiol. Behav.* 1983; 30:757–761.

Helsing KL, Szklo M, and Comstock EW: Mortality after bereavement. *Am. J. Publ. Health* 1981; 71:802–809.

Hofer MA: Relationships as regulators: a psychobiological perspective on bereavement. *Psychosom. Med.* 1984; 46:183–197.

Hofer MA and Weiner H: Psychological mechanisms for cardiac control by nutritional intake after early maternal separation in the young rat. *Psychosoc. Med.* 1975; 37:8–29.

Hofer MA: Studies of how early maternal separation produces behavioral change in young rats. *Psychosoc. Med.* 1975; 37:245–264.

Hwang D: Essential fatty acids and immune response. *IASEBJ* 1989; 3:2052–2061.

Irwin M, Daniels M, Bloom E, et al.: Life events, depression and natural killer cell function. *Psychopharmacol. Bull.* 1986a; 22:1093–1096.

Irwin M, Daniels M, Bloom E, et al.: Depression and change in T-cell subpopulations. *Psychosom. Med.* 1986b; 48:303–304.

Irwin M, Daniels M, Bloom E, et al.: Life events, depressive symptoms and immune function. *Am. J. Psychiatry* 1987a; 144:437–441.

Irwin MR, Daniels M, Bloom E, et al.: Impaired natural killer cell activity during bereavement. *Brain Behav. Immunol.* 1987b; 1:98–104.

Irwin M, Daniels M, and Weiner H: Immune and neuroendocrine changes during bereavement. *Psychiatry Clin. N. Am.* 1987c; 10:449–465.

Jacobs S and Ostfeld A: An epidemiologic review of the mortality of bereavement. *Psychosom. Med.* 1977; 39:344–357.

Jemmott JB and Locke SE: Psychosocial factors, immunologic mediation and human susceptibility to infectious diseases: how much do we know? *Psychol. Bull.* 1984; 95:78–108.

Jones DR, Goldblatt PO, and Leon DA: Bereavement and cancer: some data on deaths of spouses from the longitudinal study of Office of Population Censuses and Surveys. *Br. Med. J.* 1984; 289:461–464.

Justice A: A review of the effects of stress on laboratory animals: importance of time of stress application and type of tumor. *Psychol. Bull.* 1985; 98:108–138.

Kaprio J, Koskenvko M, and Rita HH: Mortality after bereavement: a prospective study of 96,647 widowed persons. *Am. J. Publ. Health* 1987; 77:283–287.

Keller SE, Ackerman SH, Schliefer ST, et al.: Effect of premature weaning on lymphocyte stimulation in the rat. *Psychosom. Med.* 1983; 45:75.

Kiecolt-Glazer JK, Garner W, Speicher C, et al.: Psychosocial modifiers of immunocompetence in medical students. *Psychosom. Med.* 1984; 46:7–14.

Kiecolt-Glazer JK, Fisher L, Ogrocki P, et al.: Marital quality, marital disruption and immune function. *Psychosom. Res.* 1987; 49:13.

Klerman GL and Izen JE: The effects of bereavement and grief on physical health and well being. *Adv. Psychosom. Med.* 1977; 9:66–104.

Knapp MS and Pownall R: Lymphocytes and rhythmic: Is this important? *Br. Med. J.* 1984; 28:1328.

Krauchi K and Wirt-Justice A: The four seasons: food intake frequency in seasonal affective order in the course of a year. *Psychiatr. Res.* 1988; 25:323–328.

Krauss AA and Lilienfield AM: Some epidemiological aspects of high mortality rate in the widowed group. *J. Chron. Dis.* 1959; 10:207.

Kritchovsky D and Klurfeld DM: Caloric effects in experimental mammary carcinogenesis. *Am. J. Nutr.* 1987; 45:236–242.

Kronfol Z, Silva J, Greden J, et al.: Impaired lymphocyte function in depressive illness. *Life Sci.* 1984; 33:242–247.

Kronfol Z, Nasrallah HA, Chapman S, et al.: Depression, cortisol metabolism and lymphocytopenia. *J. Affect. Dis.* 1985; 9:169–173.

Krupnick J and Horowitz MJ: Brief psychotherapy with vulnerable patients: an outcome assessment. *Psychiatry* 1985; 48:223–233.

Latimer PR: Colonic psychophysiology: implications for functional bowel disorders, in *Psychophysiology of the Gastrointestinal Tract,* Holzl R and Whitehead WW, Eds., Plenum Press, New York, 1983, pp. 263–265.

Laudenslager ML and Reite ML: Loss and separations: immunological consequences and health implications, in *Review of Personality and Social Psychology,* Shaver P, Ed., Sage, Beverly Hills, 1985, pp. 285–311.

Laudenslager ML, Ryan SM, Drugan RC, et al.: Coping and immunosuppression: inescapable but not escapable shock suppresses lymphocyte proliferation. *Science* 1983; 221:568–570.

Lazzarin A, Mella L, Trombini M, et al.: Immunological status in heroin addicts: effects on methadone maintenance treatment. *Drug Alcohol Depend.* 1984; 13:117–123.

Levav F, Canon C, Blum JP, et al.: Circadian rhythms in nine lymphocyte-related variables from periperal blood of healthy subjects. *J. Immunol.* 1985; 134:217–221.

Levav FA, Canon C, Youitous Y, et al.: Circadian rhythms in circulating T lymphocyte subtypes and plasma testosterone, total and free cortisol in five healthy men. *Exp. Immunol.* 1988; 71:329–335.

Lewis JK, McKinney WJ, Young LD, et al.: Mother-infant separation in Rhesus monkeys as a model of human depression. *Arch. Gen. Psychiatry* 1976; 133:699–705.

Lindemann E: Symptomatology and management of acute grief. *Am. J. Psychiatry* 1944; 101:141–148.

Linn MW, Linn BS, and Jensen J: Stressful events, disphoric mood and immune responsiveness. *Psychol. Rep.* 1984; 54:219–222.

Linn BL and Jensen J: Age and immune response to a surgical stress. *Arch. Surg.* 1983; 118:405–409.

Locke SE, Kraus L, Leserman J, et al.: Life change stress, psychiatric symptoms and natural killer cell activity. *Psychosom. Med.* 1984; 46:441–453.

Maddison DC and Viola A: The health of widows in the year following bereavement. *J. Psychosom. Res.* 1968; 12:296.

Melges FT and DeMaso DR: Grief resolution therapy: reliving, revising and revisiting. *Am. J. Psychother.* 1980; 34:51–61.

Miller LG, Goldstein G, Murphy M, et al.: Reversible alterations in immunoregulatory T cells in smoking. *Chest* 1982; 82:526–529.

Monjan AA and Collector MI: Stress-induced modulation of the immune response. *Science* 1977; 196:307–308.

Monk TH, Flaherty JA, Frank E, et al.: The social rhythm metric: an instrument to quantify the daily rhythm of life. *J. Nerv. Ment. Dis.* 1990; 178:120–126.

Mor V, McHorney C, and Sherwood S: Secondary morbidity among the recently bereaved. *Am. J. Psychiatry* 1986; 143:158–163.

Mormede P, Dantzer R, Michaud B, et al.: Influence of stressor predictability and behavioral control on lymphocyte reactivity, antibody responses and neuroendocrine activation in rats. *Physiol. Behav.* 1988; 43:577–583.

Moswon D, Marks I, Ramm L, et al.: Guided mourning for morbid grief: a controlled study. *Br. J. Psychiatry* 1981; 138:185–193.

Murison R, Overmier B, Hellhemmer DH, et al.: Hypothalamopituitary-adrenal manipulations and stress ulceration in rats. *Psychoneuroendocrinology* 1989; 12:331–339.

Nelson RL, Tanure JC, and Andrianopoulos GD: The effect of dietary milk and calcium on experimental colon carcinogenesis. *Dis. Colon Rectum* 1987; 30:947–949.

Nelson RL, Tanure JC, and Andrianopoulos GD: A comparison of dietary fish oil and corn oil in experimental colorectal carcinogenesis. *Nutr. Cancer* 1988; 11:215–220.

Newman HL, Wargovich MJ, and Bruce WR: Colon cancer and dietary fat, phosphate and calcium. A hypothesis. *JNCI* 1984; 72:1323–1325.

Osterweiss M, Solomon F, and Green M: *Bereavement: Responses, Consequences and Care.* National Academy Press, Washington, D.C., 1984.

Palmblad J, Petrini B, Wasserman J, et al.: Lymphocyte and granulocyte reactions during sleep deprivation. *Psychosom. Med.* 1979; 41:273–278.

Pare WP: Activity-stress ulcer in the rat: frequency and chronicity. *Physiol. Behav.* 1976; 16:699–704.

Parkes CM, Benjamin B, and Fitzgerald RG: Broken heart: a statistical study of increased mortality among widowers. *Br. Med. J.* 1969; 1:740–743.

Parkes CM and Brown PJ: Health after bereavement. *Psychosom. Med.* 1982; 34:449–461.

Parkes CM: Recent bereavement as a cause of mental illness. *Br. J. Psychiatry* 1984; 110:198–201.

Parks CM: Bereavement and mental illness. *Br. J. Med. Psychol.* 1965; 38:1–26.

Parks CM: *Bereavement: Studies of Grief in Adult Life.* International University Press, New York, 1972.

Parks CM: Bereavement counseling: does it work? *Br. Med. J.* 1980; 281:3–6.

Penn I: Malignancies associated with immunosuppressive or cytotoxic therapy. *Surgery* 1978; 83:492–502.

Penn I: The occurrence of cancer in immune deficiencies. *Curr. Probl. Cancer* 1982; 6:1–64.

Persky RW, Kempthorne-Rawson J, and Shekelle RB: Personality and risk of cancer: 20 year risk follow up of the Western Electric Study. *Psychosom. Med.* 1976; 49:435–449.

Rachmilewitz D: *Inflammatory Bowel Disease*, Vol. 3. Martinus Nijhoff, The Hague, 1980.

Raphael B and Middleton W: Current state of research in the field of bereavement. *Isr. J. Psychiatry Rel. Sci.* 1987; 24:5–21.

Rees WD and Lutkins SG: Mortality of bereavement. *Br. Med. J.* 1967; 4:13–16.

Reite M, Kaufman IC, Pandy JD, et al.: Depression in infant monkeys: physiological correlates. *Psychosom. Med.* 1974; 36:363–367.

Ritchie WS, Uswald I, Mickeam HS, et al.: Circadian variation of lymphocyte sub-population. *Br. Med. J.* 1983; 286:1773.

Rubio CA, Sveander M, and Duvander A: A model to evaluate acute and chronic stress in the colonic mucosa of rats. *Dis. Colon Rectum* 1989; 32:26–29.

Selye H: *Stress*. Acta Medical Publications, Montreal, 1950.

Schaefer C, Koyne JC, and Lazarus RS: The health related functions of social support. *J. Behav. Med.* 1981; 4:381–406.

Schleifer SJ, Keller SE, Meyerson AT, et al.: Lymphocyte function in major depressive disorder. *Arch. Gen. Psychiatry* 1984; 41:484–486.

Schleifer SJ, Keller SE, Bond RN, et al.: Major depressive disorder and immunity. *Arch. Gen. Psychiatry* 1989; 46:817.

Schleifer SJ, Keller SE, Camerino M, et al.: Suppression of lymphocyte stimulation following bereavement. *JAMA* 1983; 250:347–377.

Schleifer SJ, Keller SE, and Stein M: Stress effects on immunity. *Psychiatr. J. Univ. Ottawa* 1985; 10:125–133.

Schindler BA: Stress affective disorders and immune function. *Med. Clin. N. Am.* 1985; 69:585–597.

Schmale AH and Iker H: Hopelessness as a predictor of cervical cancer. *Soc. Sci. Med.* 1966a; 5:95–100.

Schmale A and Iker H: The psychological setting of uterine cervical cancer. *Ann. N.Y. Acad. Sci.* 1966b; 125:807–815.

Schuchter SR, Zisook S, Kirkorowiez C, et al.: The dexamethasone test in acute bereavement. *Am. J. Psychiatry* 1986; 143:879–881.

Shekelle RB, Raynor WJ, Ostfeld AM, et al.: Psychological depression and 17 year risk of death from cancer. *Psychosom. Med.* 1981; 43:117–125.

Smotherman WD, Hund LE, McGinnis LM, et al.: Mother-infant separation on group living Rhesus macaques. *Dev. Psychol.* 1979; 12:211–217.

Solomon F, Parron DL, and Dews PB, Eds.: Biobehavioral factors in sudden cardiac death, in *Summary of Institute of Medicine Conference*, Academy Press, Washington, D.C., 1982.

Solomon GF: Emotional and personality factors in the onset of and course of autoimmune disease, particularly rheumatoid arthritis, in *Psychoneuroimmunology*, Ader R, Ed., Academic Press, New York, 1981, pp. 259–280.

Stein M: A biopsychosocial approach to immune function and medical disorder. *Pediatr. Clin. N. Am.* 1981; 4:203–221.

Tannenbaum A: The genesis and growth of tumors. II. Effects of caloric restriction per se. *Cancer Res.* 1942; 2:460–467.

Tutton PJM and Barkla DH: Biogenic amines as regulators of the proliferative rate of normal and neoplastic intestinal epithelial cells. *Anticancer Res.* 1987; 7:1–12.

Vena JE, Graham S, Zielezney M, et al.: Life time occupational exercise and colon cancer. *Am. J. Epidemiol.* 1985; 122:357–365.

Watson RR, Eskelson C, and Hartman B: Severe alcohol abuse and cellular immune functions. *Ariz. Med.* 1984; 41:665–668.

Weiss JM: Somatic effects of predictable and unpredictable shock. *Psychosom. Med.* 1970; 32:397–408.

Weiss JM: Behavioral and psychological influences on gastrointestinal pathology: experimental techniques and findings. *Handb. Behav. Med.* 1984; 19:74–221.

Weiss JM: Effects of coping responses on stress. *J. Comp. Physiol. Psychol.* 1968; 65:251–260.

Werner RA: Order and disorder in human circadian rhythmicity: possible relations to mental disorders, in *Biological Rhythms and Mental Disorders,* Kupfer DJ, Monk TH, and Barchus JD, Eds., Springer-Verlag, New York, 1979, pp. 238–324.

Young M, Benjamin B, and Wallis C: The mortality of widowers. *Lancet* 1963; 2:454 456.

Zisook S, DeVaul RA, and Click MA: Measuring symptoms of grief and bereavement. *Am. J. Psychiatry* 1982; 139:1590–1593.

Zonderman AB, Costa PT, and McCrae RR: Depression of risk factor for cancer morbidity and mortality in a nationally representative sample. *JAMA* 1989; 262:1191–1195.

Depressive Disorders and Immunity

Steven J. Schleifer
and
Steven E. Keller
University of Medicine and Dentistry of New Jersey
New Jersey Medical School
Department of Psychiatry
Newark, New Jersey

INTRODUCTION

The investigation of immunity in relation to affective disorders was suggested by the neuroendocrine abnormalities in patients with depressive disorders as well as by the accumulating evidence linking both the central nervous system (CNS) and stressful life experience with immune regulation. Much of this research is reviewed elsewhere in this volume. In addition, there is evidence that depressive disorders are associated with increased medical mortality (Avery and Winokur, 1976; Murphy et al., 1987), which may be related to alterations in immune and other physiologic systems. This chapter will primarily review the authors' studies on depression and immune processes.

Research serving as the basis for our studies of immunity in depressed persons included early observations from our laboratory that symmetrical lesions placed in the anterior hypothalamus result in decreased humoral and cell-mediated immune responses (reviewed in Stein et al., 1987) as well as decreased lymphocyte proliferative activity (Keller et al., 1981). Another line of research demonstrated that major stressful life experiences that routinely elicit emotional distress can alter immune processes. Animal studies demonstrated that a variety of stressors can alter B- and T-cell processes (Ader, 1981; Monjan and Collector, 1977; Keller et al., 1981; Laudenslager and Ryan, 1983), with effects related to the nature, duration, and intensity of the stressor as well as to specific characteristics and responses of the stressed organism (e.g., Monjan and Collector, 1977; Keller et al., 1981). Research on life stress and immunity in man identified several conditions in which altered immunity occurs, including conjugal bereavement (Bartrop et al., 1977; Schleifer et al., 1983; Irwin et al., 1987), sleep deprivation (Palmblad et al., 1979), and examination stress (Kiecolt-Glaser et al., 1984; Dorian et al., 1982).

Of particular relevance to the hypothesis that depression is associated with altered immunity was the evidence, first presented by Bartrop et al. (1977), that the death of a spouse, which commonly elicits symptoms similar to major depressive disorder, is associated with decreased lymphocyte function. This association is of additional interest since conjugal bereavement is also associated with increased medical mortality (Helsing et al., 1981). We investigated the effect of bereavement on immunity in a prospective study of spouses of women with advanced breast carcinoma (Schleifer et al., 1983). Several immune system measures were obtained in 15 men before and after the death of their wives. We found that the number of circulating lymphocytes and of T- and B-cells were not significantly altered following bereavement; however, lymphocyte proliferative responses to the mitogens phytohemagglutinin (PHA), concanavalin A (ConA), and pokeweed mitogen (PWM) were significantly lower during the first 2 months post-bereavement compared with pre-bereavement responses. By the end of the post-bereavement year, mitogen responses had returned to pre-bereavement levels for the majority, but not all, of the subjects. Several of the bereaved, including the youngest members of the sample, showed delayed decrements in lymphocyte activity that persisted for at least 1 year. This study suggested that major events such as the death of a spouse induce a generalized change in the functional capacity of the lymphocyte, with differing effects for different subgroups of subjects.

MAJOR DEPRESSIVE DISORDER AND IMMUNITY

We hypothesized that changes in affective state, including the development of depression, could be involved in the effects of bereavement and other stressors on immunity. Bereavement is regularly associated with marked changes in mood state and with neurovegetative symptoms that often suggest the presence of a clinical affective disorder (Clayton et al., 1972; Parkes, 1972). Moreover, depression, like bereavement, has been reported to be associated with increased medical mortality (Odegaard, 1952; Avery and

Winokur, 1976; Murphy et al., 1987) and with immune-related disorders (Shekelle et al., 1982; Odegaard, 1952; Cappel et al., 1978). In addition, neuroendocrine functions are altered in many depressed patients (Sachar et al., 1980; Carroll et al., 1976; Whybrow and Prange, 1981), and neurohormones and hypothalamic processes have been shown to modulate immune function (reviewed in Stein et al., 1981).

In our initial studies of depression and immunity, we found significantly decreased mitogen responses in drug-free hospitalized patients with major depressive disorders (MDD) compared with healthy age- and sex-matched controls (Schleifer et al., 1984) but no differences between ambulatory MDD patients and controls (Schleifer et al., 1985). Hospitalized patients with schizophrenia also showed no immunologic changes (Schleifer et al., 1985). These observations suggested a specific link between MDD and immunity, with the psychoimmunologic effects apparently restricted to a subgroup of patients. Characteristics that distinguished the hospitalized from the ambulatory sample included, aside from hospitalization status, their being more severely depressed, as well as older and more predominantly male. These factors were investigated in a subsequent study of 91 hospitalized and ambulatory unipolar patients with MDD and 91 matched controls (Schleifer et al., 1989a). To further elucidate the nature of the immune effects, the study utilized an expanded battery of immune measures. As in our other studies, all subjects were free of acute and chronic medical disorders associated with alterations in immunity and were not taking drugs known to affect immune function. They had not been treated with antidepressants for at least the preceding 3 months.

There were no significant overall differences between the entire sample of 91 depressed patients and their controls for any of the immune measures. Significant patient-control differences were revealed, however, when age, sex, severity of depression, and hospitalization were considered. Most striking was that the relationship between age and lymphocyte function for the controls and for the patients was significantly different for each of the mitogens (ConA, PHA, and PWM). A similar difference between patients and controls in age-immune relationship was found for the number of T-helper (CD4+) cells. Specifically, the data suggested that, with increasing age in the middle and later years, patients with major depressive disorder have specific concurrent deficits in the number of T4 cells and in lymphocyte proliferative activity in response to mitogen challenge. In contrast, depressed young adults appeared to have increased T4 cells and lymphocyte activity. An additional independent finding was that severity of depressive symptoms, as measured by the Hamilton Depression Scale (Hamilton, 1967), was associated with lower mitogen responses independent of age. An effect of the Hamilton Depression Scale score on the number of T4 cells was not seen; however, there was a contribution of hospitalization status, with inpatients having significantly fewer T4 cells than less severely depressed outpatients. No significant depression-related differences were found for other aspects of immunity, including numbers of suppressor cells and natural killer cell activity.

The findings of our studies with depressed as well as bereaved samples demonstrate the need to consider a range of biological, experiential, and psychologic variables in psychoimmunologic processes. They suggest that there are several dimensions of psychoimmunologic effects, for example, age-dependent and -independent, and that these effects are linked to changes in specific aspects of the immune system (e.g., distribution of lymphocyte subsets, lymphocyte proliferative response). The clarification of these effects requires a multidimensional approach.

Our findings with depressed patients suggest an association between the diagnostic entity of depression and an age-dependent change in mitogen activity that may result from a quantitative or qualitative change in the T-helper cell subpopulation, and a second "severity" effect that may reflect an association between level of distress/symptomatology and mitogen responsivity. The age-related changes in mitogen responsivity may be of considerable importance in relation to the understanding of both affective and immunologic processes. Two types of mechanisms may be involved. First, the age-related effects on immunity in depressed patients, and possibly in states such as bereavement, may represent an interaction between processes associated with depression and those associated with aging. Thus, the suppressed mitogen reactivity in older depressed patients may be due to effects of factors associated with depression (e.g., neuroendocrine) on an immune system that is at the limits of its adaptive capacity due to normal immunosenescent processes (Weksler and Hutteroth, 1974; Weksler, 1983). The net effect of the same depression-related factors in younger patients, impacting upon an immune system with greater residual and adaptive capacity, may result in either little change or an enhanced response. It is of note that in preliminary studies of children with major depressive disorder, we found elevated lymphocyte proliferative activity in depressed compared with nondepressed 8 to 12 year olds (Bartlett et al., 1989a).

The second category of age-related mechanisms to be considered relates to the heterogeneity of the depressive disorders found in younger and older patients. Differential familial loading in older and younger onset depression (Weissman et al., 1984), for example, suggests biologically distinct disorders. Early onset depressive disorders may have biological features that contribute to elevated T4 cells and lymphocyte activity, while suppressive factors may be found in older patients, including subjects with late onset disorders. The possibility of genetic factors linking depression and immune expression is of considerable interest and would be consistent with the immune changes in depression being trait characteristics. Such immune trait changes could be demonstrable both prior to illness onset and following clinical remission.

Research in this area is important but difficult due to limitations of case-finding prior to illness onset and the difficulty in obtaining an adequate drug-free patient sample in complete remission.

Our findings of an association between severity of depression and mitogen response, independent of age, suggests that at least some component of the mitogen changes in depression are state related. The severity-related changes are also consistent with an association between affective *symptomatology* and altered immunity, an effect that may be independent of syndromal status. Affective distress and related symptomatology could thus account for the observations of altered immunity seen both in depressive disorders and in subsyndromal states of affective disturbance such as following bereavement. We have begun to address these issues in several studies.

ROLE OF AFFECTIVE STATES IN STRESS-RELATED IMMUNE CHANGES

In an ongoing study, affective states and immune function have been investigated in family members of trauma victims within 1 week of the traumatic episode. This model was designed to determine immune effects immediately following acute unanticipated major life stress in man, a paradigm not previously investigated. Preliminary analyses have been conducted for 20 otherwise healthy family members studied within 7 d of the traumatic episode (12 motor vehicle accident, 3 gunshot, and 5 other) concurrent with 20 healthy age- and sex-matched controls (Schleifer et al., 1989b). No significant overall differences were found between family members and control subjects on the immune measures. When levels of stress and depression were considered in regression analyses, however, significant contributions were found in relation to mitogen response. Extent of depressive symptoms, but not the presence of syndromal criteria for depression, were associated with decreased mitogen responsivity. Anxiety, in contrast, appeared to be associated with increased mitogen response. These observations support the association of depressive symptoms with decreased mitogen responsivity, an association that may be independent of the syndrome of major depressive disorder and found across the age range.

In another study, we have been investigating the psychoimmunology of otherwise healthy adolescents living in an inner city. Initial analyses of psychological, social, and immunologic data for more than 100 adolescents revealed that depressive symptoms were associated with decreased mitogen responses. We also found that adolescents reporting more aggressive behaviors had relatively increased lymphocyte mitogen responses (Bartlett et al., 1989b). This study provides additional support for an association of depressive affects with decreased mitogenic activity and further evidence that other affective states may be associated with differing immune effects.

DISCUSSION

Taken together, the above studies begin to suggest a pattern of psychoimmunologic relationships related to the nature and intensity of stressful conditions, biological characteristics of the individual, and affective states. One hypothesis suggested by our studies is that affective states represent a common pathway for many psychoimmunologic effects, whether associated with psychiatric disorders or life stress. It also appears that multiple components of the immune system are sensitive to psychoimmunologic processes involving a number of disparate mechanisms. This has been demonstrated most clearly using animal models. We and others (Keller et al., 1983; Blecha et al., 1982) have shown distinct mechanisms of stress-induced immune alterations in rodents. We found, for example, that stress-induced suppression of the number of circulating lymphocytes is adrenal dependent and effects on peripheral blood lymphocyte proliferation can occur independent of adrenal activity (Keller et al., 1983). Consequently, psychological states may be associated with differential activation of physiologic systems (e.g., adrenal vs. opioid; e.g., Shavit et al., 1986) and induce changes in specific components of the immune system.

In this context, the role of adrenal hormones in the psychoimmunology of depression, while of considerable interest, remains uncertain. The rationale for a primary adrenal mechanism is compelling: alterations in the hypothalamic-pituitary-adrenal (HPA) axis have been demonstrated consistently in depressed patients (Sachar et al., 1979; Stokes et al., 1984; Kocsis et al., 1985; Carroll et al., 1976) and appear to be age related (Asnis et al., 1981; Kocsis et al., 1985; Weiner et al., 1987). Corticosteroids suppress lymphocyte proliferation (Cupps and Fauci, 1982) and alter specifically the distribution of T-helper lymphocytes (Cupps et al., 1984). In our studies of major depressive disorder and immunity, plasma cortisol was significantly elevated in the morning blood samples used for the immune assays (Schleifer et al., 1989a). However, the relationships between age, severity, and the immune variables were not materially changed when cortisol level was included in the regression models. While a single measure of cortisol is only a very rough index of HPA axis function, the findings do not support a major role for cortisol in the psychoimmunology of major depressive disorder. Other pituitary and nonpituitary hormones that can influence the immune system are altered in depression and should also be considered (reviewed in Stein et al., 1987).

The complexity and variability of immune systems and of immunologic assays dictate a need for caution in the design and interpretation of psychoimmunologic studies. Ultimately, clarification of the interactions among brain, behavior, and immunity will be facilitated by the identification of more fundamental immune ''targets'' of the CNS and behavioral influences. For example, the inhibition of mitogen-induced T-cell proliferation may result from the abrogation of interleukin-2 secretion (Gillis et al., 1979; Grabstein et al., 1986), reduction of IL-2 receptors (Reed et al., 1986), or altered accessory cell functions (Strickland et al., 1986).

In conclusion, the relationship between depressive states and immune processes is not simple; however, consistent patterns of associations are emerging and provide a foundation for further systematic research.

REFERENCES

Ader R: *Psychoneuroimmunology*. Academic Press, New York, 1981.

Asnis GM, Sachar EJ, Halbreich V, Nathan RS, Novacenko H, and Ostrow LC: Cortisol secretion in relation to age in major depression. *Psychosom. Med.* 1981; 43:235–242.

Avery D and Winokur G: Mortality in depressed patients treated with electroconvulsive therapy and antidepressants. *Arch. Gen. Psychiatry* 1976; 33:1029–1037.

Bartlett JA, Schleifer SJ, and Keller SE: Immune changes in prepubescent major depressive disorder. In Annu. Meet. Society of Biological Psychiatry, San Francisco, May, 1989a (Abstr.).

Bartlett JA, Schleifer SJ, Keller SE, and Cranshaw ML: Immune change associated with aggression and depression. In 36th Annu. Meet. American Academy of Child and Adolescent Psychiatry, New York, 1989b (Abstr.).

Bartrop RW, Lazarus L, Luckherst E, and Kiloh LH: Depressed lymphocyte function after bereavement. *Lancet* 1977; 1:834.

Blecha F, Kelley KW, and Satterlee DG: Adrenal involvement in the expression of delayed-type hypersensitivity to SRBC and contact sensitivity to DNFB in stressed mice (41339). *Proc. Soc. Exp. Biol. Med.* 1982; 169:247–252.

Cappel R, Gregoire F, Thiry L, and Sprecher S: Antibody and cell mediated immunity to herpes simplex virus in psychotic depression. *J. Clin. Psychiatry* 1978; 39:266–268.

Carroll BJ, Curtis GC, and Mendels J: Neuroendocrine regulation in depression. II. Discrimination of depressed from nondepressed patients. *Arch. Gen. Psychiatry* 1976; 33:1051–1058.

Clayton PJ, Halikes JA, and Maurice WL: The depression of widowhood. *Br. J. Psychiatry* 1972; 120:71.

Cupps TR, Edgar LC, Thomas CA, and Fauci AS: Multiple mechanisms of B cell immunoregulation in man after administration of in vivo corticosteroids. *J. Immunol.* 1984; 132:170–175.

Cupps TR and Fauci AS: Corticosteroid-mediated immunoregulation in man. *Immunol. Rev.* 1982; 65:134–155.

Dorian B, Garfinkel G, Brown G, Shore A, Gladman D, and Keystone E: Aberrations in lymphocyte subpopulations and function during psychological stress. *Clin. Exp. Immunol.* 1982; 50:132–138.

Gillis S, Crabtree GR, and Smith KA: Glucocorticoid-induced inhibition of T cell growth factor production. I. The effect on mitogen-induced lymphocyte proliferation. *J. Immunol.* 1979; 123:1624.

Grabstein K, Dower S, Gillis S, Urdal, and Larsen A: Expression of interleukin 2 interferon and the IL 2 receptor by human peripheral blood lymphocytes. *J. Immunol.* 1986; 136:4503–4508.

Hamilton M: Development of a rating scale for primary depressive illness. *Br. J. Soc. Clin. Psychol.* 1967; 6:278–296.

Helsing KJ, Szklo M, and Comstock GW: Factors associated with mortality after widowhood. *Am. J. Publ. Health* 1981; 71:802.

Ilfeld FW Jr: Further validation of a psychiatric symptom index in a normal population. *Psychol. Rep.* 1976; 39:1215–1228.

Irwin M, Daniels M, Bloom ET, Smith TL, and Weiner H: Life events, depressive symptoms, and immune function. *Am. J. Psychiatry* 1987; 144:437–441.

Keller SE, Weiss JM, Schleifer SJ, Miller E, and Stein M: Stress induced suppression of lymphocyte stimulation in adrenalectomized rats. *Science* 1983; 221:1301–1304.

Keller SE, Schleifer SJ, Liotta AS, Bond RN, Farhoody N, and Stein M: Stress-induced alterations of immunity in hypophysectomized rats. *Proc. Natl. Acad. Sci. U.S.A.* 1988; 85:92–97.

Keller SE, Weiss JM, Schleifer SJ, Miller E, and Stein M: Suppression of immunity by stress: effect of a graded series of stressors on lymphocyte stimulation in the rat. *Science* 1981; 213:1397–1400.

Kiecolt-Glaser JK, Glaser R, Strain EC, Stout JC, Tarr KL, Holliday J, and Speicher C: Modulation of cellular immunity in medical students. *J. Behav. Med.* 1986; 9:5–21.

Kiecolt-Glaser JK, Garner W, Speicher C, Penn GM, Holliday J, and Glaser R: Psychosocial modifiers of immunocompetence in medical students. *Psychosom. Med.* 1984; 46:7–14.

Kocsis JH, Davis JM, Katz MM, et al: Depressive behavior and hyperactive adrenocortical function. *Am. J. Psychiatry* 1985; 142:1291–1298.

Kronfol Z, Silva J Jr, Greden J. et al: Impaired lymphocyte function in depressive illness. *Life Sci.* 1983; 33:241–247.

Laudenslager ML and Ryan SM: Coping and immunosuppression: inescapable but not escapable shock suppresses lymphocyte proliferation. *Science* 1983; 221:568.

Linn BS and Jensen JJ: Age and immune response to a surgical stress. *Arch. Surg.* 1983; 118:405–409.

Monjan AA and Collector MI: Stress-induced modulation of the immune response. *Science* 1977; 196:307.

Murphy JM, Monson RR, Olivier DC, Sobol AM, and Leighton AH: Affective disorders and mortality. *Arch. Gen. Psychiatry* 1987; 44:473–480.

Odegaard O: The excess mortality of the insane. *Acta Psychiatr. Scand.* 1952; 27:353–367.

Palmblad J, Petrini B, Wasserman J, and Ackerstedt T: Lymphocyte and granulocyte reactions during sleep deprivation. *Psychosom. Med.* 1979; 41:273–278.

Parkes CM: *Bereavement: Studies of Grief in Adult Life.* International University Press, New York (1972).

Reed JC, Abibi AH, Alpers JD, Hoover RG, Ross RJ, and Nowell PC: Effect of cyclosporin A and dexamethasone on interleukin 2 receptor gene expression. *J. Immunol.* 1986; 137:150–154.

Sachar EJ, Asnis G, Halbreich V et al: Recent studies in the neuroendocrinology of major depressive disorders. *Psychiatr. Clin. N. Am.* 1980; 3:313–326.

Sachar EJ, Hellman L, Roffwarg HP, Halpern FS, Fukushima DK, and Gallagher TF: Disrupted 24-hour patterns of cortisol secretion in psychotic depression. *Arch. Gen. Psychiatry* 1973; 134:493–501.

Schleifer SJ, Keller SE, Bond RN, Cohen J, and Stein M: Major depressive disorder and immunity: role of age, sex, severity, and hospitalization. *Arch. Gen. Psychiatry* 1989a; 46:81–87.

Schleifer SJ, Keller SE, Siris SG, Davis KL, and Stein M: Depression and immunity. Lymphocyte function in ambulatory depressed, hospitalized schizophrenic, and herniorrhaphy patients. *Arch. Gen. Psychiatry* 1985; 42:129.

Schleifer SJ, Keller SE, Scott BJ, Cottrol CH, and Vallente TJ: Familial traumatic injury and immunity. In New Research, American Psychiatric Association Annual Meeting, San Francisco, May, 1989b (Abstr.).

Schleifer SJ, Keller SE, Camerino M, Thornton JC, and Stein M: Suppression of lymphocyte stimulation following bereavement. *JAMA* 1983; 250:374.

Schleifer SJ, Keller SE, Meyerson AT, Raskin MJ, Davis KL, and Stein M: Lymphocyte function in major depressive disorder. *Arch. Gen. Psychiatry* 1984; 41:484–486.

Shavit Y, De Paulis A, Martin FC, Terman GW, Pechnick RN, Zane CJ, Gale RP, and Liebeskind JC: Involvement of brain opiate receptors in the immune-suppressive effect of morphine. *Proc. Natl. Acad. Sci. U.S.A.* 1986; 83:7114–7117.

Shekelle RB, Raynor WJ, Ostfeld AM, Garron D, Bieliauskas L, Liv S, Maliza C, and Paul O: Psychological depression and 17 year risk of death from cancer. *Psychosom. Med.* 1982; 43:1017–1022.

Stein M, Schleifer S, and Keller S: Hypothalamic influences on immune responses. In *Psychoneuroimmunology*. Ader R, Ed. Academic Press, New York (1981).

Stein M, Schleifer S, and Keller S: Psychoimmunology in clinical psychiatry. In *Annual Review of Psychiatry*. Vol. 6. American Psychiatric Association, Washington, D.C. (1987) pp. 210–234.

Stokes PE, Stoll PM, Koslow SH et al: Pretreatment DST and hypothalamic-pituitary-adrenocortical function in depressed patients and comparison groups: a multicenter study. *Arch. Gen. Psychiatry* 1984; 41:257–266.

Strickland RW, Wahl LM, and Finbloom DS: Corticosteroids enhance the binding of recombinant interferon to cultured human monocytes. *J. Immunol.* 1986; 137:1577–1580.

Weiner MF, Davis BM, Mohs RC, and Davis KL: Influence of age and relative weight on cortisol suppression in normal subjects. *Am. J. Psychiatry* 1987; 144:646–649.

Weissman M, Wickramarative P, Merikangas K et al: Onset of major depression in early adulthood: increased familial loading and specificity. *Arch. Gen. Psychiatry* 1984; 41:1136–1143.

Weksler ME and Hutteroth TH: Impaired lymphocyte function in aged humans. *J. Clin. Invest.* 1974; 53:99–104.

Weksler ME: The thymus gland and aging. *Ann. Intern. Med.* 1983; 98:105–107.

Whybrow PC and Prange AJ: A hypothesis of thyroid catecholamine receptor interaction. *Arch. Gen. Psychiatry* 1981; 38:106–113.

Stress, Depression and Immunity: Research Findings and Clinical Implications

Diana O. Perkins, Jane Leserman, John H. Gilmore,
John M. Petitto, and Dwight L. Evans,
Department of Psychiatry
University of North Carolina School of Medicine
Chapel Hill, N.C.
and
Department of Medicine
University of North Carolina School of Medicine
Chapel Hill, N.C.

INTRODUCTION

Popular enthusiasm for the idea that depression and stressful life events may impact adversely on an individual's physical health is to some extent supported by recent research findings. Technical advances in immunology and psychiatric phenomenology have paved the way for research designed to determine the existence and define the nature of such relationships. A growing body of evidence indicates that depressive illness and stressful life events are associated with (1) alterations in immune system function and (2) alterations in the neuroendocrine system. In addition, there is substantial evidence that the neuroendocrine and immune systems have bidirectional regulatory inter-actions. These converging lines of evidence suggest an intriguing biological causal model for depression and/or stress-related influences on the development or prognosis of a physical illness. In this model, environmental factors (such as stressful life events) or biological factors that may result in psychiatric illness or mood alterations (such as anxiety or depression) may result in endocrine system dysregulation. The endocrine system changes may mediate immune system alterations that then could impact on the clinical prognosis and/or development of a physical disease (Evans et al., 1990).

In this chapter, we review studies that investigate depression and stress-related changes in the immune and neuroendocrine systems, and explore the biological mechanism that could link these systems. We then review the evidence that depression and stress are associated with the development and/or progression of physical illness, using the example of cancer. In addition, we discuss the many methodological problems inherent in the study of these relationships, and explore the research implications of the proposed psycho-neuroendocrine-immune (PNEI) causal model.

DEPRESSION, STRESS, AND IMMUNE SYSTEM RELATIONSHIPS

Immune system function can be assessed in a number of ways. Frequently, blastogenesis, that is, stimulation of lymphocytes by a number of mitogens, has been used to assess cell-mediated immune system function. In addition, researchers have measured the number, proportion, and activity of various immune system cell subpopulations, (e.g., T-cell, B-cell, and natural killer [NK] cell) to indicate immune system status.

Depression and Immunity

Several studies have found that patients hospitalized for a major depressive illness have reduced lymphocyte function, as measured by mitogen stimulation. Kronfol et al. (1983) compared lymphocyte mitogen response in major depressed psychiatric inpatients with nondepressed normal controls, and found reduced lymphocyte function in the hospitalized depressed patients. These findings have been confirmed by others (Schleifer et al., 1984, 1985). Depression-associated alterations in immune system function may be state related; Cappel et al. (1978) found that lymphocyte response to mitogens increased in patients with psychotic major depressions when their depressive illness went into remission.

Immune system alterations may primarily be associated with severe depressions. In a recent study, Schleifer et al. (1989) found that lymphocyte response to mitogens was significantly lower in patients with higher scores on the Hamilton Depression Rating Scale (Hamilton, 1960) (and thus more severe depressive illness). Older age was also associated with lower mitogen response in this study. Schleifer et al. (1985) found no differences in lymphocyte response to mitogens between normal controls and psychiatric outpatients with major depression. Albrecht et al. (1985) reported similar findings for depressed psychiatric outpatients. Psychiatric outpatients presumably have, in general, less severe illness than inpatients. Thus, lower lymphocyte response to mitogens has been associated with older age and more severe depressive illness. As discussed in the next section, *Depression and Neuroendocrine System Function,* older age and more severe depression are also associated with increased likelihood of altered neuroendocrine system function (Evans et al., 1983; Evans and Nemeroff, 1987; see the latter for a review), consistent with the notion that the neuroendocrine system may mediate these immune system changes.

Recent studies also suggest that alterations in NK cell number and activity, and in B-cell and T-cell subpopulations may occur in patients with major depression. In a pilot study, we found reduced numbers of NK cells in hospitalized major depressed patients compared with psychiatric control subjects with diagnoses other than major depression (Evans et al., 1988b). Similarly, total lymphocyte number and lymphocytes as a percent of white blood cells were also reduced in the major depressed patients compared with the controls. However, no significant correlation was found between severity of depression (score on the Hamilton Depression Rating Scale [Hamilton, 1960]) or the Carroll Self Rating Scale for Depression (Carroll et al., 1981) and NK cell number. NK cell activity may be reduced in patients with major depression; Irwin et al. (1987a) reported reduced NK cell activity in psychiatric inpatients with major depression compared to matched normal controls. In this study, severity of depression was not correlated with NK cell activity. No studies have simultaneously assessed NK cell number and activity in depressed patients. Our research group is currently conducting such studies, which we hope will further our understanding of the nature and possible physiological significance of depression-related changes in cellular immunity.

Studies of T-cell subpopulations in patients with major depression have yielded varied results. Syvalahti et al. (1985) reported an increased ratio of T-helper cells to T-suppressor cells, and a decreased percentage of suppressor-cytotoxic T-cells in patients with major depression when compared with non-depressed control subjects. However, others have not found differences in numbers of helper cells or suppressor cells in depressed patients (Wahlin et al., 1984; Evans et al., 1989). Schleifer et al. (1989) did note increased T-helper cell lymphocytes in older control patients, but not in the older depressed patients. Differences in subtypes of depressive disorder, age of subjects, and severity of depressive illness may explain the discrepancies between the reported studies.

Stress and Immunity

Ongoing stressful life events, including bereavement, divorce/separation, academic stress, and unemployment have been shown to impact on immune system function. We have previously reviewed this area (Evans et al., 1989), and we will summarize here the major studies conducted to date. Altered cellular immunity has been found in bereaved individuals. Bartrop et al. (1977) observed that recently widowed women exhibited decreased lymphoprolif-erative response to mitogens compared to matched community controls. Sim-ilarly, Schleifer et al. (1983) reported reduced lymphocyte response to mi-togens in men 2 months after the death of their spouse, compared to their pre-bereavement mitogen response. NK cell activity has also been found to be reduced in recently bereaved women compared with matched controls (Irwin et al., 1987b, 1988a).

Divorce and marital separation may also affect the immune system. Kie-colt-Glaser et al. (1987) found separated or divorced women to have a lower lymphoproliferative response to mitogens, lower percentage of NK cells, and higher antibody titers to Epstein-Barr virus as compared to demographically matched married women. Poorer immune function was associated with shorter time since divorce or separation, and greater attachment to the ex-spouse.

The stress of academic examination has been associated with altered immunity in several studies. Dorian et al. (1982) found resident physicians to have a decreased mitogen response immediately prior to a competitive examination and an increased mitogen response 2 weeks following the exam, compared to matched physician controls. These findings have been confirmed in more recent studies. Medical students showed a decrease in several pa-rameters of immunity on the day of an exam compared with values 1 month prior to exam (Kiecolt-Glaser et al., 1984a, 1986; Glaser et al., 1985). De-creases were found in NK cell activity, the percentage of helper/inducer T-lymphocytes, the helper/suppressor cell ratio, and lymphocyte mitogen stim-ulation response. In an earlier study, Jemmott (1981) found that salivary immunoglobulin A levels were significantly lower for dental students during their exam period compared with prior levels.

Arnetz et al. (1987) have examined the immunological impact of the stress of unemployment. They compared unemployed women to demograph-ically matched controls in a Swedish longitudinal study. The unemployed women had decreased lymphocyte response to mitogens after 9 months of unemployment compared to controls; no other immunologic differences were found.

Attempts to relate past stressful life changes or life events to immune system function have yielded more variable findings. A possible explanation for this variability may be that how one reacts to stress (coping) may have more immunologic relevance than the "objective" stress experience. In par-ticular, coping and social support may buffer or mediate the stress and immune relationship. Kiecolt-Glaser et al. (1984a) found a significant relationship between stressful life events, as measured by the Holmes and Rahe Social Readjustment Scale (1967), and decreased NK cell activity in a group of medical students, but not in a group of psychiatric patients (Kiecolt-Glaser et al., 1984b). Locke et al. (1984) did not find an overall relationship between life-change stress and NK cell activity in student volunteers. However, among those students who had high levels of life-change stress, those with many psychological symptoms ("poor copers") had lower NK cell activity compared with those with few psychological symptoms ("good copers"). Dorian et al. (1982) showed that exam stress was more immunosuppressive among those who reacted with much distress compared to those who reacted with little distress. In addition to coping, loneliness has been associated with decreased NK cell activity among medical students (Kiecolt Glaser et al., 1984a) and decreased NK cell activity and mitogen response of T-lymphocytes among psychiatric inpatients (Kiecolt-Glaser et al., 1984b). Thus, coping and social support appear to be important concepts for future research delineating the relationship between stress and immunity. More precise definitions and measures of these concepts are needed.

Depressive symptoms in bereaved individuals have also been associated with decreases in measures of cellular immunity. Linn et al. (1984) found that a reduced lymphoproliferative response to mitogen stimulation occurred only in the bereaved subjects with depressive symptoms. Similarly, Irwin et al. (1987a) found a strong negative correlation between the severity of depressive symptoms, as measured by the Hamilton Depression Rating Scale, and NK cell activity after the death of a spouse compared to before the death. Women undergoing anticipatory bereavement demonstrated lower NK cell activity compared to matched control subjects with healthy husbands. In addition, the severity of depressive symptoms was correlated with both reduced NK cell activity and decreased numbers of suppressor/cytotoxic T-cells (Irwin et al., 1987a).

In summary, mood disorders and a range of stressful life events have been associated with decreases in measures of immunocompetence. There are methodological difficulties inherent in retrospective study designs that may contribute to the contradictory study findings. In particular, it is not possible to determine all past stressful events or control for all relevant psychological, psychosocial, and behavioral (e.g., health habits) variables that may confound study findings.

DEPRESSION AND NEUROENDOCRINE SYSTEM FUNCTION

Changes in the levels of the three primary hormones of the hypothalamic-pituitary-adrenal (HPA) axis: cortisol, adrenal corticotrophic hormone (ACTH), and cortisol-releasing factor (CRF) have been described in patients with mood disorders. Gibbons et al. (1964) found increased cortisol levels in some hospitalized depressed patients that normalized upon "relief" of the depression. Subsequent studies have confirmed this finding in adult inpatients with depression (Linkowski et al., 1985; Doig et al., 1966; McClure, 1966). Studies of ACTH levels have yielded conflicting results. Pfohl et al. (1985a, 1985b) found significantly elevated plasma ACTH in hospitalized patients with depression, while Linkowski et al. (1985, 1987) did not. Finally, CRF concentrations in cerebral spinal fluid have been found to be elevated in depressed patients (Nemeroff et al., 1984; Owen et al., 1988). Therefore, it seems clear that there is an alteration in the HPA axis that is associated with at least some forms of depression, yet it remains unclear as to the exact site or sites within the HPA axis that are responsible for the observed changes.

In addition to the static measures of HPA axis components that have been found to be altered in some depressed patients, alterations in the regulation of the HPA axis have been observed, both in a change in the rhythm of cortisol release and in response to various challenge tests (Lesch and Rupprecht, 1989). The normal daily cycle of the cortisol afternoon "trough" and morning surge is phase advanced in depressed patients (Linkowski et al., 1985; Pfohl et al., 1985). Dysregulation of the HPA axis is a frequent finding in patients with major depression; approximately 44 to 50% of such patients will show nonsuppression of cortisol levels when given a standard dose of dexamethasone, a synthetic glucocorticoid that is known to suppress cortisol release. Severity of mood disorder is related to likelihood of cortisol nonsuppression following dexamethasone. For example, in a study of hospitalized psychiatric patients, the majority with melancholic or psychotic subtypes of major depression exhibited nonsuppression (78 and 95%, respectively), whereas a lower proportion (48%) of patients with nonpsychotic, nonmelancholic subtype exhibited nonsuppression (Evans and Nemeroff, 1987). Similarly, higher concentrations of serum cortisol following dexamethasone occur in patients with melancholic or psychotic subtypes when compared with patients with non-melancholic major depression (Evans and Nemeroff, 1987). Similar findings have been reported by others (Schatzberg et al., 1983; see Arana et al., 1985 for a review). HPA axis hyperactivity, as measured by the dexamethasone challenge test, appears to be a state-related phenomenon. Normalization of HPA axis regulation, i.e., suppression of cortisol following dexamethasone administration, is associated with clinical improvement following antidepressant treatment, and may be correlated with decreased risk of relapse (Nemeroff and Evans, 1984). Further indication of depression-related HPA axis dysfunction is found in the demonstration of increased cortisol response to an ACTH challenge in depressed patients compared with normal controls (Amsterdam et al., 1983). In addition, CRF challenge studies have revealed a blunted ACTH response in some depressed patients (Gold et al., 1988b; Holsboer et al., 1988).

HPA axis changes are also found in association with psychological stress.

Rose et al. (1982a, 1982b) studied plasma cortisol levels in 416 air traffic controllers in a work environment and found higher baseline cortisol levels when compared to comparable controls in the literature, as well as higher levels within individuals on days with higher workloads and higher levels of "subjective difficulties". It is interesting to note that on days of high cortisol, the subjects also felt more "blue". Breier et al. (1987) studied ACTH responses in ten normal volunteers to the stress of a loud noise under controllable or uncontrollable conditions. They found significantly higher levels of ACTH under the uncontrollable condition; levels that were associated with higher levels of subjective stress and lower levels of happy feelings. A study by Hudgens et al. (1989) of 26 male medical students taking exams revealed higher cortisol levels associated with anxiety and, in the post-exam state, depressed feelings, when compared to controls.

There have been a few studies of the DST in stress. Baumgartner et al. (1985) studied the DST in psychiatrists around the stress of presenting at a conference, and found that 9 of 16 (56%) failed to suppress. Under non-stressful conditions, none (0%) failed to suppress. Ceulemans et al. (1985) found that of 40 patients who were hospitalized, about to have back surgery, 19 (47.5%) failed to suppress cortisol after dexamethasone. The possible contribution of depressed mood to the above findings was not studied.

In summary, both stress and depression have been associated with measurable changes in the HPA axis in some individuals. This observation is consistent with the theory that depression, at least melancholic depression, "arises from an acute generalized stress response that has escaped the usual counterregulatory restraint" (Gold et al., 1988b).

NEUROENDOCRINE AND IMMUNE SYSTEM RELATIONSHIPS

Mediation of stress or depression-related immune system alterations through the neuroendocrine system requires the immune and neuroendocrine systems to be linked. Recent findings suggest that communication between the neuroendocrine and the immune system exists, and is likely to be bidirectional. For example, Blalock et al. (1985) have suggested that the immune system may produce many, and perhaps all, of the known neuroendocrine peptide hormones. Furthermore, corticosteroids are known to modulate immune function. Experimentally induced stress in animals is associated not only with adrenocortical hypersecretion, but also with lymphocyte depletion, thymic involution, and decreases in spleen and lymph node tissue mass (Riley, 1981; Stein et al., 1981). In addition, there is now evidence that a number of stress-related hormones, including endorphins (Morley et al., 1985), enkephalins (Plotnikoff et al., 1985), and prolactin (Holaday et al., 1988), as well as corticosteroids, exert a modulatory effect on the immune system. Endorphins, enkephalins, and prolactin have been associated with immune enhancement, in contrast to the immunosuppressive effects of the corticosteroids. Thus, stress can result in activation of the hypothalamic-pituitary axes, with concomitant release of ACTH, prolactin, and endorphins from the pituitary gland, along with release of steroid hormones and enkephalins from the adrenal gland. Plotnikoff et al. (1985) have postulated that endogenous opioids (the enkephalins and the endorphins) modulate the effects of corticosteroids on immune function during times of stress, and Holaday et al. (1988) have demonstrated the ability of prolactin to reverse glucocorticoid-induced immunosuppression.

Additional evidence supporting a bidirectional interaction between the endocrine and immune systems includes the findings that the monokine, interleukin-1 (IL-1), appears to regulate the secretion of ACTH at both the hypothalamic and pituitary levels (Bernton et al., 1987; Sapolsky et al., 1987; Berkenbosch et al., 1987). Therefore, immune system peptides may regulate the activity of the HPA axis and interact with HPA axis regulation via CRF, which itself may play a role in immune system regulation (Irwin et al., 1987c).

Simultaneous study of the neuroendocrine and immune system sheds light on the potential for clinically important effects through this bidirectional communication. Lowy et al. (1984) simultaneously studied HPA axis and immune system response to a dexamethasone challenge. They found that lymphocyte response to mitogen stimulation was suppressed in patients who exhibited normal cortisol response to dexamethasone. Those patients who exhibited cortisol nonsuppression following dexamethasone administration, however, consistently exhibited suppressed mitogen response as well. Schleifer et al. (1984) found that in depressed patients high plasma cortisol concentrations were associated with decreases in measures of immune system function. Kronfol et al. (1985) found dexamethasone nonsuppression to be associated with lower lymphocyte counts and percentages of lymphocytes in depressed patients when compared with controls. However, we did not find a significant relationship between the numbers of T-cells or T-cell subpopulations and cortisol nonsuppression following dexamethasone in depressed patients (Evans et al., 1988b; Pedersen et al., 1989), nor a relationship between cell population responses to dexamethasone challenge and cortisol status. Urinary cortisol concentrations have been correlated with immune system impairments in psychiatric patients scoring high on "loneliness" on the UCLA Loneliness Scale (Kiecolt-Glaser et al., 1984b). However, no correlations were found between serum cortisol in bereavement (Bartrop et al., 1977; Irwin et al., 1988a). Thus, the relationship between various measures of HPA axis activity and various aspects of immunity has been variable in the available studies.

CLINICAL RELEVANCE—CANCER

Animal Models

A large body of basic research has accumulated over the last 3 decades documenting stress-induced alterations in immune function and cancer development in animals (Riley, 1979; Riley et al., 1981; Monjan, 1981; Sklar and Anisman, 1981; Newberry et al., 1984; Tecoma and Leighton, 1984). These models are valuable in that they permit mechanistic studies critical to the generation of testable hypotheses concerning the mediation of immune alterations that often accompany stressful life events or clinical mood disorders. Additionally, these models provide the opportunity to examine cellular changes in physiologically important immune organs, such as the spleen (see Fox, 1981 for a review).

Stress-Induced Alterations in State and Immune Function

Despite the advantages associated with animals models, the relationship between stress and immune function or stress and disease process (e.g., cancer) remains ambiguous. This stems from, in part, methodological problems such as the type of stress, its timing and duration, and how these variables interact with subject variables such as sex, age, animal strain, immune parameter being measured, and tumor type. Additionally, stressors are quite heterogeneous and their effects depend upon different neural and neuroendocrine mechanisms (e.g., opioid dependent vs. opioid independent, corticosteroid dependent vs. corticosteroid independent) that appear to regulate stress-induced immune system alterations which occur with different types of stresses (Keller et al., 1983; Shavit et al., 1986; Yirimiya et al., 1987; Weiss et al., 1989).

For example, uncontrollable stress (e.g., inescapable shock) has a far greater effect on immune function than controllable (e.g., escapable shock) stress (Laudenslager et al., 1983). Thus, availability of a "coping" response is critical even when the duration and magnitude of the stressor is held constant. The pattern of adaptation to repeated stress is also crucial. In this regard, Sklar and Anisman (1981), based on their work and a review of the literature, have described the following generalities. Typically, acute stress, and chronic stress in which adaptation to the stress does not develop, lead to depletion of norepinepherine (NE) and dopamine (DA) in some brain regions, with increased levels of acetylcholine (Ach) and some HPA axis hormones such as ACTH, β-endorphin, and corticosteroids. These changes are associated with immune suppression and enhanced tumor development in a variety of animal models. Conversely, chronic stress paradigms in which animals show adaptation to the stress most often lead to enhanced synthesis of NE and DA and a concomitant decrease from acute levels of Ach and above-HPA-axis hormones toward baseline. This adaptation or ability to effectively "cope" generally leads to enhanced immune function and deceleration of tumor growth.

Behavioral Traits and Immune Function

Much less attention has been given to the issue of the relationship between stable individual differences (e.g., emotionality) and immune function. Recently, different strains of inbred mice exposed to identical stressors exhibited strain-specific differences on some measures of brain neurochemistry (Zacharko and Anisman, 1989) and patterns of immunosuppression (Irwin et al., 1988b). While it has been established that a number of immune responses can be classically conditioned (Ader and Cohen, 1985), the recent work of Gorcynski and Kennedy (1987) suggests that a behavioral trait (open-field behavior) may be one factor which predicts immune conditionability in mice. Thus, it appears that trait-dependent factors, as well as varied life experiences, likely influence neuroimmune response patterns. Future research may define key genetic variables which may help predict coping styles and elucidate salient endocrine/immune variables that differentiate subtypes of patients with mood disorders.

Cancer Etiology

Although there is considerable support for a relationship between alterations in immune function and stress and depression, the clinical relevance of these findings remains unclear. To assess the clinical relevance, we review evidence relating psychologic and psychosocial variables to disease etiology and prognosis in cancer.

There are only a few long-term prospective studies of large, initially healthy samples designed to evaluate the role of psychologic variables on cancer etiology (Shekelle et al., 1981; Thomas, 1982; Berkman and Syme, 1979; Kaplan and Reynolds, 1988). Most studies examining the relationship between psychologic factors and cancer etiology have been retrospective or semiprospective in design. "Semiprospective" studies follow patients with an abnormal condition (e.g., breast lump) from before their condition has been diagnosed to after the outcome has been determined (usually only a few days). These studies are inherently limited by (1) the potential unreliability of psychologic measurements during a traumatic event, (2) the patients' possible ability to discern the likely biopsy outcome from physicians' comments and covert cues (Schwarz and Geyer, 1984), and (3) the subtle neuroendocrine and immune abnormalities that could be present as a consequence of the disease which theoretically could alter mental state.

In addition to the paucity of prospective studies, the design of research on psychologic and psychosocial cofactors of cancer makes comparisons between studies difficult. Some studies include patients with many different types of cancer, while others focus on only one type of malignancy. Furthermore, stage of cancer and other relevant biologic factors are rarely specified or controlled for when analyzing the effects of psychologic or psychosocial factors. Finally, questions of prognosis and etiology tend to get blurred when cancer mortality is the outcome variable (Temoshok and Heller, 1984). It is with these caveats that we analyze the findings on psychologic and psychosocial aspects of cancer etiology and prognosis.

Psychologic Variables

In a 17-year longitudinal study of men, Shekelle et al. (1981) found that depression scores on the Minnesota Multiphasic Personality Inventory (MMPI) positively correlated with subsequent cancer mortality, but were unrelated to all other causes of death. This relationship remained even when other cancer risk factors (e.g., smoking) were held constant. A relationship between depression and cancer mortality was not upheld by Kaplan and Reynolds (1988), using the 17-year longitudinal database of Alameda County adults. These researchers found a significant association between initial depressive symptoms and subsequent *noncancer* causes of mortality, but no relationship between depressive symptoms and cancer incidence or cancer mortality. However, the same Alameda County study after 9 years showed that those who scored low on life satisfaction were at greater risk for developing cancer (Berkman and Syme, 1979).

In a study utilizing MMPI data gathered initially on healthy males entering a Veterans Administration hospital domicile (Dattore et al., 1980), researchers subsequently examined two diagnostic groups of cancer and noncancer subjects (e.g., hypertension, ulcers, and no diagnosis). The cancer group had greater repression and less self-reported depression. The authors interpret this finding as cancer patients' greater tendency toward repression of emotion, especially depressive affect.

Other studies examining psychological correlates of cancer incidence have incorporated a semiprospective design, one that is limited as described above. Patients diagnosed with breast cancer were no more likely to have been treated for depressive illness or to score higher on depression rating scales than those diagnosed with benign breast disease (Greer and Morris, 1975). Furthermore, the depression and ego strength scales on the MMPI were not related to the biopsy results for uterine cervical cancer (Schmale and Iker, 1966); however, hopelessness was related to positive biopsy. Except for the Shekelle study (1981) and the lower life satisfaction in the Alameda County study, there is no other evidence that depression leads to a higher cancer incidence or cancer mortality. To the contrary, some evidence, including work by Dattore et al. (1980), indicates that emotional repression may be associated with cancer development. The predominance of excessive emotional control on Rorschach responses was correlated with later development of cancer in a prospective study of medical students (Graves and Thomas, 1981). Semiprospective studies have shown that there is a greater tendency to suppress anger and anxiety, and to deny or control emotions among those patients whose biopsies were positive for breast cancer compared to those with benign disease (Morris et al., 1981; Greer and Morris, 1975; Wirsching et al., 1982; Jansen and Muenz, 1984). On the other hand, one semiprospective study did not find a difference among those with breast cancer, benign disease, or healthy women on anger suppression or anxiety (Scherg et al., 1981).

Stressful Events

Studies assessing the role of past stressful events have, by necessity, been retrospective or semiprospective. For the most part, stressful events have not been correlated with the development of cancer. Using the semiprospective design (pre/post biopsy), studies have shown (1) no relationship between early childhood separation experiences and malignant breast biopsy results (Muslin et al., 1966), (2) greater life change scores (Holmes and Rahe, 1967) among patients with benign breast tumors compared to malignant ones (Schonfield, 1975), and (3) no relationship between experience of stressful life events (assessed via an interview) and diagnosis of cancer (Greer and Morris, 1975). In addition, two retrospective, controlled studies found no difference between those with cancer and matched controls on loss of spouse (Ewertz, 1986) or life stress (Priestman et al., 1985). To the contrary, Horne and Picard (1979) found those with cancerous lung biopsies had a recent significant loss compared to those with benign lesions. Despite (or perhaps because of) the methodologic limits in these studies, there is not much evidence that stressful events are related to cancer etiology.

Social-Psychological Variables

Two of the few prospective studies examining cancer etiology have reported significant findings relevant to social connections. Berkman and Syme (1979), in a 9-year longitudinal study of Alameda County, California residents, found that mortality (from all causes combined) was negatively related to the amount of social connections and life satisfaction. Thomas and colleagues' (1979) prospective study of male medical students examined many psychological and psychosocial variables, but found that lack of closeness to parents was the primary correlate of cancer incidence. A semiprospective study also found less closeness to parents among women with malignant biopsies compared to those with benign disease (Grassi and Molinari, 1986). Thus, the area of social connection, including social support and closeness to parents, deserves further consideration for possible etiologic significance in cancer.

Cancer Prognosis

Perhaps the most well-known study examining psychologic factors and breast cancer survival is the 5-year longitudinal study by Greer and co-workers (1979). They found the highest survival rates among those reacting to their diagnosis with "fighting spirit" or "denial" and the poorest outcome among those responding with "stoic acceptance" or "hopelessness". Following 35 breast cancer patients for 1 year, Derogatis et al. (1979) found higher psychologic distress (e.g., anxiety, depression) and poorer adjustment to illness among long-term survivors. Although clearly contrary to expectations, greater distress was interpreted as a greater ability to express feelings during a stressful life event. Stavraky and colleagues (1968) also showed a positive relationship between hostility and favorable outcome in cancer. Rogentine et al. (1979) found that patients expecting difficulty in adjusting to illness had less relapse from malignant melanoma. In a study of cancer patients, however, those with less emotional distress had longer than average survival (Weisman and Worden, 1975). Other studies have not shown a relationship of psychologic state or adjustment with cancer survival (Jamison et al., 1987; Cassileth et al., 1985).

Stressful Events and Social Support

In a 20-year longitudinal study of breast cancer patients, Funch and Marshall (1983) found stressful events (e.g., death, illness, and unemployment) were correlated with a shorter survival among older patients. Subjective stressors (e.g., tiredness, upset) were correlated with shorter survival among younger patients. Also, social involvement was found to correlate with longer survival. Weisman and Worden (1975) also found that cancer patients who had closer personal relationships had increased survival. A recent study, however, has not found a relationship between social support and length of survival (Cassileth et al., 1985).

Depression and Cancer

Many investigators have found clinical depression in a high percentage of patients with cancer (see Evans et al., 1986 and in press, a and c for reviews) and have evidence that depression in the cancer patient is characterized by a similar frequency and degree of HPA axis hyperactivity as that seen in hospitalized psychiatric patients with nonmelancholic, nonpsychotic depression. Studies of depression-related alterations of immune function in cancer patients have not been conducted, nor do we know if depression-related endocrine changes result in immune alterations. Preliminary studies suggest that depressed cancer patients benefit from antidepressant pharmacotherapy and have better psychosocial adaptation compared to depressed cancer patients who do not receive adequate antidepressant medication (Evans et al., 1988a). We are now planning studies to assess longitudinally depression-related immune alterations and the relationship to the endocrine state in and the relationship to the endocrine state in an effort to determine the possible clinical relevance of depression in the course of malignancy.

The complex methodological issues encountered in the research of psychologic and psychosocial predictors of cancer etiology and outcome complicate the interpretation of the numerous studies cited above. These issues need to be pursued further, utilizing more precise measures of emotional suppression vs. psychologic symptoms, social network, and coping responses.

SUMMARY AND CONCLUSIONS

There is substantial literature supporting the concept that depression and stress can result in altered endocrine system function and altered immune system function. Research also indicates that the endocrine and immune systems possess common regulatory substances, and thus may influence each other. The evidence that stress and depression can exert a clinical effect, influencing the development or course of a physical disease, is less certain and remains an intriguing question. Methodological problems are a major obstacle to elucidating the true impact of psychological factors on physical disease. The physiologic impact of these psychological factors is likely to be an important variable, as not all individuals respond to the same stressors in the same way. Additionally, depressive illness is a heterogenous condition, varying in clinical features and in severity, and biological subtypes may be associated with varying central nervous system, neuroendocrine, and immune profiles.

A model for a possible pathway that could explain how depression and stress impact on the development or course of a physical disease, such as cancer, involves the endocrine and the immune systems as mediating links (see Figure 1). In this model, environmental stressors may have an impact on mood state and on the development of a clinical psychiatric illness. The impact of environmental stressors is buffered by psychosocial variables such as coping and social support. Alternatively, disturbances in mood or the development of a psychiatric illness may result from biological factors, such as endocrine system disease, or from a genetic predisposition to major depressive disorders. Depressive illness or possibly altered mood state may be associated with changes in the endocrine system that in turn may result in, and interact with, specific alterations in immune function, including decreased cellular immunity. This decrease in the body's ability to mount an immune response could make the individual more vulnerable to certain illnesses, such as cancer or infectious diseases. In this model, we hypothesize that depressive illnesses or altered mood states that do not impact on the endocrine or the immune systems will not result in increased vulnerability to physical disease. This approach allows depressive illness or stress that is "immunologically

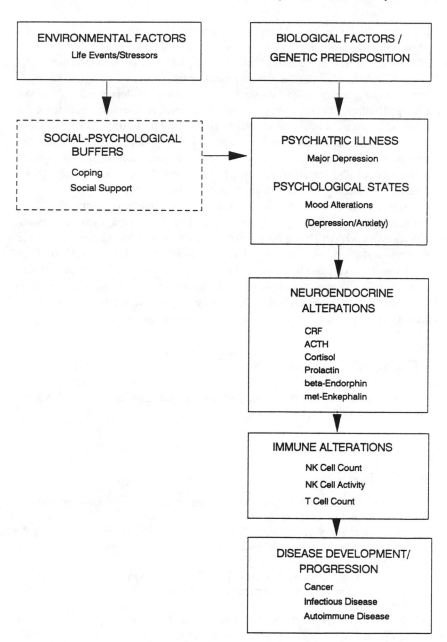

Figure 1. Psychoneuroendocrine-immune (PNEI) model.

important" to be defined. Variability in research findings related to problems in determining biologically relevant stress or depression may in this way be addressed. Thus, this model provides a systematic approach to the assessment of PNEI relationships in the development or prognosis of a physical illness. For example, cancer prognosis could be compared in depressed individuals with and without measurable neuroendocrine and/or immune system alterations. Under this model, depressed individuals with neuroendocrine and/or immune system changes would be expected to have a poorer prognosis than depressed individuals without these changes. This model could also be applied to the study of PNEI relationships in other physical illnesses, such as infectious diseases, including AIDS, and autoimmune diseases.

Considerable study will be necessary to document alterations in cellular immunity in individuals undergoing stress and in patients with depression. Additional study will then be necessary to determine the clinical relevance of stress and depression-associated alterations in immunity. Positive findings from this type of investigation would have important implications for individuals with physical diseases, such as cancer. However, negative findings are also of importance, since there is a strong popular belief that psychological state influences the development and/or course of physical illness.

ACKNOWLEDGMENTS

This work was supported in part by the National Institutes of Mental Health: MH42625, MH44618, MH33127.

REFERENCES

Ader R and Cohen N: CNS-immune system interactions: conditioning phenomena. *Behav. Brain Sci.* 1985; 8:379–394.

Albrecht J, Helderman JH, Schlesser MA, and Rush AJ: A controlled study of cellular immune function in affective disorders before and during somatic therapy. *Psychiatry Res.* 1985; 15:185–193.

Amsterdam JD, Winokur A, Abelman E, Lucki J, and Rickels K: Cosyntropin AC-$TH_{alpha-1-24}$ stimulation test in depressed patients and healthy subjects. *Am. J. Psychiatry* 1983; 140:907–909.

Arana GW, Baldessarini RJ, and Ornsteen M: The Dexamethasone suppression test for diagnosis and prognosis in psychiatry. *Arch. Gen. Psychiatry* 1985; 42:1193–1204.

Arnetz BB, Wasserman J, Petrini B, Brenner O, Levi L, Eneroth P, Salovaara H, Hielm R, Saloraara L, Theorell T, and Petterson L: Immune function in unemployed women. *Psychosom. Med.* 1987; 49:3–12.

Bartrop RW, Luckhurst E, Lazarus L, Kiloh LG, and Penny R: Depressed lymphocyte function after bereavement. *Lancet* 1977; 83:834–836.

Baumgartner A, Graf KJ, and Kurten I: The dexamethasone suppression test in depression, in schizophrenia, and during experimental stress. *Biol. Psychiatry* 1985; 20:675–679.

Berkenbosch F, Oers JV, Del Rey A, Tilders F, and Besedovsky H: Corticotropin-releasing factor-producing neurons in the rat activated by interleukin-1. *Science* 1987; 238:524–526.

Berkman LF and Syme SL: Social networks, host resistance, and mortality: a nine year follow-up study of Alameda County residents. *Am. J. Epidemiol.* 1979; 109:186–204.

Bernton EW, Beach JE, Holaday JW, Smallridge RC, and Fein HG: Release of multiple hormones by a direct action of interleukin-1 on pituitary cells. *Science* 1987; 238:519–524.

Blalock JE, Harbour-McMenamin D, and Smith EM: Peptide hormones shared by the neuroendocrine and immunologic systems. *J. Immunol.* 1985; 135:858s–862s.

Breier A, Albus M, and Pickar D: Controllable stress in humans: alterations in mood and neuroendocrine and psychophysiological function. *Am. J. Psychiatry* 1987; 144:1419–1425.

Cappel R, Gregoire F, Thiry L, and Sprecher BS: Antibody and cell-mediated immunity to herpes simplex virus in psychotic depression. *J. Clin. Psychiatry* 1978; 39:266–268.

Carroll BJ, Feinberg M, and Greden JF: A specific laboratory test for the diagnosis of melancholia. *Arch. Gen. Psychiatry* 1981; 38:15–22.

Cassileth BR, Lusk EJ, Miller DS, Brown LL, and Miller C: Psychosocial correlates of survival in advanced malignant disease? *N. Engl. J. Psychiatry* 1985; 12:1551–1555.

Ceulemans DLS, Westenberg HGM, and van Praag HM: The effect of stress on the dexamethasone suppression test. *Psychiatry Res.* 1985; 14:189–195.

Dattore PJ, Shantz FC, and Coyne L: Premorbid personality differentiation of cancer and noncancer groups: a test of the hypothesis of cancer prognosis. *J. Consult. Clin. Psychol.* 1980; 48:388–394.

Derogatis LR, Feldstein M, and Morrow G: A survey of psychotropic drug prescriptions in an oncology population. *Cancer* 1979; 44:1919–1929.

Doig RJ, Mummery RV, Willis MR, and Elkes A: Plasma cortisol levels in depression. *Br. J. Psychiatry* 1966; 112:1263–1267.

Dorian B, Garfinkel P, Brown G, Shore A, Gladman D, and Keystone E: Aberrations in lymphocyte subpopulations and function during psychological stress. *Clin. Exp. Immunol.* 1982; 50:132–138.

Evans DL, Burnett GB, and Nemeroff CB: The dexamethasone suppression test in the clinical setting. *Am. J. Psychiatry* 1983; 140(5):586–588.

Evans DL, McCartney CF, Nemeroff CB, Raft D, Quade D, Golden RN, Haggerty JJ, Holmes V, Simon JS, Droba M, Mason GA, and Fowler WC: Depression in women treated for gynecological cancer: clinical and neuroendocrine assessment. *Am. J. Psychiatry* 1986; 143:447–451.

Evans DL and Nemeroff CB: The clinical use of the dexamethasone suppression test in DSM-III affective disorders: correlation with the severe depressive subtypes of melancholia and psychosis. *J. Psychiatr. Res.* 1987; 21(2):185–194.

Evans DL and Nemeroff CB: Depression and aging: psychoneuroendocrinology and psychoneuroimmunology. *Prog. Neuroendocrinol.* 1987; 1(4):21–27.

Evans DL, McCartney CF, Haggerty JJ, Nemeroff CB, Golden RN, Simon JS, Quade D, Holmes V, Droba M, Mason GA, Fowler WC, and Raft D: Treatment of depression in cancer patients is associated with better life adaptation: a pilot study. *Psychosom. Med.* 1988a; 50:72–76.

Evans DL, Pedersen CA, and Folds JD: Major depression and immunity: preliminary evidence of decreased natural killer cell populations. *Prog. Neuropsychopharmacol. Biol. Psychiatry* 1988b; 12:739–748.

Evans DL, Golden RN, Nemeroff CB, Pedersen CA, McCartney CF, Haggerty JJ, Simon JS, and Raft D: Clinical aspects of neuropeptide research. In *Neuropsychopharmacology.* Bunney WE Jr, Hippins H, Laakmann G, and Schmauss M, Eds. Springer-Verlag, 1990; 521–528.

Evans DL, Leserman J, Pedersen CA, Golden RN, Lewis MH, Folds JA, and Ozer H: Immune correlates of stress and depression. *Psychopharmacol. Bull.* 1989; 25(3):319–324.

Evans DL, Stern RA, Golden RN, Haggerty JJ, Perkins DO, Simon JS, and Nemeroff CB: Neuroendocrine and peptide challenge tests in primary and secondary depression. In *Neuropeptides in Psychiatry.* Nemeroff CB, Ed. APA Press, Washington, D.C., 1990; 281–298.

Ewertz M: Bereavement and breast cancer. *Br. J. Cancer* 1986; 53:701–703.

Fox BH: Psychosocial factors and the immune system in human cancer. In *Psychoneuroimmunology.* Ader R, Ed. Academic Press, New York.

Funch DP and Marshall J: The role of stress, social support, and age in survival from breast cancer. *J. Psychosom. Res.* 27:77–83.

Gibbons JL: Cortisol secretion rate in depressive illness. *Arch. Gen. Psychiatry* 1964; 10:572–575.

Glaser R, Kiecolt-Glaser JK, Stout JC, Tarr KL, Speicher CE, and Holliday JE: Stress-related impairments in cellular immunity. *Psychiatr. Res.*1985; 16:233–239.

Gold PW, Goodwin FK, and Chrousos GP: Clinical and biochemical manifestations of depression: relation to the neurobiology of stress. *N. Engl. J. Med.* 1988a; 319:348–353.

Gold PW, Goodwin FK, and Chrousos GP: Clinical and biochemical manifestations of depression: relation to the neurobiology of stress. *N. Engl. J. Med.* 1988b; 319:413–420.

Gorczynski RM and Kennedy M: Behavioral trait associated with conditioned immunity. *Brain Behav. Immun.* 1987; 1:72–80.

Grassi L and Molinari S: Family affective climate during the childhood of adult cancer patients. *J. Psychosoc. Oncol.* 1986; 4:53–62.

Graves PL and Thomas CB: Themes of interaction in medical students' Rorschach responses as predictors of midlife health or disease. *Psychosom. Med.* 1981; 43:215–225.

Greer S and Morris T: Psychological attributes of women who develop breast cancer: a controlled study. *J. Psychosom. Res.* 1975; 19:147–153.

Greer S, Morris T, and Pettingale KW: Psychological response to breast cancer: effect on outcome. *Lancet* 1979; 2:785–787.

Hamilton M: A rating scale for depression. *J. Neurol. Neurosurg. Psychiatry* 1960; 23:56–62.

Holaday JW, Bryant HU, Kenner JR, and Bernton EW: Pharmacologic manipulation of the endocrine-immune axis. *Prog. Neuroendocrinimmunol.* 1988; 1(3):6–10.

Holmes TH and Rahe RH: The social readjustment rating scale. *J. Psychosom. Res.* 1967; 11:213–218.

Holsboer F, Von Bordeleben V, Heuser I, and Steiger A: Human corticotropin-releasing hormone challenge tests in depression. In *The Hypothalamic-Pituitary-Adrenal Axis: Physiology, Pathophysiology, and Psychiatric Implications.* Schatzberg AF and Nemeroff CB, Eds. Raven Press, New York (1988), pp. 79–100.

Horne RL and Picard RS: Psychosocial risk factors in lung cancer. *Psychosom. Med.* 1979; 41:503–514.

Hudgens GA, Chatterton RT, and Torre J: Hormonal and psychological profiles in response to a written examination. In *Molecular Biology of Stress.* Breznitz S and Zinder O, Eds. Alan R. Liss, New York (1989), pp. 265–275.

Irwin M, Smith TL, and Gillin JC: Low natural killer cell activity in major depression. *Life Sci.* 1987a; 41:2127–2133.

Irwin M, Daniels M, Bloom ET, Smith TL, and Weiner H: Life events, depressive symptoms, and immune function. *Am. J. Psychiatry* 1987b; 144:4.

Irwin M, Vale W, and Britton K: Central corticotropin releasing factor suppresses natural killer cell cytotoxicity. *Brain Behav. Immun.* 1987c; 1:81–87.

Irwin MR, Daniels M, Risch SC, Bloom E, and Weiner H: Plasma cortisol and natural killer cell activity during bereavement. *Biol. Psychiatry* 1988a; 24:173–178.

Irwin J, Zalcman S, and Anisman H: Strain differences in immunological responses to stress. *Soc. Neurosci.* 1988b; 14:1282.

Jamison RN, Burish TG, and Wallston KA: Psychogenic factors in predicting survival of breast cancer patients. *J. Clin. Oncol.* 1987; 5:768–772.

Jansen MA and Muenz LR: A retrospective study of personality variables associated with fibrocystic disease and breast cancer. *J. Psychosom. Res.* 1984; 28:35–42.

Jemmott JB III, Borysenko JZ, Borysenko M, McClelland DC, Chapman R, Meyer D, and Benson H: Academic stress, power motivation and decrease in secretion rate of salivary immunoglobulin. *Lancet* 1983; 11:1400–1402.

Kaplan GA and Reynolds P: Depression and cancer mortality and morbidity: prospective evidence from the Alameda County study. *J. Behav. Med.* 1988; 11(1):1–13.

Keller SE, Weiss JM, Schleifer SJ, Miller NT, and Stein M: Stress-induced suppression of immunity in adrenalectomized rats. *Science* 1983; 221:1301–1304.

Kiecolt-Glaser JK, Fisher LD, Ogrocki P, Stout JC, Speicher CE, and Glaser R: Marital quality, marital disruption, and immune function. *Psychosom. Med.* 1987; 49:1.

Kiecolt-Glaser JK, Garner W, Speicher CE, Penn G, and Glaser R: Psychosocial modifiers of immunocompetence in medical students. *Psychosom. Med.* 1984a; 46:7–14.

Kiecolt-Glaser JK, Glaser R, Strain E, Stout J, Tarr K, Holliday J, and Speicher C: Modulation of cellular immunity in medical students. *J. Behav. Med.* 1986; 9:5–21.

Kiecolt-Glaser JK, Ricker D, and George J: Urinary cortisol levels, cellular immunocompetence, and loneliness in psychiatric inpatients. *Psychosom. Med.* 1984b; 46:15–23.

Kronfol Z, Nasrallah HA, Chapman S, and House JD: Depression, cortisol metabolism and lymphocytopenia. *J. Affect. Disord.* 1985; 9:169–173.

Kronfol Z, Silva JR, Greden J, Dembinski S, Gardner R, and Carroll B: Impaired lymphocyte function in depressive illness. *Life Sci.* 1983; 33:241–247.

Laudenslager ML, Ryan SM, Drugan RC, Hyson RL, and Maier SF: Coping and immunosuppression: inescapable but not escapable shock suppresses lymphocyte proliferation. *Science* 1983; 221:568–570.

Lesch K and Rupprecht R: Psychoneuroendocrine research in depression. II. Hormonal responses to releasing hormones as a probe for hypothalamic-pituitary-end organ dysfunction. *J. Neural Transm.* 1989; 75:179–194.

Linn NW and Linn BS: Stressful events, dysphoric mood, and immunologic systems. *Psychol. Rep.* 1984; 54:219–222.

Linowski P, Mendelwicz J, Kerkhofs M, Leclercq R, Goldstein J, Brasseur M, Copinschi G, and Van Cauter E: 24-Hour profiles of adrenocorticotropin, cortisol and growth hormone in major depressive illness: effect of antidepressant treatment. *J. Clin. Endocrinol. Metab.* 1987; 65:141–152.

Linowski P, Mendlewicz J, Leclercq R, Brasseur M, Haubain P, Goldstein J, Copinschi G, and Van Cauter E: The 24-hour profile of adrenocorticotropin and cortisol in major depressive illness. *J. Clin. Endocrinol. Metab.* 1985; 61:429–438.

Locke SE, Kraus L, Leserman J, Hurst MW, Heisel JS, and Williams RM: Life change stress, psychiatric symptoms, and natural killer cell activity. *Psychosom. Med.* 1984; 46:441–453.

Lowy MT, Reder AT, Antel JP, and Meltzer HY: Glucocorticoid resistance in depression: the dexamethasone suppression test and lymphocyte sensitivity to dexamethasone. *Am. J. Psychiatry* 1984; 141:1365–1370.

McClure DJ: The diurnal variation of plasma cortisol levels in depression. *J. Psychosom. Res.* 1966; 10:189–195.

Monjan AA: Stress and immunologic competence: studies in animals. In *Psychoneuroimmunology.* Ader R, Ed. Academic Press, New York (1981), pp. 185–228.

Morley JE, Kay N, Allen J, Moon T, and Billington CJ: Endorphins, immune function, and cancer. *Psychopharmacol. Bull.* 1985; 21:485–488.

Morris T, Greer S, Pettingale KW, and Watson M: Patterns of expression anger and their psychological correlates in women with breast cancer. *J. Psychosom. Res.* 1981; 25:111–117.

Muslin HL, Gyarfas K, and Pieper WJ: Separation experience and cancer of the breast. *Ann. N.Y. Acad. Sci.* 1966; 125:802–806.

Nemeroff CB and Evans DL: Correlation between the dexamethasone suppression test in depressed patients and clinical response. *Am. J. Psychiatry* 1984; 39:1033–1036.

Nemeroff CB, Widerlov E, Bissette G, Walleus H, Karlson I, Eklund K, Kilts CD, Loosen PT, and Vale W: Elevated concentrations of CSF corticotropin-releasing factor-like immunoreactivity in depressed patients. *Science* 1984; 226:1342–1344.

Newberry BH, Leibelt AG, and Boyle DA: Variables in behavioral oncology: overview and assessment of current issues. In *Impact of Psychoendocrine Systems in Cancer and Immunity.* Fox BH and Newberry BH, Eds. Hogreffe, Toronto (1984), pp. 87–145.

Owen S, Michael J, and Nemeroff CB: The neurobiology of corticotropin releasing factor: implications for affective disorders. In *The Hypothalamic-Pituitary-Adrenal Axis: Physiology, Pathophysiology, and Psychiatric Implications.* Schatzberg AF and Nemeroff CB, Eds. Raven Press, New York (1988), pp. 1–35.

Pedersen CA, Folds J, and Evans DL: Dexamethasone effects on numbers of cells in lymphocyte subpopulations: changes associated with major depression and DST non-suppression. *Progr. Neuropsychopharmacol. Biol. Psychiatry* 1989; 13:896–906.

Pfohl B, Sherman B, Schlechte J, and Stone R: Pituitary-adrenal axis rhythm disturbances in psychiatric depression. *Arch. Gen. Psychiatry* 1985a; 42:897–903.

Pfohl B, Sherman B, Schlechte S, and Winokur G: Differences in plasma ACTH and cortisol between depressed patients and normal controls. *Biol. Psychiatry* 1985b; 20:1055–1072.

Plotnikoff NP, Murgo AJ, Miller GC, Corder CN, and Faith RE: Enkephalins: immunomodulators. *Fed. Proc.* 1985; 44:118–122.

Priestman P, Priestman SG, and Bradshaw C: Stress and breast cancer. *Br. J. Can.* 1985; 51:493–498.

Riley V: Cancer and stress: overview and critique. *Cancer Detect. Prev.* 1979; 2:163–195.

Riley V: Psychoneuroendocrine influence on immunocompetence and neoplasia. *Science* 1981; 212:1100–1109.

Riley V, Fitzmaurice MA, and Spackman DH: Psychoimmunologic factors in neoplasia: studies in animals. In *Psychoneuroimmunology.* Ader R, Ed. Academic Press, New York (1981), pp. 31–94.

Rogentine S, Boyd S, Bunney W, Doherty J, Fox B, Rosenblatt J, and Van Kammen D: Psychological factors in the prognosis of malignant melanoma. *Psychosom. Med.* 1979; 41:647–658.

Rose RM, Jenkins DC, and Hurst M: Endocrine activity in air traffic controllers at work. I. Characterization of cortisol and growth hormone levels during the day. *Psychoneuroendocrinology* 1982a; 7:101–111.

Rose RM, Jenkins DC, and Hurst M: Endocrine activity in air traffic controllers at work. II. Biological, psychological and work correlates. *Psychoneuroendocrinology* 1982b; 7:113–123.

Sapolsky R, Rivier C, Yamamoto G, Plotsky P, and Vale W: Interleukin-1 stimulates the secretion of hypothalamic corticotropin-releasing factor. *Science* 1987; 238:522–524.

Schatzberg AF, Rothchild AJ, Stahl JB, Bond TC, Rosenbaum AH, Lofgren SB, MacLaughlin RA, Sullivan MA, and Cole JO: The dexamethasone suppression test: identification of subtypes of depression. *Am. J. Psychiatry* 1983; 140:88–91.

Scherg H, Cramer I, and Blohmke M: Psychosocial factors and breast cancer: a critical reevaluation of established hypotheses. *Cancer Detect. Prev.* 1981; 4:165–171.

Schleifer SJ, Keller SE, Bond RN, Cohen J, and Stein M: Major depressive disorder and immunity. *Arch. Gen. Psychiatry* 1989; 46:81–87.

Schleifer SJ, Keller SE, Camerino M, Thornton JC, and Stein M: Suppression of lymphocyte function following bereavement. *JAMA* 1983; 250:374–377.

Schleifer SJ, Keller SE, Meyerson AT, Raskin MJ, Davis KL, and Stein M: Lymphocyte function in major depressive disorder. *Arch. Gen. Psychiatry* 1984; 41:484–486.

Schleifer SJ, Keller SE, Siris SG, Davis KL, and Stein M: Depression and immunity. *Arch. Gen. Psychiatry* 1985; 42:129–133.

Schmale A and Iker H: The psychological setting of uterine cervical cancer. *Ann. N.Y. Acad. Sci.* 1966; 125:807–813.

Schonfield J: Psychological and life experience differences between Israeli women with benign and cancerous breast lesions. *J. Psychosom. Res.* 1975; 19:229–234.

Schwarz R and Geyer S: Social and psychological differences between cancer and non-cancer patients. *Psychother. Psychosom.* 1984; 41:195–199.

Shavit Y, Terman GW, Lewis JW, Gale RP, and Liebeskind JC: Effects of footshock stress and morphine on natural killer lymphocytes in rats: studies of tolerance and cross-tolerance. *Brain Res.* 1986; 372:382–385.

Shekelle RB, Raynor WJ, and Ostfeld AM: Psychological depression and 17-year risk of death from cancer. *Psychosom. Med.* 1981; 43:117–125.

Sklar LS and Anisman H: Stress and cancer. *Psychol. Bull.* 1981; 89(3):369–406.

Stavraky K, Buck C, Lott J, and Wanklin J: Psychological factors in the outcome of human cancer. *J. Psychosom. Res.* 1968; 12:251–259.

Stein M, Keller S, and Schleifer SJ: The hypothalamus and the immune response. In *Brain, Behavior, and Bodily Disease.* Weiner H, Hofer MA, and Stunkard AJ, Eds. Raven Press, New York (1981), pp. 45–65.

Syvalahti E, Eskola J, Ruuskanen O, and Laine T: Nonsuppression of cortisol in depression and immune function. *Prog. Neuropsychopharmacol. Biol. Psychiatry.* 1985; 9(4):413–422.

Tecoma ES and Leighton HY: Psychic distress and the immune response. *Life Sci.* 1984; 36:1799–1812.

Temoshok L and Heller B: On comparing apples, oranges, and fruit salad: a methodological overview of medical outcome studies in psychosocial oncology. In *Psychosocial Stress and Cancer.* Cooper CL, Ed. John Wiley & Sons, London (1984), pp. 231–260.

Thomas CB, Duszynski KR, and Shaffer JW: Family attitudes reported in youth as potential predictors of cancer. *Psychosom. Med.* 1979; 41:287–302.

Thomas CB: *The Precursors Study.* John Hopkins University School of Medicine, Baltimore.

Wahlin A, vonKnoring L, and Ross E: Altered distribution of T lymphocyte subjects in lithium-treated patients. *Neuropsychobiology* 1984; 11:243–246.

Weisman AD and Worden JW: Psychosocial analysis of cancer deaths. *Omega* 1975; 6:61–75.

Weiss JM, Sundar SK, Becker KJ, and Cierpial MA: Behavioral and neural influences on cellular immune responses: effects of stress and interleukin-1. *J. Clin. Psychiatry* 1989; 50(Suppl.5):43–53.

Wirsching M, Stierlin H, Hoffmann F, Weber G, and Wirsching B: Psychological identification of breast cancer patients before biopsy. *J. Psychosom. Res.* 1982; 26:1–10.

Yirimiya R, Martin PG, McKinley PG, Shavit JC, and Liebeskind JC: Stress-induced immunosuppression in rats: a naltrexone-insensitive paradigm. *Soc. Neurosci. Abstr.* 1987; 12:1382.

Zacharko RM and Anisman H: Pharmacological, biochemical and behavioral analysis of depression: animal models. In *Animal Models of Depression.* Ehlers E and Kupfer D, Eds. Birkhauser, Boston.

Chapter 12

Depression and Coping Style as Modulators of the Immune Response Under Stress

Massimo Biondi and Paolo Pancheri
3rd Psychiatric Clinic,
University of Rome "La Sapienza"
Viale Universitá 30,
Rome, Italy

INTRODUCTION

Studies in the field of psychoneuroimmunology (PNI) have shown the existence of specific interactions between brain and immunity (Solomon, 1969, 1987; Stein et al., 1976; Rogers et al., 1979; Ader, 1980; Biondi and Kotsalidis, 1990). Between 1960 and 1980, several studies in animals demonstrated that conditions of emotional stress can affect immunity, with a prevalent immunosuppressive effect under acute stress (Monjan, 1981; Riley, 1981). In the early 1980s further studies consistently showed that the immune function in humans can also be highly sensitive to stressful situations (Palmblad, 1981; Biondi and Pancheri, 1987). Human research has been mainly carried out by assessing mean group modifications of immune parameters, such as reactivity to mitogens, rosette formation test, natural killer (NK) cell number and activity, helper function, and other responses, in samples of subjects exposed to stressful situations such as academic examination (Kiecolt-Glaser et al., 1984; Halvorsen and Vassend, 1987; Marchesi et al., 1989), preoperative surgical stress (Biondi et al., 1987; Tonnesen et al., 1987), bereavement and threat of loss (Bartrop et al., 1977; Schleifer et al., 1983; Calabrese et al., 1987; Irwin et al., 1988), forced wakefulness (Palmblad et al., 1976, 1979), unemployment (Arnetz et al., 1987), and accumulation of life stress events (Locke et al., 1984). Findings derived from mean group modifications have clearly shown statistically significant alterations of immune response under stress. Mean group values are, however, obscuring the role of individual variability. Studies in the psychobiology of human stress have actually shown that neurovegetative and psychoneuroendocrine modifications under emotionally stressful conditions can differ widely according to the personality characteristics, coping styles, and psychological defense mechanisms of different subjects when confronted with stressful stimuli and conditions (Frankenhaeuser, 1971; Mason, 1975; Biondi and Pancheri, 1984; Biondi and Brunetti, 1988). The interindividual variability of the stress response is a key factor for the understanding of individual susceptibility to somatic and psychosomatic diseases (Lazarus and Folkman, 1984). As in the case of neurovegetative and psychoneuroendocrine studies, an interesting further perspective of psychoneuroimmunological studies will be the investigation of the role of personality and coping styles on stress-induced immune modifications. To our knowledge, little is known about the role of personality and coping styles as possible mediators of the immune modification under stress. Loneliness (Locke et al., 1984) and lowest scores on the personality profile of the Minnesota Multiphasic Personality Inventory has been associated with lower NK cell activity (Heisel et al., 1986). At the Psychiatric Clinic of the University of Rome, our group is investigating the relationship between stress, personality, coping, and psychobiological responses (neuroendocrine and immune responses). We report here findings from a past investigation; another study on the effect of chronic life stress, personality, and coping on immunity is now in progress (Biondi et al., 1989), but will not be reviewed here.

AIM AND DESIGN

The purpose of this study was to evaluate the relationship between emotional reactivity and immune reactivity in a group of patients waiting for a surgical intervention for a life-threatening disease. According to the experimental design, the preoperative setting represents a powerful real-life stressor capable of generating differential emotional reactions according to individual personalities and coping styles. The sample of subjects under stress was dichotomized into two subgroups, according to their immune reactivity to the *in vitro* and *in vivo* tests. The two subgroups were then compared for personality profile, coping styles, and previous life events.

METHODOLOGY

The sample consisted of (1) 22 breast cancer patients (mean age 40.3, S.D. 8.2) with a clinical and histopathological diagnosis of breast carcinoma in the beginning phase of development, classifiable at T1a, T2a (without fixation to the underlying pectoral fascia or muscle, or skin compromission), with or without axillary lymph node involvement (N0, N1), and without distant metasases (M0), and (2) 20 fibrocystic disease patients (mean age 39.1, S.D. 9.8). Only subjects under 65 years of age, having a minimum of 5 years of formal education, belonging to the lower or middle socioeconomic classes, and without other concomitant somatic pathology were included in the study. The patients were hospitalized in the same hospital in Rome. The psychological interview, and the psychometric and immune assessments were carried out within 3 d before surgery; at that time, the patients were not aware of their exact diagnoses, but were merely informed that a surgical intervention was imminent. The exact diagnoses were given only after post-surgical histopathological examination. At the time of assessment, the psychological and environmental conditions of the two groups were similar. They were inpatients of the same ward, had a therapeutic relationship with the same medical staff, and received the same or similar diagnostic and routine laboratory procedures. The condition of undergoing breast surgery put both groups at a similar level of emotional reaction and somatic concern.

Psychometric Assessment

The psychometric evaluation was carried out by means of the Minnesota Multiphasic Personality Inventory (MMPI) (Dahlstrom et al., 1972), the State and Trait Anxiety Inventory (STAI) (Spielberger et al., 1970), and the Reaction Scheme Test (RST) for the assessment of coping styles. The RST, designed at the 3rd Psychiatric Clinic of the University of Rome (Pancheri and Biondi, 1979) consists of the description of 38 stressful situations which could generate a state of anxiety and conflict. The subject is requested to indicate her or his most probable behavioral reaction among five alternatives. The alternatives are (1) projection (P), assessing the tendency toward an extrapunitive response, with projection of guilt, (2) self-blaming (C), assessing the tendency toward introjection of aggressiveness and assumption of guilt, (3) repression-denial (N), assessing the tendency to minimize or annul the impact and significance of the stimulus, (4) rationalization (R), assessing the tendency to confront the situation on the basis of rationalizing, and actively searching for an adequate response to the stimulus, and (5) blocked projection (PB), assessing the tendency toward inhibition of an overt behavioral reaction, in spite of the wish to be emotionally expressive or extrapunitive.

The assessment of life stress events was carried out by means of the Life Experience Survey (Sarason et al., 1978), in its Italian translation.

Immune Evaluation

Before surgery and while patients were for the last 48 h free of any kind of therapy, and under a common standard diet, immune cell function was assessed by means of (1) the PHA lymphocyte transformation test, with assessment of the percent increase of glycolysis of PHA-stimulated lymphocytes, as compared to unstimulated lymphocytes, according to Cordiali Fei et al. (1980), (2) the E-rosette formation test, assessed on the basis of the count of E-rosette-forming cells (n.v., 55 + 10%) (Sega et al., 1980), and (3) skin tests by means of intradermic PPD (Sclavo), 50 U Varidase (Lederle), and 1:1000 Candida solution (Pasteur). The skin tests were classified as positive if erythema and induration appeared from 24 to 48 h later, with the following response degrees: negative (−), no reaction or erythema only 0 to 5 mm; positive (+), erythema and induration 5 to 9 mm; positive (+ +), erythema and induration 10 to 20 mm; positive (+ + +), erythema and induration greater than 20 mm or vesicle formation. The overall skin test reactivity was classified on the following scale: from 7 to 9 + , high reactivity; from 4 to 6 + , medium reactivity; from 0 to 3 + , low reactivity (Sega et al., 1978). All the immune assessments were performed between 8 and 10 a.m.

Dichotomization of the Sample

Normoreactive and hyporeactive subgroups were identified for each of the two *in vitro* immune assessments (PHA, E-rosette formation) and for the *in vivo* assessment (skin test reactivity). No significant differences in the clinical diagnoses (early breast cancer, mastopathy) were found between the two normoreactive (N) and hyporeactive (H) subgroups (PHA test: cancer group, 12 N and 11 H; mastopathy group, 11 N and 9 H: E-rosette test: 12 N and 11 H; mastopathy group, 14 N and 6 H; skin tests: cancer group, 10 N and 13 H; mastopathy group, 7 N and 13 H). The absence of significant differences between breast carcinoma and mastopathy is consistent with previous findings in the literature concerning immune asset in the early phase of breast cancer (Nemoto et al., 1974). Finally, no significant differences were found between mean age in the two subgroups.

RESULTS

At the PHA test, hyporeactive subjects had significantly higher MMPI Depression ($p < 0.02$) and Social Introversion ($p < 0.05$) scores (Figure 1). Hyporeactive subjects also had significantly higher repression-denial scores on the Reaction Scheme Test ($p < 0.01$) (Figure 2). State anxiety was significantly lower in the hyporeactive subgroup (STAI X1: hyporeactive subgroup 45.71, SD 6.32; normoreactive group 59.72, SD 9.2, $p < 0.01$). Finally,

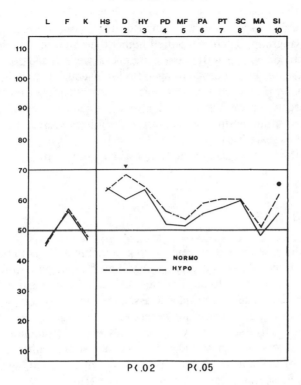

Figure 1. Mean personality profiles on the Minnesota Multiphasic Personality Inventory. Immunohyporeactive subjects on the PHA lymphocyte transformation test have significantly higher scores on the Depression and Social Introversion scales. (From Pancheri and Biondi, 1987. With permission.)

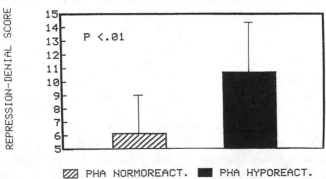

Figure 2. Mean Repression-Denial scores of the hyporeactive and normoreactive PHA groups on the Reaction Scheme Test. PHA hyporeactive subjects have a significantly higher repression of emotional expression score under stressful situations. (From Pancheri and Biondi, 1987. With permission.)

hyporeactive subjects more frequently reported a higher Total Change Score on the Life Experience Survey, relative to the last year: in the hyporeactive group, 11 subjects scored higher than 5 (with 4 subjects under 5); in the normoreactive group, 3 subjects scored higher than 5 (with 9 subjects under 5) (chi-square 6.23, p <0.01). No differences were found for life event frequencies or for the frequency of specific life events, such as loss events.

Subjects with reduced skin test reactivity scored higher on the MMPI Depression scale: in the hyporeactive group, 18 subjects scored above 65, and 11 below; in the normoreactive group, 2 subjects scored above 65, and 11 below (chi-square 7.84, p <0.01).

No significant differences were found with respect to rosette E formation test.

DISCUSSION

The findings of this study seem to suggest that not all the subjects under a severe emotional stress, but only a subgroup of them, may show immune modifications. According to our findings, decreased functional reactivity of immune parameters under stress may be associated with psychological factors. In a sample of women subject to the stress of undergoing breast surgery, immune hyporeactive subjects had significantly higher depression and social introversion scores, higher attitude to cope with stress with psychological mechanisms of the repression-denial type, lower anxiety, and higher subjective life change scores in the last year.

Although suggestive, these findings have several limitations. Due to the transversal experimental design of the study, it cannot be ruled out that both depression and immune hyporeactivity exist prior to the stressor exposure, and are not related to it. Again, we can only report an association between psychological status (MMPI, STAI) and coping style (RST), but we cannot exclude that both depression and immune hyporeactivity, for instance, could be dependent upon a third, unknown, factor.

The association between *in vitro* (PHA transformation test) and *in vivo* (skin tests) immune hyporeactivity and higher depression scores seems consistent with recent reports of immunosuppression in psychiatric pathologies such as major depression (Solomon, 1981; Kronfrol et al., 1983; Denman, 1985; Schleifer et al., 1984). Our patients, however, were not suffering from major depression. They came from a "normal" general population; data from clinical interviews with patients revealed no diagnosis of major depression. Moreover, psychometric data excluded the role of "psychiatric depressions" because the mean MMPI Depression score of the immune hyporeactive group was within normal ranges (not exceeding a score of 70, the upper limit of the norm). These data seem more suggestive of an effect of the stress situation, rather than of a preexistent, severe psychopathological condition. In any case, if confirmed by further and larger studies, it would seem that under acute emotional stress, moderate or "subclinical" depression could be associated with alterations in immune reactivity.

Regarding coping styles, the higher repression-denial scores in the hyporeactive subgroup are interesting. Stress literature shows a growing interest in the mechanisms of individual coping as a key factor for the negative consequences of stress (Lazarus and Folkman, 1984). Clinical and experimental investigations of the psychobiology of human stress recognized repression-denial schemes of confronting stress as modalities associated with a major risk of some somatic stress-dependent and psychosomatic pathology (Alexander, 1950; Bahnson, 1969; Esler et al., 1977; Pancheri, 1978; Laborit, 1980). Our findings are consistent with this line of evidence.

Finally, the lower mean values of state anxiety in the hyporeactive group are not surprising. The STAI is a self-administered questionnaire; the final score is representative of the self-report of perceived anxiety. High deniers can also deny the feeling of anxiety, which will be underestimated in a self-report scale. The low levels of self-report of anxiety can thus be interpreted as a proof of the efficacy with which high-denier patients were (apparently) coping with acute stress: the psychological repression-denial mechanisms protected them very well from the discomfort and suffering of excessive anxiety. And, in fact, subjects from the hyporeactive subgroup have also higher mean scores of repression-denial on the RST.

ACKNOWLEDGMENTS

For the assessment and laboratory procedure of immune responses, we thank Prof. E. Sega (Director, Immune Laboratory of the Regina Elena Institute of Rome), Dr. ssa P. Cordiali Fei and M. C. Apollonj (Immune Laboratory, Regina Elena Institute), and Dr. F. M. Sega (Clinical Assistant, Regina Elena Institute); for the clinical and psychometric assessment, Dr. ssa C. Conti.

REFERENCES

Ader R: Psychosomatic and psychoimmunologic research. *Psychosom. Med.* 1980; 42:307.

Alexander F: *Psychosomatic Medicine.* WW Norton, New York, 1950.

Arnetz BB, Wasserman J, Petrini B, Brenner SO, Levi L, Eneroth P, Salovaara H, Hjelm R, Salovaara L, Theorell T, and Petterson L: Immune function in unemployed women. *Psychosom. Med.* 1987; 49:3.

Bahnson CB: Psychophysiological complementarity in malignancies: past work and future vistas. *Ann. N.Y. Acad. Sci.* 1969; 164:319.

Bartrop RW, Lazarus L, Luckhurst E, and Kiloh LG: Depressed lymphocyte function after bereavement. *Lancet* 1977; 1:834.

Biondi M and Pancheri P: *Psicobiologia del Sistema Neurovegetativo*. Pancheri P, Ed., Trattato di Medicina Psicosomatica, Firenze, USES, 1984.

Biondi M and Pancheri P: Mind and immunity. *Adv. Psychosom. Res.* 1987; 17:234.

Biondi M, Pancheri P, and Cotugno A: Personalitá e coping styles nella risposta immunitaria dei linfociti T in condizioni di stress emozionale. In *Stress, Emozioni e Cancro*. Pancheri P and Biondi M, Eds., Il Pensiero Scientifico, Roma, 1987.

Biondi M and Brunetti G: Stress e sistema endocrino: rassegna degli studi 1980–1988. *Med. Psicosom.* 1988; 33:317.

Biondi M, Zuccaro P, Pierantozzi L, Pacifici R, Di Carlo S: Chronic stress, personality and immune function. Paper presented at the Int. Conf. Molecular Aspects of Immune Response and Infectious Diseases. Rome, July 25 to 28, 1989.

Biondi M and Kotzalidis GD: Human psychoneuroimmunology today. *J. Clin. Lab. Anal.* In press.

Calabrese JR, Kling MA, and Gold PW: Alterations in immunocompetence during stress, bereavement, and depression: focus on neuroendocrine regulation. *Am. J. Psychiatry* 1987; 144:1123.

Cordiali Fei P, Floridi A, Apollonj MC, and Natali PG: Estimation of PHA induced transformation in peripheral lymphocytes through the measurement of their increased glycolysis. *Immunol. Commun.* 1980; 9:210.

Dahlstrom WG, Welsch SG, and Dahlstrom LE: *An M.M.P.I. Handbook*. University of Minnesota Press, Minneapolis, 1972.

Denman AM: Immunity and depression. *Br. Med. J.* 1985; 1:293.

Esler M, Julius S, Zweifler A, Randall O, Harburg E, Gardiner A, and De Quatro V: Mild high renin essential hypertension: neurogenic human hypertension? *N. Engl. J. Med.* 1977; 296:405.

Frankenhaeuser M: Behaviour and circulating catecholamines. *Brain Res.* 1971; 31:241.

Halvorsen R and Vassend O: Effects of examination stress on some cellular immunity functions. *J. Psychosom. Res.* 1987; 31:693.

Heisel JS, Locke SE, Kraus LJ, and Williams M: Natural killer cell activity and MMPI scores of a cohort of college students. *Am. J. Psychiatry* 1986; 143:1382.

Irwin M, Daniels M, Risch SC, Bloom E, and Weiner H: Plasma cortisol and natural killer cell activity during bereavement. *Biol. Psychiatry* 1988; 24:173.

Kiecolt-Glaser JK, Garner W, and Speicher C: Psychosocial modifiers of immunocompetence in medical students. *Psychosom. Med.* 1984; 46:7.

Kronfol Z, Silva J, and Greden J: Impaired lymphocyte function in depressive illness. *Life Sci.* 1983; 33:241.

Laborit H: *L'Inhibition de l'Action*. Masson, Paris, 1980.

Lazarus RS and Folkman S: *Stress, Appraisal and Coping*. Springer-Verlag, New York, 1984.

Locke SE, Kraus L, Leserman J, Hurst MW, Heisel JS, and Williams RM: Life change stress, psychiatric symptoms and natural killer cells activity. *Psychosom. Med.* 1984; 46:441.

Mason JW: In *Emotions as Reflected in Patterns of Endocrine Integration*. Levi L, Ed., Raven Press, New York, 1975.

Marchesi GF, Cotani P, Santone G, Di Giuseppe S, Bartocci C, and Montroni M: Psychological and immunological relationship during acute academic stress. *New Trends Exp. Clin. Psychiatry* 5, 1989.

Monjan AA: Stress and immunologic competence: studies in animals. In *Psychoneuro-immunology*. Ader R, Ed., Academic Press, New York, 1981, pp. 185–228.

Nemoto T, Han T, Minowada J, Angkur V, Chamberlain A, and Dao TL: Cell-mediated immune status of breast cancer patients: evaluation by skin tests, lymphocyte stimulation, and counts of rosette-forming cells. *J. Natl. Cancer Inst.* 1974; 53:64.

Palmblad J, Cantell K, Strander H, Froberg J, Carlsson C, Levi L, Granstrom M, and Unger P: Stressor exposure and immunological response in man: interferon producing capacity and phagocytosis. *J. Psychosom. Res.* 1976; 20:193.

Palmblad J, Petrini B, Wasserman J, and Akerstedt T: Lymphocyte and granulocyte reactions during sleep deprivation. *Psychosom. Med.* 1979; 41:273.

Palmblad J: Stress and immunologic competence: studies in man. In *Psychoneuro-immunology*. Ader R, Ed., Academic Press, New York, 1981, pp. 229–256.

Pancheri P: Stress, personality and interacting variables. An interpretative model for psychoneuroendocrine disorders. In *Clinical Psychoneuroendocrinology in Repro-duction*. Carenza L, Pancheri P, and Zichella L, Eds., Academic Press, New York, 1978.

Pancheri P and Biondi M: *Psicologia e Psicosomatica dei Tumori*. La Goliardica, Roma, 1979.

Riley V: Psychoneuroendocrine influences on immunocompetence and neoplasia. *Science* 1981; 212:1100.

Rogers M, Dubey D, and Reich P: The influence of the psyche and the brain on immunity and disease susceptibility: a critical review. *Psychosom. Med.* 1979; 41:147.

Sarason IG, Johnson JH, and Siegel JM: Assessing the impact of life change: development of the Life Experience Survey. *J. Cons. Clin. Psychol.* 1978; 46:432.

Schleifer SJ, Keller SE, Camerino M, Thornton JC, and Stein M: Suppression of lymphocyte stimulation following bereavement. *JAMA* 1983; 250:374.

Schleifer SJ, Keller SE, Meyerson AT, et al: Lymphocyte function in major depressive disorder. *Arch. Gen. Psychiatry* 1984; 41:484.

Sega E and Sega FM: *Il Ruolo dell' Immunologo nella Caratterizzazione Clinica-Biologica (Statica-Dinamica) dei Tumori. Corso Nazionale di Terapia Antiblastica dell' Ospedale Malpighi*. Editrice Universitaria, Bologna, 1978.

Sega E, Rinaldi M, Mottolese M, Cordiali Fei P, Apollonj MC, De Santis M, Gionfra T, Casali A, Gianciotto A, and Dallo Curcio C: Immunologic monitoring during combined radiochemoimmunotherapy in inoperative lung cancer. *Oncology* 1980; 37:390.

Solomon GF: Emotions, stress, central nervous system and immunity. *Ann. N.Y. Acad. Sci.* 1969; 124:335.

Solomon GF: Immunologic abnormalities in mental illness. In *Psychoneuroimmunol-ogy*. Ader R, Ed., Academic Press, New York, 1981, pp. 259–280.

Solomon GF: Psychoneuroimmunology: interactions between central nervous system and immune system. *J. Neurosci. Res.* 1987; 18:1.

Spielberger CD, Gorsuch RL, and Lushene RE. *Manual for the State and Trait Anxiety Inventory.* Consulting Psychologist Press, Palo Alto, 1970.

Stein M, Schiavi RC, and Camerino M: Influence of brain and behavior on the immune system. *Science* 1976; 191:436.

Tonnesen E, Brinklov MM, Christensen NJ, Olesen AS, and Madsen T: Natural killer cell activity and lymphocyte function during and after coronary artery bypass grafting in relation to the endocrine stress response. *Anesthesiology* 1987; 67:526.

Psychological Factors, Immune Processes, and the Course of Herpes Simplex and Human Immunodeficiency Virus Infection

Margaret E. Kemeny
Department of Psychiatry and Biobehavioral Sciences
University of California,
Los Angeles School of Medicine

INTRODUCTION

Psychological factors have long been believed to influence the etiology and progression of immunologically related diseases such as infections, autoimmune diseases, and cancers. More recently, research findings have been reported indicating that certain immune processes can be altered following exposure to stressful circumstances and in association with certain psychological states, such as depression (see Chapters 1, 8, and 10, this volume). However, the health implications of these immune changes remain unclear. There is only limited evidence that the immune changes found to be associated with psychological factors alter the probability of developing an immunologically related disease or alter the course of such a disease. Human studies have tended to evaluate the relationship between psychological factors and either disease processes or measures of immune status, but not both. And most of the human studies of psychological factors and immune processes have found relatively small changes in immune parameters that have remained well within the normal range. Thus, the role of the immune system as a mediator of the relationship between psychosocial factors and specific disease processes has not been established.

Latent viral infections may serve as useful models for studying the relationships among psychological factors, immune changes, and disease progression. Nonlatent viruses (such as the rhino virus that can cause the common cold) are cleared from the host by the effector arm of the immune system. Studying the relationship between psychological factors and the onset and course of such viral infections is difficult, unless the timing and nature of the exposure is known. Other viruses, such as the herpesviruses (e.g., herpes simplex, cytomegalovirus), are capable of latency and remain in the host for life. In a latent infection, the virus enters certain host cells but does not immediately replicate or cause cell injury. However, the genome of the virus is conserved, latency can become interrupted, and viral replication can occur. Viral replication can result in recrudescence of the infection (e.g., lesion formation in the case of herpes simplex) (Blyth and Hill, 1984). Host factors, including the functioning of certain aspects of the immune system, are believed to play a role in controlling viral reactivation and/or recrudescence. Thus, psychological factors in individuals with latent viral infections can be studied as they impact relevant immune processes and the course of infection.

PSYCHOLOGICAL FACTORS, IMMUNE PROCESSES, AND GENITAL HERPES RECURRENCE

There are a number of reasons to believe that psychological factors could influence the course of herpes simplex virus (HSV) infection via changes in the immune system. Wide variability in the timing of herpes recurrences exists both within individuals across time and between individuals. A number of factors have been suggested to activate a herpes recurrence and account for this variability, including sunlight, a cold or infection, trauma to the skin, the menstrual cycle, and emotional stress (Hill, 1985). Persons with herpes often report that lesions develop following times of distress, and there is some research support for this notion (e.g., Friedman et al., 1977). In addition, the immune system is believed to play a role in preventing herpes recurrences, possibly by controlling viral multiplication when a low level of virus is being chronically produced by infected cells. While the importance of the immune system in HSV recurrence remains to be substantiated (Rouse, 1985), there have been studies linking changes in specific immune parameters, such as natural killer cell activity and lymphocyte subset levels, with herpes recurrences (e.g., Lopez et al., 1983; Sheridan et al., 1982).

A study was conducted of 36 individuals with genital herpes (30 females, 6 males; mean age of 33.4) to determine the relationship between certain psychological and immunological processes and outbreaks of the disease (Kemeny et al., 1989). All subjects had chronic recurrent HSV infections (two or more recurrences in the last 6 months), and were free from immunologically related diseases or medical treatments that could influence the immune system or viral infection (e.g., acyclovir).

All subjects participated in a stress and coping interview once a month for 6 months and filled out a series of psychosocial questionnaires at the time of each interview. Questionnaires assessed stressful life experiences (major life change events, herpes-related events, chronic ongoing stressors, and anticipated life events) and negative mood (anxiety, depression, and hostility). In addition, all subjects were asked to go to a participating physician for documentation of herpes recurrences that occurred during the 6-month period and to report recurrences at the monthly interviews. Nineteen of the subjects had blood drawn at the time of each interview; the proportion of CD4 helper/inducer and CD8 suppressor/cytotoxic T-lymphocytes was determined on the basis of these monthly blood samples.

The results of the study indicated that increased levels of stressful life experience or negative mood over the 6-month period did not predict the timing of herpes outbreaks. The stress and mood measures also did not predict changes in the proportion of CD4 or CD8 cells. Thus, fluctuations in monthly levels of stressful experience or mood did not predict the timing of recurrences or alterations in the levels of the major lymphocyte subsets.

Second, the study determined whether individuals who reported more stressful life experience or negative mood over the study period had a greater HSV recurrence rate. We eliminated from these analyses individuals with a large number of other types of infections (e.g., colds), since we found a relationship between symptoms of other infections and the number of herpes recurrences in these subjects. And colds and other infections are believed to be capable of triggering HSV out of the latent state (Hill, 1985). Results indicated that the mean level of stressful life experience was uncorrelated with HSV recurrence rate. However, depressed mood was significantly correlated with HSV recurrence rate ($r = 0.34$, $p < 0.05$). The most depressed individuals in the sample (the top one third) had twice as many herpes recurrences as the less depressed subjects. On the basis of further analyses, it was determined that this relationship was not due to changes in health behaviors (sleep disturbance, exercise, or alcohol consumption) that may occur in depressed individuals.

We then evaluated whether the relationship between depressed mood and HSV recurrence might be mediated by the percent of CD4 or CD8 lymphocytes. Depressed mood over the 6 months was significantly and negatively correlated with CD8 levels ($r = -0.49$, $p < 0.05$). Individuals who had greater levels of depressed mood over the 6 months also had lower levels of CD8 cells. In addition, CD8 levels averaged over the 6 months and herpes recurrence rate were significantly and negatively correlated with each other (r = −0.45, p <0.03). Thus, depressed mood was associated with lower levels of CD8 cells and lowered levels of CD8 cells were associated with a higher rate of HSV recurrences.

These cross-sectional analyses could not determine the direction of causality among these variables, however. In order to explore the timing of these changes, a further analysis was conducted to determine if CD8 levels decreased prior to HSV recurrences. Five phases of HSV recurrence were defined (e.g., recurrence, convalescence) and we evaluated the level of CD8 cells at each phase with available blood samples. We found that CD8 levels were significantly lower during the 1 to 2 weeks prior to a recurrence and during convalescence, compared to quiescence (t[39] = 3.02, p <0.01). These data suggest the possibility that CD8 cells or an associated immune parameter may mediate the relationship between depressed mood and HSV recurrences in this sample.

The results of the study support the notion that persistently high levels of depressed mood may be associated with recurrences of genital herpes, possibly via aspects of immune status, although this particular pathway must be confirmed in further longitudinal investigations. These data are consistent with prior studies indicating that unhappy mood (Katcher et al., 1973; Friedman et al., 1977) and negative psychological symptoms (Goldmeier and Johnson, 1982) precede herpes recurrences. The high depression scores over the 6 months may represent chronic depression or a stable tendency to experience high levels of negative affect (referred to as negative affectivity by Watson and Clark, 1984).

In this study, we also assessed the relationship between methods of coping, immune parameters, and herpes recurrences (Kemeny et al., 1986). Structured interviews were conducted on a monthly basis to assess the coping processes used to handle stressful situations. The interview protocol was based on the structured interview format developed by Cohen (Cohen, 1975; Cohen and Lazarus, 1973) which has been used in a number of contexts (e.g., Cohen et al., 1986). Ratings of tapes or transcripts have demonstrated high interrater reliability and good predictive validity. Subjects were asked to describe two stressful situations that had occurred over the past month, their thoughts and feelings in response to each situation, and how they handled each situation. Both open-ended and close-ended questions were used to elicit the modes of coping described by Cohen and Lazarus (1973, 1979) as well as a variety of sub-modes (see Kemeny, 1985). A total of 12 modes were elicited and combined into four coping factors based on a factor analysis (see Table 1). A structured coding method was used to code the interviews. During this study, an agreement of 88% was reached between coders across the coping modes.

TABLE I.
Factor Analysis of Coping Modes

Problem Orientation
Problem focused action
Gathering information
Make a plan
Suppress emotion
Accept situation

Emotion Regulation
Emotion-focused action (eating more, sleeping more, etc.)
Express feelings
Amplify feelings

Problem Analysis
Analyze problem
Inhibit action

Avoidance
Suppress thoughts/
Distract self

Note: An oblique rotation was used with a principal components analysis in order to allow for correlations between the factors.

TABLE II.
Pearson Correlations Between Coping Factors, CD8 Levels, and HSV Recurrence Rate[a]

Coping Mode Factor	CD8 (%)	HSV Recurrences
Problem Orientation	0.07	−0.17
Emotion Regulation	−0.73[b]	0.14
Problem Analysis	0.17	−0.13
Avoidance	−0.20	0.33

[a]Subjects were eliminated who had a large number of symptoms of other infections over the 6 months (the top one third of the sample).
[b]$p < 0.005$

The correlations between each of the coping mode factors averaged over the 6 months and the immune parameters and number of herpes recurrences are presented in Table 2. As can be seen, Emotion Regulation (e.g., expressing or amplifying feelings, eating more, sleeping more) was significantly correlated with CD8 level, such that individuals who used a greater degree of Emotion Regulation over the course of the 6 months had a lower percent of CD8 cells. Emotion Regulation was also associated with higher levels of depression ($r = 0.58$, $p < 0.001$), anxiety ($r = 0.75$, $p < 0.001$), and hostility ($r = 0.42$, $p < 0.05$). The other coping mode factors were not significantly correlated with mood scores.

In an exploratory analysis, we divided the sample into four groups in order to define a group of active problem-oriented individuals and a group of less problem-oriented individuals who tended to use Emotion Regulation exclusively. The coping groups were as follows: those who used a high level (above the sample median) of both Problem Orientation and Emotion Regulation, those who used a low level of both of these coping strategies, those who used a high level of Problem Orientation and a low level of Emotion Regulation, and those who used a high level of Emotion Regulation and a low level of Problem Orientation. We compared these groups on CD4 and CD8 levels as well as the number of herpes recurrences experienced over the 6 months. The four groups did not differ on CD4 or CD8 levels. However, there was a significant difference across the four groups in the number of herpes recurrences experienced (F = 3.72, df = 3, p <0.05). The differences across the groups were primarily a result of the difference between the group that used predominantly Emotion Regulation and the three other groups. This Emotion Regulation group had more than twice as many recurrences as the other three groups (see Table 3). Aspects of this pattern of coping have been described by coping researchers as "passive-avoidant coping" in that they involve passive activities (e.g., sleeping or drinking alcohol) that allow individuals to avoid the stressful situation, rather than active behaviors aimed at changing the situation. Unfortunately, there were very few subjects in our sample who consistently reported this particular pattern of coping with stressful experience, so this analysis must be viewed as exploratory.

We have recently completed a study of 58 women with chronic, recurrent genital herpes evaluated over a 6-month period (Cohen et al., 1990). The aim of this study was to increase the sensitivity of our methodology in order to detect possible associations between fluctuations in mood and a subsequent increased risk for a herpes recurrence. In order to do this, we assessed mood at weekly rather than monthly intervals and eliminated factors that might contribute to variability in immune values (e.g., individuals who smoke). Our results indicate that extreme levels of negative mood (i.e., anxiety) were

TABLE III.
Mean Number of HSV Recurrences in Groups Defined by Coping Modes

Coping Mode Factor Group	Mean HSV Recurrences[a]
High problem and emotion orientation (n = 10)	0.33
Low problem and emotion orientation (n = 8)	0.39
High problem and low emotion orientation (n = 3)	0.39
Low problem and high emotion orientation (n = 3)	0.98

[a]Per month.

associated with a greater likelihood of an HSV recurrence over the next month period. The possible mediation of various immune parameters are currently being investigated.

PSYCHOLOGICAL FACTORS AND IMMUNE CHANGES IN HIV INFECTION

The clinical course of infection with the human immunodeficiency virus (HIV) is remarkably variable. Some individuals remain symptom free for years following infection while others develop AIDS-related symptomatology or AIDS rapidly (Curran et al., 1988). The course of HIV infection appears to depend on the extent of damage to the immune system caused by HIV. HIV-seropositive individuals vary in the sequence and magnitude of these immune changes. For example, HIV can selectively infect and kill CD4 helper/inducer T-lymphocytes. HIV-seropositive individuals vary in the rapidity with which they lose CD4 cells over time (Detels et al., 1988). A rapid decrease in CD4 cells has been shown to be a strong predictor of the development of AIDS (Fahey et al., 1987). This variability in the immunological, and consequently the clinical, course of HIV infection may be due exclusively to the properties of the virus itself (e.g., the strain). Or environmental or host factors, called cofactors, may contribute to the progression of HIV infection. Several cofactors (e.g., contracting another sexually transmitted disease) have been found to be associated with HIV progression.

It is believed that some cofactors influence HIV progression by activating latently infected CD4 cells. It appears that HIV can remain latent in CD4 cells for long periods of time. Activation signals are believed to transform a latently infected cell into a cell that actively produces virus. A productive infection can then accelerate the killing of CD4 cells (Fauci, 1988), and thus hasten the development of AIDS. The link between immune activation and HIV progression to AIDS is supported by evidence that increased levels of serum markers of immune activation, such as neopterin, are prognostic for the development of AIDS (Melmed et al., 1989).

CD4 cells latently or chronically infected with HIV can be converted to an active productive state when the cells are exposed to other viruses (Fauci, 1987). Hirsch and colleagues (1984) have proposed that interactions between HIV and other viruses may contribute to the progression of disease. Since HSV, cytomegalovirus (CMV), and human herpesvirus-6 (HHV-6) can activate a release of HIV from CD4 cells, Fauci and colleagues (Rosenberg and Fauci, 1989) and Gallo and Montagnier (1988) have hypothesized that these viruses may act as cofactors contributing to the development of AIDS.

The AIDS epidemic has resulted in exposure to a number of profound stressors among gay men, such as the risk of developing a deadly disease, repeated bereavement as friends and lovers die of AIDS, stigmatization, and alterations in sexual practices and lifestyle. There are a variety of biological pathways that might allow such stressors and other psychological factors to act as cofactors, influencing immune or viral processes associated with HIV progression (see Solomon et al., 1990). Many of these factors will be discussed in other chapters of this book.

First, psychological factors may reactivate other latent viral infections (such as HSV or CMV) which could then activate CD4 cells infected with HIV, contributing to the development of AIDS. Particular stressors, such as medical student exams, marital separation, and caring for a spouse with Alzheimers disease, have been associated with increased levels of antibody to latent viruses (i.e., HSV, EBV, and CMV), suggesting reactivation of these latent viruses under stressful conditions (Glaser et al., 1985; Kiecolt-Glaser et al., 1987a, 1987b). In addition, the data discussed above indicate that psychological factors, such as depressed mood, may be capable of either reactivating latent HSV or altering immune responses to chronic low-level production of HSV.

Second, changes in hormone or neuropeptide levels due to stressor exposure could alter the distribution of lymphocyte subsets, like CD4 cells, exacerbating immune impairment due to HIV. For example, cortisol levels are increased following exposure to some stressors and in association with depression, and increases in cortisol level have been shown to be associated with decreases in circulating lymphocytes, including CD4 cells (Parillo and Fauci, 1979; Ritchie et al., 1983).

Third, stressor exposure may influence components of the immune system that play a role in the host response and containment of HIV infection, such as natural killer (NK) cell or T-cell cytotoxicity. Research has documented changes in a variety of immune functions, such as NK activity and proliferative response to mitogenic stimulation, in association with stressful life experiences such as bereavement, or psychological states such as depression in healthy individuals (e.g., Schleifer et al., 1983). In addition, more recent studies have shown that stress exposure alters receptor expression for important lymphokines that regulate immune activity, such as the interleukin-2 (IL-2) receptor (Glaser et al., 1989). HIV also alters the expression of the IL-2 receptor on lymphocytes (Prince et al., 1984). Again, distress could exacerbate the immune changes that occur as a result of HIV infection.

We are currently conducting studies to determine if the stressors prevalent in gay men as a result of the AIDS epidemic (e.g., bereavement) and psychological responses to those stressors can act as cofactors in HIV progression, via the biological pathways described above. In the first study, we selected from among participants in the Multi-Center AIDS Cohort Study (MACS) at UCLA HIV-seropositive and -seronegative individuals who had been repeatedly bereaved over the past year as a result of the death of close friends to

AIDS (Kemeny et al., 1988; Kemeny et al., 1990). We compared them to nonbereaved individuals matched on age and HIV serostatus. Immune assessment focused on lymphocyte subsets, including the percent of CD4 cells, measures of immune activation, and one measure of immune function that is associated with advanced stages of HIV infection, the proliferative response to the mitogen, phytohemagglutinin (PHA). It was hypothesized that repeatedly bereaved individuals would show changes in the immune system consistent with HIV progression, particularly those reporting higher levels of depressed mood.

Among the HIV seropositive men, results indicated that bereaved individuals did not differ from matched controls on the immune parameters assessed. However, we found that individuals with higher levels of depressed mood who were not bereaved showed the following immune pattern: a lower percent of CD4 helper/inducer T-cells, a higher percent of CD8 cells with activation markers, and a lower proliferative response to the mitogen PHA. The strong correlations between depression and immune parameters were found not to be due to neuropsychological dysfunction in the depressed men nor to health behaviors that depressed men may engage in (i.e., recreational drug use, alcohol consumption, altered sleep patterns, and reduced exercise).

A second study of bereavement and depression was then conducted (Kemeny et al., 1989). HIV seropositive men who were bereaved of an intimate partner over the past year showed evidence of increased immune activation and decreased lymphocyte proliferation within the year following the death of the partner. In addition, higher levels of depressed mood were associated with a lower percentage of T-lymphocytes and indications of immune activation among the nonbereaved men. Thus, both studies suggest that depressed mood in nonbereaved men is associated with immune parameters relevant to HIV progression.

In a third study (Kemeny et al., 1991), preliminary data suggested that chronic depression preceded a decline in CD4 cells over a 5-year period in HIV seropositive men. If these results are confirmed, the results of these three studies would suggest that a particular form of depression may act as a cofactor for certain HIV seropositive individuals, contributing to the variable decline in CD4 cells and therefore, potentially, the course of HIV infection.

CONCLUSION

Certain latent viral infections, such as HSV and HIV, may serve as useful models for testing the clinical significance of psychologically mediated changes in the immune system, for two reasons. First, the clinical course of these infections is often quite variable and the immune system is believed to be important in contributing to this variability by influencing viral latency and/

or containment of chronically produced virus. And, second, there is anecdotal and some research support for a role for psychological factors in the course of these infections. Our research to date supports the hypothesis that certain psychological factors, particularly depressed mood, may influence immune processes relevant to the course of HSV and HIV infection. Specifically, depressed mood has been shown to be associated with the rate of HSV recurrences and certain lymphocyte subsets in individuals with chronic recurrent genital herpes. And depressed mood has been found to be associated with immune parameters relevant to the course of HIV infection in sub-groups of gay men who are HIV positive but relatively asymptomatic. Current work is underway (1) to determine whether depression precedes these immune changes (the direction of causality), (2) to pinpoint the form of depression that is most relevant to disease course, and (3) to determine the biological pathways that may underlie these relationships.

ACKNOWLEDGMENTS

The research on herpes simplex was supported in part by a grant from the Research, Evaluation and Allocation Committee (2-444949-35110-3), School of Medicine, University of California, San Francisco (UCSF), and from a Biomedical Research Support Grant (570071-30102), Langley Porter Institute, UCSF. The research on HIV infection was supported in part by the National Institute of Mental Health (NIMH) (MH42918) and the National Institute of Allergy and Infectious Diseases (N01-AI-72631). The author was supported by a Research Scientist Development Award from NIMH (MH00820).

REFERENCES

Blyth W and Hill T: Establishment, maintenance, and control of herpes simplex virus (HSV) latency. In *Immunobiology of Herpes Simplex Virus Infection,* Rouse B and Lopez C, Eds. CRC Press, Boca Raton, FL 1984.
Cohen F and Lazarus RS: Active coping processes, coping dispositions, and recovery from surgery. *Psychosom. Med.* 1973; 35:375–389.
Cohen F: Psychological Preparation, Coping, and Recovery from Surgery. Ph.D. thesis. University of California, Berkeley, 1975.
Cohen F and Lazarus RS: Coping with the stresses of illness. In *Health Psychology: A Handbook.* Stone GC, Cohen F, Adler NE, et al., Eds. Jossey-Bass, San Francisco 1979, pp. 217–254.
Cohen F and Lazarus RS: Coping and adaptation in health and illness. In *Handbook of Health, Health Care, and the Health Professions.* Mechanic D, Ed. Free Press, New York 1983, pp. 608–635.

Cohen F, Reese LB, Kaplan GA, and Riggio RE: Coping with the stresses of arthritis. In *Arthritis and the Elderly,* Moskowitz RW and Haug M, Eds. Springer-Verlag, New York 1986, pp. 47–56.

Cohen F, Kemeny M, Kearney K, Zegans L, Neuhaus J, Conant M, and Stites D: Psychological states, immunity, and genital herpes recurrence: stress, mood and personality as predictors. Submitted, 1991.

Curran JW, Jaffe HW, Hardy AM, Morgan WM, Selk RM, and Dondero TJ: Epidemiology of HIV infection and AIDS in the United States. *Science* 1988; 239:610–616.

Detels R, English PA, Giorgi JV, Visscher BR, Fahey JL, Taylor JMG, Dudley JP, Nishanian P, Munoz A, Phair JP, Polk BF, and Rinaldo CR: Patterns of CD4+ cell changes after HIV-1 infection indicate the existence of a co-determinant of AIDS. *J. AIDS* 1988; 1:390–395.

Fahey JL, Giorgi JV, Martinez-Maza O, Detels R, and Taylor JMG: Immune pathogenesis of AIDS and related syndromes. *Ann. Inst. Pasteur Immunol.* 1987; 138:245–252.

Fauci A: AIDS: Immunopathogenic mechanisms and research strategies. *Clin Res.* 1987; 35:503–510.

Fauci A: The human immunodeficiency virus: infectivity and mechanisms of pathogenesis. *Science* 1988; 239:617–622.

Friedman E, Katcher A, and Brightman V: Incidence of recurrent herpes labialis and upper respiratory infection: a prospective study of the influence of biologic, social, and psychologic predictors. *Oral Surg.* 1977; 43:873–878.

Gallo RC and Montagnier L: AIDS in 1988. *Sci. Am.* 1988; 259:40–48.

Glaser R, Kiecolt-Glaser JK, Speicher CE, and Holliday JE: Stress, loneliness, and changes in herpesvirus latency. *J. Behav. Med.* 1985; 8:249–260.

Goldmeier D and Johnson A: Does psychiatric illness affect the recurrence rate of genital herpes? *Br. J. Vener. Dis.* 1982; 54:40–43.

Hill TJ: Herpes simplex virus latency. In *The Herpes Viruses,* Roizman B, Ed. Plenum Press, New York 1985, pp. 175–240.

Hirsch MS, Schooley RT, Ho DD, and Kaplan JC: Possible viral interactions in the acquired immunodeficiency syndrome (AIDS). *Rev. Infect. Dis.* 1984; 6:726–731.

Katcher A, Honori A, Brightman B, Luborsky L, and Ship I: Prediction of the incidence of recurrent herpes labialis and systemic illness from psychological measurements. *J. Dent. Res.* 1973; 52:49–58.

Kemeny ME: Psychological and Immunological Predictors of Genital Herpes Recurrence. Ph.D. thesis. University of California, San Francisco 1985.

Kemeny M, Cohen F, and Zegans L: The relationship of coping strategies to immunity and genital herpes recurrence. Paper presented at Society of Behavioral Medicine Annu. Conf. San Francisco March, 1986.

Kemeny M, Fahey JL, Schneider S, Weiner H, Taylor S, and Visscher B: Bereavement associated alterations in phenotypes of lymphocytes in HIV+ and HIV− homosexual men. Paper presented at 4th Int. Conf. AIDS. Stockholm June, 1988.

Kemeny M, Fahey JL, Schneider S, Taylor S, Weiner H, and Visscher B: Psychosocial cofactors in HIV infection: bereavement, depression and immune response in HIV+ and HIV− homosexual men. Paper presented at Federation of American Societies of Experimental Biologists Conf. New Orleans March, 1989.

Kemeny M, Duran R, Weiner H, Taylor S, Visscher B, and Fahey JL: Bereavement of partner and immune processes in HIV seropositive and negative homosexual men. Paper presented at 7th Int. Conf. AIDS. Florence, Italy 1991.

Kemeny ME, Weiner H, Taylor SE, Schneider S, Visscher B, and Fahey JL: Repeated bereavement, depressed mood, and immune response in HIV seropositive and seronegative homosexual men. Submitted, 1991.

Kiecolt-Glaser JK, Fisher LD, Ogrocki P, Stout JC, Speicher CE, and Glaser R: Marital quality, marital disruption, and immune function. *Psychosom. Med.* 1987a; 49:13–34.

Kiecolt-Glaser JK, Glaser R, Shuttleworth EC, Dyer CS, Ogrocki P, and Speicher CE: Chronic stress and immunity in family caregivers of Alzheimer's disease victims. *Psychosom. Med.* 1987b; 49:523–535.

Lopez C, Kirkpatrick D, Read S, Fitzgerald P, Pitt J, Pahwa S, Ching C, and Smithwick E: Correlation between low natural killing of fibroblasts infected with herpes simplex virus type 1 and susceptibility to herpes virus infections. *J. Infect. Dis.* 1983; 147:1030–1035.

Melmed RN, Taylor JMG, Detels R, Bozorgmehri M, and Fahey JL: Serum neopterin changes in HIV infected subjects: indicators of significant pathology, CD4 T cell changes and the development of AIDS. *J. AIDS* 1989; 2:70–76.

Parillo JE and Fauci AS: Mechanisms of gluccocorticoid action on immune processes. *Annu. Rec. Pharmacol. Toxicol.* 1979; 19:179–201.

Prince H, Kermani-Arab V, and Fahey J: Depressed interleukin-2 receptor expression in acquired immune deficiency and lymphadenopathy syndromes. *J. Immunol.* 1984; 133:1313–1317.

Ritchie AW, Oswald I, Micklem HS, Boyd JE, Elton RA, Jazwinska E, and James K: Circadian variation of lymphocyte sub-populations: a study with monoclonal antibodies. *Br. Med. J.* 1983; 286:1773–1775.

Rosenberg ZF and Fauci AS: Mini-review: induction of expression of HIV in latently or chronically infected cells. *AIDS Res. Hum. Retroviruses* 1989; 5:1.

Rouse BT: Cell-mediated immune mechanisms. In *Immunobiology of Herpes Simplex Virus Infection*, Rouse B and Lopez C, Eds. CRC Press, Boca Raton, FL 1985, pp. 107–120.

Schleifer SJ, Keller SE, Camerino M, Thornton JC, and Stein M: Suppression of lymphocyte stimulation following bereavement. *JAMA* 1983; 250:374–377.

Sheridan J, Donnerberg A, Aurelian L, and Elpern D: Immunity to herpes simplex virus type 2. IV. Impaired lymphokine production during recrudescence correlates with an imbalance in T lymphocyte subsets. *J. Immunol.* 1982; 129:326–331.

Solomon GF, Kemeny ME, and Temoshok L: Psychoneuroimmunologic aspects of human immunodeficiency virus infection. In *Psychoneuroimmunology II*. Ader R, Felten DL, and Cohen N, Eds. Academic Press, Orlando 1991.

Watson D and Clark LA: Negative affectivity: the disposition to experience aversive emotional states. *Psychol. Bull.* 1984; 96:465–490.

Physical Exercise and Immunity

Robert C. Hickson
and
James B. Boone, Jr.
College of Kinesiology
University of Illinois at Chicago
Chicago, Illinois,

INTRODUCTION

Regularly performed exercise is associated with a number of physiological, biochemical, psychological, and health-related benefits. These include improved fitness, exercise capacity, and cardiovascular function, metabolic changes within muscle that are geared to the type of training performed, feelings of well-being, decreased coronary risk factors, retardation of the age-related decline in exercise performance, improvement in the quality of life, and possibly increased longevity. Because of the widespread effects physical training has been shown to exhibit, it is possible that the beneficial effects of exercise would also carry over to the immune system. Several reports and reviews give the impression of an improved immune state with exercise (cf., Green et al., 1981; Simon, 1984; Nash, 1986), while others suggest there is an increased susceptibility or a decreased resistance to minor infections in athletes (cf., Asgeirsson and Bellanti, 1987; Tomasi et al., 1982; Jokl, 1974; Roberts, 1986; Nash et al., 1986; Peters and Bateman, 1983; Lewicki et al., 1987). Additionally, the stress hormones (catecholamines and glucocorticoids), which are released during exercise, are known to generate an environment conducive to immunosuppression (cf., Hedman, 1980; Balow et al., 1975; Eriksson and Hedfors, 1977).

In attempting to further determine whether exercise can produce immunostimulation or immunosuppression, evaluation of the available information has been classified into several sections. The first two sections will examine whether there is a specific range of exercise durations or exercise intensities that are associated with positive or negative immune responses. The third category will investigate whether the immune responses to exercise are short-lived, long-lasting, or even delayed. Another section will evaluate the role of training on immune adaptations at rest and during exercise. Finally, consideration is given to the known mechanisms that may regulate the exercise effects. Since lymphocyte and natural killer responses to exercise have received considerable attention as well as the fact that mounting of the immune response is a function of the lymphocytes, a major portion of the review is directed at evaluating these parameters.

EXERCISE DURATION

Previous studies that have examined the influence of single bouts of exercise on the immune system have employed a wide variety of durations, from just a few minutes of cycling or stairclimbing to several hours of exercise such as marathon running. Consequently, an attempt was made to distinguish short-term from medium- and long-term responses. The exercise durations were arbitrarily classified into three durations of 5 to 25, 35 to 65, and 118 to 240 min based on the available data in the literature. The purpose was to determine if a specific duration or range of durations might enhance immune functioning, as well as to evaluate what durations are more conducive to immunosuppression.

As shown in Table I, short-duration exercise generally results in an increase in the absolute levels of total lymphocytes, total T-cells, T-helper (T_4) cells, T-suppressor (T_8) cells, B-cells, and natural killer cells. Natural killer cytotoxicity is also increased. When evaluated on a relative basis, the data indicate an increase in total lymphocytes, a decrease in total T-cells and T-helper cells, no change in T-suppressor cells (a reduction in the T_4/T_8 ratio is generally found), an increase in the percentage of B-cells, although no change or a decrease has also been observed, and an increase in natural killer cells.

A similar pattern can be seen with exercise of medium duration (35 to 65 min), although studies have reported no changes in the relative amount of total lymphocytes, and no increase in T- or B-cell numbers (Table I). With 2 h of exercise or more, total lymphocyte number, the number of total T-cells, and T_4 and T_8 cells have been observed to remain unchanged. A decrease in B-cell number may also be observed with long-term exercise (Table I).

Since the data were somewhat more limited, *in vitro* lymphocyte functioning in the presence of some commonly studied mitogens was classified into two rather than three exercise-duration categories of 5 to 36 and 118 to 240 min (Table II). When exercise lasts from 5 to 36 min, lymphocyte proliferation is either unchanged or decreased immediately after exercise. Generally, with long-term exercise of at least 2 h, there is a depressed blastogenic response to the various mitogens. In examining spontaneous blastogenesis, which is determined in the absence of specific mitogens and is thought to reflect *in vivo* stimulation of lymphocytes, Nieman et al. (1989a) found increased activity during 3 h of treadmill running to exhaustion.

One of the main conclusions of this section appears to be that long-term exercise may predispose an individual to more of an immunosuppressive state than short-term exercise. The data in Table I suggest that the mobilization of lymphocytes, T-cells, and the lymphocyte subpopulations following a short-term exercise bout can become reversed with longer exercise durations. In support of this observation, Nieman et al. (1989b) have observed both an increase and later a reduction in total lymphocytes with prolonged physical activity. In contrast to the possible lymphocyte suppression by exercise, the consensus findings show that the natural killer cell responses, number, and cytotoxicity appear to be increased by most exercise durations reported to date. The discrepancies seen with *in vitro* mitogenesis vs. spontaneous blastogenesis require further investigation.

EXERCISE INTENSITY

There is some evidence that moderate exercise intensity may be optimal for immune stimulation (cf., Mackinnon and Tomasi, 1986). Nevertheless, the role of exercise intensity was evaluated by separating the results of previous studies into four categories (Table III). Three of the categories are based on specific ranges of maximal oxygen uptake ($\dot{V}O_2$max) and were obtained directly or estimated from other measurements (i.e., heart rate) within the individual investigations. Since several studies used a protocol where exercise intensity was progressively increased to maximum, this format is included in the table as the fourth category.

Based on the data in Table III exercise intensities at 30% of $\dot{V}O_2$max or less may not change the various lymphocyte parameters. At 50 to 70% of $\dot{V}O_2$max, there are decreases in the percentage of T-cells and T_4 cells, while the percentage of T_8 cells remains unchanged or increases, B-cells are unchanged, and natural killer cells are increased. On an absolute level, exercise at 50 to 70% of VO_2max generally increases total lymphocyte, T-cell, B-cell, and T_4, T_8, and natural killer cell numbers. At 70 to 90% of $\dot{V}O_2$max, and during progressive exercise to exhaustion, somewhat similar lymphocyte effects are observed as found at 50 to 70% of VO_2max. However, the absence

TABLE I.
Peripheral Blood Total Lymphocyte, Lymphocyte Subpopulation, and Natural Killer Cell Responses Following Exercise of Various Durations

References	Time of Exercise	Total Lymphocytes Rel	Abs	T-cells Rel	Abs	T-Helper Rel	Abs	T-Suppressor Rel	Abs	B-Cell Rel	Abs	NK Cells Rel	Abs	NK Cytotoxic Activity
	5–25 min													
Steel et al., 1974			↑	→	NC					↑				↑
Hedfors et al., 1976		↑	↑	→	↑					↑	↑			NC
Hedfors et al., 1978		↑		→						↑	↑			↑
Targan et al., 1981														↑
Soppi et al., 1982		↑	↑	NC						NC				
Edwards et al., 1984		↑	↑	→	↑	NC	↑			↑	↑		↑	
Landmann et al., 1984				→	↑		↑		↑	↑	↑	↑	↑	
Brahmi et al., 1985		↑	↑	→		→	→	NC				↑		↑
Masuhara et al., 1987				→		→		NC	↑	→	↑	↑	↑	
Deuster et al., 1988		↑	↑	→	↑	→				→	NC	↑	↑	↑
Fiatarone et al., 1988												↑	↑	↑
Lewicki et al., 1988		↑	↑	→	↑	→	↑	NC	↑	NC	↑		↑	
Ferry et al., 1990		↑												↑
	35–65 min													
Eskola et al., 1978		NC												
Hanson and Flaherty, 1981											NC			↑
Robertson et al., 1981		→	↑	→	NC									
Pedersen et al., 1988		↑		→		→		NC				↑		↑

118–240 min

	118–240 min						
Eskola et al., 1978	NC						
Moorthy and Zimmerman, 1978							
Gmunder et al., 1988	↑	NC	NC		↑		
Nieman et al., 1989	NC	NC	NC	NC	NC	↑	
	NC	NC	NC	NC	NC	→	
Oshida et al., 1988	↑	→	→	↑NC	NC	↑	↑

NC = no change, Rel = relative, Abs = absolute.

TABLE II.
In Vitro Lymphocyte Mitogenesis Following Exercise of Various Durations

References	Exercise Duration (min)	Phytohemagglutinin PHA (T-, B-cells)	Concanavalin A ConA (T-cells)	Pokeweed Mitogen PWM (T-, B-cells)	Lipopolysaccharide LPS (B-cells)
	5–36 min				
Hedfors et al., 1976		→	→	→	NC
Eskola et al., 1978		NC	NC		
Robertson et al., 1981		→	NC	NC	
Soppi et al., 1982		→	→→		
Edwards et al., 1984			NC		
	118–240 min				
Eskola et al., 1978		→ NC	→		
Moorthy and Zimmerman, 1978					
Gmunder et al., 1988			→		
Oshida et al., 1988		→			

NC = no change, Rel = relative, Abs = absolute.

of change in lymphocytosis seen in several of these studies, particularly at 70 to 90% of $\dot{V}O_2$max, may also in large part be attributed to interaction of the long-term duration component of the exercise.

Natural killer cell cytotoxicity is seen to increase at most exercise intensities (Table III). Lymphocyte functioning of selected mitogens generally appears to remain unchanged or decreased at all exercise intensities (Table IV). From the data in Tables III and IV there does not appear to be any singular exercise intensity range that is more favorable or harmful to the immune system than any other. If exercise intensity at 50 to 70% of $\dot{V}O_2$max can be considered moderate, then the responses to moderate exercise are very similar in direction to high-intensity exercise protocols to exhaustion. In a number of the moderate- and high-intensity exercise protocols examined, the similar responses were obtained at similar exercise durations. Keast et al. (1988) have proposed that a more accurate measure of the role of various types of exercise is possible based on a selective stressing of various energy metabolism systems. Nonetheless, an immunological distinction based on acute exercise of moderate vs. high intensity has not yet been clearly delineated.

RAPID VS. LONG-LASTING EFFECTS OF EXERCISE ON THE IMMUNE SYSTEM

Another of the major questions that requires consideration in determining the positive or counterproductive effects of exercise on the immune system is the length of time in which these responses are expressed, or even if certain effects are delayed and are expressed later on. Of the studies that have followed a time course of circulatory changes after exercise, total lymphocytes and relative changes in T_3, T_4, T_8, and natural killer cells returned to pre-exercise values within 24 h (Robertson et al., 1981; Brahmi et al., 1985; Pedersen et al., 1988; Oshida et al., 1988). Several studies examined earlier time points and observed that lymphocyte subpopulations returned within 15 min (Robertson et al., 1981), 1 h (Deuster et al., 1988), 2 h (Brahmi et al., 1985; Pedersen et al., 1988), or even during exercise (Nieman et al., 1989a).

The increased natural killer cell cytotoxicity with exercise has been reported to be still elevated 24 h after an 8-mile run at 72% $\dot{V}O_2$max (Hanson and Flaherty, 1981). In contrast, two cycling studies (Brahmi et al., 1985; Pedersen et al., 1988) of 12 to 18 min to exhaustion or 60 min at 80% of $\dot{V}O_2$max show that the increased natural killer cytotoxicity then decreases by 120 min post-exercise and returns to pre-exercise levels by 24 h. The post-exercise reversal of natural killer cytotoxicity is thought to be related to inhibition by prostaglandins that are released by monocytes (Pedersen et al., 1988).

Lymphocyte functioning, which is depressed immediately after exercise,

TABLE III.
Peripheral Blood Total Lymphocyte, Lymphocyte Subpopulation, and Natural Killer Cell Responses Following Exercise of Various Intensities

References	Intensity	Total Lymphocytes		T-cells		T-Helper		T-Suppressor		B-Cell		Natural Killer (NK) Cells		NK Cytotoxic Activity
		Rel	Abs	Rel	Abs	Rel	Abs	Rel	Abs	Rel	Abs	Rel	Abs	
Pedersen et al., 1988	≤30% of $\dot{V}O_2$ max			NC		NC		NC				NC		
Hedfors et al., 1976	~50–70% of $\dot{V}O_2$ max	↑	↑	↓	↑					↑	↑			↑
Hedfors et al., 1978		↑	↑	↓	↑					↑	↑			NC ↑
Targan et al., 1981		↑	↑		↑						↑		↑	
Landmann et al., 1984		↑	↑	↓		↓	↑		↑	↑	↑		↑	
Oshida et al., 1988	70–90% of $\dot{V}O_2$ max							↑NC		NC		↑		
Steel et al., 1974			↑	↓	NC						↑			
Eskola et al., 1978		NC			NC									
Moorthy and Zimmerman, 1978			↑	NC							↑			
Hanson and Flaherty, 1981				NC	↑					NC				
Edwards et al., 1984			↑	NC		NC	NC	↑	NC	NC	↑ ↓		↑	↑
Gmunder et al., 1988		NC	NC	NC							↓			↑

Increasing to Exhaustion (≤20 min)

Study											
Pedersen et al., 1988	←		↓		←		NC		←		↑
Nieman et al., 1989	NC		NC		NC	NC	NC	↑		↑	
Robertson et al., 1981	←		→						↑		↑
Soppi et al., 1982	←		NC	↑							
Brahmi et al., 1985	←		→	←		NC	NC		↑		
Masuhara et al., 1987	←		→	←	↑	NC	NC	→	←	←	
Deuster et al., 1988			→					→		←	
Fiatarone et al., 1988	←					←	←	NC	←	←	←
Lewicki et al., 1988	←		←	←	←	←			←	←	←
Ferry et al., 1990	←	←	→		←	NC	NC	←	←	↑	←

NC = no change, Rel = relative, Abs = absolute.

TABLE IV.
In Vitro Lymphocyte Mitogenesis Following Exercise of Various Intensities

References	Exercise Intensity (min)	Phytohemagglutinin PHA (T-, B-cells)	Concanavalin A ConA (T-cells)	Pokeweed Mitogen PWM (T-, B-cells)	Lipopolysaccharide LPS (B-cells)
Hedfors et al., 1978	50–70% of $\dot{V}o_2$ max	↓	↓	↓	NC
Oshida et al., 1988		↓			
Eskola et al., 1978	70–90% of $\dot{V}o_2$ max	↓NC	↓NC		
Moorthy and Zimmerman, 1978		NC			
Edwards et al., 1984			NC↓		
Gmunder et al., 1988					
Robertson et al., 1981	Increase to Exhaustion (<20 min)	↓	NC↓	NC	
Soppi et al., 1982		↓			

NC = no change, Rel = relative, Abs = absolute.

has been shown to remain depressed 3 h after a marathon (Eskola et al., 1978), but returned to pre-exercise values by 24 h. Several other studies observed a return to pre-exercise levels by 24 or 48 h (Oshida et al., 1988; Gmunder et al., 1988), as earlier time points were not measured. Robertson et al. (1981) showed that the reduction in concanavalin A (ConA) and phytohemagglutinin (PHA) mitogenesis was reversed within 15 min following short-duration exercise. The increased spontaneous blastogenesis observed during a 3-h run still remained elevated when measured 24 h later (Wieman et al., 1989a).

There is a precedent for immunostimulatory responses to be refractory or delayed following the introduction of various stimuli. Short-term daily stress (auditory) in mice induced an initial depression of splenic B- (lipopolysaccharide [LPS]) and T-cell (ConA) functions and natural killer activity over several days (Monjan and Collector, 1977). With longer exposure to the same stress, an enhancement of these variables was observed. Additionally, epinephrine injections resulted in a decline in the peripheral blood mononuclear cell T_4/T_8 ratio 60 min after injection (Crary et al., 1983b). But, by 2 h post-injection, there was approximately a 50% increase above baseline levels in this ratio. The data from several exercise investigations also exhibit a similar phenomenon. Gmunder et al. (1988) observed that total T-cells and T_4 cells had increased above baseline levels 48 h after a marathon run. Similarly, the T_4/T_8 ratio was elevated (due to a decrease in T_8 cells) 1.5 and 21 h after an exhausting 3-h treadmill run (Nieman et al., 1989a).

Overall, the studies that have reported various forms of apparent immunosuppression accompanying an acute exercise bout demonstrate a return to baseline conditions over several minutes to hours. The susceptibility to increased infection is greater during these "transient immune depressive" periods and would seemingly represent an opportune time for the initiation of infection. Moreover, it is encouraging that several acute exercise studies have shown a positive, persistent effect on some immune variables. Furthermore, the fact that immunostimulation can appear later on, rather than initially, indirectly suggests that exercise training on a regular basis has the potential for improving immune functions.

TRAINING AND IMMUNE RESPONSES

Comparison of Trained Vs. Untrained Individuals

In evaluating the positive or negative effects of regular exercise on immunity, Green et al. (1981) measured selected immune parameters and administered a questionnaire to male marathon runners. They subjectively expressed an increased resistance to infection, but no differences in leukocyte function or in quantitative immunoglobulins were seen out of the normal range. Nieman et al. (1989b) also did not find any differences in immuno-globulins before or after a graded maximal exercise test in marathoners and controls. However, resting and post-exercise complement levels were lower in the athletes than in the controls (Nieman et al., 1989b). Salivary IgA concentrations were demonstrated to be lower in cross-country skiers than in age-matched controls (Tomasi et al., 1982).

Brahmi et al. (1985) observed no differences in the percent of total T-lymphocytes, T_4, T_8, and natural killer cells, and natural killer cytotoxicity following progressive exercise to exhaustion (12 to 18 min) in males who endurance trained regularly vs. untrained males or females. Oshida et al. (1988) observed no endurance training differences in blastogenesis using PHA, or in total lymphocytes, or in the percentage of T- or B-lymphocytes, and T_4, T_8, and natural killer cells at rest. In this study, cycling at 60% $\dot{V}O_2$max for 2 h doubled the percentage of natural killer cells in the circulation in the athletes, but not in the nonathletes. The data of Pedersen et al. (1989) provide further support for an endurance training effect on natural killer cells. The percentage of natural killer cells and natural killer cytotoxicity at rest were higher in highly trained cyclists than in untrained individuals.

Until recently, the influence of strength training on the immune system has received no attention. Strength and endurance training for the most part produce completely diversified adaptations. In general terms, the former results in increased muscle strength, muscle enlargement, and ability to rapidly resynthesize ATP from immediate sources of energy (cf., Hickson, 1980; Hickson et al., 1980). The latter results in an increased maximal oxygen uptake, ability to sustain prolonged intense exercise, and increased capacity to generate energy aerobically without any increase in muscle size or strength (cf., Holloszy and Booth, 1976). In studying strength-trained individuals, Calabrese et al. (1989) did not find any differences in resting total lymphocytes, total T-cells, or T_4 and T_8 cells among anabolic-steroid-using and steroid-free bodybuilders as well as sedentary controls. B-cell mitogenesis was increased in the steroid users. Natural killer cell activity was also elevated in the steroid users, but not in the steroid-free group, while serum immunoglobin, IgA, was lower in the steroid users than in the controls.

Responses to Endurance Training Regimens

Generally positive effects of training have been observed following two human training studies in which the subjects had not previously been exercising on a regular basis. Soppi et al. (1982) did not find any effects of the Finnish 6-week naval training program on total blood lymphocyte number at rest. However, following a progressive cycling test to exhaustion in approximately 20 min, there was a smaller increase after training than prior to training, although the percent of T-cells was not different. Lymphocyte transformation using PHA and ConA at rest was higher after training. Furthermore, on a per cell basis, the cycling test decreased mitogenesis using PHA and ConA to a smaller extent after than before training. Similarly, Watson et al. (1986) observed increased T-cell mitogenesis and an increased percentage of T-lymphocytes in peripheral blood at rest following a program of walk-jog-run 45 to 60 min/d, 5 d/week, for 15 weeks. However, natural killer cell lysis was reduced, perhaps due to increased formation of mature T-lymphocytes, while β-blockade did not alter these training responses. The reason for the disparity between these data and the higher natural killer cell activity observed in cyclists (Pedersen et al., 1989) is not known.

In a training study of a population of highly conditioned cyclists, Ferry et al. (1990) examined immune responses before and following a 5-month interval of training. They observed no changes in resting relative lymphocyte subpopulation differences, although relative and total lymphocytes were higher in the cyclists than in a separate control group. Lymphocyte mobilization of T_4, T_8, and T_{11} cells to maximal exercise was reduced after training, a finding similar to that of Soppi et al. (1982). However, Gimenez et al. (1987) has reported similar lymphocytosis following strenuous exercise in trained and untrained subjects.

In training studies using rodents, Hoffman-Goetz et al. (1986) reported that 4 weeks of treadmill running in mice reduced total splenic lymphocytes from those in untrained animals, when examined 30 min after the last training session. When trained rats were rested 48 h, these differences were eliminated. Splenic proliferative responses using ConA were reduced in trained rats, even when compared with exercising untrained animals. On the other hand, Mahan and Young (1989) found that the reduction in splenic mitogenesis using ConA was less in swim-trained (for 10 weeks) than in untrained rats when both groups were swum to exhaustion. ConA blastogenesis was reduced in sedentary and untrained-exhausted rats but stimulated in trained-exhausted rats when splenic macrophage fractions were added to spleen cells. Indomethacin, a cyclooxygenase inhibitor, attenuated the macrophage-mediated suppression in sedentary and untrained-exhausted rats (Mahan and Young, 1989). The addition of prostaglandin E_2 inhibited the ConA blastogenic responses in sedentary and untrained-exhausted rats, but not in the trained-exhausted rats (Mahan and Young, 1989). The discrepancy between these two studies could be related to the extent of training (4 vs. 10 weeks) and even the type of training. The reduced mitogenic responses in the trained animals may be related to the fact that the animals may not undergo immunological adaptation to the running in just 4 weeks, whereas, with swim training, the 10-week exercise period was sufficient to detect differences between trained and untrained mice.

Other evidence for beneficial effects of endurance training on immunity are the increased antibody levels after immunization in trained mice (Liu and

Wang, 1987). Endurance training has also been shown to retard tumor growth (Rusch and Kline, 1944; Hoffman et al., 1962; Good and Fernandes, 1981), increase survival times in mice infected with bacteria (Cannon and Kluger, 1984) and tumor inoculation (Rashkis, 1952), and increase phagocytic activity of peritoneal macrophages (Fehr et al., 1988). In epidemological studies, job-related activity was found to be associated with a reduction in colon cancer (Garabrant et al., 1984; Vena et al., 1985; Gerhardsson et al., 1986); and former female college athletes were associated with a lower incidence of breast and reproductive system cancers (Frisch et al., 1985). On the negative side, weanling mice who were exercised by swimming and infected with a virus displayed reduced serum interferon activity and neutralizing antibodies when compared with infected sedentary mice (Reyes and Lerner, 1976).

POTENTIAL MODULATORS OF THE IMMUNE RESPONSES TO EXERCISE

Lymphocyte Responses

Both circulating catecholamines and glucocorticoids have been considered to participate in the regulation of lymphocyte responsiveness to exercise. Epinephrine administration at rest is known to increase blood lymphocytes (Martin, 1932; Eriksson and Hedfors, 1977; Samuels, 1951). The lymphocytosis induced by epinephrine did not change the percentage of total T-cells, T_8 cells, or B-cells, but reduced T_4 cells (Crary et al., 1983b).

Elevated levels of blood glucocorticoids are known to cause lymphocytopenia (Clarke et al., 1977; Fauci and Dale, 1974). Pretreatment with glucocorticoids in humans *in vivo* is known to suppress the exercise-induced rise in the absolute numbers of T- and B-lymphocytes, with the depression more marked in T-cells (Yu et al., 1974). Introduction of a swimming stress to mice results in elevated corticosterone and depression of thoracic duct T-lymphocytes (Hedman, 1980).

Plasma catecholamines are known to be secreted during moderate to strenuous exercise (cf., Winder et al., 1978, 1979), while circulating cortisol concentrations generally increase with long-term rather than short-term exercise (Eskola et al., 1978; Robertson et al., 1981; Landmann et al., 1984). Consequently, the increases in total lymphocytes, total T-cells, the percentage decrease in T-helper, and increases in T-suppressor and B-cells following short-duration exercise (and in the early phase of long-duration activity) are consistent with the known catecholamine effects on lymphocytes in resting individuals. Several studies show good correlations of exercise-induced lymphocytosis with plasma levels of epinephrine (Masuhara et al., 1987) and norepinephrine (Nieman et al., 1989b). The absence of changes or decreases in total lymphocytes, total T-cells, T_4, T_8, and B-cell numbers that have been observed following long-duration exercise (see Table I) are also compatible with the actions of glucocorticoid hormones. Nevertheless, Gmunder et al. (1988) observed both epinephrine and cortisol to be elevated along with reduced lymphocyte responsiveness following a marathon run. Thus, the control of lymphocyte action may be more complex than through dual hormonal regulation.

Another mechanism by which the lymphocytosis of exercise may become down-regulated is through the training state of the individual. It has been shown that the elevated catecholamine response to submaximal exercise is blunted by endurance training (Winder et al., 1979). Therefore, the smaller rise in catecholamines may produce a smaller lymphocytosis, as has been observed following a training program (Soppi et al., 1982). On the other hand, the increase in O_2 uptake during exercise may represent a nonhormonal factor in the up-regulation of lymphocytosis following short-term strenuous exercise. Masuhara et al. (1987) observed that the increase in percent of $\dot{V}O_2$max during exercise was correlated with the lymphocytosis.

Glucocorticoids, catecholamines, and opioids are also known to alter lymphocyte proliferative responses. Glucocorticoid treatment, both *in vitro* and *in vivo,* generally shows an inhibition of lymphocyte proliferation using ConA, PHA, and pokeweed mitogen (PWM) to varying degrees (Heilman et al., 1973; Fauci and Dale, 1974; Blomgren, 1974; Balow et al., 1975; Clemmensen et al., 1976; Fauci, 1976; Clarke et al., 1977). The magnitude of effects is also related to the type of steroid administered (Heilman et al., 1973; Blomgren, 1974; Fauci and Dale, 1974; Barlow et al., 1975; Fauci, 1976; Clarke et al., 1977). *In vivo* administration of epinephrine also reduces ConA, PWM, and PHA at various time points in mononuclear cells up to 60 min post-injection (Crary et al., 1983a). *In vitro* treatment by epinephrine at pharmacologic doses had no effect on PHA or PWM (Crary et al., 1983b). β-endorphins have been found to increase *in vitro* mitogenesis of ConA and PHA when presented to rat splenic lymphocytes in physiological concentrations (Gilman et al., 1982).

The depression of lymphocyte mitogenesis following a number of short- and long-term exercise protocols may be regulated, in part, by catecholamine and glucocorticoid suppression of activity, while opioid involvement, perhaps acting as a counterbalancing hormone with positive effects, requires additional study. Epinephrine inhibition may play a larger role than cortisol in humans, since its effects appear more rapid. Another previously suggested possibility (Landmann et al., 1984) is that the decline in the T_4/T_8 ratio immediately following exercise might explain the reduced T-lymphocyte functioning at this time, although this reduction may be secondary to the catecholamine- or glucocorticoid-induced suppression of T_4 cells. Whole blood vs. isolated lymphocytes in the assay may also be related to the responses. Eskola et al. (1978) reported no change in ConA and PHA after 35 min using whole blood;

whereas, other studies of similar duration (see Table II) have reported decreases in mitogenesis when isolated lymphocytes were used.

Other components within the circulation, such as androgenic compounds (Calabrese et al., 1989) and prolactin (Drago et al., 1989), may also be involved in lymphocyte responsiveness. Androgens have been found to be immunosuppressive (Hirota et al., 1976), although the results of Calabrese et al. (1989) in stength-trained individuals suggest otherwise. The action of prolactin may serve to counteract the responses to the stress hormones. In particular, prolactin may antagonize the adrenocorticotropin hormone (ACTH)-glucocorticoid hormone activation (Drago et al., 1989).

Natural Killer Activity

Unlike the exercise responses, other forms of stress, including thermal injury, trauma, acute myocardial infarction, inescapable foot shock, and tail electroshock, are associated with suppressed natural killer cell activity (Kraut and Greenberg, 1986; Aarstad et al., 1983; Shavit et al., 1984; Blazar et al., 1986; Irwin et al., 1986; Klarlund et al., 1987). Stress is associated with a decreased interferon production by leukocytes along with the decline in natural killer activity (Glaser et al., 1986). Shavit et al. (1984) reported that one type of inescapable foot-shock procedure, which induced opioid analgesia, reduced splenic natural killer activity. The suppression of natural killer activity was reversed by the opioid antagonist naltrexone. However, these data were obtained after a 4-d treatment period and may indicate that repeated exposure to opioids may lead to a reversal of the initial stimulatory effects. By contrast, Kraut and Greenberg (1986) found that the suppression of splenic natural killer activity 30 and 60 min after onset was reversed by naltrexone or naloxone. However, morphine or β-endorphin injection enhanced splenic natural killer activity (Kraut and Greenberg, 1986).

In general, opioid compounds (β-endorphins, methionine- and leucine-enkephalins) have been shown to increase the *in vitro* natural killer activity of human peripheral blood mononuclear cells (Mathews et al., 1983; Kay et al., 1984; Froelick and Bankhurst, 1984; Faith et al., 1984; Morley et al., 1987; Mandler et al., 1986). β-endorphin also can increase the interferon production of large granular lymphocytes (Mandler et al., 1986). The β-endorphin action appears to occur by the nonopioid fragments of this compound (Kay et al., 1987). Besides these blood constituents, both interferon and interleukin-2 can also up-regulate natural killer activity in humans (Herberman et al., 1979; Henney et al., 1981; Pedersen et al., 1988). Interleukin-2 production may be stimulated through interleukin-1 (Lewicki et al., 1988).

Epinephrine administration can increase peripheral blood natural killer activity *in vivo* within 15 to 30 min of injection, with the rise in activity correlated with plasma epinephrine levels (Tønneson et al., 1984). *In vitro* studies also indicate that epinephrine treatment stimulates natural killer cell activity at 10^{-7} and 10^{-9} M (Hellstrand et al., 1985), whereas pharmacologic levels ($\sim 10^{-6}$ M) of epinephrine can reduce natural killer activity (Brahmi et al., 1985; Hellstrand et al., 1985). Evidence for a β-adrenergic-mediated regulation was present for both dual effects (Hellstrand et al., 1985).

Glucocorticoid treatment has been reported to enhance natural killer cy-totoxicity after 4 h when given intravenously (Onsrud and Thorsby, 1981; Katz et al., 1984). However, this effect is mediated by a reversible redistri-bution (depletion) of nonnatural killer cells from the circulation, as natural killer cells appear to be glucocorticoid resistant (Katz et al., 1984; Onsrud and Thorsby, 1981). Long-term glucocorticoid therapy depresses natural killer activity (Pedersen et al., 1984). Glucocorticoid inhibition of natural killer cell activity is well established, when studied *in vitro* (Pedersen and Beyer, 1986; Gatti et al., 1987).

Thus far, interleukin-1, interferon, catecholamines, and opioids may in-dividually or cumulatively have a role in the enhanced natural killer activity associated with exercise. Brahmi et al. (1985) observed no *in vitro* stimulation of natural killer activity by epinephrine in cells at all exercise time points. However, based on the data from *in vivo* effects of catecholamines on natural killer activity, they still remain as a possible regulator of natural killer action. Interferon is known to increase after moderate (70% of $\dot{V}O_2$max) exercise of 1 h duration (Viti et al., 1985). Furthermore, several studies (Brahmi et al., 1985; Targan et al., 1981; Pedersen et al., 1988) have shown an α- or β-interferon enhancement of the increased natural killer activity associated with exercise. However, the fact that interferon and exercise produced additive effects on natural killer activity also raises the possibility that they are op-erating through different mechanisms.

Interleukin-1 activity in plasma has been found to increase 3 h after 1 h of exercise at 60% of $\dot{V}O_2$max, but not as an immediate response (Cannon et al., 1986). This effect is not consistent with the natural killer activities seen after exercise. Lewicki et al. (1988) did, however, observe an increase in the *in vitro* production of interleukin-1 and decrease in interleukin-2 pro-duction from peripheral blood mononuclear cells following 19 min of intense exercise to fatigue. From this information, the relationship of interleukin-1 with the natural killer responses to exercise remains uncertain.

Opioid peptides (β-endorphin, met-enkephalin) are known to increase in response to moderate and strenuous exercise and return to basal levels within 30 to 50 min after exercise (Fraioli et al., 1980; Carr et al., 1981; Grossman et al., 1984). This pattern is consistent with the observed natural killer re-sponses to exercise. Fiatarone et al. (1988) observed an inhibition of natural killer activity by β-endorphin addition to cells after exercise. This finding does not support an opioid suppressive effect, but is actually compatible with a change in opioid responsiveness resulting from the initial opioid stimulation during exercise. In this study (Fiatarone et al., 1988), naloxone attenuated the natural killer activity increases following exercise, thereby giving further support to opioid involvement.

CONCLUSIONS AND RECOMMENDATIONS

Based on the available evidence, single bouts of exercise may create an immunosuppressive state within the circulation, particularly following long-term exercise. The immunosuppression appears transient and can return to pre-exercise levels within minutes or hours, depending on the study. There is presently no strong evidence to indicate exercise intensity has a key role in either immunosuppression or immunostimulation. Several studies have demonstrated several positive immune responses, and in particular, natural killer activity increases with most durations of exercise reported to date. Additionally, several investigations have reported a delayed immunostimulation following exercise.

Several positive immune system effects of endurance training have been demonstrated. They include increased *in vitro* mitogenesis and T-cell formation at rest. Highly trained individuals may also have greater natural killer cell activity. Endurance training can also result in a smaller reduction of certain immunosuppressive responses (i.e., *in vitro* mitogenesis on a parallel basis) to exercise. Another major area of physical activity, strength training, has only begun to receive attention regarding its action on the immune system. Much of this work remains to be completed.

Various mechanisms have been proposed to explain the exercise-immune interplay. Catecholamines and glucocorticoids may exert positive and negative effects, respectively, on lymphocyte responsiveness following exercise. Opioids may have a pivotal role in the regulation of natural killer cell activities. However, the number of potential modulators of immune system action suggests a vast participation by a number of compounds. Further in-depth investigations of the specific mechanisms involved in the exercise-related immune responses would appear to represent a wide-open topic for future research.

Another area in which exercise may have positive effects is in immunosuppressed individuals. Following this line of reasoning, the absence of stimulation observed in many of the exercise studies might be attributed to the fact that the normal immune system is already functioning at or near optimal levels. Whether regular exercise training is capable of reversing immunosuppression remains an important unanswered question.

REFERENCES

Aarstad HJ, Gaudernack G, and Seljelid R: Stress causes reduced natural killer activity in mice. *Scan. J. Immunol.* 1983; 18:461.

Anderson R, Gatner EMS, Imkamp FMJH, and Kok SH: *In vivo* effects of propranolol on some cellular and humoral immune functions in a group of patients with lepromatous leprosy. *Lepr. Rev.* 1980; 51:137.

Asgeirsson G and Bellanti JA: Exercise, immunology, and infection. *Semin. Adolescent Med.* 1987; 3:199.

Balow JE, Hurley DL, and Fauci AS: Immunosuppressive effects of glucocorticosteroids: differential effects of acute vs. chronic administration on cell-mediated immunity. *J. Immunol.* 1975; 114:1072.

Blazar BA, Rodrick ML, O'Mahony JB, Wood JJ, Bessey PQ, Wilmore DW, and Mannick JA: Suppression of natural killer-cell function in humans following thermal and traumatic injury. *J. Clin. Immunol.* 1986; 6:26.

Blomgren H: Steroid sensitivity of the response of human lymphocytes to phytohemagglutinin and pokeweed mitogen: role of phagocytic cells. *Scand. J. Immunol.* 1974; 3:655.

Brahmi Z, Thomas JE, Park M, Park M, and Dowdeswell IRG: The effect of acute exercise on natural killer-cell activity of trained and sedentary human subjects. *J. Clin. Immunol.* 1985; 5:321.

Calabrese LH, Kleiner SM, Barna BP, Skibinski CI, Kirkendall DT, Lahita RG, and Lombardo JA: The effect of anabolic steroids and strength training on the human immune system. *Med. Sci. Sports Exercise* 1989; 21:386.

Cannon JG, Evans WJ, Hughes VA, Meredith CN, and Dinarello CA: Physiological mechanisms contributing to increased interleukin-1 secretion. *J. Appl. Physiol.* 1986; 61:869.

Cannon JG and Kluger MJ: Exercise enhances survival rate in mice infected with salmonella typhimurium (41830). *Proc. Soc. Exp. Biol. Med.* 1984; 175:518.

Carr DB, Bullen BA, Skrinar GS, Arnold MA, Rosenblatt M, Beitins IZ, Martin JB, and McArthur JW: Physical conditioning facilitates the exercise-induced secretion of β-endorphin and β-lipotropin in women. *N. Engl. J. Med.* 1981; 305:560.

Clarke JR, Gagnon RF, Gotcha FM, Heyworth MR, Maclennan ICM, Truelove SC, and Waller CA: The effect of prednisolone on leucocyte function in man. *Clin. Exp. Immunol.* 1977; 28:292.

Clemmenson O, Andersen V, Hansen NE, Karle H, Koch C, Søborg M, and Weeke B: Sequential studies of lymphocytes, neutrophils and serum proteins during prednisone treatment. *Acta Med. Scand.* 1976; 199:105.

Crary B, Borysenko M, Suitherland DC, Kutz I, Borysenko JZ, and Benson H: Decrease in mitogen responsiveness of mononuclear cells from peripheral blood after epinephrine administration in humans. *J. Immunol.* 1983a; 130:694.

Crary B, Hauser SL, Borysenko M, Kutz I, Hoban C, Ault KA, Weiner HL, and Benson H: Epinephrine-induced changes in the distribution of lymphocyte subsets in peripheral blood of humans. *J. Immunol.* 1983b; 131:1178.

Deuster PA, Curiale AM, Cowan ML, and Finkleman FD: Exercise-induced changes in populations of peripheral blood mononuclear cells. *Med. Sci. Sports Exercise* 1988; 20:276.

Drago F, D'Agata V, Iacona T, Spadaro F, Grassi M, Valerio C, Raffaele R, Astuto C, Lauria N, and Vitetta M: Prolactin as a protective factor in stress-induced biological change. *J. Clin. Lab. Anal.* 1989; 3:340.

Edwards AJ, Bacon TH, Elms CA, Verardi R, Felder M, and Knight SC: Changes in the population of lymphoid cells in human peripheral blood following physical exercise. *Clin. Exp. Immunol.* 1984; 58:420.

Eriksson B and Hedfors E: The effect of adrenaline, insulin and hydrocortisone on human peripheral blood lymphocytes studied by cell surface markers. *Scand. J. Haematol.* 1977; 18:121.

Eskola J, Ruuskanen O, Soppi E, Viljanen MK, Järvinen M, Toivonen H, and Kouvalainen K: Effect of sport stress on lymphocyte transformation and antibody formation. *Clin. Exp. Immunol.* 1978; 32:339.

Faith RE, Liang HJ, Murgo AJ, and Plotnikoff NP: Neuroimmunomodulation with enkephalins: enhancement of human natural killer (NK) cell activity *in vitro*. *Clin. Immunol. Immunopathol.* 1984; 31:412.

Fauci AS: Mechanisms of corticosteroid action on lymphocyte subpopulations. II. Differential effects of *in vivo* hydrocortisone, prednisone and dexamethasone on *in vitro* expression of lymphocyte function. *Clin. Exp. Immunol.* 1976; 24:54.

Fauci AS and Dale DC: The effect of *in vivo* hydrocortisone on subpopulations of human lymphocytes. *J. Clin. Invest.* 1974; 53:240.

Fehr H-G, Lotzerich H, and Michna H: The influence of physical exercise on peritoneal macrophage functions: histochemical and phagocytic studies. *Int. J. Sports Med.* 1988; 9:77.

Ferry A, Picard F, Duvallet A, Weill B, and Rieu M: Changes in blood leukocyte populations induced by acute maximal and chronic submaximal exercise. *Eur. J. Appl. Physiol.* 1990; 59:435.

Fiatarone MA, Morley JE, Bloom ET, Benton D, Makinodan T, and Solomon GF: Endogenous opioids and the exercise-induced augmentation of natural killer cell activity. *J. Lab. Clin. Med.* 1988; 112:544.

Fraioli F, Moretti C, Paolucci D, Alicicco E, Crescenzi F, and Fortunio G: Physical exercise stimulates marked concomitant release of β-endorphin and adrenocorticotropic hormone (ACTH) in peripheral blood in man. *Experientia* 1980; 36:987.

Frisch RE, Wyshak G, Albright NL, Albright TE, Schiff I, Jones KP, Witschi J, Shiang E, Koff E, and Marguglio M: Lower prevalence of breast cancer and cancers of the reproductive system among former college athletes compared to non-athletes. *Br. J. Cancer* 1985; 52:885.

Froelich CJ and Bankhurst AD: The effect of β-endorphin on natural cytotoxicity and antibody dependent cellular cytotoxicity. *Life Sci.* 1984; 35:261.

Garabrant DH, Peters JM, Mack TM, and Bernstein L: Job activity and colon cancer risk. *Am. J. Epidemiol.* 1984; 119:1005.

Gatti G, Cavallo R, Sartori ML, del Ponte D, Masera R, Salvadori A, Carignola R, and Angeli A: Inhibition by cortisol of human natural killer (NK) cell activity. *J. Steroid Biochem.* 1987; 26:49.

Gerhardsson M, Norell SE, Kiviranta H, Pedersen NJ, and Ahlbom A: Sedentary jobs and colon cancer. *Am. J. Epidemiol.* 1986; 123:775.

Gilman SC, Schwartz JM, Milner RJ, Bloom FE, and Feldman JD: β-endorphin enhances lymphocyte proliferative responses. *Proc. Natl. Acad. Sci. U.S.A.* 1982; 79:4226.

Gimenez M, Mohan-Kumar T, Humbert JC, De Talance N, Teboul M, and Ariño Belenguer FJ: Training and leucocyte, lymphocyte and platelet response to dynamic exercise. *J. Sports Med.* 1987; 27:172.

Glaser R, Rice J, Speicher CE, Stout JC, and Kiecolt-Glaser JK: Stress depresses interferon production by leukocytes concomitant with a decrease in natural killer cell activity. *Behav. Neurosci.* 1986; 100:675.

Gmunder FK, Lorenzi G, Bechler B, Joller P, Muller J, Ziegler WH, and Cogoli A: Effect of long-term physical exercise on lymphocyte reactivity: similarity to space-flight reactions. *Aviat. Space Environ. Med.* 1988; 59:146.

Good RA and Fernandes G: Enhancement of immunologic function and resistance to tumor growth in balb/c mice by exercise. *Fed. Proc.* 1981; 40:1040.

Green RL, Kaplan SS, Rabin BS, Stanitski CL, and Zdziarski U: Immune function in marathon runners. *Ann. Allergy* 1981; 47:73.

Grossman A: Opioids and stress in man. *J. Endocrinol.* 1988; 119:377.

Grossman A, Bouloux P, Price P, Drury PL, Lam KSL, Turner T, Thomas J, Besser GM, and Sutton J: The role of opioid peptides in the hormonal responses to acute exercise in man. *Clin. Sci.* 1984; 67:483.

Hanson PG and Flaherty DK: Immunological responses to training in conditioned runners. *Clin. Sci.* 1981; 60:225.

Hedfors E, Biberfeld P, and Wahren J: Mobilization to the blood of human non-T and K lymphocytes during physical exercise. *Clin. Lab. Immunol.* 1978; 1:159.

Hedfors E, Holm G, and Ohnell B: Variations of blood lymphocytes during work studied by cell surface markers, DNA synthesis and cytotoxicity. *Clin. Exp. Immunol.* 1976; 24:328.

Hedman LA: The effects of steroids on the circulating lymphocyte population. *Lymphology* 1980; 13:34.

Heilman DH, Gambrill MR, and Leichner JP: The effect of hydrocortisone on the incorporation of tritiated thymidine by human blood lymphocytes cultured with phytohaemagglutinin and pokeweed mitogen. *Clin. Exp. Immunol.* 1973; 15:203.

Hellstrand K, Hermodsson S, and Strannegård O: Evidence for a β-adrenoreceptor-mediated regulation of human natural killer cells. *J. Immunol.* 1985; 134:4095.

Henney CS, Kuribayashi K, Kern DE, and Gillis S: Interleukin-2 augments natural killer cell activity. *Nature* 1981; 291:335.

Herberman RR, Ortaldo JR, and Bonnard GD: Augmentation by interferon of human natural and antibody-dependent cell-mediated cytotoxicity. *Nature* 1979; 277:221.

Hickson RC: Interference of strength development by simultaneously training for strength and endurance. *Eur. J. Appl. Physiol.* 1980; 45:255.

Hickson RC, Rosenkoetter MA, and Brown MM: Strength training effects on aerobic power and short-term endurance. *Med. Sci. Sports Exercise* 1980; 12:336.

Hirota Y, Suzuki T, Chayano Y, and Bito Y: Hormonal immune responses characteristic of testosterone-proprinate-treated chickens. *Immunology* 1976; 30:341.

Hoffman SA, Paschkis KE, DeBias DA, Cantarow A, and Williams TL: The influence of exercise on the growth of transplanted rat tumors. *Cancer Res.* 1962; 22:597.

Hoffman-Goetz L, Keir R, Thorne R, Houston ME, and Young C: Chronic exercise stress in mice depresses splenic T lymphocyte mitogenesis *in vitro*. *Clin. Exp. Immunol.* 1986; 66:551.

Holloszy JO and Booth FW: Biochemical adaptations to endurance exercise in skeletal muscle. *Annu. Rev. Physiol.* 1976; 38:273.

Irwin M, Daniels M, Bloom ET, and Weiner H: Life events, depression, and natural killer cell activity. *Psychopharmacol. Bull.* 1986; 22:1093.

Jokl E: The immunological status of athletes. *J. Sports Med.* 1974; 14:165.

Katz P, Zaytoun AM, and Lee JH Jr: The effects of *in vivo* hydrocortisone on lymphocyte-mediated cytotoxicity. *Arthritis Rheum.* 1984; 27:72.

Kay N, Allen J, and Morley JE: Endorphins stimulate normal human peripheral blood lymphocyte natural killer activity. *Life Sci.* 1984; 35:53.

Kay N, Morley JE, and van Ree JM: Enhancement of human lymphocyte natural killing function by non-opioid fragments of β-endorphin. *Life Sci.* 1987; 40:1083.

Keast D, Cameron K, and Morton AR: Exercise and the immune response. *Sports Med.* 1988; 5:248.

Klarlund K, Pedersen BK, Theander TG, and Andersen V: Depressed natural killer cell activity in acute myocardial infarction. *Clin. Exp. Immunol.* 1987; 70:209.

Kraut RP and Greenberg AH: Effects of endogenous and exogenous opioids on splenic natural killer cell activity. *Nat. Immunol. Cell Growth Regul.* 1986; 5:28.

Landmann RMA, Muller FB, Perini CH, Wesp M, Ernie P, and Buhler FR: Changes of immunoregulatory cells induced by psychological and physical stress: relationship to plasma catecholamines. *Clin. Exp. Immunol.* 1984; 58:127.

Lewicki R, Tchorzewski H, Majewska E, Norwak Z, and Baj Z: Effect of maximal physical exercise on T-lymphocyte subpopulations and on interleukin 1 (IL 1) and interleukin 2 (IL 2) production *in vitro*. *Int. J. Sports Med.* 1988; 9:144.

Lewicki R, Tchorzewski H, Denys A, Kowalska M, and Golinska A: Effect of physical exercise on some parameters of immunity in conditioned sportsmen. *Int. J. Sports Med.* 1987; 8:309.

Liu YG and Wang SY: The enhancing effect of exercise on the production of antibody to *salmonella typhi* in mice. *Immunol. Lett.* 1987; 14:117.

Mackinnon LT and Tomasi TB: Immunology of exercise. *Ann. Sports Med.* 1986; 3:1.

Mahan MP and Young MR: Immune parameters of untrained or exercise-trained rats after exhaustive exercise. *J. Appl. Physiol.* 1989; 66:282.

Mandler RN, Biddison WE, Mandler R, and Serrate SA: β-endorphin augments the cytolytic activity and interferon production of natural killer cells. *J. Immunol.* 1986; 136:934.

Martin HE: Physiological leucocytosis. The variation in the leucocyte count during rest and exercise, and after the hypodermic injection of adrenaline. *J. Physiol.* 1932; 75:113.

Masuhara M, Kami K, Umebayasi K, and Tatsumi N: Influences of exercise on leukocyte count and size. *J. Sports Med.* 1987; 27:285.

Mathews PM, Froelich CJ, Sibbitt WL Jr, and Bankhurst AD: Enhancement of natural cytotoxicity by β-endorphin. *J. Immunol.* 1983; 130:1658.

Monjan AA and Collector MI: Stress-induced modulation of the immune response. *Science* 1977; 196:307.

Moorthy AV and Zimmerman SW: Human leukocyte response to an endurance race. *Eur. J. Appl. Physiol.* 1978; 38:271.

Morley JE, Kay NE, Solomon GF, and Plotnikoff NP: Neuropeptides: conductors of the immune orchestra. *Life Sci.* 1987; 41:527.

Nash HL: Can exercise make us immune to disease? *Physician Sports Med.* 1986; 14:250.

Nieman DC, Berk LS, Simpson-Westerberg M, Arabatzis K, Youngberg S, Tan SA, Lee JW, and Eby WC: Effects of long-endurance running on immune system parameters and lymphocyte function in experienced marathoners. *Int. J. Sports Med.* 1989a; 10:317.

Nieman DC, Tan SA, Lee JW, and Berk LS: Complement and immunoglobulin levels in athletes and sedentary controls. *Int. J. Sports Med.* 1989b; 10:124.

Onsrud M and Thorsby E: Influence of *in vivo* hydrocortisone on some human blood lymphocyte subpopulations. *Scand. J. Immunol.* 1981; 13:573.

Oshida Y, Yamanouchi K, Hayamizu S, and Sato Y: Effect of acute physical exercise on lymphocyte subpopulations in trained and untrained subjects. *Int. J. Sports Med.* 1988; 9:137.

Pedersen BK, Tvede N, Christensen LD, Klarlund K, Kragbak S, and Halkjaer-Kristensen J: Natural killer cell activity in peripheral blood of highly trained and untrained persons. *Int. J. Sports Med.* 1989; 10:129.

Pedersen BK, Tvede N, Hansen FR, Andersen V, Bendix T, Bendixen G, Bendtzen K, Galbo H, Haahr PM, Klarlund K, Sylvest J, Thomsen BS, and Halkjaer-Kristensen J: Modulation of natural killer cell activity in peripheral blood by physical exercise. *Scand. J. Immunol.* 1988; 27:673.

Pedersen BK and Beyer JM: Characterization of the *in vitro* effects of glucocorticosteroids on NK cell activity. *Allergy* 1986; 41:220.

Pedersen BK, Beyer JM, Rasmussen A, Klarlund K, Pedersen BN, and Helin P: Methylprednisolone pulse therapy induced fall in natural killer cell activity in rheumatoid arthritis. *Acta Pathol. Microbiol. Immunol. Scand. Sect. C* 1984; 92:319.

Peters EM and Bateman ED: Ultramarathon running and upper respiratory tract infections. *S. Afr. Med. J.* 1983; 64:582.

Rashkis HA: Systemic stress as an inhibitor of experimental tumors in Swiss mice. *Science* 1952; 116:169.

Reyes MP and Lerner AM: Interferon and neutralizing antibody in sera of exercised mice with coxsackievirus B-3 myocarditis (39204). *Proc. Soc. Exp. Biol. Med.* 1976; 151:333.

Roberts JA: Viral illnesses and sports performance. *Sports Med.* 1986; 3:296.

Robertson AJ, Ramesar KCRB, Potts RC, Gibbs JH, Browning MCK, Brown RA, Hayes PC, and Beck JS: The effect of strenuous physical exercise on circulating blood lymphocytes and serum cortisol levels. *J. Clin. Lab. Immunol.* 1981; 5:53.

Rusch HP and Kline BE: The effect of exercise on the growth of a mouse tumor. *Cancer Res.* 1944; 4:116.

Samuels AJ: Primary and secondary leucocyte changes following the intramuscular injection of epinephrine hydrochloride. *J. Clin. Invest.* 1951; 30:941.

Shavit Y, Lewis JW, Terman GW, Gale RP, and Liebeskind JC: Opioid peptides mediate the suppressive effect of stress on natural killer cell cytotoxicity. *Science* 1984; 223:188.

Simon HA: The immunology of exercise. *JAMA* 1984; 252:2735.

Soppi E, Varjo P, Eskola J, and Laitinen LA: Effect of strenuous physical stress on circulating lymphocyte number and function before and after training. *J. Clin. Lab. Immunol.* 1982; 8:43.

Steel CM, Evans J, and Smith MA: Physiological variation in circulating B cell: T cell ratio in man. *Nature* 1974; 247:387.

Targan S, Britvan L, and Dorey F: Activation of human NKCC by moderate exercise: increased frequency of NK cells with enhanced capability of effector-target lytic interactions. *Clin. Exp. Immunol.* 1981; 45:352.

Tomasi TB, Trudeau FB, Czerwinski D, and Erredge S: Immune parameters in athletes before and after strenuous exercise. *J. Clin. Immunol.* 1982; 2:173.

Tønnesen E, Tønnesen J, and Christensen NJ: Augementation of cytotoxicity by natural killer (NK) cells after adrenaline administration in man. *Acta Pathol. Microbiol. Immunol. Scand. Sect. C* 1984; 92:81.

Vena JE, Graham S, Zielezny M, Swanson MK, Barnes RE, and Nolan J: Lifetime occupational exercise and colon cancer. *Am. J. Epidemiol.* 1985; 122:357.

Viti A, Muscettola M, Paulesu L, Bocci V, and Almi A: Effect of exercise on plasma interferon levels. *J. Appl. Physiol.* 1985; 59:426.

Watson RR, Moriguchi S, Jackson JC, Werner L, Wilmore JH, and Freund BJ: Modification of cellular immune function in humans by endurance exercise training during β-adrenergic blockade with atenolol or propranolol. *Med. Sci. Sports Exercise* 1986; 18:95.

Winder WW, Hagberg JM, Hickson RC, Ehsani AA, and McLane JA: Time course of sympathoadrenal adaptation to endurance exercise training in man. *J. Appl. Physiol.* 1978; 45:370.

Winder WW, Hickson RC, Hagberg JM, Ehsani AA, and McLane JA: Training-induced changes in hormonal and metabolic responses to submaximal exercise. *J. Appl. Physiol.* 1979; 46:766.

Yu DTY, Clements PJ, Paulus HE, Peter JB, Levy J, and Barnett EV: Human lymphocyte subpopulations: effect of corticosteroids. *J. Clin. Invest.* 1974; 53:565.

Yu DTY, Clements PJ, and Pearson CM: Effect of corticosteroids on exercise-induced lymphocytosis. *Clin. Exp. Immunol.* 1977; 28:326.

Catecholamine and Leukocyte Phenotype Responses to Mental Stress in Subjects with Anxiety or Suppressed Aggression

Regine M.A. Landmann, Charles Perini,
Franco B. Müller, and Fritz R. Bühler
Department of Research and Department of Medicine
University Hospital
Basel, Switzerland

INTRODUCTION

Psychosocial stressors have been related to the incidence and progression of neoplastic and infectious diseases (Glaser et al., 1987; Grossharth-Maticek et al., 1985; Borysenko, 1982; Cox and Mackay, 1982; Plaut and Friedman, 1981) via immunological mechanisms (Arnetz et al., 1987; Schleifer et al., 1987; Kiecolt-Glaser et al., 1987, 1984; Jemott et al., 1983; Bartrop et al., 1977). The sympathetic nervous system may provide a common link between psychological factors and immune response (Solomon and Amkraut, 1981; Locke, 1982). In man, psychological or pharmacological activation of the sympathetic nervous system leads *ex vivo* to an increase of natural killer (NK) cell activity and to a reduction of the mitogen-induced lymphocyte proliferation and immunoglobulin secretion (Tonnesen et al., 1987, 1984; Targan et al., 1981; Crary et al., 1983; Hedfords et al., 1983). In normal subjects, standardized sympathetic activation by short-term mental stress changes the proportions of blood leukocyte subpopulations and this is related to changes in plasma catecholamines (Landmann et al., 1984). Thus, monocytes, surface immunoglobulin-positive B-cells and NK cells increase during sympathetic stimulation, and a reduced CD4 to CD8 T-cell ratio relates to a high plasma adrenaline concentration before and during the stress test. These results suggest a differential leukocyte mobilization which contributes to the immuno-modulation *in vitro* known to occur following sympathetic stimulation *in vivo* (Tvede et al., 1989; Tonnesen et al., 1987; Schlesinger and Yodfat, 1987; Targan et al., 1981; Crary et al., 1983; Hedfords et al., 1983). It is well known that during periods of high psychological stress, immune reactions are modulated by emotional and behavioral factors (Workman and Mariano, 1987; Kiecolt-Glaser et al., 1984; Jemott et al., 1983). Therefore, the present study investigates the plasma catecholamine and leukocyte responses to short-term mental stress relative to the individual's anxiety, depression, and aggressive behavior.

METHODS

Psychological Tests

Fifteen healthy subjects, 11 males and 4 females, 17 to 25 years of age, without a family history of cardiovascular disease, were given the following tests. The German translation (Laux et al., 1981) of the State-Trait Anxiety Inventory of Spielberger (Spielberger et al., 1970) was applied to assess an individual's present level of, and tendency toward, anxiety. It consists of 20 statements requesting subjects to describe how they feel at a particular moment (state scale) and another 20 statements that ask subjects to describe how they generally feel on a 4-point scale (trait scale) (Table I). The Rosenzweig Picture-Frustration test (Rosenzweig, 1950) consists of 24 cartoons, each of which displays two or more persons in various situations, one of whom frustrates or describes the frustration of another person in an everyday situation. The test subject has to identify him- or herself with the person being frustrated in the cartoon and to express their response in writing. Standard values are defined between one and nine ("stanine"), adjusted for age and sex (Rauchfleisch, 1979) (Table I). Subjects were also asked to mark the level of their depressive feelings on a visual analog scale of 100 mm (Table I).

Stress Testing

In a second session, studies were performed between 10:00 and 12:00 a.m., adapting a previously described protocol (Landmann et al., 1984a). After an initial resting period of 20 min and during the final 30 s of an 8-

TABLE I.
Results of Depression Score and Psychological Tests

Subject	Depression Self-Rating Scale (mm)	Anxiety		Aggression				
		State	Trait	E	I	Cat. I	np	Cat. M + *I*
		(raw values)				(stanine values)		
1	0	35	30	6	5	5	5	5
2	2	33	30	1	9	9	7	8
3	0	40	42	4	4	5	3	6
4	27	31	39	3	5	5	7	6
5	32	44	39	6	6	6	5	5
6	11	41	43	3	5	6	7	9
7	0	27	29	3	6	7	7	6
8	0	46	34	6	5	6	6	2
9	3	46	37	5	3	4	7	4
10	0	34	47	5	8	6	3	5
11	0	26	23	5	4	8	7	3
12	0	30	21	1	4	7	9	9
13	71	40	39	7	3	2	5	4
14	19	32	35	8	2	1	5	3

[a]E, externalized aggression; I, internalized aggression, Cat. I, (Category I) autoaggression, actions directed inwardly; np, need to solve problems; Cat M + *I*, guilt denial (= tendency to avoid confrontation).

minute mental stress test, blood samples were taken for leukocyte analyses and determination of plasma catecholamines. The mental stress test was comparable to Bjorkvall's modification (Bjorkvall, 1966) of the Stroop word conflict test (Stroop, 1935), where four color words (red, green, blue, and yellow), each presented in a different color, were displayed for 0.8 to 1.5 s. At the same time, subjects were aurally exposed (by earphones) to the name of a color that was again different from the one shown on the screen. Subjects had to unravel the name of the color, the color of the word, and the color heard.

Leukocyte and Hormone Measurements

Leukocytes were counted in blood and buffy coat. Phenotypes of lymphocyte subpopulations from buffy coat were determined by indirect or direct immunofluorescence (Landmann et al., 1984a). Purified or biotinylated monoclonal antibodies directed against CD5 on T-cells (Leu-1), CD4 on T-inducer cells (Leu-3a), CD8 on cytotoxic cells (Leu-2a), and against CD11b (the C3bi receptor on monocytes and NK cells, identified with OKM1) were used. Cells were stained with avidin-coupled fluorescein isothyocyanate (FITC) or rabbit antimouse immunoglobulin (Ig) FITC. B-cell staining was performed with FITC coupled F(ab')$_2$ fragment of goat-antihuman-Ig. These measurements were performed on cells which were not devoid of cytophilic Ig and therefore included enumeration of absorbed Ig on B- and NK cells.

Light scatter (indicative of cell size allowing differentiation of monocytes and lymphocytes) and fluorescence of the cells were analyzed in a Cytofluorograf 50HH (Ortho Instruments, Westwood, Maine). CD11b, on monocytes and NK cells, was differentiated by scatter analysis (Breard et al., 1981; Wright et al., 1983). Catecholamines were measured by radioenzymatic assay (Da Prada and Zürcher, 1976) in the supernatant of the buffy coat preparation, and plasma cortisol was determined by radioimmunoassay (Travenol, Boston).

Statistical Methods

Relationships between the results of the psychological tests and hormonal or cellular changes were calculated with the Spearman rank correlation test.

Results

During the color-word conflict test, the mean values of plasma catecholamines remained unchanged, whereas the numbers of monocytes, surface Ig-positive B-cells, and NK cells increased (Table 2). Changes in monocytes and lymphocytes, although variable, were correlated inversely with the individual's anxiety and depressive state. Thus, subjects with a high anxiety score both before and during the mental stress test had lower monocyte

TABLE II.
Plasma Catecholamines and Leukocyte Subpopulations in Buffy Coat of 10 ml of Blood Before and During Mental Stress

		Mental Stress	
		Before	During
Noradrenaline (pg/ml)		279 + 21	288 + 20
Adrenaline (pg/ml)		46 + 5	52 + 5
Cell subtypes ($\times 10^6$)			
Granulocytes		5.2 ± 0.05	5.6 ± 0.05
Monocytes	Scatter	0.37 ± 0.04	0.40 ± 0.03
	CD11b	0.11 ± 0.02	0.14 ± 0.02[b]
Lymphocytes		6.9 ± 0.08	7.4 ± 0.07
T-cells	CD5	4.9 ± 0.07	5.1 ± 0.05
T-inducer cells	CD4	3.1 ± 0.04	3.1 ± 0.03
T-cytotoxic cells	CD8	1.8 ± 0.03	1.9 ± 0.02
B- + NK cells	(sIg)	1.4 ± 0.01	1.8 ± 0.02[b]
NK cells	(CD11b)	0.3 ± 0.05	0.47 ± 0.07[c]

[a] n = 15, mean ± SEM. $p < 0.01$, comparing stress with control values.

numbers than those expressing weak anxiety (r = $-0.77, p = 0.004$, Figure 1A, and $p = 0.017$ during mental stress, respectively). These relationships were independent of the method used to quantify monocytes (i.e., by light scatter analysis or C3bi receptor counting).

Changes in monocyte numbers during mental stress were variable, ranging from no change to a threefold change. In those subjects who showed a score greater than 10 on the self-report depression scale, monocyte numbers either did not increase or decreased in some. In contrast, in subjects who were not depressed, a clear increase in monocyte numbers was seen (Figure 1B).

When aggressive behavior was quantified by the Rosenzweig picture frustration test, subjects with suppressed or internalized aggression had a marked change in the concentration of plasma adrenaline and numbers of lymphocytes as compared to those with externalized aggression. In particular, the autoaggressive behavior score related directly to plasma adrenaline concentration during mental stress (r = $0.67, p = 0.011$, Figure 2). Similarly, suppressed aggression was associated with the numerical changes of sIg-positive B- and NK cells during mental stress (Figure 3). Guilt denial was related to the stress-induced increase in lymphocyte numbers (Figure 4, r = $0.62, p = 0.010$), and this held true for separate analysis of all T-cells (r = $0.73, p = 0.007$) as well as for the subtypes of T-helper (r = $0.66, p = 0.013$) and T-cytotoxic phenotype (r = $0.70, p = 0.009$). This correlation remained significant when the one subject with a very strong increase of lymphocytes was excluded from the analysis. No relationship was found between the number of NK cells, as defined by OKM1 labeling in the lymphocyte cluster, and the subject's anxiety, depression, or reaction to frustration.

Discussion

The present study demonstrates that anxiety and depression relate to low monocyte numbers and weak adrenergic mobilization of these cells, whereas subjects with autoaggression and a tendency to avoid confrontation—as assessed by the parameter called "guilt denial"—had a marked mobilization of lymphocytes following mental stress together with greater adrenaline responses. These data lend support to the psychological factors directly influencing the adrenaline-modulated distribution of circulating blood cells involved in immune response.

In previous studies, adrenergic activation was achieved by short-term standardized exercise or adrenaline infusion. In both conditions, similar changes of blood leukocyte subsets were induced (Landmann et al., 1984a, 1989). β-adrenergic specificity of the cellular effects was assessed by conducting the studies in the presence or absence of propranolol (Landmann et al., 1985, 1989). Exercise and adrenaline lead to an increase in numbers of monocytes, of CD8+ and Leu7/OKM1+ lymphocytes (Landmann et al., 1988, 1989). The changes were reversible after stop of adrenergic stimulation (Landmann

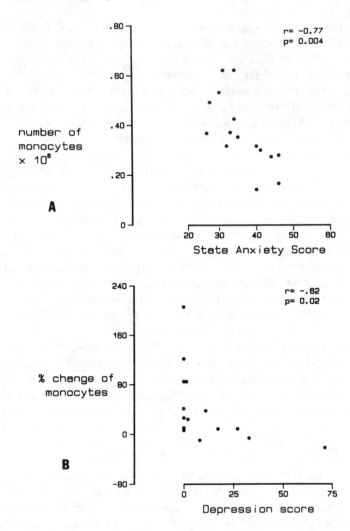

Figure 1. The upper panel (**a**) shows the relationship between state anxiety and number of monocytes before the mental stress test and the lower panel (**b**), the relationship between depression score and percent change of monocytes (as defined by OKM1) during mental stress.

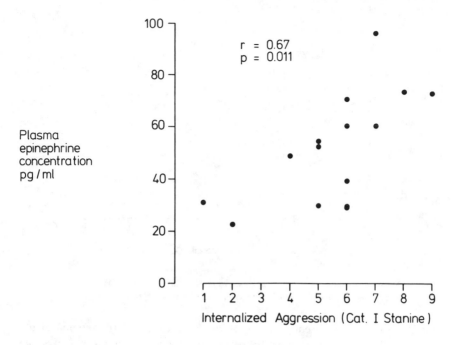

Figure 2. Relationship between Rosenzweig test variable "Cat. I" (internalized aggression) and plasma epinephrine concentration during mental stress.

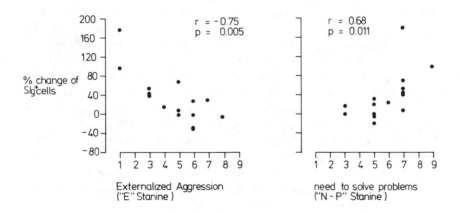

Figure 3. Relationship between Rosenzweig test variables "E" (externalized aggression) and "n-p" (need to solve problems) and percent change of SIg positive B and NK cells during mental stress test.

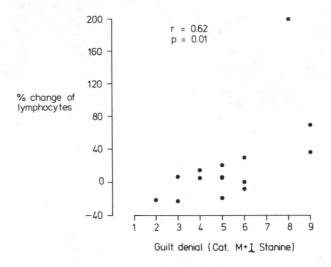

Figure 4. Relationship between Rosenweig test variable "Cat. M + *I*" (guilt denial) and percent change of lymphocytes during mental stress.

et al., 1988), and absent in the presence of propanolol (Landmann et al., 1985, 1989). They were most probably due to demargination of leukocytes upon binding of adrenaline to β-adrenergic receptors on different cell subsets (Landmann et al., 1984b). It is at present still unclear whether the differential mobilization of leukocytes favors or impairs immune responses *in vivo*. Adrenaline-induced cell movements may alter the availability of effector cells in different compartments of the lymphoid system. Therefore, an ongoing immune response may be enhanced or reduced according to when and where cell traffic is influenced by adrenaline.

In the present study, a model of short-lasting mental stress was used to elicit adrenergic activation. This stimulation was weak and caused only slight changes in the mean plasma adrenaline concentration. We nevertheless postulate that the observed increase of monocytes and of cells with the NK cell phenotype was due to adrenergic stimulation for the following reasons. First, mental stress and the abovementioned strong sympathetic stimuli lead to enrichment of the same leukocyte subpopulations. Second, the rapid appearance of leukocyte changes during mental stress makes it unlikely that other hormones participated in the effect.

The tool of the present investigation was not to quantify phenotype changes, but to define psychological factors which modulate adrenaline and leukocyte response to short-term stress. In fact, hormonal and cellular reactions were related both to emotional and behavioral factors: anxiety and depression were associated with reduced monocyte numbers and a lack of stress-induced mobilization. In earlier studies, anxiety and depression have both been related to impaired immune response: during bereavement and in major depressive disorders, lymphocyte mitogen responses were found to be lower as compared to healthy controls (Schleifer et al., 1989, 1987). Monocyte function has not yet been studied; however, reduced monocyte numbers or ineffective monocytes may have been at the origin of the decreased mitogen response in depression, because there is no lymphocyte proliferation without monocytes. The observed lower monocyte numbers and mobilization during mental stress in anxious subjects may be related to reduced β-adrenoceptor sensitivity, as this has been described for mononuclear leukocytes of patients with depression (Mann et al., 1985).

Autoaggressive behavior and a tendency to avoid confrontation, as assessed with the parameter ''guilt denial'' in the Rosenzweig test, was associated with strong adrenaline and lymphocyte responses to mental stress. No previous studies were conducted to evaluate the impact of behavioral factors on a short-term stress response. In a chronic stressful situation like examination, two groups described suppressed immune parameters as related to personality characteristics: impaired salivary IgA secretion and lymphocyte proliferation were more pronounced in subjects during academic stress, who presented with an ''inhibited power motive syndrome'' or intrusion stress-response style (Workman and Mariano, 1987; Jemott et al., 1983). Probably, the adrenergic nervous system contributed little to suppressed immune functions observed during long-lasting stress. Therefore, similarities between previous data and the present study are restricted to the observation that stress controllability by personality characteristics rather than stress itself modulates immune response (Schlesinger and Yodfat, 1988).

SUMMARY

In summary, specific effective and behavioral states which are known to influence disease risk were found to be associated with qualitative and quantitative differences in the adrenaline and leukocyte reactions to short-term mental stress.

In the future, further investigations are needed to confirm that psychological variables influence acutely induced changes of immunological parameters.

REFERENCES

Arnetz BB, Wasserman J, Petrini B, Brenner SO, Levi L, Eneroth P, Salovaara H, Hjelm R, Salovaara RN, Theorell T, and Petterson IL: Immune function in unemployed women. *Psychosom. Med.* 1987; 49:3–12 (1987).

Bartrop RW, Lazarus L, Luckhurst E, Kiloh LG, and Penny R: Depressed lymphocyte function after bereavement. *Lancet* 1977; 1:834–836.

Bjorkvall CA: *A Note on Inducing Stress by an Audiovisual-Conflict Test.* Psychol. Lab. Rep. 210.

Borysenko JZ: Behavioral-physiological factors in the development and management of cancer. *Gen. Hosp. Psychiatry* 1982; 4:69–74.

Breard J, Reinherz E, O'Brien C, and Schlossman SF: Delineation of an effector population responsible for natural killing and antibody dependent cellular cytotoxicity in man. *Clin. Immunol. Immunopathol.* 1981; 18:145–150.

Cox T and Mackay C: Psychosocial factors and psychophysiological mechanisms in the aetiology and development of cancers. *Soc. Sci. Med.* 1982; 16:382–396.

Crary B, Borysenko M, Sutherland DC, Kutz I, Borysenko JZ, and Benson H: Decrease in mitogen responsiveness of mononuclear cells from peripheral blood after epinephrine administration in humans. *J. Immunol.* 1983; 130:694–697.

Da Prada M and Zürcher G: Simultaneous radioenzymatic determination of plasma and tissue adrenaline, noradrenaline and dopamine within the femtomole range. *Life Sci.* 1976; 19:1161–1174.

Glaser R, Rice J, Sheridan J, Fertel R, Stout J, Speicher C, Pinsky D, Kotur M, Post A, and Beck M: Stress-related immune suppression: health implications. *Brain Behav. Immun.* 1987; 1:7–20.

Grossharth-Maticek R, Bastiaans J, and Kanazir DT: Psychosocial factors as strong predictors of mortality from cancer, ischemic heart disease and stroke. The Yugoslav prospective study. *J. Psychosom. Res.* 1985; 29:167–176.

Hedfords E, Holm G, Ivansen M, and Wahren J: Physiological variation of blood lymphocyte reactivity: T-cell subsets, immunoglobulin production, and mixed-lymphocyte reactivity. *Clin. Immunol. Immunopathol.* 1983; 27:9–14.

Jemott JB, Borysenko M, Chapman R, Borysenko JZ, McClelland DC, Meyer D, and Benson H: Academic stress, power motivation, and decrease in secretion rate of salivary secretory immunoglobulin A. *Lancet* 1983; 1:1400–1402.

Kiecolt-Glaser JK, Fisher LD, Ogrocki P, Stout JC, Speicher CE, and Glaser R: Marital quality, marital disruption, and immune function. *Psychosom. Med.* 1987; 49:13–34.

Kiecolt-Glaser JK, Garner W, Speicher C, Penn GM, Holliday J, and Glaser R: Psychosocial modifiers of immunocompetence in medical students. *Psychosom. Med.* 1984; 46:7–14.

Landmann RMA, Müller FB, Perini C, Wesp M, Erne P, and Bühler FR: Changes of immunoregulatory cells induced by psychological and physical stress: relationship to plasma catecholamines. *Clin. Exp. Immunol.* 1984a; 58:127–135.

Landmann RMA, Bürgisser E, Wesp M, and Bühler FR: Beta-adrenergic receptors are different in subpopulations of human circulating lymphocytes. *J. Recept. Res.* 1984b; 4:47–50.

Landmann RMA, Dürig M, Gudat F, Wesp M, and Harder F: Beta-adrenergic regulation of the blood lymphocyte phenotype distribution in normal subjects and splenectomized patients. In *Microenvironments in the Lymphoid System*. Klaus GGB, Ed, Plenum Press, New York (1985), pp. 1051–1062.

Landmann RMA, Portenier M, Staehelin M, Wesp M, and Box R: Changes in beta-adrenoceptors and leucocyte subpopulations after physical exercise in normal subjects. *Naunyn Schmiedebergs Arch. Pharmacol.* 1988; 337:261–266.

Landmann RMA, Wesp M, Box R, Keller U, and Bühler FR: Distribution and function of beta-adrenergic receptors in human blood lymphocytes. In *Interactions Among CNS, Neuroendocrine and Immune Systems*. Hadden JW, Masek K, and Nistico G, Eds. Pythagora Press, Rome (1989), pp. 251–264.

Laux L, Glanzmann P, Schaffner P, and Spielberger CD: *State-Trait-Angstinventar*. Beltz Testgesellschaft, Weinheim (1981).

Locke St E: Stress, adaptation, and immunity: studies in humans. *Gen. Hosp. Psychiatry* 1982; 4:49–58.

Mann JJ, Brown RP, Halper JP, Sweeney JA, Kocsis JH, Stokes PE, and Bilezikian JP: Reduced sensitivity of lymphocyte beta-adrenergic receptors in patients with endogenous depression and psychomotor agitation. *N. Engl. J. Med.* 1985; 313:715–720.

Plaut SM and Friedman St B. In *Psychoneuroimmunology*. Ader R, Ed. Academic Press, New York (1981), pp. 3–30.

Rauchfleisch U: *Handbuch zum Rosenzweig Picture-Frustration Test. Band 1 + 2*. Hans Huber, Bern (1979).

Rosenzweig S: *Manual for the Rosenzweig Picture-Frustration Study. Adult Form*. Privately published, St. Louis, MO (1950).

Schleifer SJ, Keller SE, and Stein M: Conjugal bereavement and immunity. *Isr. J. Psychiatry Relat. Sci.* 1987; 24:111–123 (1987).

Schleifer SJ, Keller SE, Bond RN, Cohen J, and Stein M: Major depressive disorder and immunity. Role of age, sex, severity and hospitalization. *Arch. Gen. Psychiatry* 1989; 46:81–87.

Schlesinger M and Yodfat Y: Effect of psychosocial stress on natural killer cell activity. *Cancer Detect. Prev.* 1988; 12:9–14.

Solomon GF and Amkraut AA: Psychoneuroendocrinological effects on the immune response. *Annu. Rev. Microbiol.* 1981; 35:155–184.

Spielberger CD, Gorsuch RL, and Lushene RH, Eds. *State-Trait Anxiety Inventory*. Consulting Psychologists Press, Palo Alto (1970).

Stroop JR: Interference in serial verbal reactions. *J. Exp. Psychol.* 1935; 18:643–662.

Targan S, Britvan L, and Dorey F: Activation of human NKCC by moderate exercise: increased frequency of NK cells with enhanced capability of effector-target lytic interactions. *Clin. Exp. Immunol.* 1981; 45:353–360.

Tonnesen E, Tonnesen J, and Christensen NJ: Augmentation of cytotoxicity by natural killer cells after adrenaline administration in man. *Acta Pathol. Microbiol. Immunol. Scand. Sect. C* 1984; 92:81–83.

Tonnesen E, Christensen NJ, and Brinklov MM : Natural killer activity during cortisol and adrenaline infusion in healthy volunteers. *Eur. J. Clin. Invest.* 1987; 17:497–503.

Tvede N, Pedersen BK, Hansen FK, Bendix T, Christensen LD, Galbo H, and Halkjaer-Kristensen J: Effect of physical exercise on blood mononuclear cell subpopulations and *in vitro* proliferative responses. *Scand. J. Immunol.* 1989; 29:383–389.

Workman EA and Mariano F: T-lymphocyte polyclonal proliferation: effects of stress and stress response style on medical students taking national board examinations. *Clin. Immunol. Immunopathol.* 1987; 43:308–313.

Wright SD, Rao PE, Talle MA, Westberg EF, Goldstein G, and Silverstein SC: Identification of the C3bi receptor of human monocytes and macrophages by using monoclonal antibodies. *Proc. Natl. Acad. Sci. U.S.A.* 1983; 80:5699–5703.

Assessment of Stress-Induced Immune Function in Chronic Fatigue Syndrome Patients

H. G. Gratzner, T. S. Johnson
DNA Sciences, Inc.
8058 El Rio,
Houston, Texas

W. J. Hermann, T. L. Steinbach
Memorial Medical Center
920 Frostwood
Houston, Texas

Regina De Herrera
DNA Sciences, Inc.
8058 El Rio,
Houston, Texas

INTRODUCTION

In this chapter, we discuss the use of flow cytometry methodology for assessing the immune function response of chronic fatigue syndrome (CFS) patients using peripheral blood lymphocytes. In the context of this discussion, immune function will refer to the *in vitro* blastogenesis response of T-lymphocytes to mitogens such as phytohemagglutinin (PHA) and concanavalin A (ConA) as measured by quantitative and objective flow cytometric detection of the lymphocyte DNA replication activity. The basic underlying assumption of the methodology is that the peripheral blood lymphocytes (PBLs) are sensitive "barometers" of each person's immune status and general health condition, which would include stress-induced immune alterations such as observed in CFS patients (Holmes et al., 1988; Straus, 1988).

By measuring the *in vitro* blastogenic (DNA replication) response to selected mitogen(s), useful information can be obtained to characterize PBL immune function at patient workup, during therapy, and for follow-up evaluation. Since the flow cytometric method for blastogenic assay of PBL is based on immunocytochemical staining and rapid, cell-by-cell analysis of 25,000 to 50,000 cells for each specimen, high signal-to-noise and sensitivity can be achieved to detect stress-induced inhibition or suppression of PBL immunofunction heretofore not possible using the radioisotope method which employs scintillation counting or radiography. The use of radioisotopic thymidine also can result in lymphocyte cell cycle perturbation (Pollack et al., 1979). The emphasis in this chapter will be placed on the flow cytometric immune function *in vitro* assay technique, with examples presented for normal donor and CFS PBL specimens to demonstrate the utility of the methodology.

Current scientific dogma is that stress-induced immune suppression is an important underlying cause of CFS (Straus, 1988). Complex biological interrelationships exist between the immune system and the central nervous system. Feedback loops link the immune system and brain via biological response modifiers, neuropeptides, and other physiological regulatory molecules. Prolonged stress induces functional alterations in the lymphocytes and other cells of the immune system, and these factors serve as messengers between the immune and central nervous systems. Figure 1 shows a simplistic, schematic diagram of this feedback loop. In this model, lymphocytes have receptors for endorphins, and produce factors such as the interferon(s), interleukin-1, interleukin-2, and others. It should be emphasized, however, that "neurohormones" are not exclusively produced by the neuroendocrine system. Immune cells are known to secrete endorphins (Smith and Blalock, 1981), and neurological cells have been shown to have receptors for insulin (Pert et al., 1985). Importantly, in the case of CFS (and other viral-associated conditions), the stress-induced immune suppression or inhibition is thought to provide the opportunity for latent viral particles to actively replicate and subsequently cause the classical clinical symptoms. Intuitively, one would predict that the intrinsic ability of the lymphocytes to mount an effective immune defense against Epstein-Barr virus (or other virus) would be compromised by prolonged stress. The general concept for CFS etiology is consistent with both the scientific and clinical data reported to date in that the viral infection and related clinical symptoms represent secondary and tertiary sequellae. The primary etiology is more likely not the virus per se, but rather the stress-induced immune suppression, which provides opportunistic viruses favorable conditions for replicating. Presently, the mechanisms underlying

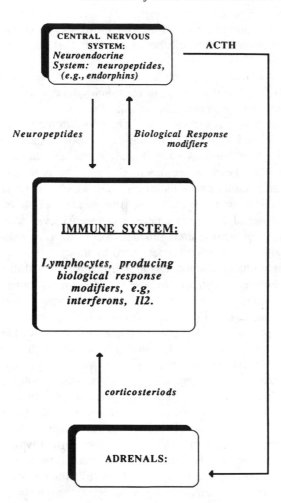

Figure 1. Interrelationship between the immune system, exemplified by T- and B-lymphocytes and the central nervous system. Cells of the immune system possess receptors for neuropeptides, and neurological cell receptors for the BRMs produced by immune cells. It should also be emphasized that immune cells also produce endorphins and possess receptors for these factors.

stress-induced immune suppression are not well understood and additional experimental and clinical data will be needed to further elucidate the cause-and-effect relationships.

Clinically, the biologic effects of stress may best be expressed in the newly defined CFS. The syndrome closely mimics the effects of other "high lymphokine" states such as that seen as side effects during administration of interferon or interleukin-2 intravenously. The flow cytometric immune function assay can be used to monitor immune suppression in these patients prior to and following regulation. A careful analysis of many hundreds of these patients reveals that the most prominent characteristic is the presence of a high level of stress, either emotional or physical, which was previously manageable, but becomes unmanageable; the patients are not able to recover by the usual psychological defense mechanisms that were previously functioning. The predominance of women among patients (3:1) may have a biologic basis. A cycle of events is commonly experienced by these individuals, in which fatigue overwhelms them, and frustration compromises their ability to perform in perceived critical circumstances in their career, business, or personal stress situations. Importantly, one cannot help but be impressed with the hard-driving, aggressive nature of these individuals seeking treatment for CFS. Commonly, these patients may not be primarily depressed, but develop a secondary depression due to a long-standing frustration with themselves and a perceived ineffective medical profession which is frequently seen. This leads to a vicious cycle which creates more stress. The second most common "trigger" of CFS is the stress of allergic reaction. Allergies, known and unknown, to common molds and pollens, or the more obscure factors such as foods, seem to be common in CFS patients. Aside from the need for immune modulation therapy to biologically restore normal lymphocyte function, variable degrees of behavioral and stress management are considered essential to successful treatment. The most effective immune modulator will be rendered useless if a patient does not modify, manage, or eliminate the stress trigger.

CFS, a recently described, debilitating phenomenon, is characterized by lethargy, myalgia, painful lymph nodes, sore throat, depression, and other symptoms. The syndrome has been linked to Epstein-Barr virus (EBV) because many of the affected individuals display a high titer to EBV (Holmes et al., 1988). There is considerable controversy, however, concerning the association of EBV as the causative agent of CFS (Straus et al., 1988). Cytomegalovirus (CMV) as well as other viral etiologies have been implicated (Holmes et al., 1988; Straus, 1988). Recent studies suggest that the syndrome might be due to physiological manifestations of neurological influences on immune function, by neurohormones, or other immunomodulators of T-lymphocyte function. Previous laboratory studies have reported various test results for CFS patients, e.g., alterations in IgG subclasses (Komaroff et al., 1988), and abnormalities in distributions of natural killer (NK) cells (Caligiuri et al.,

1987). A significant problem encountered in the diagnosis and treatment of CFS has been the absence of a test which reliably can be employed to facilitate diagnosis and to assess patient treatment response. Making a diagnosis on the basis of viral serology, blood chemistry, or CBC hasn't proved satisfactory.

Relevant to this discussion, one study indicated that immune function is depressed with regard to interleukin-2 (IL-2) and interferon production subsequent to stimulation with a mitogen and phorbol ester (Kibler et al., 1985). This observation suggests that mitogen stimulation, which induces the synthesis of IL-2 and IL-2 receptors among other phenomena, should provide a test of the immune competency of CFS patient lymphocytes on a more generalized basis than the individual assessment of lymphokine or immunoglobulin production. The question of the cause and effect relationship of stress on immune function in CFS patients has been addressed recently (Straus, 1988). Studies of the effects of stress in non-CFS individuals demonstrate that immune function is altered by stressful situations (Kibler et al., 1985). As discussed below, our immune function test appears, in preliminary studies, to be effective in monitoring CFS patients and predicting disease outcome.

FLOW CYTOMETRIC ASSESSMENT OF IMMUNE STATUS

Flow cytometric techniques have proved to be powerful analytical tools to study immune status, immune competence, and immune function (Lovett et al., 1984; Reinherz, 1980). Flow cytometry can be used to assay cell surface markers, which identify specific subsets of immune cells, and monoclonal antibodies can be rapidly used to quantitatively detect B- and T-cell markers of differentiated functions on a cell-by-cell basis. The reader is referred to several review articles and books which have been published on the subject (Melamed et al., 1979; Loken et al., 1979; Johnson et al., 1988). The flow cytometric immunofunction test which we employ is based on the use of BrdUrd/IdUrd labeling and detection of mitogen-stimulated DNA replication by a two-color flow immunofluorescent method (Gratzner, 1982; Dolbeare et al., 1983). The method measures DNA replication by means of a monoclonal antibody which detects the incorporation of halogenated deoxyuridine analogs (BrdUrd and IdUrd) of thymidine into DNA. The DNA *content* is simultaneously measured, correlated with replication on a cell-by-cell basis. This provides a powerful method to rapidly quantify DNA replication in relation to cell cycle and other biological properties.

The lymphocyte immune function (LIF) test measures the *in vitro* response of patient PBLs to lectin (PHA) in short-term culture. The assay is based on the method originally developed by Gratzner (1982). After 72 h of culture, of which the final 2 h are in the presence of the thymidine analog iododeoxyuridine (IdUrd), the cells are fixed in cold ethanol and stained for the incorporation of IdUrd into DNA. The IdUrd is detected by a monoclonal antibody which is highly specific for IdUrd. A DNA-specific fluorochrome, propidium iodide (PI), is applied in order to stoichiometrically stain lymphocyte DNA (Dolbeare et al., 1983). The cells are then analyzed in the flow cytometer. An argon laser excites both the fluorescein and PI for the measurement of DNA replication and DNA content, respectively. Representative examples of the LIF test results are shown in Figure 2. Figure 3 illustrates the basic two-color fluorescence analysis method to be used for the LIF tests to assess the lymphocyte immune function of age- and sex-matched controls (n = 30), immunomodulator-treated patients (n = 10), and patients treated with a placebo (n = 10). Figure 2 illustrates how the bivariate plots are computer windowed to extract the LIF test parameters: DNA replication rate, labeling index, and stimulation index.

Based on the analysis of PBL from more than 50 control donors and 300 CFS patients to date, it is apparent that this LIF test affords a quantitative,

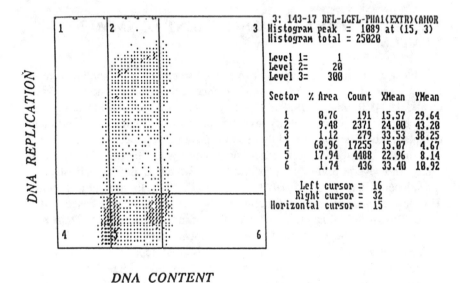

DNA CONTENT

Figure 2. Method for "windowing" analysis of bivariate plots for the extraction of immune function parameters. The histogram represents a culture that has been stimulated with PHA. Unstimulated cultures ordinarily have very few labeled cells in Sectors 1, 2, and 3. In order to derive the labeling index and mean Y-fluorescence, the vertical cursors are placed at the midpoints of G1 and G2M peaks on the x-axis, and the horizontal cursor is placed at 2SD above the G1 peak. The region, *sector* 2, then contains the S-phase-labeled cells. In the figure, LI = 9.48 and mean Y-fluorescent = 43.20. The *DNA replication rate,* DNAR, for this example is thus calculated as LI × (mean Y-fluorescence), or 9.8 × 43.20 = 423.4.

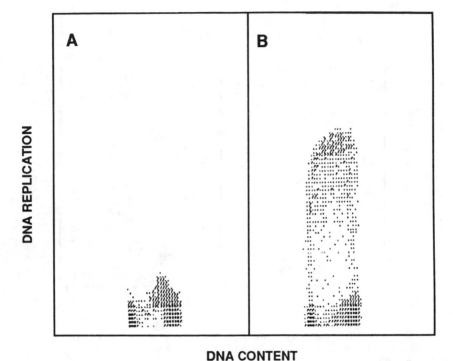

DNA CONTENT

Figure 3. DNA replication patterns of lymphocyte immune function assay, from a normal individual. Pattern showing positions on the bivariate plots for G1, S, and G2M phases of the cell cycle. Cells were incubated with 10 μM IdUrd for 120 min, and stained for IdUrd incorporation by the indirect technique. A: Control, no PHA; B: 5 μg/ml PHA.

objective flow cytometric test to assess a patient's PBLs; the test has application for the initial workup and for monitoring CFS patient treatment response using PBL. Importantly, the flow cytometric test has advantages over the radioisotope method which employs tritiated thymidine: it is rapid, requires no radioisotopes, and measures both the *percentage* of labeled cells in the S-phase and the *rate* of replication.

Our studies to date for representative "normal" donor blood specimens vs. blood specimens obtained from clinically symptomatic CFS patients lead to several conclusions: (1) that "normal" PBL immune function as measured by short-term mitogen (PHA) stimulation is characterized by a reproducible DNA content/DNA replication pattern and stimulation index. "Normal" PBL specimens invariably display a predictable dot-plot pattern in about 95% of normal donors (Figure 3). The unstimulated cultures, i.e., those without PHA, show no detectable replication (Figure 3A), whereas those cultures which have added PHA display a replication pattern as shown in Figure 3B. PBL specimens obtained from symptomatic CFS patients display DNA content/

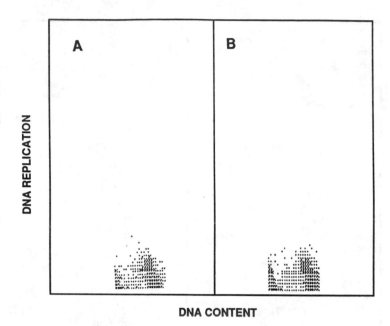

Figure 4. DNA replication patterns of lymphocytes from a patient with chronic fatigue syndrome inhibited for immune function. A: control, no PHA; B: 5 μg/ml PHA.

DNA replication patterns ranging from completely inhibited immunofunction to partially inhibited patterns, as illustrated in Figure 4. Comparison of tests of immune function for symptomatic CFS patients prior to and following an initial course of therapy with an immune modulator, Kutapressin, which is a liver extract containing a mixture of polypeptides with bradykinin-like activity, has indicated that the PBL DNA content and DNA replication patterns revert to the normal patterns in patients clinically responding to the therapy, as illustrated for three CFS patients in Figure 5. Generally, if the lymphocyte immune function progresses from the pre-treatment, "inhibited" condition to post-treatment, "normal" status, the patients invariably were reported to be "responding". Clinical response to the injections is demonstrated by the increase in blastogenic response, which is manifested by increases in DNA replication. Patients prior to therapy display the inhibited pattern; subsequent to multiple injection of the immunomodulator, they exhibit the "normal" response, which is manifested in patterns such as that shown in Figure 5. Patients not responding to the therapy or relapsing show the abnormal, inhibited patterns. The test appears to be an effective method to facilitate the clinical diagnosis of CFS (i.e., identification of patients with inhibited/suppressed PBL) and to objectively assess CFS patient response.

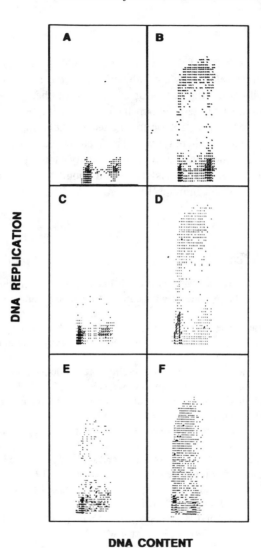

DNA CONTENT

Figure 5. Increase in immune response of CFS patients after treatment with an immunomodulator. PHA-stimulated DNA replication patterns of three patients with chronic fatigue syndrome. (A) Patient #1, pre-treatment; inhibited (anergic) pattern, with no observable DNA synthesis; (B) same patient, post-treatment, subsequent to multiple injections; (C) patient #2, pre-treatment; (D) patient #2, post-treatment; (E) patient #3, pre-treatment; (F) patient #3, post-treatment.

CONCLUSIONS

The basic problem of following patients with syndromes such as CFS, presumably stress-related, is the subjectivity of the assessment. Patient interviews usually form the basis for evaluation of therapy or degree of involvement. Most of the tests which have been attempted for the workup of CFS patients are inconsistent or inconclusive, including, as shown in this report, surface marker phenotyping. The measurement of immune response by the IdUrd/DNA method described in this study should provide an objective, independent technique which is useful for monitoring the course of those conditions which affect immune function.

REFERENCES

Caligiuri MC, Murray D, Buchwald, et al: Phenotypic and functional deficiency of natural killer cells in patients with chronic fatigue syndrome. *J. Immunol.* 1987; 139:10.

Dolbeare F, Gratzner HG, Pallavicini MG, and Gray JW: Flow cytometric measurement of total DNA content and incorporated bromodeoxyuridine. *Proc. Natl. Acad. Sci. U.S.A.* 1983; 80:5573.

Gratzner HG: Monoclonal antibody to 5-bromo- and 5-iododeoxyuridine: a new reagent for the detection of DNA replication. *Science* 1982; 218:474.

Holmes G, Kaplan JE, Ganz NM, et al: Chronic fatigue syndrome: a working case definition. *Ann. Intern. Med.* 1988; 108:387.

Johnson TS, Katz RL, and Pershouse M: Flow cytometric applications in cytopathology. *Anal. Quant. Cytol. Histol.* 1988; 10:423.

Kibler R, Lucas DO, Hicks MJ, Paulos BT, and Jones JT: Immune function in chronic active Epstein Barr virus infection. *J. Clin. Immunol.* 1985; 5:46.

Komaroff A, Geiger A, and Wormsley S: IgG subclass deficiency in chronic fatigue syndrome. *Lancet* June 4:1288–1289.

Loken ML, Stout RD, and Herzenberg LA: Lymphoid cell analysis and sorting. In *Flow Cytometry and Sorting.* Melamed MR, Mullany PF, and Mendelsohn ML, Eds. John Wiley & Sons, New York (1979), pp. 505–528.

Meehan R: Operation Everest. II. Alterations in the immune system at high altitudes. *J. Clin. Immunol.* 1988; 8:1.

Melamed MR, Mullany PF, and Mendelsohn ML, Eds. *Flow Cytometry and Sorting.* John Wiley & Sons, New York (1979).

Pert CB, Ruff MR, Weber RJ, and Herkenham M: Neuropeptides and their receptors: a psychosomatic network. *J. Immunol.* 1985; 135:820s.

Pollack ACB, Bagwell GL, and Irwin III: Radiation from tritiated thymidine perturbs the cell cycle progression of stimulated lymphocytes. *Science* 1979; 203:1025.

Reinherz EL and Schlossman SF: The differentiation and function of human T lymphocyte: a review. *Cell* 1980; 19:821.

Smith EM and Blalock JE: Human lymphocyte production of ACTH and endorphin-like substances: association with leucocyte interferon. *Proc. Natl. Acad. Sci. U.S.A.* 1981; 78:7530.

Straus SE: The chronic mononucleosis syndrome. *J. Infect. Dis.* 1988; 157:405.

Straus SE, Dale JK, Tobi M, Lawley T, Preble O, Blaese RM, Hallahan C, and Henle W: Acyclovir treatment of the chronic fatigue syndrome. *N. Engl. J. Med.* 1988; 319:1692.

Chapter

17

Psychosocial Stress and Breast Cancer

C. L. Cooper and E. B. Faragher
University of Manchester
Institute of Science and Technology
Manchester, England

INTRODUCTION

The notion that a link may exist between psychosocial stress and a subsequent diagnosis of cancer has exercised the attention of medical researchers for many centuries. Publications investigating the possibility of a relationship can be traced back as far as Galen's treatise on tumors, *De Tumoribus,* in which he observed a greater incidence of cancer in "melancholic" than in "sanguine" women. The eminent physicians Grey and Paget both furnished further anecdotal evidence during the 18th and 19th centuries, but it was not until 1893 that the first empirical evidence connecting emotional stress and cancer appeared. In his book *Cancer and the Cancer Process,* Herbert Snow reported a series of 250 successive patients studied at the London Cancer Hospital between 1883 and 1893 in whom there had been "immediate antecedent trouble" in 62%.

Similar findings by other researchers during the early part of the 20th century led to the suggestion by Evans, in her book *A Psychological Study of Cancer* (1926), that the loss of an important emotional relationship or a love object was a common precursor to cancer. Her work with cancer patients led her to believe that some people, when experiencing grief, directed their psychic energy inward, against their own natural body defenses.

Research into this area has accelerated during the past 50 years. An early contemporary historical review by LeShan (1959) again observed that the loss of a major emotional relationship occurred frequently in the years immediately preceding the diagnosis of cancer. Subsequent research has focused considerable attention on establishing the exact nature of the connection between illness, antecedent psychosocial stress, and personality. Much of this work has been concentrated in the area of cardiovascular disease (Cooper, 1983), particularly myocardial infarction, angina pectoris, and hypertension. However, associations have also been reported between stress and low birthweight (Newton and Hunt, 1984), and between antecedent stress, personality, and several types of malignancy, including gastric carcinoma (Lehrer, 1980), pediatric carcinoma (Jacobs and Charles, 1980), lung cancer (Eysenck, 1984), and breast cancer (Cooper, 1988). Until recently, very little research has been published investigating the link between breast cancer and psychosocial stress, which is surprising given the absence of any known major environmental precursors of this form of malignancy. The findings of the small number of studies in the literature vary from similar to totally contradictory.

STRESS AND PATHOLOGY

Underpinning all research into the relationship between illness and psychosocial stress is the widely held belief that a person's emotional state can directly affect their physical well being. This belief is supported by empirical evidence demonstrating that a variety of personality traits and stressful life events are correlated with both the provocation and the increased incidence of many psychosomatic disorders (Ader, 1980; Locke, 1982; Rogers et al., 1979; Solomon and Amkraut, 1981; Stein, 1981). Adverse psychological conditions have now also been implicated in the onset and exacerbation of pathological conditions in which the function of the immune system is central (Irwin and Anisman, 1984). However, the role of the immune system in cancer is poorly understood and several different theories have been put forward to explain how stress may cause disease.

Fox (1978) hypothesizes two primary cancer-causing mechanisms. The first, "carcinogenesis", involves an agent or mechanism which produces cancer by overpowering the existing natural resistance of the body, while the second, "lowered resistance to cancer", permits a potential carcinogen normally insufficient to produce cancer to do so due to, for example, a weakened emotional state. The latter mechanism involves the immunosuppression system of the body, with an "immune-deficient" individual *at risk* of one form of cancer or another, depending on the vulnerability of particular organs.

Conversely, Selye (1979) suggests that all organisms pass through a three-stage "general adaptation syndrome." The first stage, "alarm reaction", consists of a *shock phase* (defined as the initial and immediate reaction to a noxious agent) and a *countershock phase* (defined as a mobilization of defenses phase in which the adrenal cortex becomes further enlarged and secretes more corticoid hormones). The second stage, "stage of resistance", involves the individual adapting to the stressor stimulus, but decreasing his ability to cope with subsequent stimuli. The final stage, "stage of exhaustion", follows a period of prolonged and severe adaptation. Selye concludes that the hormonal attack (particularly of adrenocorticotropic hormone, ACTH) on the body may well be the ultimate cancer-producing weapon should it be activated at a frequent, continuous, and high level.

In contrast, others have concentrated on the psychological processes that may predispose to cancer. Kissen (1969) has argued that adverse life events and loss of a love object can lead to cancer by the psychological mechanisms of "despair, depression and hopelessness". Haney (1977) hypothesizes that personality predispositions may not be directly linked to cancer, but will help to determine "which psychic and somatic insults to which the individual will be exposed and the meaning these exposures will have for the individual". This suggests a high likelihood that a psychocarcinogenic process will be in operation, working to cause the stressor and bodily predispositions to interact and to covary in the production of a carcinoma, one feeding the other.

The exact bodily and psychological mechanisms are clearly not understood, but the evidence increasingly points to a link between psychosocial/personality factors and certain forms of cancer. The absence of properly established environmental factors makes the study of this link in breast cancer a potentially fertile area of research. However, relatively few research papers have been published, and those that have exhibit important methodological weaknesses, making it difficult to evaluate the strength of the associations so far reported. Research into psychosocial stress and breast cancer can be conveniently subdivided into two categories—those studies which focus on the relationship between various psychometric predispositions and breast cancer, and those which examine the emotional history or adverse life events and the pathogenesis of cancer.

PERSONALITY PREDISPOSITIONS AND BREAST CANCER

In one of the earliest studies, Tarlau and Smalheiser (1951) found negative attitudes towards sexuality, rejection of the female role, and patterns of mother dominance in a small personality study of 11 women with malignant breast tumors and 11 women with similar tumors in the cervix. Similar findings were reported by Bacon et al. (1952) in a psychoanalytic case history study of 40 breast cancer patients. The major behavioral characteristics of this group included inhibition of both sexuality and motherhood, and a tendency toward unresolved hostile conflict with their mothers. This group of women exhibited masochistic characteristics and an inability to discharge or deal appropriately with anger, aggressiveness, or hostility covered over by a facade of pleasantness. A general delay in securing medical treatment for the symptoms of their condition was also noted.

The first large study was published by LeShan and Worthington (1955), who compared 152 breast cancer patients with a group of 125 control patients who were suffering from some other illness or were healthy, using a projective test developed by Worthington. Relative to the controls, the cancer women were found to have had difficulty in expressing hostile feelings, showed greater potential anxiety about the death of a parent, and had suffered the death of a loved one prior to diagnosis.

In a study of 47 breast cancer patients, Coppens and Metcalfe (1963) used the Maudsley Personality Inventory to investigate levels of extroversion. They found that their group of women with breast cancer had significantly raised extroversion scores and that this was a constitutionally determined characteristic, as opposed to a temporary reaction to their illness.

Greer and Morris (1975) reported a consecutive series of 160 women attending for a breast biopsy, of whom 69 were subsequently diagnosed histologically as having breast cancer and the remaining 91 were found to have benign breast disease. The two groups were found to be comparable with respect to both social class and marital status, but the cancer women were significantly older. There was a nonsignificant trend for the cancer group to have a less satisfactory sexual adjustment than the benign group, but there were no other differences in terms of previous psychiatric history, severity of depression (Hamilton rating scale), social adjustment, verbal intelligence (Mill Hill test), hostility (HDHQ), and extroversion and neuroticism (EPI). The mean Lie scores were over two standard deviations above the Eysenck reported norms in both diagnosis groups. Over 30% of the subjects in both groups reacted to life stresses by use of denial, and this was significantly correlated with delay in seeking treatment after the first appearance of their breast symptoms. A significantly increased proportion of the cancer patients manifested extreme suppression of both anger and other emotions, while the ability to release emotions was found to be positively correlated with age. The cancer and benign subjects reported similar amounts and types of stress, both within the preceding 5 years and during their whole lives.

Pettingale et al. (1977) studied 69 women with breast cancer and a control group of 91 women with benign breast disease. Ability to express emotions, particularly anger, was assessed using the Caine and Foulds HDHQ1 at biopsy and then at 3, 12, and 24 months after surgery. Serum IgA levels were measured at the same times. IgA levels were found to be significantly higher, in both the cancer and benign groups, among those women who were able to express anger. Over the 2-year postoperative follow-up period, serum IgA levels remained consistently higher in all patients found to suppress anger, with this relationship achieving statistical significance in the breast cancer patients at 3 and 24 months after surgery. A similar relationship with anger suppression was found by Bageley (1979), who found a significant correlation between breast cancer and a chronic behavior pattern of abnormal emotional expression, specifically, concealment of emotions and bottling up of anger, in a study of 45 women with breast cancer and 68 women with benign breast problems admitted for a breast biopsy. Bageley also reported a significantly higher incidence of subjectively stressful events during the 15 years preceding the appearance of a breast lump in the cancer group.

In a study of 71 women awaiting a breast biopsy, Morris et al. (1981) administered a battery of psychological tests and found that patients subsequently diagnosed as having cancer reported experiencing "feelings of anger" or "losing control in anger" less frequently than those patients found to have benign disease. Similarly, Wirsching et al. (1982) administered a structured interview to 56 women attending for a breast biopsy: 18 and 38 cases were subsequently diagnosed as malignant and benign lumps, respectively. The cancer patients were found to have difficulty in expressing anger, tended to avoid trouble and conflict, were less accessible or aloof, and were less anxious about the likely diagnosis of their lump, but were also less realistic about the clinical outcome, compared with the benign group. The cancer patients claimed to be more self-sufficient and altruistic, but less aggressive, than the benign group, with 70% being extremely optimistic, tending to sacrifice themselves (particularly for their family). An identified psychological syndrome was found in all of the cancer patients and about 30% of those diagnosed as having benign nodes.

A group of 121 women undergoing breast lesion biopsy (46 of which were subsequently diagnosed as cancer and 75 as benign disease) were studied by Cheang and Cooper (1985). An additional control cohort of 42 women with no palpable breast lump was drawn at random from a well-woman clinic. All the patients were assessed on the day preceding their biopsy. The cancer group was older on average, but otherwise demographic factors were well-balanced across all three groups. No significant differences were found between the groups with respect to their overall mean Type A behavior scores, but significant differences were found on 7 of the 13 individual items making up the scale. The cancer group emerged as being less pressured by time and by busy schedules, was easygoing, and tended to suppress their feelings, whereas the benign group was pressured by time and busy schedules, was fast in doing things, competitive in nature, prone to try to do many things at once, thought about what to do next, was expressive, and generally handled their emotions in a different manner from the cancer group. The control group had some of the personality traits of both lesion groups. In addition, the cancer patients had recently experienced significantly more life events than the other subjects overall. The types of events experienced differed, the cancer group reporting proportionally less low-stress events, but an increased proportion of loss-related and/or illness-related events.

Jansen and Muenz (1984) studied 69 women with breast cancer, 82 with fibrocystic disease, and 71 healthy controls drawn from other outpatient clinics prior to the subjects being made aware of their diagnosis. Relative to the benign and control groups, the cancer patients recorded significantly lower aggression and exhibition scores, but higher depression scores. The healthy controls had significantly lower order scores, but high understanding scores. Group differences were also identified for ten of the MAACL items: the healthy group was relaxed, calm, outgoing, and able to express their anger; the fibrocystic group was tense, restless, outgoing, and able to express their anger; the cancer group was timid, nonassertive, noncompetitive, calm, easy-going, and suppressed their anger. These findings held even after statistical adjustment for significant differences between the groups with respect to age, race, education level, socioeconomic status, and marital status.

Finally, Priestman et al. (1985) studied 100 women presenting at a surgical clinic with a new benign breast lump and 100 women attending a radiotherapy department for treatment of stage I/II breast cancers diagnosed within the previous 3 months; 93 of the cancer patients and 66 of the benign group were aware of their diagnosis at the time of assessment. A group of 100 "control" women were drawn from paramedical and ancillary staff at the study hospital, from members of the general public, and from friends and relatives of the women attending the study clinics. The cancer group was significantly older than the other two groups, and the control group had a significantly higher socioeconomic status, but neither imbalance was found to significantly affect the study findings. No differences were found between the groups in terms of personality (standard EPI). The control group had experienced significantly more life events in total than both the cancer and benign groups, although the types of events reported were similar in all of the groups.

LIFE EVENTS AND CANCER

The second category of studies has focused on the relationship between recent stressful life events and the diagnosis of breast cancer. Much of the published work has used the Holmes and Rahe (1967) Social Readjustment Rating Scale or a similar instrument as the main measurement tool. There are several well-documented problems with this type of rating scale which have probably contributed to the absence of any overall consistency in the findings of the studies so far published. In general, each scale consists of a list of life events, and subjects are required to indicate which of the events they have experienced in a given time period immediately prior to the study. Opinions differ over the optimum length of this time period, but most researchers have used between 2 and 5 years. Unfortunately, a number of the events listed on these instruments may be symptoms or consequences of illness rather than critical incidents (e.g., change in number of marital arguments, redundancy from work, sex difficulties, etc.). Also, the illness itself may affect recollection, impeding or preventing the patient from accurately recalling past events (Napier et al., 1972). In some instances, an extra degree of sophistication is added whereby subjects are asked to indicate the severity of the impact of each life event experienced, using a Likert-type scale. This only partially overcomes the final problem, that each event listed has differential meaning for each subject, yet they are rigidly enumerated in scoring.

Despite these problems, a small number of interesting studies have been published. In LeShan's (1959) early review of 75 studies on psychological factors in the development of malignant disease, he concluded that "the most consistently reported, relevant psychological factor has been the loss of a major emotional relationship prior to the first noted symptoms of neoplasm." In a later, large-scale epidemiological study into mortality rates among different groups of people likely to be affected by the loss of a close emotional relationship, LeShan (1966) went on to predict that cancer mortality rates would be highest for widowed and divorced persons and lowest for married and single subjects, if the theory relating to the loss of emotional relationships was valid. He age adjusted the mortality rates from a series of epidemiological studies and discovered that the results were indeed consistent with the hypothesis.

Muslin et al. (1969) interviewed and administered a life-events questionnaire to 165 women awaiting a breast biopsy. Assessments were completed prior to diagnosis, but they managed to match 37 pairs of malignant and benign patients. Relative to the benign group, twice as many diagnosed cancer patients had "a permanent loss of a first degree relative or other person whom the subject specifically stated was emotionally important to her". The same phenomenon was found by Schmale and Iker (1966), this time in a group of women reporting for a cone biopsy as the result of a positive Pap test. Conversely, however, in an investigation of social trauma in 352 women with breast cancer and 670 women with cancer and nonneoplastic diseases of organs other than the breast, Snell and Graham (1971) found no relationship between diagnosis and life events experienced during the 5 years prior to the onset of illness.

Schofield (1975) interviewed 112 Israeli women with suspicious breast lesions on the day prior to their biopsy; 85 were found to have benign tumors, but the remaining 27 subsequently had a histological diagnosis of cancer. The Minnesota Multiphasic Personality Inventory (MMPI) Lie Scale was administered and found to be both culture and age dependent. The cancer women were found to score significantly higher than the equivalent benign patients of European or American origin, but not those born in North Africa or Asia. Furthermore, the difference between the Lie scores for the cancer and benign groups was significantly more marked among the younger patients. The MMPI depression and well-being scales produced no statistically significant differences. The cancer patients had significantly higher covert anxiety scores than the benign patients, but this finding was restricted to those women under 42 years of age. No significant differences were found on the measure of overt anxiety. An examination of five items relating specifically to loss and separation showed no difference between the two diagnosis groups, but overall the cancer women had significantly lower life change unit scores than the benign group.

Finally, Becker (1978) reported a study of 49 breast cancer patients who had undergone surgery followed by post-irradiation. The youngest 25 women were defined as a "young" group (mean age, 40 years) and the remaining 24 as an "older" group (mean age, 61 years). The study revealed a high incidence of early childhood loss-related events, a low incidence of positive family atmosphere, high proportions of immunological defense system related-illnesses and surgery, a high incidence of psychosomatic symptoms prior to the diagnosis of cancer, poor marriage and sexual relations, a less positive attitude toward offspring, a high proportion of pregnancy and breast-feeding complications, a high degree of ambition and activity within marriage, a high incidence of loss and loss-related life events in the years immediately preceding diagnosis, and feelings of both disgrace and shame as a reaction to the cancer diagnosis. Most of these findings were accentuated in the "young" group. The most frequent coping strategies observed were projection, denial, and transfer to others. A high proportion of the subjects attributed their illness to psychic stress. It must be strongly emphasized, however, that the overall reliability of this study is difficult to assess as no control levels were provided for the variables studied.

PROSPECTIVE CLINICAL STUDY

Although previously published studies can be broadly divided into the two categories detailed above, in reality this dichotomy is likely to be purely academic. It is more likely that a complex intercorrelation exists between the three elements of psychosocial stress, personality, and the diagnosis of breast cancer. A large-scale prospective study was thus conducted in the U.K. to examine in depth the relationship between breast disease diagnosis, antecedent stressful life events, coping skills, and personality.

In total, 2163 women were studied at three centers; 1324 were attending as outpatients at the University Hospital of South Manchester Breast Unit and 272 were attending as outpatients at the St. Lukes Hospital Breast Clinic in Huddersfield, England. All 1596 outpatients had originally presented to their general practitioner complaining of either breast lumpiness or tenderness and had been subsequently referred for specialist assessment. Thus, on attendance at the clinic, each woman was aware that her general practitioner considered the problem sufficiently serious for referral to a specialist center, but no diagnostic tests had been carried out and no diagnosis had been made at the time she was studied. The remaining 567 women were undergoing a general medical checkup, which included a breast examination, at the BUPA Medical Centre in London, and had not complained of a breast condition in the recent past. On arriving at her clinic, each woman was asked to complete a questionnaire and to return it to the receptionist *before* her examination. The completed questionnaire was placed in the patient's clinic notes until a definitive diagnosis was available, at which time it was coded and passed on for data processing. When the final diagnoses were completed, the women were classified into four categories. Group 1 contained those women with the most severe condition, a Stage I or Stage II breast malignancy having been detected; more advanced cases were excluded from the study. Group 2 contained those women diagnosed as having a cyst; this group was created as there is some medical evidence indicating that cysts may be a precursor to a malignancy (Davies et al., 1964). All women found to have a benign condition (e.g., fibroadenosis, fibroadenoma, or nonspecific pain) were combined into a third group as there was no statistical evidence of any important differences between these benign diagnostic groupings. The fourth group was considered to be a form of control group, containing all those women found to have normal breasts.

Demographic Data

The same questionnaire was used for all 2163 women in the study. The first section of this sought background demographic details, including age, marital status, occupation, cigarette smoking history, alcohol consumption, and contraceptive pill usage (Table I). The cancer group was older on average than the cyst group, which was in turn older than the benign and normal groups. The cancer and cyst women were more likely to be married; there was a considerably greater proportion of widowed women in the cancer group relative to the remaining three groups. The cancer group women were more likely to be retired and less likely to be in either full-time or part-time employment: women in the cancer group who were in jobs were more likely to be in only part-time employment. Work pattern differences between the groups were unaffected by age.

The benign group contained proportionally more cigarette smokers in total than the other three diagnostic groups; this finding was age-related, the differences in smoking habit being much more pronounced among the younger women in the study sample. Alcohol consumption decreased as severity of diagnosis increased for all age groups. As could be expected, contraceptive

TABLE I.
Demographic Data

	Cancer	Cyst	Benign	Normal	p
	\multicolumn{4}{c}{Diagnosis Group (All Women)}				
N	171	155	1110	727	—
Age (year) mean	55	44	38	39	
(S.D.)	(14)	(9)	(11)	(11)	<0.001
Marital status (%)					
Married	75	78	67	71	<0.001
Single	6	8	17	17	
Div./sep.	5	9	13	9	
Widowed	14	5	3	3	
Occupation (%)					
Full-time	23	45	42	45	<0.001
Part-time	19	31	28	23	
Unemployed	4	2	3	1	
Retired	14	1	1	1	
Housewife	40	21	26	30	
Cigarette smokers (%)	28	32	40	26	<0.001
Alcohol consumers (%)	61	71	77	85	<0.001
Ever used contraceptive pill (%)	39	53	72	75	<0.001

pill usage (both current and previous) fell markedly with increasing age in all four diagnostic groups; pill usage also decreased as the severity of diagnosis increased among the younger women studied.

Life Events Data

The second part of the questionnaire consisted of a 42-item life events inventory devised for a U.K. female sample (Cheang and Cooper, 1985). Each woman was asked to indicate which of the listed events had been experienced during the preceding 2 years and then to score each event experienced for degree of upset or stressfulness using a 10-point, Likert-type rating scale (a score of 1 indicated minimal impact, while a score of 10 represented the worst imaginable level of upset).

The proportions of women in each group who had experienced each listed life event in the relevant time period were computed. A breakdown of these proportions by age showed that the occurrence of many of the events (e.g., retirement) were age related. Thus, as group comparisons were likely to be affected by this confounding age effect, multiple logistic regression methods were applied to each individual life event: the dependent variable was presence/absence of the life event, and the independent variables were diagnostic group and age. Since diagnostic group was a categorical variable, it was analyzed as a factor, whereas age, being a continuous variable, was treated as a covariate. To ensure that group comparisons were correctly adjusted for age effects, age was forced into the regression model before the significance of the diagnostic group was determined. A secondary analysis was then carried out, again for each life event individually, using the severity scores from those women who had experienced an event. In this instance, standard multiple regression methods were applied using severity rating as the dependent variable; age and diagnostic group were again the independent variables, with age forced into the regression model ahead of diagnostic group as before. The computations were done using the GLIM 3.77 computer program, using the procedures described by Aitken et al. (1989). Normal probability plots were constructed to verify the adequacy of each regression model (Draper and Smith, 1981).

Table II summarizes the proportions who had experienced each individual life event in the checklist. The mean numbers of life events reported by the women in the cancer, cyst, benign, and normal groups were 4.1, 4.7, 5.3, and 5.5, respectively, and these differences were highly significant ($p < 0.001$). Although the benign and normal women reported more events, these tended to be more "minor" events such as buying/moving house, pet-related problems, etc. The events recorded by the cancer and/or cyst women tended to be loss or illness related, most notably retirement, redundancy, increased nursing responsibilities, death of husband/family member/close friend, serious illness of self requiring hospitalization, and surgical operation on self (although not all of these differences reached the conventional level of statistical significance).

Table III summarizes the mean severity ratings for each life event separately. Perception of the severity of events was the reverse of incidence, with women diagnosed as having a malignancy rating most life events as producing a greater impact relative to the women in the remaining three groups. The mean severity scores over all reported events for the cancer, cyst, benign, and normal groups were 6.7, 5.4, 5.4, and 5.2, respectively. The differences were most marked for illness-related events affecting the woman personally and death-related events (with the exception of death of husband, which was rated as extremely severe by all of the women who experienced that loss). Particularly pronounced was the increased incidence, coupled with a high severity rating, among the women in the cancer group of the death of a close friend.

In an attempt to unify these findings, the 42 life events were factor analyzed to identify intercorrelated events. A severity rating of zero was allocated to all events not experienced. The number of statistical factors was determined by a varimax rotation and subsequent examination of the eigen values (only factors with eigen values greater than 1.5 were accepted). Separate factor analyses were carried out using just the presence or absence of

TABLE II.
Percentages of Women Experiencing Life Events in the Last 2 Years
(Adjusted for Age Differences)

Life Event	Cancer	Cyst	Group Benign	Control	Significance
N	171	155	1110	727	
Bought house	14.2	20.8	17.1	21.0	**
Sold house	11.2	11.7	11.9	15.7	
Moved house	13.7	9.8	15.5	20.2	**
Major house renovation	11.8	16.3	13.2	22.0	
Separation from loved one	7.4	9.0	9.5	10.5	
End of a relationship	2.5	2.1	3.8	4.4	
Got engaged	0.9	0.7	1.5	1.4	
Got married	3.7	1.1	2.3	2.6	
Marital problem	4.2	8.7	11.6	11.0	
Awaiting divorce	0.0	1.5	2.8	3.2	
Divorce	1.7	4.4	3.6	1.7	
Child started school/ nursery	5.2	1.9	6.9	9.3	
Nursing responsibility	13.3	20.3	15.8	12.2	**
Problems with relatives	14.8	16.3	23.5	24.3	
Problems with friends	4.8	6.8	9.4	8.4	
Pet-related problems	6.2	4.8	5.8	11.6	
Work-related problems	8.7	18.5	18.1	19.2	**
Change in work	8.3	10.5	12.9	14.1	
Threat of redundancy	5.2	6.3	6.0	3.3	**
Changed job	5.3	6.6	9.4	7.7	**
Made redundant	5.2	5.3	3.5	2.8	**
Unemployed	2.5	6.1	5.2	2.9	
Retired	7.7	2.3	3.1	2.5	**
New loan or mortgage	6.6	23.6	14.9	16.4	**
Financial problem	9.3	18.0	15.2	11.7	
Insurance problem	3.0	2.1	1.9	1.0	
Legal problem	0.2	5.9	8.8	5.3	
Illness to family member	26.2	23.2	32.8	30.2	
Family member in hospital	28.8	24.5	23.6	22.2	
Family member had surgery	16.2	20.3	16.5	19.1	
Death of husband	2.4	2.9	2.1	2.0	
Death of family member	32.0	28.6	23.7	26.0	

(Continued)

TABLE II (Cont.).
Percentages of Women Experiencing Life Events in the Last 2 Years (Adjusted for Age Differences)

Death of close friend	11.7	7.8	7.7	5.5	**
Illness of self	26.5	26.6	28.5	20.6	
Self in hospital	8.9	7.0	8.1	2.5	
Self had surgery	27.0	17.1	24.5	17.5	
Pregnancy	2.9	1.0	1.7	3.3	**
Birth of baby	0.4	0.9	1.9	2.6	**
Birth of grandchild	11.3	6.5	6.8	10.2	**
Family left home	8.0	21.3	13.7	15.6	**
Difficulties with children	4.7	12.4	14.1	14.2	**
Difficulties with parents	2.5	4.8	6.5	7.8	

** $p < 0.05$.

TABLE III.
Mean Severity Scores for Life Events Experienced in the Last 2 Years (Adjusted for Age Differences)

Life Event	Group				S.D.[a]	Significance
	Cancer	Cyst	Benign	Control		
Bought house	2.5	3.1	3.3	3.5	2.3	
Sold house	3.5	4.3	4.5	4.3	2.7	
Moved house	3.3	4.2	4.1	4.1	2.6	
Major house renovation	4.1	5.0	4.0	4.3	2.5	
Separation from loved one	7.0	7.7	7.9	7.2	2.4	
End of a relationship	7.5	6.2	7.2	7.0	2.5	
Got engaged	6.8	4.8	3.0	2.9	2.3	*
Got married	5.7	4.8	3.8	3.5	2.5	
Marital problem	6.2	7.4	7.4	7.0	2.4	
Awaiting divorce	6.2	6.6	7.0	7.3	3.0	
Divorce	7.4	8.4	6.4	5.4	3.0	
Child started school/ nursery	3.3	4.2	2.9	2.7	2.1	
Nursing responsibility	7.8	6.0	6.8	6.0	2.5	**
Problems with relatives	7.1	6.2	6.3	6.1	2.3	
Problems with friends	4.8	6.1	5.4	4.6	2.5	*
Pet-related problems	6.0	6.8	5.6	5.5	2.6	

(Continued)

TABLE III (Cont.).
Mean Severity Scores for Life Events Experienced in the Last 2 Years
(Adjusted for Age Differences)

Work-related problems	6.1	5.2	5.6	5.8	2.4	
Change in work	4.0	4.9	4.0	4.1	2.6	
Threat of redundancy	5.8	4.7	6.1	6.9	3.0	
Changed job	4.8	3.7	3.6	4.1	2.5	
Made redundant	6.4	7.7	5.8	5.4	3.1	
Unemployed	6.6	7.2	5.8	5.8	2.7	
Retired	6.1	3.5	4.5	3.5	3.0	
New loan or mortgage	3.9	3.7	3.7	3.6	2.3	
Financial problem	5.3	7.0	5.7	5.8	2.5	*
Insurance problem	4.4	6.0	4.0	4.4	2.3	
Legal problem	3.3	7.1	6.5	5.9	2.4	
Illness to family member	7.4	6.8	7.0	6.7	2.3	
Family member in hospital	8.0	7.3	7.5	7.2	2.2	
Family member had surgery	6.5	6.9	6.2	6.3	2.7	
Death of husband	9.7	9.5	10.0	10.0	0.5	
Death of family member	8.1	7.4	7.8	7.3	2.5	
Death of close friend	9.1	7.7	6.9	7.0	2.1	**
Illness of self	7.5	6.3	6.2	6.5	2.5	**
Self in hospital	7.7	6.2	6.8	6.1	2.5	
Self had surgery	7.1	5.5	5.6	5.3	2.5	**
Pregnancy	5.5	3.0	4.2	4.3	3.0	
Birth of baby	6.0	4.0	4.1	4.4	2.9	
Birth of grandchild	3.9	3.1	3.7	4.3	2.6	
Family left home	3.9	4.8	5.4	5.2	2.9	
Difficulties with children	6.3	4.7	5.6	5.8	2.6	
Difficulties with parents	7.2	3.6	5.3	5.6	2.6	

* $p < 0.10$; ** $p < 0.05$.
[a] Pooled standard error.

TABLE IV.
Factor Analysis of Life Event Severity Ratings

Factor	Factor Scores Mean (S.E.)				*p*
	Cancer	Cyst	Benign	Normal	
1	0.43 (0.08)	0.76 (0.13)	0.81 (0.05)	1.07 (0.07)	<0.001
2	0.56 (0.06)	0.81 (0.12)	1.00 (0.05)	0.89 (0.05)	<0.002
3	0.57 (0.08)	0.93 (0.13)	1.01 (0.04)	1.03 (0.05)	<0.001
4	2.21 (0.20)	1.84 (0.22)	1.86 (0.08)	1.86 (0.09)	<0.412
5	0.22 (0.08)	0.14 (0.06)	0.25 (0.03)	0.24 (0.04)	<0.597

Factor 1
  Bought house; sold house; moved house; major house renovation; increased or new bank loan/mortgage
Factor 2
  Separation from loved one; end of relationship; marital problem; awaiting divorce; divorce; financial difficulty; legal problem; emotional or physical illness of yourself
Factor 3
  Problem with relatives; work-related problems; change in nature of work; threat of redundancy; changed job; made redundant; unemployed; increased or new bank loan/mortgage; financial difficulty
Factor 4
  Increased nursing responsibilities; problem with relatives; emotional or physical illness of close family or relative; serious illness of close family or relative requiring hospitalization; surgical operation experienced by family members or relatives; death of family member or relative
Factor 5
  Got married; pregnancy; birth of a baby

each event and then using the actual severity rating. Factor scores were computed for each of the 2163 women in the study and then the mean factor scores were compared across the four diagnostic groups (without age adjustment) using a one-way analysis of variance and Tukey multiple comparison tests. The severity ratings revealed five factors (Table IV), defined as "property related", "personal relationship problems", "work/employment related", "serious illness of a close family member", and "marriage/birth". Only the first three of these factors produced any significant differences between the diagnostic groups, with mean scores tending to decrease as the severity of illness increased (i.e., the largest scores were found in the normal and benign groups, and the smallest scores in the cancer group). The cancer group recorded the highest mean score for the "illness of a close family member" factor, although the differences between the four diagnostic groups failed to reach a conventional level of statistical significance. The factor analysis of the incidence data was less satisfactory, mainly due to the non-normal form of the data (Table V). Four factors emerged, defined as "personal relationship/work-related problems", "property related", "marriage/birth", and "serious illness of a close family member". Significant differences in mean scores were achieved only by the first two of these factors, the mean score tending to decrease as diagnostic severity increased.

Coping Skills Data

The third section of the questionnaire was an adopted and shortened ways of coping inventory of 36 items (Folkman and Lazarus, 1980). The women in the cancer and cyst groups recorded significantly fewer "coping skills" in total than the benign and normal subjects (Table VI). The actual skills reported by the cancer and cyst groups tended to be "negative", in the sense that they indicated a tendency to bottle up feelings combined with a reluctance to show/express their emotions even in private.

Personality Data

The fourth section of the questionnaire was a Type A behavior inventory of 14 personality traits, each self-related on an ll-point, Likert-type scale, with high scores indicating type A behavior. The mean scores for each of the 14 traits are summarized in Table VII. The cancer women tended to be less casual about appointments than other subjects, but for virtually all the other measures of behavior, the cancer group was substantially less type A in nature. The cumulative effect of these differences was that the total behavior score was significantly lower (i.e., type B) in the cancer group than in the remaining three diagnostic groups. The statistical significance of these differences was

TABLE V.
Factor Analysis of Life Event Incidence

Factor	Factor Scores Mean (S.E.)				p
	Cancer	Cyst	Benign	Normal	
1	0.12 (0.01)	0.18 (0.02)	0.23 (0.01)	0.22 (0.01)	<0.001
2	0.14 (0.02)	0.21 (0.03)	0.21 (0.01)	0.28 (0.01)	<0.001
3	0.04 (0.01)	0.04 (0.02)	0.06 (0.01)	0.06 (0.01)	<0.588
4	0.27 (0.02)	0.25 (0.93)	0.25 (0.01)	0.27 (001)	<0.802

Factor 1
  Separation from loved one; end of relationship; marital problem; awaiting divorce; divorce; problem with relatives; problems with friends/neighbors; work-related problems; change in nature of work; changed job; unemployed; financial difficulty; legal problem; emotional or physical illness of yourself; difficult relationship with parents
Factor 2
  Bought house; sold house; moved house; major house renovation; increased or new bank loan/mortgage
Factor 3
  Pregnancy; birth of a baby
Factor 4
  Increased nursing responsibilities for elderly or sick person; problem with relatives; emotional or physical illness of close family or relative; serious illness of close family or relative requiring hospitalization; surgical operation experienced by family member or relative; death of family members or relative

TABLE VI.
Coping Skills

	Diagnosis Group									
	All Women					Women 50 Years of Age or More				
	Cancer	Cyst	Benign	Normal	p	Cancer	Cyst	Benign	Normal	p
Cry on my own (%)	30	34	41	40	0.030	27	29	31	30	0.895
Bottle it up, then break down (%)	24	17	23	18	0.024	19	17	17	13	0.664
Tearful when relaxed (%)	9	17	15	19	0.014	8	14	5	19	0.003
Eat more (%)	13	17	23	27	<0.001	9	20	20	20	0.082
Get angry (%)	10	14	25	21	<0.001	10	11	14	15	0.646
Let feelings out (%)	39	38	47	49	0.027	32	34	39	46	0.213
Treat myself (%)	11	9	18	27	<0.001	11	3	13	13	0.353
Wish could change what happened (%)	27	29	39	43	<0.001	23	34	39	40	0.024
Fantasize (%)	9	11	21	22	<0.001	47	11	16	14	0.229
Feel learned something (%)	20	27	28	33	0.002	16	20	23	31	0.073
No. of coping skills mean	7.9	7.7	9.1	9.2	<0.001	7.0	6.8	7.7	7.8	0.490
(S.D.)	(5.3)	(5.0)	(5.4)	(5.0)		(5.1)	(5.2)	(5.4)	(4.8)	

TABLE VII.
Personality Traits Constituting Behavior Inventory Factors

Factor 1: Time Consciousness
   Never feels rushed (even under pressure)/always rushed
   Can wait patiently/impatient while waiting
   Takes things one at a time/tries to do many things at once, thinks
      about what will do next
   Slow deliberate talker/emphatic speech, fast and forceful

Factor 2: Personal Drive
   Not competitive/very competitive
   Easy going/hard driving (pushing yourself and others)
   Unambitious/ambitious

Factor 3: Satisfaction/Contentedness
   Casual about appointments/never late
   Cares about satisfying self no matter what others may think/wants
      good job, wants to be recognized by others
   Slow doing things/fast (eating, talking)
   Casual/eager to get things done

Interpersonal Relations
   Good listener/anticipates what others are going to say (nods, attempts
      to finish for them)
   Expresses feelings/hides feelings
   Many outside interests/few interests outside work and home

evaluated using one-way analyses of variance to compare the mean values for the low diagnostic groups.

Numerically, the overall differences between the four subject groups were smaller than might have been expected if type A/B personality traits were an important precursor to susceptibility to breast cancer. This raised the possibility that a straight dichotomy of individuals into either type A or type B personality types was too crude, and that much subtler differences in personality traits existed between the diagnostic groups. To examine this hypothesis, the behavior inventory data for all the subjects combined were subjected to a principal components analysis with a single varimax rotation. This identified four separate factors with eigen values greater than 1.5. The personality traits making up each factor are listed in Table VIII.

The first factor was made up of four personality traits relating to time consciousness (i.e., rushing/"hurry sickness"). The cancer, cyst, and benign groups all scored significantly lower than the normal group, indicating that the women diagnosed as having breast problems tended to have more "laid back" lifestyles, being less rushed, more deliberate, and more patient than the control women. The cancer women scored lower on average for this factor than the benign and cyst groups, although these differences did not reach an acceptable level of statistical significance.

The second factor consisted of three personality traits relating to personal drive (i.e., levels of ambition and competitiveness). As with factor 1, the cancer and benign groups all scored significantly lower than the normal group, indicating that the women with breast pathologies were much less competitive, ambitious, and hard driving than the women with normal breasts.

The third factor included four personality traits relating to levels of personal satisfaction and contentedness with one's own activities. The cancer and benign groups scored significantly lower on this factor than the cyst and normal groups. Low scores in this instance were indicative of a slow and casual approach to activities and an increased desire to gain personal satisfaction irrespective of the reaction of others.

The final factor was made up of three personality traits describing interpersonal relations. The cancer group scored significantly higher (indicating a tendency to suppress feelings and to have few interests involving personal relationships outside of the home and work environments) than both the benign and normal groups.

These findings confirm those obtained by many other researchers on the relationship between personality traits and breast pathology, the most prominent effects being observed among the women with malignancies. Relative to the normal group, the women with breast pathologies tended to be more "laid back", deliberate, and patient, were measurably less competitive, ambitious, and hard-driving, had a slow and casual approach to activities, and showed an increased level of introversion.

Social Support Data

The final section of the questionnaire was a social support inventory listing the people to whom a subject could turn with a major personal problem or crisis and their relationship to the patient. Overall, the total amount of social support was the same for the four diagnostic groups, although the

TABLE VIII.
Mean (S.D.) Personality Factor Scores

	Cancer	Cyst	Benign	Normal	*p*
Factor 1	27.1	28.5	28.4	29.4	0.002
	(7.4)	(7.0)	(7.2)	(7.2)	
Factor 2	18.4	18.6	18.9	19.7	0.014
	(6.5)	(6.0)	(6.0)	(6.2)	
Factor 3	31.4	32.6	31.9	32.7	0.020
	(5.8)	(5.8)	(5.9)	(5.8)	
Factor 4	21.5	20.9	19.8	19.8	0.002
	(5.5)	(5.8)	(5.9)	(5.8)	

women with cancer were found to have significantly less access to a parent, counterbalanced by significantly more access to their children.

METHODOLOGICAL DIFFICULTIES

Many of the studies described above contain serious methodological flaws, making interpretation difficult and the existence of apparently contradictory findings incvitable.

The most glaring weakness is the inadequacy of the sample sizes used in many studies. With few notable exceptions, total samples are less than 200, with individual group sizes of considerably below 100 commonplace. Under such circumstances, it is questionable whether the study samples are particularly representative of the population as a whole. The findings on personality predispositions are less affected by sample size, so are generally more consistent than those on life events. Personality measures can be taken from all subjects in a study allowing an overall picture to be built up on relatively small numbers. Sample size is a much more acute problem when studying life events, particularly when the types of events most closely related to the diagnosis of breast cancer are loss and illness related, which tend to occur relatively infrequently in a normal population over a short (2 to 3-year) time period. For theoretical statistical reasons, the less frequent the event, the larger the sample required, both to obtain an accurate estimate of the true population frequency and to establish statistical significance at conventional levels between diagnosis groupings.

Many studies also employ weak experimental designs, particularly with respect to the choice of a control group. A common fault is the use of only a cancer and a benign breast disease group. The discovery of breast lumpiness or tenderness may conceivably alter some personality factors (notably anxiety) and attitude to other life events, so it is unreasonable to assume that a benign lump group is an adequate control for breast cancer patients. For this reason, either a group of normal "healthy" subjects drawn randomly from the general population, or a group of normal subjects drawn randomly from a nonbreast disease clinic, should also be included. This would provide an ideal of two control groups, one of subjects who have some chronic, nonmalignant breast problem sufficient to cause anxiety about their health, and the other a group of "healthy" subjects. Great care should be taken to balance these groups (as far as logistically possibly) with respect to important confounding factors such as age, smoking history, and alcohol consumption so that the study findings can be fitted into a proper conceptual or theoretical framework.

Several reported studies have been retrospective and have used patients who are aware of their diagnosis. If the presence of a breast problem may affect the measurement of personality and life events, the effect of the knowledge of the histological diagnosis will have an even greater effect. Indeed, there is already evidence available (Craig and Abeloff, 1974) suggesting that the awareness of having cancer can alter various personality measures. It is vital, therefore, that subjects are assessed certainly prior to diagnosis and, if at all possible, prior to biopsy.

Choice of measurement scales is clearly important when designing a study, particularly for the assessment of life events. A great deal of research in the stress field has been conducted using life event scales which include generic weightings which may bias or distort research results. Such scales list events which may be either symptoms or consequences of illness rather than critical incidents; the illness itself may impede or prevent the patient from accurately recalling past events and then rating the severity of their impact; and individual perceptions of the events are rarely taken into proper account. A full critique of stress and life event methodology has been compiled by Cooper et al. (1985).

In addition to design flaws, there are considerable concerns relating to the methods of statistical analysis used in many studies. Specifically, it is commonly assumed that the variables measured are statistically independent, with no interrelationships present, despite clear evidence that this is not the case. As already stated, it is important that groups of patients to be compared in a statistical analysis are comparable with respect to their demographic characteristics. However, when diagnosis is not known until after the study assessments have been completed, this is not always possible. Thus, a finding common to many published studies is that breast cancer patients tend to be older than the benign lump patients and the healthy controls. Age is clearly an important confounding factor, particularly when important outcome measures are themselves age dependent. It has been established that a number of personality measures and the frequency of major impact life events (particularly loss and illness-related events) change with increasing age. It is grossly inadequate, therefore, to analyze such data univariately; statistical adjustment for age and other confounding factors present using multivariate methods is essential.

Finally, it is becoming increasingly obvious that the relationship between psychosocial factors and breast cancer is both clinically and mathematically extremely complex. If the intricacies of the interrelationships are to be untangled, future studies must be large (probably multicenter) if they are to achieve adequate samples of breast cancer patients. The objectives of such studies may also need to be rethought. While it may be interesting to establish statistically significant differences between diagnostic groups, this is of limited clinical interest. A more probabilistic approach may have more relevance, whereby combinations of psychosocial factors are sought which can be formed into a multivariate statistical algorithm for predicting the relative risks of each diagnosis (cancer, benign, and normal) for an individual patient. Such an approach would then lead naturally into the next era of longitudinal studies; these would be designed to investigate the effects of treating/manipulating psychosocial factors found to be statistically related to diagnosis, with the long-term aim of reducing the population incidence of breast cancer.

DISCUSSION

Although the results of published studies have been contradictory in detail, a number of recurrent findings are beginning to emerge which fit into a definable theoretical framework. Many studies report an increase in major impact life events in the years immediately preceding the diagnosis of breast cancer. An increased incidence of recent bereavement is a particularly frequent finding, and this link need not necessarily be limited to the death of the patient's husband or a close family member. The study described in detail above further implicates the death of a close (nonfamily) friend. This would imply that it is not simply the loss of a loved family member which can, for some women, act as a precursor to breast malignancy, but, rather, the loss of any very close personal relationship through bereavement. The effects on individuals of a death within the family are well known and support is often available both from within the family and from outside support agencies such as the family medical practitioner. Such support may not be forthcoming, however, when the death occurs outside the confines of the standard family grouping, suggesting that the impact of such an event may be generally underestimated. Outward visible signs of grief and distress are socially acceptable in the wake of the death of a family member. Indeed, such behavior is often encouraged as a vital part of the healing process in these circumstances, but it is much less regarded when a nonfamily friend dies. Following the latter, therefore, grief is less likely to be openly expressed and may be bottled up, to the detriment of the individual concerned, particularly as hiding the signs of grief will minimize the chances of the required social/family support being mobilized. It is probably not coincidence that personality factors identified by many studies as being related to breast cancer are of an introverted nature, a tendency to bottle up feelings and a decreased ability to express emotions such as anger.

Other major impact life events found to be related to breast cancer were major personal illness (particularly if this involved hospitalization and/or surgery), retirement, and redundancy. Illness of a close family member appears to be related primarily when the illness involves much increased responsibility for nursing that family member. All other life events generally show either no differences between diagnostic groups or a decreased incidence in women with breast cancer.

In our own study, however, examination of the severity ratings recorded by those women who experienced each life event revealed a completely different picture. Virtually all of the events in a 42-item checklist showed a similar trend, mean ratings tending to increase with the severity of the diagnosis. Clearly, irrespective of incidence rates, the cancer group was *perceiving* the impact of events as being most severe, with the "normal" women producing the lowest mean severity scores. A factor analysis of these results grouped together combinations of relatively minor events, but noticeably excluded all of the major events such as bereavement, serious personal illness, and retirement. This would suggest that each major event was having sufficient impact on its own to be correlated with diagnosis, whereas the more minor events were having a measurable effect only when occurring in combination. Furthermore, some of these minor event factors emerged as negatively related to diagnosis severity; being relatively minor, it is possible that these events were being suppressed subconsciously due to the presence of one or more major events, causing some under reporting. Certainly, it is possible that, for example, house renovations in the past 2 years will pale into insignificance relative to a bereavement.

The degree of impact of the life events also appeared to be related to the degree of *control* the individuals had over them. Thus, the events with a minor and/or negative relationship with diagnosis were largely within the control of the patient, who could be reasonably expected to have some personal responsibility for them occurring. Conscious individual decisions usually precipitate a house move or major renovation. Interrelationship problems with family, friends, or neighbors can often be resolved with the necessary will. Positively related problems, conversely, were generally outside of personal control. Bereavement and personal illness are events which invariably strike unexpectedly without prior warning. Similarly, for most women, retirement and redundancy are often imposed events over which they have little, if any, control. In the presence of the appropriate coping skills, their impact may be controllable, but their occurrence is not. Unfortunately, another feature of many studies in this area is that women diagnosed as having breast cancer tend not have the requisite coping skills and tend to have personality facets which decrease, rather than increase, their ability to control their situation adequately. These women tend to use fewer coping skills than other groups, utilizing "negative" skills such as crying on their own, bottling up their emotions, failing to get angry or to let their feelings out, and are less adept at learning from their experiences. They also tend to have a more "laid back" and less rushed lifestyle, to have reduced personal drive (i.e., unambitious and noncompetitive), to be less contented and satisfied with their activities, and to have fewer personal relationships outside of their own home and work environments.

CONCLUSIONS

It is becoming increasingly clear that some (but not all) major life events are related to both the incidence and the severity of breast disease. If a major impact event occurs which is outside the personal control of the individual experiencing it, it is much more likely to be a precursor, particularly to a breast malignancy. It is not simply the occurrence of the event which is implicated, but also (and probably more importantly) the individual's perception of its effect on them. The greater the perceived impact, the higher the risk of breast disease and the severity of that disease. However, the degree to which the individual is equipped to deal with the situation she finds herself in also correlates significantly with diagnosis: the evidence suggests that a positive, well-integrated lifestyle allied to appropriate and varied coping skills may act as mediators.

It is unlikely, from the evidence available, that a major impact life event can cause breast cancer, but it may well accelerate an already existing disease process because of the reduction in the effectiveness of the immunological system due to a switching of resources to cope with the impact of the life event. It is now possible to hypothesize that personality and coping skills moderate this process, reducing the strain on the immune processes. The implications of this hypothesis on the etiology of breast cancer is immense and should produce much exciting future research in the whole area of the effect of stress perception on breast cancer and other illnesses.

REFERENCES

Ader R: Psychosomatic and psychoimmunologic research. *Psychosom. Med.* 1980; 42:307–321.

Aitken M, Anderson A, Francis B, and Hinde J: *Statistical Modelling in GLIM.* Clarendon Press, Oxford, 1989.

Bacon CL, Renneker R, and Cutler M: A psychosomatic survey of cancer of the breast. *Psychosom. Med.* 1952; 14(6):453–460.

Bageley C: Control of events, remote stress and emergence of breast cancer. *Am. J. Clin. Psychol.* 1979; 6:213–220.

Becker H: Psychodynamic aspects of breast cancer: differences in younger and older patients. *Psychother. Psychosom.* 1978; 32:287–296.

Cheang A and Cooper CL: Psychosocial factors in breast cancer. *Stress Med.* 1985; 1:61–66.

Cooper CL, Ed: *Stress Research: Issues for the Eighties.* John Wiley & Sons, Chichester, 1983.

Cooper CL, Ed. *Psychosocial Stress and Cancer.* John Wiley & Sons, Chichester, 1984.

Cooper CL, Ed. Stress and Breast Cancer. John Wiley & Sons, Chichester, 1988.

Cooper CL, Cooper R, and Faragher EB: Stress and life event methodology. *Stress Med.* 1985; 1:287–289.

Coppens A and Metcalfe M: Cancer and extroversion. *Br. Med. J.* 1963; 18–19.

Davies HH, Simons M, and Davie JB: Cystic disease of the breast: relationship to carcinoma. *Cancer* 1964; 17:957–978.

Draper NR and Smith H: *Applied Regression Analysis.* John Wiley & Sons, New York (1981).

Evans E: *A Psychological Study of Cancer.* Dodd-Mead, New York (1926).

Eysenck HJ: Lung cancer and stress personality inventory. In *Psychosocial Stress and Cancer.* Cooper CL, Ed. John Wiley & Sons, Chichester 1984; 49–72.

Folkman S and Lazarus RS: An analysis of coping in a middle-aged community sample. *J. Health Soc. Behav.* 1980; 21:219–239.

Fox BH: Premorbid psychological factors as related to cancer incidence. *J. Behav. Med.* 1978; 1(1):45–133.

Greer S and Morris T: Psychological attributes of women who develop breast cancer: a controlled study. *J. Psychosom. Res.* 1975; 19:147–153.

Haney CA: Illness behaviour and psychosocial correlates of cancer. *J. Soc. Sci. Med.* 1977; 11(4):223–228.

Holmes TH and Rahe RH: The social readjustment rating scale. *J. Psychosom. Res.* 1967; 11:218–231.

Irwin T and Anisman H: Stress and pathology: immunological and central nervous system interactions. In *Psychosocial Stress and Cancer.* Cooper CL, Ed. John Wiley & Sons, Chichester, 1984.

Jacobs TJ and Charles E: Life events and the occurrence of cancer in children. *Psychosom. Med.* 1980; 42:11.

Jansen MA and Muenz LR: A retrospective study of personality variables associated with fibrocystic disease and breast cancer. *J. Psychosom. Res.* 1984; 28:35.

Kissen D: The present status of psychosomatic cancer research. *Geriatrics* 1969; 24:129.

Lehrer S: Life changes and gastric cancer. *Psychosom. Med.* 1980; 42:499.

LeShan L: Psychological states as factors in the development of malignant disease: a critical review. *J. Natl. Cancer Inst.* 1959; 22:1–18.

LeShan L: An emotional life-history pattern associated with neoplastic disease. *Ann. N.Y. Acad. Sci.* 1966; 125:780–793.

LeShan L and Worthington RE: Some psychological correlates of neoplastic disease: preliminary report. *J. Clin. Exp. Psychopathol.* 1955; 16:281.

Locke SE: Stress, adaptation and immunity: studies in humans. *Gen. Hosp. Psychiatry* 1982; 4:49–58.

Morris T, Greer S, Pettingale KW, and Watson M: Patterns of expression of anger and their psychological correlates in women with breast cancer. *J. Psychosom. Res.* 1981; 25:111–117.

Muslin HL, Gyarfas K, and Pieper WJ: Separation experience and cancer of the breast. *Ann. N.Y. Acad. Sci.* 1966; 125:802–806.

Napier JS, Metzner H, and Johnson BC: Limitations of morbidity and mortality data obtained from family histories: a report from the Tecumseh studies. *Am. J. Publ. Health* 1972; 62:30–35.

Newton RW and Hunt LP: Psychosocial stress in pregnancy and its relation to low birth weight. *Br. J. Med.* 1984; 288:1191.

Pettingale KW, Greer S, and Dudley E: Serum IgA and emotional expression in breast cancer patients. *J. Psychosom. Res.* 1977; 21:395–399.

Priestman TJ, Priestman SG, and Bradshaw C: Stress and breast cancer. *Br. Med. J.* 1985; 51:493–498.

Rogers MP, Dubey D, and Reich P: The influence of the psyche and the brain on immunity and disease susceptibility: a critical review. *Psychosom. Med.* 1979; 41:147–164.

Schmale AH and Iker HP: The effect of hopelessness and the development of cancer. *J. Psychosom. Med.* 1966; 28:714–721.

Schofield J: Psychological and life experience differences between Israeli women with benign and cancerous breast lesions. *J. Psychosom. Res.* 1975; 19:229–234.

Selye H: Correlating stress and cancer. *Am. J. Proctol. Gastroenterol. Colon Rect. Surg.* 1979; 30(4):18–28.

Snell L and Graham S: Social trauma as related to cancer of the breast. *Br. J. Cancer* 1971; 25:271.

Snow H: *Cancer and the Cancer Process.* J. & A. Churchill, London (1983).

Solomon GF and Amkraut AA: Psychoneuroendocrinological effects on the immune response. *Annu. Rev. Microbiol.* 1981; 35:155–184.

Stein M: A biopsychosocial approach to immune function and medical disorders. *Psychiatr. Clin. N. Am.* 1981; 4:203–221.

Tarlau M and Smalheiser I: Personality patterns in patients with malignant tumours of the breast and cervix. *Psychosom. Med.* 1951; 13(2):117–121.

Wirssching M, Stierlin H, Hoffman F, Weber G, and Wirsching B: Psychological identifications of breast cancer patients before biopsy. *J. Psychosom. Res.* 1982; 26:1–10.

e Role of Stress Hormones in the Modulation the Immune Response

Interactions Between the Immune System and the Nervous System*

Robert E. Faith
Center for Comparative Medicine
Baylor College of Medicine
Houston, Texas

Anthony J. Murgo
Food and Drug Administration
Rockville, Maryland

Nicholas P. Plotnikoff
Department of Pharmacodynamics
College of Pharmacy
University of Illinois at Chicago
Chicago, Illinois

*This Chapter was co-authored by Dr. Murgo in his private capacity. No official support or endorsement by the Food and Drug Administration is intended or should be inferred.

Stress is a complex concept that has both mental and physiological components. Some forms of stress are predominately psychological but result in a variety of physiological changes, including modulation of immune function. This indicates a link between the nervous and immune systems, and data supporting this link is reviewed in this chapter. The subject matter to be covered in this chapter, while considered to be a relatively new area of investigation by some, actually covers a sizable body of information. Due to the volume of information which relates to interactions between the central nervous system and the immune system, this chapter will review representative information indicating the extent of these interactions.

The science of immunology has come a long way in its relatively brief history. Earlier, the immune system and immune responses were viewed in rather simple terms. The immune system was viewed to be rather autonomous in its functions and to be a primarily internally regulated system. This view was supported by the fact that various elements of the immune system are capable of functioning in *in vitro* systems and by the natural antibody selection theory (Jerne, 1955). As our knowledge of immunity and the immune system has grown, it has become increasingly clear that the immune system is quite complex in its makeup, functions, and interactions with other physiological systems.

As the complexity of the immune system has become increasingly clear, it has also become apparent that the immune system interacts with other bodily systems, especially the endocrine system and the nervous system. Research is now being done which examines the relationships and interactions between other systems and the immune system. In fact, it has recently been suggested that perhaps the immune system should be viewed as an internal sensory organ recognizing noncognitive stimuli such as bacteria, viruses, antigens, etc. and relaying information to the neuroendocrine system by lymphocyte-derived hormones (Blalock, 1984). The field of immunology is being expanded to include interactions with the nervous system and the endocrine system. This field of investigation is being viewed as a new discipline which is currently being called neuroimmunology by N.H. Spector or, with more emphasis on the behavioral aspects, psychoneuroimmunology by R. Ader.

Observations linking the central nervous system and host defense mechanisms are not all recent. Clinicians have been making observations for more than 2000 years indicating that mood states may affect susceptibility to physical illness (Kronfol et al., 1983). Studies have shown that severe depression and other mental illnesses may result in suppression of host defense mechanisms (Kronfol et al., 1983; Solomon, 1981, Tecoma and Huey, 1985). Kronofol et al. (1983) have shown depressed patients to have suppressed lymphocyte responsiveness to *in vitro* stimulation by mitogens. Tecoma and Huey (1985) have reviewed a number of studies relating mood state to immune function. Studies with bereaved patients have shown that while bereavement results in no change in absolute T- and B-cell numbers, it does result in significant suppression in the ability of T-lymphocytes to respond to mitogen stimulation. Patients hospitalized for major depressive disorders were found to have significantly depressed lymphocyte responses to mitogens, lymphocytopenia, and relative hypercortisolemia compared to nondepressed controls. Studies of medical students and nonpsychotic psychiatric inpatients indicate that loneliness may result in a suppression of natural killer (NK) cell activity. Finally, a number of immunologic abnormalities have been shown in schizophrenics (Solomon, 1981). Findings in schizophrenics include abnormalities in levels of immunoglobulins, abnormal heterophile antibodies, the presence of autoantibodies to a variety of self components, including the presence of antibrain antibodies, deficient immune responsitivity, and morphologic and functional abnormalities of immunologically competent cells.

There have been preliminary studies which indicate that survival time for some patients with cancer and AIDS seem to be prolonged in association with a positive mental state (Derogatis et al., 1979; Solomon et al., 1987; Solomon, 1985). Personality-type models of patients have been developed which correlate with the length of time that patients might survive (Fox et al., 1987). Often, therapy of patients with chronic diseases now includes measures aimed at improving the mental state of the patient.

The observations of changes in immunological functions associated with changes in mental state provide one body of indirect evidence showing interactions between the immune system and the central nervous system. Other indirect evidence comes from studies which indicate that behavioral conditioning techniques may be used to modify immune responses. In a series of fairly recent studies, Ader and co-workers have investigated conditioning suppressive effects on immune functions (Ader and Cohen, 1981). These investigators used an illness-induced taste aversion conditioning paradigm in which consumption of distinctively flavored drinking solution, saccharin, was paired with an injection of an immunosuppressive drug, cyclophosphamide. Conditioned animals subsequently reexposed to saccharin drinking water and immunized showed a lessened antibody response when compared to control animals or conditioned animals not reexposed to the saccharin drinking water. The investigators interpreted these results ''to reflect a conditioned immunosuppressive response in the experimental group''. This result has been successfully repeated under a variety of conditions and has been replicated by others (Rogers et al., 1976; Wayner, et al., 1987). Conditioned immunosuppressive responses have been observed in rats and mice, with T-independent antigens as well as T-dependent antigens, and with cell-mediated immune responses as well as humoral responses. The possibility of elevated corticosteroids resulting from the aversive stimuli has been ruled out as the cause of the observed immunosuppression.

Ader (1981) has recently reviewed the history of conditioned immunobiologic responses. The first report of conditioned regulation of leukocyte reactions appears to have been in 1926 in the Russian literature. Since that time, there have been a number of reports of conditioned regulation of leukocyte reactions. The phagocytosis of foreign protein has been reported to be subject to conditioning effects. Other nonspecific immune functions are also subject to conditioning. Both complement and lysozyme activity have been shown to be subject to conditioning. These responses are assumed to be mediated via hypothalamic-pituitary-adrenocortical mechanisms. Additionally, a number of studies have shown that antibody responses are subject to conditioning.

The lymphoid organs, like other organs, are innervated by elements of the autonomic nervous system, and there is a growing body of data that indicate that the autonomic nervous system can have immunomodulatory effects. The data include the location of nerves in lymphoid tissues, the effect of the sympathetic nervous system on immune responses, the identification of neurotransmitter receptors on lymphocytes, and the effect of neurotransmitters on lymphocyte activity. Each of these areas is discussed in some detail in the following paragraphs.

There are several reviews which discuss the innervation of the immune system (Bullock, 1985; Felten et al., 1987; Steal et al., 1987; Walker and Codd, 1985). Both primary (thymus and bone marrow) and secondary (spleen, lymph nodes, and gut-associated lymphoid tissue [GALT]) is supplied by mesenteric ganglia. In the thymus, the noradrenergic (NA) fibers are distributed almost exclusively in the thymic cortex. Both the outermost zone of the cortex and vasculature at the cortico-medullary junction receive dense innervation. Developing thymocytes, which have been shown to possess β-adrenoceptors and to respond to catecholamines with altered expression of T-cell surface alloantigens, are the suspected target of this innervation. There are several compartments of lymph nodes which receive NA innervation, including the medullary cords, the paracortex and subcapsular cortex, the parafollicular areas in the cortex/paracortex, the subcapsular sinus, and the capsule.

The NA innervation of the spleen has been extensively studied, and these studies will be reviewed in some depth to illustrate the interrelations between the autonomic nervous system and lymphoid organs. The NA innervation of the spleen is distributed with the vascular and trabecular systems, and is associated mainly with the central artery and its branches, the periarteriolar lymphatic sheath (PALS), the marginal sinus, and the parafollicular zone, with occasional delicate fibers also present in follicles (Felten et al., 1987). There are several regions of contact between nerves and lymphocytes or macrophages. The nerve fibers in the PALS and in the plexuses around the central arterial system are present among T-lymphocytes (both T-helper and T-suppressor cells) and interdigitating cells. In other areas of the spleen, nerve fibers run adjacent to macrophages, T-cells, B-cells, and intensely IgM-positive cells. A direct interaction between norepinephrine released from the nerves and the lymphocytes and macrophages associated with them is indicated by these relationships. This indicates the potential neural modulation of related functions. In the splenic white pulp, nerve endings have been shown abutting lymphocytes of nearby PALS, with no intervening cell processes between the terminals and the lymphocytes. Felten and Olschowka (1987) conclude "that lymphocytes in the splenic white pulp have direct associations with noradrenergic fibers of the sympathetic nervous system. This association provides a route by which the autonomic nervous system could directly influence specific immune system effector cells."

One of the normal aspects of aging is a dimunition of immune responsiveness. Bellinger et al. (1987) reported an interesting study wherein they compared noradrenergic sympathetic innervation of the spleens of adult and aged rats. They found the NA innervation of the white pulp was diminished in the aged rats. These authors propose "that a causal relationship may exist between diminished innervation and diminished immune function in aged rats."

One mechanism for direct effects of neurotransmitters on immune function would be a direct effect of these chemicals on immune competent cells (lymphocytes and macrophages) mediated via receptors for the neurotransmitters on these cells. Lymphocytes (both T- and B-cells) and macrophages have been shown to possess β-adrenergic receptors (Abras et al., 1985; Bishopric et al., 1980). Hall and Goldstein (1981) have recently reviewed the effects of both central and peripheral neurotransmitters on immune functions. Both epinephrine and norepinephrine have been implicated as being able to modulate immune functions. These implications come from indirect evidence such as the observations that splenic norepinephrine levels decrease significantly during the course of an immune response (Besedovsky et al., 1979). Both B- and T-lymphocytes possess β-adrenergic receptors. However, B-cells do not display their receptors unless they are actively producing antibody, while T-cells display the receptors at a much earlier stage of differentiation (they have been found on thymic stem cells).

There is also an indication that the cholinergic system is involved in modulating immune functions (Hall and Goldstein, 1981). Acetylcholine receptors have been demonstrated on thymic epithelial cells, and the possibility that these receptors also exist on thymocytes has been suggested. The presence of these receptors on thymic epithelial cells, which produce thymic hormones, suggests that cholinergic receptors may indirectly affect the immune system by modifying the elaboration of thymic hormones. Bone marrow stem cells have also been shown to possess cholinergic receptors, and these receptors appear to be involved in the activation of these precursor cells. Terentyeva and Kakhetelidze (1956) reported a study wherein they treated feline bone marrow cells *in vitro* with acetylcholine or epinephrine. Acetylcholine treatment decreased the number of both lymphocytes and macrophages in the marrow cell populations, while epinephrine treatment decreased the number of lymphocytes and increased the number of macrophages.

Animals can be chemically sympathectomized by treatment with the drug 6-hydroxydopamine. Chemical sympathectomy has been shown to result in modulations of immune functions. Treatment with 6-hydroxydopamine has been shown to both enhance and suppress the antibody response to immunization with sheep red blood cells (SRBCs). Besedovsky et al. (1979) reported that treatment of neonatal rats with 6-hydroxydopamine, or surgical denervation of the spleen of adult animals, resulted in enhancement in the number of plaque-forming cells (PFCs) in response to immunization. These authors also reported that noradrenaline levels in the splenic pulp are decreased just preceding the exponential phase of the immune response to SRBCs (days 3 and 4). It was also reported that noradrenaline added to murine *in vitro* splenic lymphocyte cultures strongly suppressed the response of these cells to immunization with SRBCs. In contrast, Hall et al. (1982) reported that treatment of adult mice with 6-hydroxydopamine resulted in suppression of the primary immune response to SRBCs.

Another set of interesting studies have shown that central treatment with 6-hydroxydopamine also results in modulation of immune functions. Injection of 6-hydroxydopamine via the cisterna magna of mice resulted in decreased levels of norepinephrine in the midbrain, pons-medulla, and hypothalamus, accompanied by decreased antibody responses to SRBC immunization (Cross et al., 1986). It was shown that a secondary antibody response is not diminished by this treatment. Treated animals showed a marked increase in plasma corticosterone levels, but displayed normal antibody responses; thus, these steroid increases do not account for the suppression of the antibody response. Further studies demonstrated that depletion of central nervous system catecholamines by injection of 6-hydroxydopamine into the cisterna magna in conjunction with immunization results in enhanced activity of splenic suppressor T-cells (Cross et al., 1987). 6-Hydroxydopamine treatment alone does not induce increased suppressor cell activity. The suppressor cells were not antigen specific. Interestingly, hypophysectomy abrogates the enhancement of suppressor cell activity by treatment with 6-hydroxydopamine.

Complementing the above studies are studies which have demonstrated a reduction in noradrenaline levels of lymphoid organs and decreased noradrenaline turnover in the hypothalamus following immunization with SRBCs (del Rey et al., 1983). It was also shown that chronic exposure to environmental antigens results in a reduction of noradrenaline levels in lymphoid organs (del Rey et al., 1981). The decrease in noradrenaline turnover in the hypothalamus could be induced by injection of soluble mediators released by *in vitro* cultures of activated rat spleen cells.

Attention will now be turned toward studies investigating the effects of brain lesioning on immune functions. While there is a fairly sizable body of literature dealing with this subject, only a few representative reports will be reviewed here. Hypothalamic lesioning results in changes in the number of cells in lymphoid organs and modulates immune functions. Lesioning of the anterior hypothalamus, ventromedial hypothalamus, and mamillary bodies results in a decrease in the number of nucleated spleen cells and thymocytes (Brooks et al., 1982; Roszman and Brooks, 1985). Lesions in the anterior hypothalamus result in a reduction of mitogen- or antigen-drive lymphocyte proliferation, while lesions in the mamillary bodies, hippocampus, and amygdaloid complex result in a marked enhancement of lymphocyte proliferative responses. Both the suppressive and enhancive effects have returned to normal by 14 d following lesioning. Hippocampal lesioning also resulted in an increased number of thymocytes. Further studies have revealed that the immune changes noted above are not mediated via changes in corticosterone levels (Roszman and Brooks, 1985). Further, it appears that the change in lymphocyte reactivity results from enhancement or suppression of splenic macrophage suppressor cells which follows lesioning of the central nervous system. It is interesting to note that hypophysectomy abrogates both the inhibitory and facilitory effects of neural lesioning (Roszman and Brooks, 1985), indicating that neuroendocrine hormones are involved in the observed immune modulations.

Other immune changes observed following neural lesioning include an impairment of host defense mechanisms against tumors. Destruction of the tuberoinfundibular region of the hypothalamus results in a significant increase of tumor growth in rodents. Destruction of the ventromedial, dorsomedial, and arcuate nuclei of the hypothalamus abrogates NK cell activity in mice (Forni et al., 1983). These neural lesions did not significantly affect the functions of macrophages and lymphocytes (both B and T).

Jankovic and Spector (1986) have recently reviewed the effects of brain lesioning and stimulation on the immune system. Their review covered studies similar to and including those cited above. In addition, they discussed studies of lesioning or removal of portions of the brain of developing chick embryo. These lesions of the developing chick embryo brain resulted in the modulation of immune cell populations and immune functions. The secretory activity of thymic epithelial cells (those cells which produce thymic hormones) was also altered by these manipulations of the developing brain. The result of these studies indicates that communication between the nervous system and the immune system is functional during embryogenesis.

The review by Jankovic and Spector (1986) also included a review of studies on the effects of stimulation of neural sites on immune functions. Stimulation of the hypothalamic dorsomedial nucleus and sensorimotor cortex results in a moderate increase in thymic lymphocytes. Similarly, stimulation of the hypothalamus was shown to cause an increase in hematapoiesis. Other studies have described increases of antibody production resulting from stimulation of the hypothalamic tubal region, dorsomedial nucleus, and sensorimotor cortex, the mamillary bodies, and various structures of the mesencephalon. Stimulation of other areas of the brain results in modulations of other aspects of immune functions.

To this point, this chapter has dealt mainly with effects of the nervous system on the immune system. The other side of this coin will now be briefly discussed. There is considerable evidence that an active immune response results in alterations in neuronal activity in certain areas of the brain. It has been demonstrated that antigenic stimulation results in modification of neuronal firing rates in specific nuclei of the hypothalamus (Besedovsky and Sorkin, 1977; Besedovky et al., 1977). In these studies, the activity of individual neurons in the ventromedial nucleus and the anterior nucleus of the hypothalamus was studied following immunization of rats with either SRBCs or TNP-hemocyanin. One day following the immunization, there were no detectable antibody-forming cells (AFCs) in the spleen and no measurable change in the firing rates of the neurons in the nuclei being monitored. However, on day 5 following immunization with SRBCs, the peak number of AFCs were demonstrated in the spleen of immunized animals and a threefold increase in firing rates of neurons in the ventromedial nucleus of the hypothalamus was observed. There was no observable change in the firing rate of neurons in the anterior nucleus of the hypothalamus. A greater than twofold increase in firing rates of neurons in the ventromedial nucleus was observed in animals immunized with TNP-haemocyanin. Interestingly, animals not responding immunologically to these immunizations showed no observable change in neuronal activity. The authors interpret these results to indicate that the hypothalamus is intimately linked to the process of immunoregulation in a manner external to the immune system.

As interesting as the above studies are, they are not without problems. The recording of neuronal activity was performed while the animals were under the influence of a general anesthetic. It is possible for an anesthetic agent to influence neuronal activity. However, similar studies have been performed in fully awake animals recently with similar results (Saphier et al., 1987). In these studies, neuronal activity was monitored in the preoptic area of the anterior hypothalamus and the hypothalamic paraventricular nucleus in awake rats following immunization with SRBCs. Multiunit activity increased significantly in the preoptic area to a maximum 5 d following SRBC injection, which correlated with the initial appearance of anti-SRBC serum antibodies. Significant decreases in preoptic area multiunit activity were observed on days 3 and 8 following immunization. Multiunit activity was observed to decrease significantly in the paraventricular nucleus for the first 3 d following immunization. This activity then returned to basal rate before increasing on day 6. On the ninth and tenth days following immunization, activity in both areas had returned to baseline levels.

Complementing the above studies are results reported by Felten et al. (1987). These investigators studied mice immunized with SRBCs. They observed a significant decrease in norepinephrine levels in the paraventricular nucleus of the hypothalamus, but not in the supraoptic nucleus, coincident with the peak of the splenic AFC response (day 4 following immunization), but not earlier (day 2) or later (day 8). No monoamine changes were observed in several other nuclei on day 4 following immunization. However, on day 2 after immunization, both norepinephrine and serotonin were decreased in the hippocampus, and serotonin was increased in the nucleus solitarious. In their discussion, the authors considered it important that "norepinephrine changes were localized to a key control autonomic nucleus that regulates both neuroendocrine and autonomic outflow from the CNS."

The brief review presented above has clearly shown that the nervous system can exert regulatory influence on the immune system and, conversely, that the immune system can influence functions of the nervous system. This indicates that the immune system may interrelate with the nervous system in a manner similar to other systems, such as the endocrine system, and that regulatory feedback loops are involved in this interrelationship. The influence of the two systems on each other implies bidirectional lines of communication between both systems. Communication from the nervous system to the immune system may occur via innervation of lymphoid tissues, neurohormones, endocrine hormones influenced by neurohormones, or neuropeptides such as the enkephalins and endorphins. The reverse lines of communications, immune system to nervous system, are presumably mediated via cellular products of immune cells such as lymphokines and monokines. The final paragraphs of this chapter will review lines of evidence indicating communication in both directions via the above-mentioned molecules.

If molecular products of the cells of the nervous and immune systems provide a means of communication between the two systems (as we believe they do), then cells of the two systems must possess receptors for these molecules. Indeed, receptors for a number of these molecules have been demonstrated on cells of both systems. Cells of the immune system have been demonstrated to possess receptors for catecholamines, noradrenalin, adrenalin, ACTH, cholycytokinin, and the neuropeptides methionine-enkephalin, leucine-enkephalin, β-endorphin, neurotensin, substance P, vasoactive intestinal polypeptide, and dopamine (Blalock et al., 1985; Hall and Goldstein, 1981; Jankovic and Spector, 1986; Ovadia and Abramsky, 1987; Weidermann, 1987; Weigent and Blalock, 1987). While the list of molecular receptors for products of the immune system in the nervous system is not as extensive as that above, presumably all or most of the immune system products that modulate nervous system function do this via receptors in the nervous system. A number of immune molecules which modulate nervous system functions are briefly discussed below. Receptors for both interleukin-1 (IL-

1) and interleukin-3 (IL-3) have been demonstrated in the brain (Farrar et al., 1987). Widespread binding sites for IL-1 were observed throughout the rat brain, detectable in numerous discrete brain areas, including the ventromedial hypothalamus (an area of the brain which has been implicated in immune system-nervous system interrelationships, as described earlier in this chapter). Additionally, specific areas of the brain have been shown to possess binding sites for IL-3.

A number of molecules produced by cells of the nervous system have been shown to have the ability to modulate immune functions. ACTH has been shown to be a potent direct inhibitor of antibody production, as demonstrated in the *in vitro* plaque-forming cell assay (Blalock et al., 1985; Weigent and Blalock, 1987). T-cell and macrophage functions have also been shown to be modified by ACTH, and there seems to be no correlation between the steroidogenic and immunoregulatory properties of ACTH (Weigent and Blalock, 1987). One of the first neuroendocrine hormones recognized to play a role in immunologic regulation *in vivo* was thyrotropin (TSH) (Pierpaoli et al., 1969). TSH has been shown to enhance the *in vitro* PFC response of mouse spleen cells to SRBCs in a dose-dependent manner (Weigent and Blalock, 1987). Additional studies showed that T-cells appeared to be the target cells for the TSH effect. Other pituitary hormones which have been shown to influence the immune system are growth hormone and prolactin. Growth hormone has been shown to be involved in the development of the thymus and to be enhansive of immune functions, especially those mediated by T-cells (Arezzini et al., 1972; Fabris et al., 1971; Pandian and Talwar, 1971; Pierpaoli et al., 1971). More recently, growth hormone has been demonstrated to augment T-cell proliferative responses to mitogen stimulation and NK cell activity in aged Fischer rats (Davila et al., 1987). Chemical blockade of prolactin release has been shown to inhibit adjuvant arthritis, experimental allergic encephalitis, and delayed cutaneous hypersensitivity (Nagy et al., 1983) and to severely inhibit the *in vivo* tumoricidal activation of peritoneal macrophages (Bernton et al., 1986).

Recent studies have demonstrated a number of neuropeptides to be capable of altering immune functions. The following is by no means an all-inclusive description of these studies. Dynorphin has been observed to increase phytohemaglutinin (PHA)-induced lymphocyte proliferation when added to cultures 48 h following mitogenic stimulation, but not when added prior to or simultaneously with mitogenic stimulation (Berreca et al., 1987). Dopamine was shown to have a number of negative effects on immune functions, including depression of delayed-type hypersensitivity reactions, mixed lymphocyte reactions, the generation of cytotoxic T-cells, and the number of spleen T-cell populations (Kouassi et al., 1987). The opioid peptides, endorphins and enkephalins, have been fairly extensively studied as regards their effects on immune functions. These molecules have been shown to have a number of immune effects, including, but not necessarily limited to, suppression of *in vitro* antibody responses, enhancement of T-cell rosettes, enhancement of T-cell responses to mitogen stimulation, enhancement of NK cell activity, and suppression of tumor growth and tumor metastasis (Faith et al., 1984a, 1984b, 1987a, 1987b; Faith and Murgo, 1988; Fischer and Falke, 1984; Jankovic, 1987; Jankovic and Maric, 1987; Johnson et al., 1982; Kukain et al., 1982; Mathews et al., 1983; McCain et al., 1982; Miller et al., 1983; Murgo et al., 1986; Wybran and Schandene, 1986).

If the nervous system exerts control on immune functions in the normal manner, and the preponderance of evidence is that it does, then feedback mechanisms should exist. There is a growing body of evidence that immune system products can modulate nervous system functions, and thus complete the regulatory loop. It has been observed that blood levels of glucocorticoids are increased about the time of the peak of the immune response following antigen injection (Shek and Sabiston, 1983). This increase in glucocorticoids occurs only in animals showing a strong immune response, which indicates that a threshold needs to be reached to elicit the glucocorticoid response. The steroid levels reached are known to be immunosuppressive. Several recent studies have been performed which show that several products of immune cells can lead to increases in blood corticosteroid levels. Besedovsky et al., (1986) showed that supernatants from activated lymphocyte cultures injected into rats resulted in significant corticosterone increases. The factor was shown not to be IL-2, IL-1, pyrogen, endotoxin, or γ-interferon. This factor appears to act on the pituitary, since ACTH levels are increased. This factor was named glucocorticoid-increasing factor (GIF), and intracerebroventricular injections of GIF have been demonstrated to result in increased glucocorticoid blood levels, suggesting that at least one pathway of action of this factor is via the hypothalamus. Other immune products have also been shown to increase blood glucocorticoid levels. IL-1 and thymosin fraction 5 (TSN-5) have both been shown to cause increases in blood glucocorticoid levels (Besedovsky et al., 1986; Besedovsky and del Rey, 1987; Hall et al., 1986). Both factors have been shown to induce release of ACTH and corticotropin-releasing factor (CRF) (Besedovsky and del Rey, 1987; Hall et al., 1986). In turn, glucocorticoids at increased, but still physiological levels inhibit the production of IL-1 and IL-2 (Besedovsky et al., 1986). Other observed effects of immune cell products include a decrease in insulin levels following injection of supernatants from activated lymphocyte cultures in rats (Besedovsky et al., 1986). TSN-5 and a component peptide, thymosin β4, have been shown to be capable of stimulating lutenizing hormone-releasing hormone (LHRH) and the release of lutenizing hormone (Hall et al., 1986); TSN-5 is capable of inducing the release of prolactin (Hall et al., 1986). IL-1 has been observed to induce elevations of plasma levels of growth hormone and prolactin and a decline in plasma levels of thyroid-stimulating hormone, TSH (Bettori et al., 1987); complement factor C3a has been reported to be able to mimic the effects of dopamine in hypothalamic pathways (Hall and Goldstein, 1981); IL-2 was shown to be capable of inducing proliferation of rat oligodendrocytes *in vitro* (Benveniste et al., 1986); and supernatants from activated lymphocyte cultures have been shown to stimulate both DNA and RNA synthesis in undifferentiated glioblasts *in vitro* (Hall and Goldstein, 1981).

Complementing the above findings are reports that cells of the nervous and immune systems may be capable of producing regulatory molecules of the other system. Astrocytes have been shown to produce IL-1 and IL-3 (Farrar et al., 1987). Evidence indicates that the cells of the immune system may produce a wide variety of neuropeptides and neuroendocrine hormones, including proopiomelanocortin, preproenkephalin, ACTH, endorphins, vasoactive intestinal peptide, somatostatin, thyrotropin, chorionic gonadotropin, growth hormone, follicle-stimulating hormone, lutenizing hormone, oxytocin, and neurophysin (Blalock et al., 1985; Farrar et al., 1987; Geenen et al., 1986; Martin et al., 1987; Weigent and Blalock, 1987).

There is now a considerable body of evidence drawn from various lines of investigation that indicate intimate relationships between the nervous system and the immune system. Much work lies ahead to fully understand these interrelationships and later manipulate them for therapeutic purposes. While not reviewed here in any detail, the endocrine system is also very interrelated with nervous and immune system function, making the supersystem suggested by Peasall (1987) an attractive concept.

REFERENCES

Abrass CK, O'Conner W, Scarpace PJ, and Abrass IB: Characterization of the β-adrenergic receptor of the rat peritoneal macrophage. *J. Immunol.* 1985; 135:1338–1341.

Ader R: A historical account of conditioned immunobiologic responses. In *Psychoneuroimmunology*. Ader R, Ed. New York, Academic Press (1981).

Ader R and Cohen N: Conditioned immunopharmacologic responses. In *Psychoneuroimmunology*. Ader R, Ed. New York, Academic Press (1981).

Arezzini C, DeGori V, Tarli P, and Neri P: Weight increase of body and lymphatic tissues in dwarf mice treated with human chorionic somatomammotropin (HCS). *Proc. Soc. Exp. Biol. Med.* 1972; 141:98–100.

Barreca T, Di Benedetto G, Corsini G, Lenzi G, and Puppo F: Effects of dynorphin on the PHA-induced lymphocyte proliferation *in vitro*. *Immunopharmacol. Immunotoxicol.* 1987; 9:467–475.

Berton E, Hartmann D, Gilbreath M, Holaday J, and Meltzer MS: Inhibition of macrophage *in vivo* activation by pharmacologic blockade of prolactin release. In *Leukocytes and Host Defense*. Oppenheim JJ and Jacobs DM, Eds. Alan R. Liss, New York (1986).

Bellinger DL, Felten SY, Collier TJ, and Felton DL: Noradrenergic sympathetic innervation of the spleen. IV. Morphometric analysis in adult and aged F344 rats. *J. Neurosci. Res.* 1987; 18:55–63.

Benveniste EN, Kutsunae S, and Merrill JE: Immunoregulatory molecules modulate cell growth. In *Leukocyte and Host Defense.* Oppenheim JJ and Jacobs DM, Eds. Alan R. Liss, New York (1986).

Besedovsky H and Sorkin E: Network of immune-neuroendocrine interaction. *Clin Exp. Immunol.* 1977; 27:1–12.

Besedovsky H, Sorkin E, Felix D, and Hass H: Hypothalamic changes during the immune response. *Eur. J. Immunol.* 1977; 7:323–325.

Besedovsky HO, del Rey A, Sorkin E, Da Prada M, and Keller HH: Immunoregulation mediated by the sympathetic nervous system. *Cell. Immunol.* 1979; 48:346–355.

Besedovsky H, del Rey A, Sorkin E, Da Prada M, Burri R, and Honegger C: The immune response evokes changes in brain noradrenergic neurons. *Science.* 1983; 221:564–566.

Besedovsky HO, del Rey A, and Sorkin E: Intergration of activated immune cell product in immune-endocrine feed-back circuits. In *Leukocytes and Host Defense.* Oppenheim JJ and Jacobs DM, Eds. Alan R. Liss, New York (1986).

Besedovsky H and del Rey A: Neuroendocrine and metabolic responses induced by interleukin-1. *J. Neurosci. Res.* 1987; 18:172–178.

Bishopric NH, Cohen HJ, and Lefkowitz RJ: Beta adrenergic receptors in lymphocyte subpopulations. *J. Allergy Clin. Immunol.* 1980; 65:29–33.

Blalock JE: The immune system as a sensory organ. *J. Immunol.* 1984; 132:1067–1070.

Blalock JE, Bost KL, and Smith ME: Neuroendocrine peptide hormones and their receptors in the immune system production, processing and action. *J. Neuroimmunol.* 1985; 10:31–40.

Brooks WH, Cross RJ, Roszman TL, and Markesbery WR: Neuroimmunomodulation: neural anatomical basis for impairment and facilitation. *Ann. Neurol.* 1982; 12:56–61.

Bulloch K: Neuroanatomy of lymphoid tissue: a review. In *Neural Modulation of Immunity.* Guillemin R et al., Eds. Raven Press, New York (1985).

Cross RJ, Jackson JC, Brooks WH, Sparks DL, Markesbery WR, and Roszman TL: Neuroimmunomodulation: impairment of humoral immune responsiveness by 6-hydroxydopamine treatment. *Immunol.* 1986; 57:145–152.

Cross RJ, Brooks WH, and Roszman TL: Modulation of T-suppressor cell activity by central nervous system catecholamine depletion. *J. Neurosci. Res.* 1987; 18:75–81.

Davila DR, Brief S, Simon J, Hammer RE, Brinster RL, and Kelly KW: Role of growth hormone in regulating T-dependent immune events in aged, nude, and transgenic rodents. *J. Neurosci. Res.* 1987; 18:108–116.

del Rey A, Besedovsky HO, Sorkin E, Da Prada M, and Arrenbrecht S: Immunoregulation mediated by the sympathetic nervous system. *Cell. Immunol.* 1981; 63:329–334.

Derogatis LR, Abeloff MD, and Melisaratow M: Psychological coping mechanisms and survival time in metastic breast cancer. *JAMA* 1979; 242:1504–1509.

Fabris N, Pierpaoli W, and Sorkin E: Hormones and the immunological capacity. IV. Restorative effects of developmental hormones or of lymphocytes on the immunodeficiency syndrome of the dwarf mouse. *Clin. Exp. Immunol.* 1971; 9:227–240.

Faith RE, Plotnikoff NP, and Murgo AJ (1984): Effects of opiates and neuropeptides on immune functions. In *Mechanisms of Tolerance and Dependence.* NIDA Res. Monogr. 54. Sharp CW, Ed. (1984a).

Faith RE, Liang HJ, Murgo AJ, and Plotnikoff NP: Neuroimmunomodulation with enkephalins: enhancement of human natural killer (NK) cell activity *in vitro. Clin. Immunol. Immunopathol.* 1984b; 31:412–418.

Faith RE, Liang HJ, Plotnikoff NP, Murgo AJ, and Nimeh NF: Neuroimmunomodulation with enkephalins: *in vitro* enhancement of natural killer cell activity in peripheral blood lymphocytes from cancer patients. *Nat. Immun. Cell Growth Regul.* 1987a; 6:88–98.

Faith RE, Murgo AJ, Clinkscales CW, and Plotnikoff NP: Enhancement of host resistance to viral and tumor challenge by treatment with methionine-enkephalin. *Ann. N.Y. Acad. Sci.* 1987b; 496:137–145.

Faith RE and Murgo AJ: Inhibition of pulmonary metasteses and enhancement of natural killer cell activity by methionine-enkephalin. *Brain Behav. Immun.* 1988; 2:114–122.

Farrar WL, Hill JM, Harel-Bellan A, and Vinocour M: The immune logical brain. *Immunol. Rev.* 1987; 100:361–378.

Felten DL, Ackerman KD, Wiegand SJ, and Felten SY: Noradrenergic sympathetic innervation of the spleen. I. Nerve fibers associate with lymphocytes and macrophages in specific compartments of the splenic white pulp. *J. Neurosci. Res.* 1987; 18:28–36.

Felten SY and Olschowka J: Noradrenergic sympathetic innervation of the spleen. II. Tyrosine hydroxylase (TH) — positive nerve terminals from synapticlike contacts on lymphocytes in the splenic white pulp. *J. Neurosci. Res.* 1987; 18:37–48.

Felten DL, Felten SY, Bellinger DL, Carlson SL, Ackerman KD, Madden KS, Olschowski JA, and Livnat S: Noradrenergic sympathetic neural interactions with the immune system: structure and function. *Immunol. Rev.* 1987; 100:225–260.

Fischer EG and Falke NE: B-endorphin modulates immune functions. *Psychother. Psychosom.* 1984; 42:195–204.

Forni G, Bindoni M, Santoni A, Bellvardo N, Marchese AE, and Giovarelli M: Radio frequency destruction of the tuberinfundibular region of hypothalamus permanently abrogates NK cell activity in mice. *Nature.* 1983; 306:181–184.

Fox BH, Ragland DR, Brand RJ, and Rosenman RH: Type A behavior and cancer mortality: theoretical considerations and preliminary data. *Ann. N.Y. Acad. Sci.* 1987; 496:620–629.

Geenen V, Legros JJ, Francimont P, Baudrihaye M, Defresne MP, and Boniver J: The neuroendocrine thymus: coexistence of oxytocin and neurophysin in the human thymus. *Science.* 1986; 232:508–511.

Ghanta VK, Hiramoto NS, Solvason HB, Tyring SK, Spector NH, and Hiramoto RN: Conditioned enhancement of natural killer cell activity, but not interferon, with camphor or saccharin-LiCl conditioned stimulus. *J. Neurosci. Res.* 1987; 18:10–15.

Hall NR and Goldstein AL: Neurotransmitters and the immune system. In *Psycho-neuroimmunology*. Ader R, Ed. Academic Press, New York (1981).

Hall NR, McClure E, Hu SK, Tare NS, Seals CM, and Goldstein AL: Effects of 6-hydroxydopamine upon primary and secondary thymus dependent immune response. *Immunopharmacol.* 1982; 5:39–48.

Jankovic BD and Spector NH: Effects on the immune system of lesioning and stimulation of the nervous system: neuroimmunomodulation. In *Enkephalins, Endorphins, Stress and the Immune System*. Plotnikoff NP, Faith RE, Murgo AJ, and Good RA, Eds. Plenum Press, New York (1986).

Jankovic BD: Neuroimmune interactions: experimental and clinical strategies. *Immunol. Lett.* 1987; 16:341–354.

Jankovic BD and Maric D: Enkephalins and autoimmunity: differential effect of methionine-enkephalin on experimental allergic encephalomyelitis in Wistar and Lewis rats. *J. Neurosci. Res.* 1987; 18:88–94.

Jerne NK: The natural selection theory of antibody formation. *Proc. Natl. Acad. Sci. U.S.A.* 1955; 41:849–855.

Johnson HM, Smith EM, Torres BA, and Blalock JE: Regulation of the *in vitro* antibody response by neuroendocrine hormones. *Proc. Natl. Acad. Sci. U.S.A.* 1982; 79:4171–4174.

Kouassi E, Bopukhris W, Descotes J, Zukervar P, Li YS, and Revillard JP: Selective T cell defects induced by dopamine administration in mice. *Immunopharmacol. Immunotoxicol.* 1987; 9:477–488.

Kronfol Z, Silva J, Jr., Greden J, Denbinski S, Gordner R, and Carroll B: Impaired lymphocyte function in depressive illness. *Life Sci.* 1983; 33:241–247.

Kukain EM, Muceniece RK, and Klusha VE: Comparison of neuro and immunomodulator properties of low molecular-weight neuropeptides. *Bull. Exp. Biol. Med.* 1982; 94:1105–1108.

Martin J, Prystowsky MB, and Angeletti RH: Preproenkephalin mRNA in T-cells, macrophages, and mast cells. *J. Neurosci. Res.* 1987; 18:82–87.

Mathews PM, Froelich CJ, Sibbitt WL, Jr., and Bankhurst AD: Enhancement of natural cytotoxicity by B-endorphin. *J. Immunol.* 130:1658–1662 (1983).

McCain HW, Lamster JB, Bozzone JM, and Gabic JT: B-endorphin modulates human immune activity via non-opiate receptor mechanisms. *Life Sci.* 1982; 31:1619–1624.

Miller GC, Murgo AJ, and Plotnikoff NP: Enkephalins — enhancement of active T-cell rosettes from lymphoma patients. *Clin. Immunol. Immunopathol.* 1983; 26:446–451.

Murgo AJ, Faith RE, and Plotnikoff NP: Enkephalins: mediators of stress-induced immunomodulation. In *Enkephalins, Endorphins, Stress and the Immune System*. Plotnikoff NP, Faith RE, Murgo AJ, and Good RA, Eds. Plenum Press, New York (1986).

Nagy E, Berezi J, Wren G, Asa S, and Kovacs K: Immunomodulation by bromocryptine. *Immunopharmacology*. 1983; 6:231–243.

Ovadia H and Abramsky O: Dopamine receptors on isolated membranes of rat lymphocytes. *J. Neurosci. Res.* 1987; 18:70–74.

Pandian MR and Talwar GP: Effect of growth hormone on the metabolism of thymus and on the immune response against sheep erythrocytes. *J. Exp. Med.* 1971; 134:1095–1113.

Pearsall P: *Super Immunity*. Fawcett, New York (1987).

Pierpaoli W, Baroni C, Fabris N, and Sorkin E: Hormones and the immunological capacity. II. Reconstitution of antibody production in hormonally deficient mice by somatotropic hormone, thyrotropic hormone and thyroxin. *Immunology*. 1969; 16:217–231.

Pierpaoli W, Bianchi E, and Sorkin E: Hormones and the immunological capacity. V. Modification of growth hormone-producing cells in the adenohypophysis of neonatally thymectomized germ-free mice: an electron microscopical study. *Clin. Exp. Immunol.* 1971; 9:889–901.

Rettori V, Jurcovicova J, and McCann SM: Central action of interleukin-1 in altering the release of TSH, growth hormone, and prolactin in the male rat. *J. Neurosci. Res.* 1987; 18:179–183.

Rogers MP, Reich P, Strom TB, and Carpenter CB: Behaviorally conditioned immunosuppression: replication of a recent study. *Psychosom. Med.* 1976; 38:447–454.

Roszman TL and Brooks WH: Neural modulation of immune functions. *J. Neuroimmunol.* 1985; 10:59–69.

Saphier D, Abramsky O, Mor G, and Ovadia H: Multiunit electrical activity in conscious rats during an immune response. *Brain Behav. Immun.* 1987; 1:40–51.

Shek PN and Sabiston BH: Neuroendocrine regulation of immune processes: change in circulating corticosterone levels induced by the primary antibody response in mice. *Int. J. Immunopharmacol.* 1983; 5:23–33.

Solomon GF: Immunologic abnormalities in mental illness. In *Psychoneuroimmunology*. Ader R, Ed. Academic Press, New York (1981).

Solomon G: The emerging field of psychoneuroimmunology with a special note on AIDS. *Advances*. 1985; 2:6–19.

Solomon GF, Temoshik L, O'Leary A, and Zich J: An intensive psychoimmunologic study of long-surviving persons with AIDS. *Ann. N.Y. Acad. Sci.* 1987; 496:647–655.

Solvason HR, Ghanta VK, and Hiramoto RN: Conditioned augmentation of natural killer cell activity. Independence from nociceptive effect and dependence on interferon-B. *J. Immunol.* 1988; 140:661–665.

Stead RH, Bienenstock J, and Stanisz M: Neuropeptide regulation of mucosal immunity. *Immunol. Rev.* 1987; 100:333–359.

Stein M, Schiavi RC, and Camerino M: Influence of brain and behavior on the immune system. *Science*. 1976; 191:435–440.

Tecoma ES and Huey LY: Psychic distress and the immune response. *Life Sci.* 1985; 36:1799–1812.

Terentyeva EI and Kakhetelidze MC: Influence of acetylcholine and adrenaline on the hematopoietic cells of the bone marrow in a tissue culture. *Bull. Exp. Biol. Med.* 1956; 41:1054–1058.

Walker RF and Codd EE: Neuroimmunomodulatory interactions of norepinephrine and serotonin. *J. Neuroimmunol.* 1985; 10:41–58.

Wayner EA, Flannery GR, and Singer G: The effects of taste aversion conditioning on the primary antibody response to sheep red blood cells and *Brucella abortus* in the albino rat. *Physiol. Behav.* 1987; 21:995–1008.

Wiedermann CJ: Shared recognition molecules in the brain and lymphoid tissues: the polypeptide mediator network of psychoneuroimmunology. *Immunol. Lett.* 1987; 16:371–378.

Weigent DH and Blalock JE: Interactions between the neuroendocrine and immune systems: common hormones and receptors. *Immunol. Rev.* 1987; 100:79–108.

Wybran J and Schandene L: Some immunological effects of methionine-enkephalin in man: potential therapeutical use. In *Leukocytes and Host Defense.* Oppenheim JJ and Jacobs DM, Eds. Alan R. Liss, New York (1986).

Chapter

19

Production of Opioid Peptides by Immunocompetent Cells and the Potential Role of These Cytokines in the Stress Response

Stephen J. Lolait
*Laboratory of Cell Biology,
National Institute of Mental Health,
Bethesda, MD*

INTRODUCTION

The known endogenous opioid peptides are generated from larger precursor polypeptides by posttranslational enzymatic processing. Three opioid peptide precursors encoded by different genes have been identified to date: the β-endorphin (β-EP)/ACTH precursor, proopiomelanocortin (POMC), the enkephalin precursor, proenkephalin A, and the dynorphin/neo-endorphin precursor, proenkephalin B (for a review, see Akil et al., 1984). Peptides derived from these precursors are present in high concentrations in the pituitary, adrenal medulla, and brain; in all these tissues, *de novo* synthesis has been demonstrated (Gee et al., 1983; Bloch et al., 1984; Morris et al., 1986; Shivers et al., 1986). Recently, opioid-peptide immunoreactivity, and in some instances mRNA encoding the precursor proteins, have also been detected in a number of peripheral tissues, including testis (Tsong et al., 1982; Chen et al., 1984; Pintar et al., 1984), ovary (Lim et al., 1983; Melner et al., 1986; Douglass et al., 1987), and heart (Howells et al., 1986).

The three opioid peptide families are implicated as modulators of a spectrum of biological responses, particularly in systems that regulate the body's response to stress (for a review, see Akil et al., 1984). Indeed, various forms of opioid peptides are actively secreted from the pituitary and adrenal glands into the circulation in response to stressful and/or painful stimuli. It is well established that stress is associated with alterations in the humoral and cellular arms of the immune system. While the specific mechanisms that mediate these stress effects have not been fully elucidated, it has been suggested that opioid peptides directly modulate immune responsiveness, both *in vivo* and *in vitro* (for a review, see Plotnikoff et al., 1986). Implicit in an interpretation of many of these studies is that opioid peptides released from neuroendocrine tissues (e.g., pituitary) into the circulation act on immune effector cells. It has also been proposed, however, that activated and quiescent immune cells themselves are capable of synthesizing endorphins and ACTH (Blalock and Smith, 1980; Lolait et al., 1984). We have suggested that such cells in the spleen may secrete the peptides to act in the immediate immune microenvironment (Lolait et al., 1984).

EVIDENCE FOR OPIOID PEPTIDE SYNTHESIS BY IMMUNOCOMPETENT CELLS

In concert with the prevailing techniques at the time, initial attempts to detect opioid peptides in immune tissue focused on immunochemical methods. The most thoroughly studied opioid peptides were those originating from POMC. Using immunocytochemistry, Grube (1980) localized immunoreactive (ir)-α-endorphin (α-EP is the first 16 N-terminal amino acid residues of β-EP) to a subpopulation of immunoglobulin A-containing plasma cells present in the lamina propria of the canine colonic mucosa. However, since the cells did not contain immunoreactivity for other POMC-derived peptides (e.g., ACTH), it was suggested that cross-reactivity between α-EP and an unrelated polypeptide (possibly immunoglobulins) accounted for the positive immunocytochemical findings. Other studies based on immunocytochemistry and radioimmunoassay (RIA) (DiAugustine et al., 1980; Jahnke et al., 1981) have demonstrated ir-β-EP and ir-ACTH in mast cells; in these cases, the immunoreactivity present was attributed to a mast cell proteolytic enzyme. In addition, while specific immunoreactivity for met-enkephalin is reported to be present in adult rat thymic and circulating lymphocytes (Zagon et al., 1986), others have been unable to reproduce this observation using antisera from an identical source (S.J. Lolait and A.T. Lim, unpublished observations). In immune tissue, many factors compound the inherent problems of demonstrating immunocytochemical specificity (Swaab et al., 1977). For example, T-lymphocytes can internalize surface-bound endorphin (Schweigerer et al., 1985), B-lymphocytes possess cell surface and/or cytoplasmic immunoglobulins, and macrophages have "notorious" phagocytic and proteolytic activities. The studies cited above emphasized the need to verify by other techniques results based solely on antigen-antibody interactions.

Inferential evidence that immune cells are a source of ACTH is provided by the study of Dupont et al. (1984), which showed that removal of inflammatory tissue from a patient with ectopic ACTH syndrome resulted in the normalization of basal plasma ACTH levels. In another investigation, ir-β-EP, -ACTH, and -met-enkephalin (with chromatographic profiles identical to the corresponding authentic peptides) were detected in cells from bone marrow aspirates of children affected by acute lymphocytic leukemia (Sardelli et al., 1986). An extensive series of experiments by Blalock and co-workers has demonstrated the presence of ACTH, α-EP, and γ-endorphin (γ-EP is the first 17 N-terminal amino acid residues of β-EP) immunoreactivity in human peripheral blood lymphocytes and mouse spleen mononuclear cells that had been virus infected or transformed with bacterial lipopolysaccharide (Blalock and Smith, 1980, 1985; Smith et al., 1982; Blalock et al., 1985; Harbour-McMenamin et al., 1985; Harbour et al., 1987). The lymphocyte-derived ACTH and endorphins behaved like their pituitary gland counterparts in a number of characteristics, including antigenicity, molecular weight on size-exclusion chromatography, retention time on reversed phase high-pressure liquid chromatography (RP-HPLC), and bioactivity or receptor-binding properties. Nonstimulated lymphocytes did not appear to contain immunoreactivity for α-melanocyte-stimulating hormone (α-MSH is N-acetyl ACTH $_{1-13}$amide) or γ-endorphin. Further studies by the same group showed that lymphocyte ir-ACTH and ir-β-EP could be biosynthetically labeled, and that this immunoreactivity was released in a time-dependent manner by corticotropin-releasing factor (CRF) and arginine-vasopressin, both pituitary endorphin/ACTH secretagogues, and blocked by dexamethasone (Smith et al., 1986).

Unlike lymphocytes, macrophages do not appear to require "stimulation" to elaborate POMC-related peptides. We have demonstrated low levels of radioimmunoassayable ACTH and β-EP in splenic tissue from normal (but not "germ-free") mice (Lolait et al., 1984: Table 1). Subsequently, ir-POMC peptides have been detected in human spleen extracts (DeBold et al., 1988). The amounts of immunoreactivity in mouse spleen tissue are reflected by the positive cells (less than 1% of total spleen cells) sparsely distributed in non-lymphocytic regions of the tissue (Figure 1). In dissociated spleen cells, the immunoreactivity is restricted to a subpopulation of adherent cells expressing the macrophage differentiation marker, Mac-1 (Lolait et al., 1984). Levels of ir-β-EP and ir-ACTH in cultured macrophages closely paralleled each other and appeared to increase with time in culture (Figure 2), evidence for net

TABLE I.
POMC-Related Peptide Immunoreactivity in the Spleen and Thymus[a]

	ir-β-EP[c]	ir-ACTH	ir-β-MSH
Balb/c mouse spleen[b]	14.8 ± 1.2 (6)	15.2 ± 1.4 (6)	ND
S/D rat thymus	1.53 ± 0.16 (8)	1.09 ± 0.24 (3)	0.51 ± 0.08 (14)
Balb/c mouse thymus	ND	15.6 ± 0.79 (5)	ND

[a]Results are ng/g wet weight, mean ± SEM.
[b]Values taken from Lolait et al. (1984).
[c]The radioimmunoassays (RIA) for β-EP and ACTH have been described previously (Lolait et al., 1984). The β-MSH antiserum (R67) was raised against synthetic porcine β-MSH (β-lipotropin$_{41-58}$); it cross-reacts 100% with porcine β-MSH, 13.3% with human β-lipotropin (β-LPH), and 7.3% with camel β-LPH on a molar basis, but demonstrates less than 0.01% cross-reactivity with porcine ACTH, α-MSH, and γ-MSH. It appears to be directed to the N-terminal end of the β-MSH molecule. The final antiserum dilution used in the RIA was 1:50,000.

Note: ND = not determined; values in parentheses are the number of different adult tissues assayed.

synthesis of the ir-peptides. No immunoreactivity was detectable in peripheral blood or splenic lymphocytes, nor in peripheral blood monocytes. It is possible that circulating monocytes express opioid-like peptides once they reside (and differentiate into macrophages) in an immune microenvironment.

The profiles of macrophage β-EP- and ACTH-like immunoreactivity on gel chromatography strongly suggest the presence of 3.5K β-EP (β-EP$_{1-31}$), 4.5K ACTH (ACTH$_{1-39}$), and relatively minor amounts of higher molecular weight forms of both (Figure 3). The larger immunoreactive form(s) may include a common β-EP/ACTH precursor. Further characterization of the β-EP immunoreactivity by RP-HPLC (Lolait et al., 1986) showed β-EP$_{1-31}$ to be the major ir-species in splenic macrophages, with smaller amounts of acetylated endorphin forms also present (Figure 4). This ir-β-EP profile is different from those found in other peripheral tissues (noticeably pituitary, thyroid, and testis; see Smith and Funder, 1988 for a review), suggesting a tissue-specific POMC processing mechanism(s) in the macrophage.

The normal thymus also contains immunoreactivity for POMC-related peptides (Tables I and II). Using antisera to three different regions of the POMC molecule, we have detected low levels of ir-β-EP, ir-ACTH, and ir-β-MSH in rat and mouse thymus extracts. The major ir-endorphin species present is β-EP$_{1-31}$, and no acetylated endorphin forms are detectable (S.J. Lolait, C. Cheng, A.I. Smith, and J.W. Funder, unpublished observations). As in splenic tissue, the immunoreactivity appears confined to nonlymphocytic cells, perhaps macrophages or dendritic cells (Figure 1). Furthermore, ir-β-EP levels in the thymus are altered by manipulations of the pituitary-thyroid and hypothalamus-pituitary-adrenal axis (Table II). Adrenalectomy and administration of thyroid hormones or propylthiouracil (PTU), but not ovariectomy or treatment with estrogen or the dopaminergic agents bromocriptine and haloperidol (S.J. Lolait and J.W. Funder, unpublished observations), dramatically reduce thymic ir-β-EP concentrations. Whether these changes reflect a direct or indirect effect on the synthesis and/or release of thymic ir-POMC-related peptides remains to be established.

Numerous recent studies utilizing recombinant DNA technology (summarized in Table III) reinforce the assertion, based principally on immunochemical criteria, that immunocompetent cells actually synthesize opioid peptides. Messenger RNA encoding POMC has been localized by *in situ* hybridization histochemistry to a small number of lymphocytes in the tunica propria of the rat gut (Endo et al., 1985). We have demonstrated, by blot

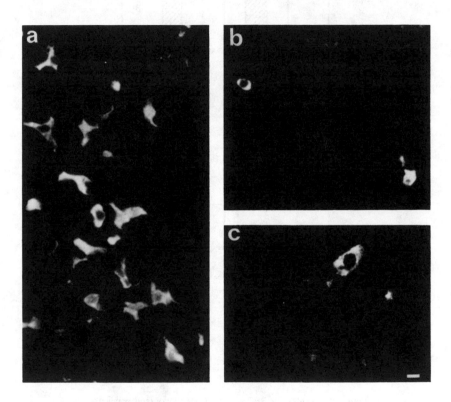

Figure 1. Indirect immunofluorescence microscopy of 4-μm sections of adult male S/D rat (a) anterior pituitary, (b) spleen, and (c) thymus reacted with an ACTH antiserum (details of method and antiserum specificity are as in Lolait et al., 1984). Approximately 3% of anterior pituitary corticotrophs and <1% of spleen or thymic cells show cytoplasmic staining. Comparison hematoxylin and eosin staining of adjacent sections (not shown) indicated that cells stained in the spleen are in the venous sinusoidal region of the red pulp, while thymic cells containing ACTH immunoreactivity are found predominantly in the cortex and cortico-medullary border. Lymphocytes are not stained in either lymphoid tissue. Scale bar = 10 μm.

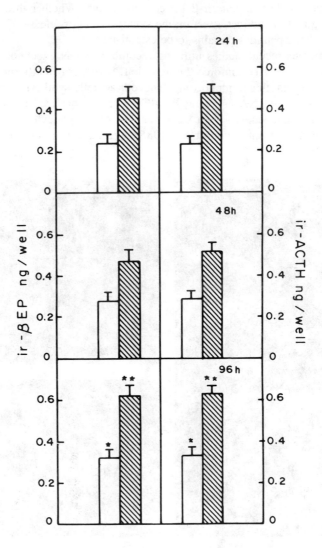

Figure 2. Levels of ir-βEP and ir-ACTH (nanograms per well) in adherent spleen leukocytes cultured for 24, 48, and 96 h. Open bars show values for 1.25×10^5 cells per well, and hatched bars 2.5×10^5 cells per well. Values shown are mean ± SEM, n = 6. (From Lolait et al., 1984. With permission.)

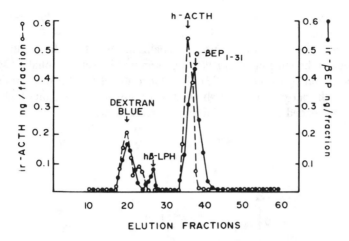

Figure 3. Size exclusion (Sephadex G-50) chromatographic profiles of ir-βEP (closed circles) and ir-ACTH (open circles) from adherent spleen cell extracts. The column was calibrated with blue dextran (void volume), purified human βLPH, synthetic ovine βEP, and purified human ACTH$_{1-39}$. (From Lolait et al., 1984. With permission.)

hybridization analysis, POMC mRNA in normal rat and mouse spleen (Lolait et al., 1986) and rat thymus (S.J. Lolait, J.A. Clements, and J.W. Funder, unpublished observations). While the major POMC transcript in these tissues is the same size (~1.1Kb) as that found in the anterior pituitary (Civelli et al., 1982), the relative abundance is at least 1000-fold less than that found in the pituitary, consistent with the ~1000-fold difference in levels of ir-endorphin in the three tissues. The presence of POMC-like mRNA has also been demonstrated in normal human thymus (Lacaze-Masmonteil et al., 1987) and spleen (DeBold et al., 1988). In addition, viral infection of rat splenocytes (Westly et al., 1986) or human B-lymphocytes (Oates et al., 1988) and mitogen stimulation of human T-lymphocytes (Farrar et al., 1987) increases the level of POMC transcripts in the cells.

Cells of the immune system also appear to synthesize enkephalins. Proenkephalin A mRNA has been detected in leukocytes from leukemia patients (Monstein et al., 1986) and in T-cell and macrophage cell lines as well as normal rat macrophages and mast cells (Martin et al., 1987). While observations of immune tissue mRNA hybridizing to POMC or proenkephalin A DNA (or RNA) probes do not constitute definitive proof that the transcripts detected code for the authentic opioid peptides, two recent findings based on cDNA cloning and nucleotide sequence analysis provide conclusive evidence that immunocytes do express genes encoding opioid peptide precursors. Zurawski et al. (1986) reported that proenkephalin A mRNA is present in mitogen-activated, but not resting, mouse T-helper cells. The mRNA was relatively abundant (~0.1 to 0.5% of total cellular mRNA) and had 93% nucleotide sequence identity with rat brain proenkephalin mRNA. In addition, the cells that produced the enkephalin mRNA also secreted ir-met-enkephalin. Moreover, Kwon and co-workers (1987) also cloned the cDNA for proenkephalin A from a T-helper cell line and showed that mitogen (but not interleukin-2) stimulation induced the levels of the proenkephalin transcript.

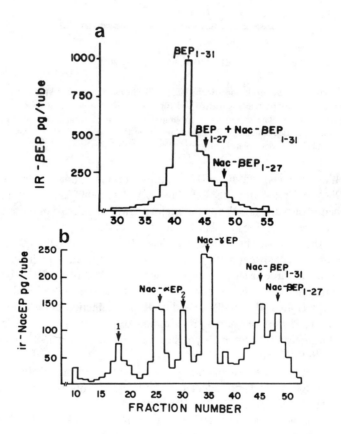

Figure 4. Profiles of βEP (a) and NacEP (b) immunoreactivity after reverse-phase HPLC of spleen adherent cell extracts. The elution positions of synthetic standards are marked. In profile b, peaks 1 and 2 correspondent to the methionine sulfoxide forms of NacαEP and nacγEP, respectively. (From Lolait et al., 1986. With permission.)

TABLE II.
βEP-Immunoreactivity in the Adult S/D Rat Thymus

| | Thymic ir-β-EP[a] | |
	pg/Thymus	ng/g Thymus
Control (8)[b]	874.4 ± 81.9	1.53 ± 0.16
Adrenalectomy		
−2d (8)	860.6 ± 86.4	1.4 ± 0.19
−4d (8)	777.4 ± 61.7	1.21 ± 0.11
−8d (8)	185.4 ± 14.6[e]	0.26 ± 0.02[e]
Control (8)[c]	829.2 ± 46.9	1.31 ± 0.13
Propylthiouracil (PTU)		
−0.03% (8)	111.4 ± 7.9[e]	0.28 ± 0.03[e]
−0.01% (8)	185.8 ± 9.8[e]	0.36 ± 0.02
−0.003% (7)	742.4 ± 44.3	1.15 ± 0.08
Control (8)[d]	843.1 ± 89.2	1.58 ± 0.18
T4 −2d (7)	204.6 ± 11.5[e]	0.41 ± 0.02[e]
−4d (7)	227.7 ± 48.5[e]	0.41 ± 0.07[e]

Note: Values in parentheses are the number of animals studied.
[a] Results are mean ± S.E.M.; the β-EP radioimmunoassay has been described previously (Lolait et al., 1984).
[b] Thymuses were removed 2, 4, and 8 d following adrenalectomy; control animals were sham operated and sacrificed after 8 d.
[c] Animals were given PTU in drinking water and sacrificed 4 d later.
[d] T4 (10 μg/100 g body weight) was injected i.m. daily for 2 and 4 d; controls received normal saline injections.
[e] $p < 0.001$, compared with controls; unpaired two-tailed Student's t-tests.

STRESS AND EFFECTS OF OPIOID PEPTIDES ON IMMUNE FUNCTION

Challenges to the body's homeostasis, collectively referred to as "stress", are classically produced by physical trauma, strenuous exercise, metabolic disturbances, and anxiety. During stress, many hormones are released into the bloodstream as a consequence of activation of the hypothalamus-pituitary-adrenal and sympatho-adrenomedullary axis. Foremost among these are ACTH, adrenal corticosteroids and catecholamines, and endogenous opioid peptides from the pituitary and adrenal glands. Some stressors (e.g., exercise, hypoglycemia) are typically associated with the stimulation of corticotropin-releasing factor (CRF) release from the hypothalamus, which, in turn, stimulates the synthesis and release of both ACTH and endorphins from the pituitary. Circulating ACTH subsequently causes an adrenal gland steroidogenic response and the resultant glucocorticoid hormone negative feedback on ACTH production. In addition, stressors such as hypoglycemia cause the release of catecholamines and enkephalins from the adrenal medulla. Many studies have shown that various stressors are also associated with profound changes in

TABLE III.
Detection of Opioid Peptide-Related Genes in the Immune System

Opioid Peptide	Species/Tissue	Technique	Findings	Reference
mRNA				
POMC	Rat gut	*in situ* hybridization	mRNA in scattered lymphocytes	Endo et al., 1985
POMC	Rat/mouse spleen and thymus	Northern blots	mRNA levels ~1000-fold lower than those in pituitary	Lolait et al., 1986 (unpublished)
POMC	Mouse spleen, leukocytes	Northern blots	mRNA in NDV-infected cells	Westley et al., 1986
POMC	Human thymus	Northern blots	Low levels of mRNA compared to pituitary and testis	Lacaze-Masmonteil et al., 1987
POMC	Human spleen	Northern blots	mRNA levels lower than those in testis, thyroid, and ovary	De Bold et al., 1988
POMC	Human T/B lymphocyte cell lines	Northern blots	mRNA in both cells; highest in EBV-transformed B-cell lines	Oates et al., 1988
POMC	Human T-lymphocytes	Northern blots	Mitogen stimulation increases mRNA levels	Farrar et al., 1987
Proenkephalin	Mouse T-helper cells	cDNA cloning; Northern blots	mRNA (93% identity with brain mRNA) in mitogen-activated cells	Zurawski et al., 1986
Proenkephalin	Mouse T-helper cells	cDNA cloning, Northern blots	mRNA induced by mitogen stimulation	Kwon et al., 1987
Proenkephalin	Human leukemic B-lymphocytes	Northern blots	mRNA in normal and leukemic cells	Monstein et al., 1986
Proenkephalin	Human T/B/mast/macrophage cell lines; normal human mast cells and macrophages	RNA dot blots	mRNA present in all cells except B-cell lines	Martin et al., 1987

immune system function, including the depression of lymphocyte responsiveness to mitogens, natural killer (NK) cell activity, and antibody production. These alterations invariably lead to (or are a consequence of) the production of intercellular chemical mediators (e.g., lymphokines, prostaglandins, bioactive amines, etc.) by leukocytes, macrophages, and other cell types. Glucocorticoids are one participant in stress-induced changes in immune function; the antiinflammatory and immunosuppressive properties of these steroids are largely due to a direct effect on the production and/or metabolism of many of the cellular byproducts that constitute a first line of defense against stress (for a review, see Munck et al., 1984).

Circulating opioid peptides may act on CNS and neuroendocrine target tissues to subserve their postulated roles in the control of niciception and blood pressure, and in modulation of reproductive function. Considering the effects of stress on immunocompetence and the elevated levels of opioid peptides during stress, they are also prime candidates as mediators of stress-induced immunomodulation. The large body of evidence suggesting that opioid peptides can directly modulate immune function has been the subject of a number of recent reviews (Shavit et al., 1985; Wybran, 1985; Murgo et al., 1986; Payan et al., 1986; Morley et al., 1987; Fischer, 1988; Sibinga and Goldstein, 1988; Blalock, 1989) and will only be briefly discussed here. A major impetus for research in this area was the demonstration of met-enkephalin and β-EP receptors on human T- and B-lymphocytes, respectively (Wybran et al., 1979; Hazum et al., 1979). Since these initial reports, there have been very few unequivocal direct ligand-binding studies. However, based primarily on pharmacological evidence, the number of immune cells thought to possess opioid peptide receptors (some of which appear to be "classical", naloxone-reversible binding sites) has expanded to include macrophages (Foris et al., 1984, 1986), polymorphonuclear leukocytes (PMNLs) (Falke and Fischer, 1985), mast cells (Liu et al., 1983; Yamasaki et al., 1983), and NK cells (Mathews et al., 1983; Mandler et al., 1986). In addition, ACTH receptors are reported to be present on lymphocytes (Johnson et al., 1982, 1984; Smith et al., 1987).

The presence of "opioid" receptors on immunocytes suggests a possible role for opioid peptides in regulating immune function. This appears to be the case, since opioid peptides directly modulate a wide range of functions of cultured T- and B-lymphocytes, PMNLs, macrophages, mast cells, and NK cells. Many of the assays (e.g., lymphocyte proliferation) in which the effects of opioid peptides have been described are often used as indices of immune function. Some studies have yielded conflicting results (e.g., β-EP is reported to enhance [Gilman et al., 1982] and inhibit [McCain et al., 1982] the proliferation of mitogen-activated T-lymphocytes), while others have noted response variability (e.g., Gilman et al. [1982] observed β-EP-enhancement of mitogen-induced lymphocyte proliferation in 10/18 separate experiments).

These apparent irregularities may be attributed to a number of factors, including differences in opioid peptide concentrations used, existence of multiple types of opioid receptors with perhaps different binding affinities, presence of a subpopulation of responding cells, or "simply" inherent differences in immune responsiveness between each subject. There is a general consensus, however, that endorphins and enkephalins stimulate mononuclear and polymorphonuclear leukocyte adherence and chemotaxis (Foris et al., 1984, 1986; Brown and Van Epps, 1985; Falke and Fischer, 1985; Van Epps and Kutvirt, 1987), regulate the release of inflammatory mediators such as superoxide radicals, serotonin, and lymphokines (e.g., γ-interferon) from macrophages, mast cells, and lymphocytes (Yamasaki et al., 1983; Sharp et al., 1985; Brown and Van Epps, 1986), and augment the spontaneous activity of NK cells (Mathews et al., 1983). Interestingly, different opioid peptides derived from the same precursor sometimes appear to have opposite effects on lymphocyte activity *in vitro*. For instance, depending on the time of peptide addition to the assay, ACTH (in an action divorced from its steroidogenic properties) and α-EP suppress, while β-EP enhances, the synthesis of immunoglobulins from antigen-activated B-lymphocytes (Johnson et al., 1982; Heijnen and Ballieux, 1986; Heijnen et al., 1986). It should be emphasized that many of the effects of opioid peptides occur only if immunocytes have been activated with antigen or mitogens, and/or primed by soluble immune mediators.

Is it possible to extrapolate from *in vitro* experiments to say that opioid peptides influence the cellular and humoral events of inflammatory responses, tissue repair, and general immune surveillance *in vivo?* A number of studies have investigated the effects of morphine and opioid peptide administration in the intact organism. The primary immune (antibody) response to sheep red blood cells in mice is inhibited by morphine, an effect which is blocked by naloxone (Güngör et al., 1980) and enhanced by low doses (20 mg/kg) of leu-, but not met-, enkephalin (Kukain et al., 1982; Murgo et al., 1986). In addition, macrophages from morphine-treated mice may be less effective at phagocytosis and killing of *Candida albicans* (Tubaro et al., 1983). Clinical studies of met-enkephalin in normal volunteers and patients with Kaposi's sarcoma (AIDS) revealed significant increases in T-cell activity (Plotnikoff et al., 1986a, 1986b). At an organ level, thymic size is increased by enkephalins, depending on the concentration used, age of animals, and species involved (Plotnikoff et al., 1984), contrasting the thymic involution associated with aging, stress, and injection of corticosteroids (Riley, 1981). Opioid peptides have also been implicated in tumor development. In an elegant series of experiments, Shavit and co-workers demonstrated that the activity of NK cells in spontaneously recognizing and killing tumor cells is suppressed by an opioid, but not nonopioid, form of footshock stress (intermittent vs. prolonged exposure, respectively), and that the same opioid stressor enhanced mammary tumor growth (Lewis et al., 1983; Shavit et al., 1984, 1985, 1986).

As pointed out by these investigators, the exact mode of action of opioid peptides *in vivo* is difficult to interpret since the peptide(s) may also interact with the brain (e.g., by stimulating sympathetic outflow) and neuroendocrine system besides directly on immunocytes. Notwithstanding this reservation, it is clear from *in vitro* and *in vivo* studies that opioid peptides alter immune function in some situations, especially when their levels are elevated (e.g., during stress).

POSSIBLE ROLE(S) OF IMMUNOCYTE-DERIVED OPIOID PEPTIDES IN THE STRESS RESPONSE

Stress-induced modulation of immunity is complex and includes a vast range of enhancing and inhibitory mechanisms. Pituitary- and adrenal-dependent and independent effects on various parameters of immune function have been noted (Keller et al., 1983, 1988). There have also been studies reporting changes in the activity of noradrenergic neurons in the hypothalamus (Besedovsky et al., 1977) and alterations in catecholamine metabolism in the hypothalamus and secondary immune tissue (e.g., spleen) (Besedovsky et al., 1983, 1985) following antigenic challenge, as well as the demonstration of sympathetic innervation to lymphoid organs (Felten et al., 1985) which implicate the autonomic nervous system in regulating immune processes in normal and stressful situations. In the intact, stressed animal, the pituitary and adrenal medulla are considered to be the major source of *circulating* endorphins and enkephalins, respectively (Rossier et al., 1977; Lewis et al., 1982; Akil et al., 1984, 1985), whereas in most peripheral tissues where low levels of opioid peptide-like material has been detected (e.g., ovary, testis), an *autocrine* or *paracrine* role has been postulated (Tsong et al., 1982; Lim et al., 1983). It is generally recognized that some immunogens [e.g., sheep erythrocytes, Newcastle disease virus (NDV)] cause a marked elevation in circulating ACTH and corticosterone levels. In this sense, antigenic challenge results in a classical stress response. Soluble immune cell factors other than opioid peptides are believed to be the prime mediators of this reponse. For example, the monokine interleukin-1 has been shown to act at the level of the hypothalamus to stimulate CRF synthesis and subsequent ACTH release from the pituitary (Besedovsky et al., 1986; Berkenbosch et al., 1987; Sapolsky et al., 1987). It is also possible that interleukins-1 and -2 have a direct action on the synthesis, processing, and release of pituitary POMC-related peptides (Woloski et al., 1985; Bernton et al., 1987; Zakarian et al., 1989). Figure 5 depicts some of the factors that may be involved in the interplay between stress and the immune system.

The studies outlined in the preceding section do not directly address the source of endogenous opioid peptides that interact with immunocompetent

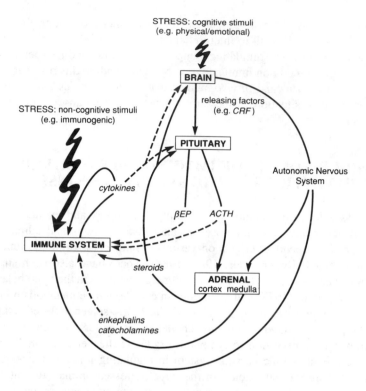

Figure 5. Summary of neural, neurohumoral, and immune mechanisms by which stress might affect the immune system. Dashed lines signify putative feedback mechanisms, e.g., immune cytokines (e.g., interleukin-1) may feed back to alter opioid peptide production by the pituitary. Circulating endorphins and enkephalins released from the pituitary and adrenal, respectively, may alter immune function. It is also possible that opioid peptides synthesized by immune cells themselves interact with the immune system.

cells. In order for immunocyte-derived opioid peptides to affect the CNS, endocrine tissue or blood-borne (e.g., other immune effector cells) targets, they would have to be released by immunocytes in quantities sufficient to significantly increase their levels in blood above "normal" circulating levels. Although there are few reports on endorphins, enkephalins, or dynorphins in this regard, one study suggests that immunocyte-derived ACTH may indeed act on classic neuroendocrine systems. Experiments by Blalock and co-workers (Smith et al., 1982) indicated that hypophysectomized (pituitary-less) mice demonstrated an increase in plasma corticosterone, and an increase in the number of splenic lymphocytes containing ir-ACTH, following administration of NDV. Synthesis (rather than the presence of ACTH immunoreactivity by immunofluorescence) of immunocyte ACTH was not demonstrated in this study, nor was the potential contribution of ACTH from other peripheral sources (e.g., gonads) eliminated. The authors postulate that lymphocyte-derived ACTH initiates a stress response (i.e., increased corticosterone secretion) by acting directly on the adrenal gland. However, this observation has not been replicated in more recent studies using similar experimental paradigms (Dunn et al., 1987; Dunn, 1988). In addition, others (Besedovsky et al., 1985) have failed to detect ir-ACTH in supernatants from NDV-infected lymphocytes. Furthermore, supernatants devoid of ACTH immunoreactivity obtained from unstimulated mononuclear cells directly enhance corticosteroid secretion from adrenal cells *in vitro* (Whitcomb et al., 1988). While resolution of this contentious issue awaits further experimentation, it appears unlikely that the immunocyte equivalents to pituitary/adrenal opioid peptides contribute substantially to circulating levels in the intact animal.

The precise role(s) of immunocyte-derived opioid peptides during stress/ antigen challenge remains obscure. *In vivo,* the integration of the complex cellular interactions which are the foundation of the immune response occurs within the organized architecture of secondary lymphoid tissue, and not the bloodstream. Tissue such as lymph nodes, spleen, and unencapsulated tissue lining the respiratory, alimentary, and urogenital tracts exhibit discrete cellular compartmentalization, e.g., T- and B-lymphocyte-enriched regions. This immune milieu facilitates cell-to-cell communication at short range, interactions that may be subject to modulation by opioid peptides released in the immediate vicinity. Given the low levels of opioid peptide immunoreactivity (and POMC-like mRNA) in unstimulated spleen macrophages, and the fact that these peptides are unlikely to make a significant impact on circulating levels, we have proposed that macrophage opioid peptide-like material, upon release by an appropriate stimuli, may act in an autocrine or paracrine manner within the specialized immune microenvironment of the spleen (Lolait et al., 1984, 1986). While β-EP$_{1-31}$ is the predominant processed endorphin form in macrophages, significant amounts of long (β-EP$_{1-31}$ and β-EP$_{1-27}$) and short (α-EP and γ-EP) N-acetylated endorphin species are also present (Lolait et al., 1986). *In vitro,* endorphins suppress B-lymphocyte antibody responses by an action on opiate-specific receptors (Johnson et al., 1982), whereas the augmentation of T-lymphocyte mitogenesis by β-EP is neither mimicked by opiates or enkephalins nor blocked by nalaxone, and hence does not appear to be mediated by classical opiate receptors (Gilman et al., 1982). Since N-acetylation renders endorphins opiate receptor-inactive, it may be (in the simplest sense) that macrophage β-EP$_{1-31}$ and enkephalins (Martin et al., 1987) have a role in regulating B-cell functions, while macrophage N-acetylated endorphins are involved in modulating T-cell responses to mitogens. The presence of specific opiate and nonopiate receptors on spleen cells (Ovadia et al., 1989) and in spleen tissue (Dave et al., 1985) is consistent with this proposal. There is also potential for a bidirectional relationship between macrophages and activated lymphocytes, whereby opioid peptides released by these cells could interact with the "opposite" cell type to affect further opioid peptide synthesis and/or act in concert with lymphokines, monokines, or other mediators of inflammatory processes. For example, the action of interleukin-1 in augmenting thymocyte proliferation is inhibited by α-MSH (Cannon et al., 1986), presumably through a direct action on specific α-MSH receptors (Tatro and Reichlin, 1987).

The ability of immunocytes to release and respond to opioid peptides appears to be well conserved in the course of evolution. Immunocompetent hemocytes of the mollusc have the capacity to release ir-enkephalins and respond to opioids by enhanced adherence and migration *in vitro* while "stress" (in the form of branchial nerve lesions) in this invertebrate evokes a cellular immune response in which opioids participate (Stefano et al., 1989). This opioid responsiveness as a first-line defense against stress appears to have been maintained at the cellular level in higher animals as more sophisticated neuroendocrine responses to stress, e.g., activation of the hypothalamic-pituitary-adrenal axis, evolved. As discussed earlier, the mobility of mammalian phagocytes is influenced by opioid peptides *in vitro*. In addition, lymphocyte traffic through peripheral lymph nodes is increased by met-enkephalin in sheep (Moore, 1984). These responses would ideally be generated by opioid peptides released locally by immunocytes (and by peptidergic nerves innervating immune tissue (Felten et al., 1985)) as responding cells follow a peptide "concentration gradient". We can envisage a state where an immune cell undergoes "hormone-dependent selection" in response to a specific antigenic stimulus accompanied by opioid peptide binding. Differential synthesis, processing, or release of opioid peptides, e.g., enkephalins rather than endorphins, N-acetylated over nonacetylated endorphins, as a consequence of exposure to unique antigens would dictate which immune cell type and function will be affected. Immunocyte opioid peptides may also modulate the phenotype of lymphoid cells, as has been shown for met-enkephalin on thymocyte Thy 1.2 antigen expression (Chakir et al., 1989), with subsequent immunological consequences such as altered lymphocyte maturation. Conversely, the phenotype of the opioid peptide-synthesizing immunocyte may also be functionally relevant; only a small percentage (<20%) of spleen macrophages contain ir-β-EP and ir-ACTH (Lolait et al., 1984), and some of these cells may express class II histocompatibility antigens (e.g., Ia), thereby having antigen-presenting capabilities, while the same or others could possess membrane receptors for CRF (Webster and De Sousa, 1988) and be subject to neurohormonal regulation of POMC expression during stress.

CONCLUSION AND FUTURE DIRECTIONS

Endogenous regulation of the humoral and cellular arms of the immune response to antigens is classically mediated by circulating immunoglobulins, products of activated immune cells and subpopulations of T-lymphocytes and "supporting" cells (e.g., macrophages). There is increasing evidence suggesting that immunocytes synthesize and respond to opioid peptides, providing additional mechanisms by which modulation of immune system components could be achieved. It is our bias that this regulation would optimally occur in the specialized microenvironment of immune tissue.

The precise identity of the opioid receptors present on immunocytes and the molecular nature of the opioid peptide-like material produced by some immune cells is currently unknown. Methods are available to isolate relatively pure populations of lymphoid cells (e.g., using fluorescence-activated cell sorting with cell-specific antibodies) that should allow investigators to ascertain the type and amount of opioid receptors (see Sibinga and Goldstein, 1988) present on a particular cell type. No one has yet isolated and sequenced an opioid peptide from cells of the immune system. The application of molecular genetic tools should permit a more rigorous identification of the types of opioid peptides produced by immune cells (by cDNA cloning) and the sites of synthesis (by *in situ* hybridization histochemistry). These studies may require the use of more sensitive methods than those employed to characterize the high levels of opioid peptides (and in most cases high levels of mRNA encoding the peptides) found in tissues like the pituitary and adrenal, e.g., utilizing the polymerase chain reaction (PCR) method to amplify rare genes from libraries made from enriched populations of opioid peptide-synthesizing immune cells. Sequence and subsequent expression data obtained from these efforts may allow us to ask some fundamental questions concerning the regulation of opioid peptide synthesis in, and by immune cells, e.g., does the POMC gene in immune cells respond to the same regulatory elements as its neural or neuroendocrine counterparts, or are there antigen-specific ones? Such studies will also help to determine whether aberrant levels of immunocyte-opioid peptides and their corresponding receptors play a role in the normal hemostatic mechanisms of stress or in the pathophysiology of immune or endocrine disease states.

ACKNOWLEDGMENTS

I thank Dr. J.W. Funder and members of the Medical Research Centre, Prince Henry's Hospital, Melbourne, Australia, for their scientific contributions, and Drs. A.-M. O'Carroll and M.J. Brownstein for critically reading the manuscript. This work was supported, in part, by Grants from the National Health and Medical Research Council of Australia, and the McKnight Foundation, U.S.A.

REFERENCES

Akil H, Watson SJ, Young E, Lewis ME, Khachaturian H, and Walker JM: Endogenous opioids: biology and function. *Annu Rev Neurosci* 1984; 7:223.

Akil H, Shiomi H, and Mathews J: Induction of the intermediate pituitary by stress: synthesis and release of a nonopioid form of β-endorphin. *Science* 1987; 227:424.

Berkenbosch F, van Oers J, del Rey A, Tiders F, and Besedovsky H: Corticotropin-releasing factor-producing neurons in the rat activated by interleukin-1. *Science* 1987; 238:524.

Bernton EW, Beach JE, Holaday JW, Smallridge RC, and Fein HG: Release of multiple hormones by a direct action of interleukin-1 on pituitary cells. *Science* 1987; 238:519.

Besedovsky HO, Sortin E, Felix D, and Haas H: Hypothalamic changes during the immune response. *Eur J Immunol* 1977; 7:325.

Besedovsky HO, del Rey A, Sorkin E, Da Prada M, Burri R, and Honegger C: The immune response evokes changes in brain noradrenergic neurons. *Science* 1983; 221:564.

Besedovsky HO, del Rey AE, and Sorkin E: Immune-neuroendocrine interactions. *J Immunol* 1985; 135 (Suppl):750.

Besedovsky HO, del Rey A, Sorkin E, and Dinarello A: Immunoregulatory feedback between interleukin-1 and glucocorticoid hormones. *Science* 1986; 233:652.

Blalock JE and Smith EM: Human leukocyte interferon: structural and biological relatedness to adrenocorticotropic hormone and endorphins. *Proc Natl Acad Sci USA* 1980; 77:5972.

Blalock JE and Smith EM: A complete regulatory loop between the immune and neuroendocrine systems. *Fed Proc* 1985; 44:108.

Blalock JE, Harbour-McMenamin D, and Smith EM: Peptide hormones shared by the neuroendocrine and immunologic systems. *J Immunol* 1985; 135 (Suppl):858.

Blalock JE: A molecular basis for bidirectional communication between the immune and neuroendocrine systems. *Physiol Rev* 1989; 69:1.

Bloch BR, Milner J, Baird A, Gubler U, Reymond C, Bohlen P, le Guellec D, and Bloom FE: Detection of the messenger RNA coding for preproenkephalin A in the bovine adrenal by *in situ* hybridization. *Regul Pept* 1984; 8:345.

Brown SL and Van Epps DE: Suppression of T lymphocyte chemotactic factor production by the opioid peptides β-endorphin and met-enkephalin. *J Immunol* 1985; 134:3384.

Brown SL and Van Epps DE: Opioid peptides modulate production of interferon γ by human mononuclear cells. *Cell Immunol* 1986; 103:19.

Cannon JG, Tatro JB, Reichlin S, and Dinarello CA: α Melanocyte stimulating hormone inhibits immunostimulatory and inflammatory actions of interleukin 1. *J Immunol* 1986; 137:2232.

Chakir J, Rouabhia M, and Deschaux P: *In vitro* effects of methionine-enkephalin and thymosin on murine expression of thy 1–2 antigen. *Immunopharmacology* 1989; 17:31.

Chen C-LC, Mather JP, Morris PL, and Bardin CW: Expression of proopiomelanocortin-like gene in the testis and epididymis. *Proc Natl Acad Sci USA* 1984; 81:5672.

Civelli O, Birnberg N, and Herbert E: Detection and quantitation of pro-opiomelanocortin mRNA in pituitary and brain from different species. *J Biol Chem* 1982; 257:6783.

Dave JR, Rubinstein N, and Eskay RL: Evidence that β-endorphin binds to specific receptors in rat peripheral tissues and stimulates the adenylate cyclase-adenosine 3', 5' monophosphate system. *Endocrinology* 1985; 117:1389.

DeBold CR, Menefee JK, Nicholson WE, and Orth DN: Proopiomelanocortin gene is expressed in many normal human tissues and in tumors not associated with ectopic adrenocorticotropin syndrome. *Mol Endocrinol* 1988; 2:862.

DiAugustine RP, Lazarus LH, Jahnke G, Khan MN, Erisman MD, and Linnoila RI: Corticotropin/β-endorphin immunoreactivity in rat mast cells. Peptide or protease? *Life Sci* 1980; 27:2663.

Douglass JE, Cox B, Quinn B, Civelli O, and Herbert E: Expression of the prodynorphin gene in male and female mammalian reproductive tissues. *Endocrinology* 1987; 120:707.

Dunn AJ, Powell ML, and Gaskin JM: Virus-induced increases in plasma corticosterone. *Science* 1987; 238:1423.

Dunn AJ: Nervous system-immune system interactions: an overview. *J Rec Res* 1988; 8:589.

Dupont AG, Sommers G, Van Steirteghem AC, Warson F, and Vanhaelst L: Ectopic adrenocorticotropin production: disappearance after removal of inflammatory tissue. *J Clin Endocrinol Metab* 1984; 58:654.

Endo Y, Sakata T, and Watanabe S: Identification of proopiomelanocortin-producing cells in the rat pyloric antrum and duodenum by *in situ* mRNA-cDNA hybridization. *Biomed Res* 1985; 6:253.

Plotnikoff NP, Faith RE, Murgo AJ, and Good RA, Eds. *Enkephalins and Endorphins: Stress and the Immune System* 1986; Plenum Press, New York.

Falke NE and Fischer EG: Cell shape of polymorphonuclear leukocytes is influenced by opioids. *Immunobiology* 1985; 169:532.

Farrar WL, Hill JM, Harel-Bellan A, and Vinocour M: The immune logical brain. *Immunol Rev* 1987; 100:361.

Felten DL, Felten SY, Carlson SL, Olschowka JA, and Livnat S: Noradrenergic and peptidergic innervation of lymphoid tissue. *J Immunol* 1985; 135 (Suppl):755.

Fischer EG: Opioid peptides modulate immune function. A review. *Immunopharmacol Immunotoxicol* 1988; 10:265.

Foris GG, Medgyesi A, Gyimesi E, and Hauck M: Met-enkephalin induced alterations of macrophage functions. *Mol Immunol* 1984; 21:747.

Foris G, Medgyesi A, and Hauck M: Bidirectional effect of met-enkephalin on macrophage effector functions. *Moll Cell Biochem* 1986; 69:127.

Gee CE, Chen C-LC, Roberts JL, Thompson R, and Watson SJ: Identification of proopiomelanocortin neurones in rat hypothalamus by *in situ* cDNA-mRNA hybridization. *Nature (London)* 1983; 306:374.

Gilman SC, Schwartz JM, Milner RJ, Bloom FE, and Feldman JD: β-endorphin enhances lymphocyte proliferative responses. *Proc Natl Acad Sci USA* 1982; 79:4226.

Grube D: α-Endorphin-like immunoreactivity in plasma cells of the canine colonic mucosa. *Histochemistry* 1980; 69:157.

Güngör ME, Genç H, Sağduyu L, Eroğlu L, and Koyuncuoğlu H: Effect of chronic administration of morphine on primary immune response in mice. *Experentia* 1980; 36:1309.

Harbour DV, Smith EM, and Blalock JE: Novel processing pathway for proopiomelanocortin in lymphocytes: endotoxin induction of a new prohormone-cleaving enzyme. *J Neurosci Res* 1987; 18:95.

Harbour-McMenamin D, Smith EM, and Blalock JE: Bacterial lipopolysaccharide induction of leukocyte-derived corticotropin and endorphins. *Infect Immun* 1985; 48:813.

Hazum E, Chang KJ, and Cuatrecasas P: Specific nonopiate receptors for β-endorphin. *Science* 1979; 205:1033.

Heijnen CB and Ballieux RE: Influence of opioid peptides on the immune system. *Inst Adv Health Sci* 1986; 3:114.

Heijnen CB, Bevers C, Kavelaars A, and Ballieux RE: Effect of α-endorphin on the antigen-induced primary antibody response in human blood B cells *in vitro. J Immunol* 1986; 136:213.

Howells RD, Kilpatrick DL, Bailey LC, Noe M, and Udenfriend S: Proenkephalin mRNA in rat heart. *Proc Natl Acad Sci USA* 1986; 83:1960.

Jahnke GD, Lazarus LH, DiAugustine RP, Soldato CM, and Erisman MD: peptide hormone degradation by a rat mast cell chymase-heparin complex. *Life Sci* 1981; 29:397.

Johnson HM, Smith EM, Torres BA, and Blalock JE: Regulation of the in vitro antibody response by neuroendocrine hormones. *Proc Natl Acad Sci USA* 1982; 79:4171.

Johnson HM, Torres BA, Smith EM, Dion LD, and Blalock JE: Regulation of lymphokine (γ interferon) production by corticotropin. *J Immunol* 1984; 132:246.

Keller SE, Weiss JM, Schleifer SJ, Miller NE, and Stein M: Stress-induced suppression of immunity in adrenalectomized rats. *Science* 1983; 221:1301.

Keller SE, Schleifer SJ, Liotta AS, Bond RN, Farhoody N, and Stein M: Stress-induced alterations of immunity in hypophysectomized rats. *Proc Natl Acad Sci USA* 1988; 85:9297.

Kukain EM, Muceniece RK, and Klusha VE: Comparison of neuro- and immunomodulator properties of low-molecular-weight neuropeptides. *Bull Exp Biol Med* 1982; 94:1105.

Kwon BS, Kim GS, Prystowsky MB, Lancki DW, Sabath DE, Pan J, and Weissman SM: Isolation and initial characterization of multiple species of T-lymphocyte subset cDNA clones. *Proc Natl Acad Sci USA* 1987; 84:2896.

Lacaze-Masmonteil T, de Keyzer Y, Luton J-P, Kahn A, and Bertagna X: Characterization of proopiomelanocortin transcripts in human nonpituitary tissues. *Proc Natl Acad Sci USA* 1987; 84:7261.

Lewis JW, Tordoff MG, Sherman JE, and Liebeskind JC: Adrenal medullary enkephalin-like peptides may mediate opioid stress analgesia. *Science* 1982; 217:557.

Lewis JW, Shavit Y, Terman GW, Nelson LR, Gale RP, and Liebeskind JC: Apparent involvement of opioid peptides in stress-induced enhancement of tumor growth. *Peptides* 1983; 4:635.

Lim AT, Lolait S, Barlow JW, Zois WSOI, Toh BH, and Funder JW: Immunoreactive β-endorphin in sheep ovary. *Nature (London)* 1983; 303:709.

Liu JS, Garrett KM, Lin S-CC, and Way EL: The effects of opiates on calcium accumulation on rat peritoneal mast cells. *Eur J Pharmacol* 1983; 91:335.

Lolait SJ, Lim ATW, Toh BH, and Funder JW: Immunoreactive β-endorphin in a subpopulation of mouse spleen macrophages. *J Clin Invest* 1984; 73:277.

Lolait SJ, Clements JA, Markwick AJ, Cheng C, McNally M, Smith AI, and Funder JW: Pro-opiomelanocortin messenger ribonucleic acid and posttranslational processing of beta endorphin in spleen macrophages. *J Clin Invest* 1986; 77:1776.

McCain HW, Lamster IB, Bozzone JM, and Grbic JT: β-Endorphin modulates human immune activity via non-opiate receptor mechanisms. *Life Sci* 1982; 31:1619.

Mandler RW, Biddison WE, Mandler R, and Serrate SA: β-Endorphin augments the cytolytic activity and interferon production of natural killer cells. *J Immunol* 1986; 136:934.

Martin J, Prystowsky MB, and Angeletti RH: Preproenkephalin mRNA in T-cells, macrophages, and mast cells. *J Neurosci Res* 1987; 18:82.

Mathews PM, Froelich CJ, Sibbitt WL, Jr, and Bankhurst AD: Enhancement of natural cytotoxicity by β-endorphin. *J Immunol* 1983; 130:1658.

Meiner MH, Young SL, Czerwiec FS, Lyn D, Puett D, Roberts JL, and Koos RD: The regulation of granulosa cell proopiomelanocortin messenger ribonucleic acid by androgens and gonadotropins. *Endocrinology* 1986; 119:2082.

Monstein H-J, Folkesson R, and Terenius L: Proenkephalin A-like mRNA in human leukemia leukocytes and CNS-tissues. *Life Sci.* 1986; 39:2237.

Moore TC: Modification of lymphocyte traffic by vasoactive neurotransmitter substances. *Immunology* 1984; 52:51.

Morley JE, Kay NE, Solomon GF, and Plotnikoff NP: Neuropeptides: conductors of the immune orchestra. *Life Sci* 1987; 41:527.

Morris BJ, Haarmann I, Kempter B, Höllt V, and Herz A: Localization of prodynorphin messenger RNA in rat brain by *in situ* hybridization using a synthetic oligonucleotide probe. *Neurosci Lett* 1986; 69:104.

Munck A, Guyre PM, and Holbrook NJ: Physiological functions of glucocorticoids in stress and their relation to pharmacological actions. *Endocr Rev* 1984; 5:25.

Murgo AJ, Faith RE, and Plotnikoff NP: *Enkephalins and Endorphins: Stress and the Immune System* Plenum Press, New York, (1986) pp. 221–239.

Oates EL, Allaway GP, Armstrong GR, Boyajian RA, Kehrl JH, and Prabhakar BS: Human lymphocytes produce pro-opiomelanocortin gene-related transcripts. *J Biol Chem* 1988; 263:10041.

Ovadia H, Nitsan P, and Abramsky O: Characterization of opiate binding sites on membranes of rat lymphocytes. *J Neuroimmunol* 1989; 21:93.

Payan DG, McGillis JP, and Goetz EJ: Neuroimmunology. *Adv Immunol* 1986; 39:299.

Pintar JE, Schachter BS, Herman AB, Durgerian S, and Krieger DT: Characterization and localization of proopiomelanocortin messenger RNA in the adult rat testis. *Science* 1984; 225:632.

Plotnikoff NP, Murgo AJ, and Faith RE: Neuroimmunomodulation with enkephalins: effects on thymus and spleen weights in mice. *Clin Immunol Immunopathol* 1984; 32:52.

Plotnikoff NP, Miller GC, Solomon S, Faith RE, Edwards L, and Murgo AJ: *Enkephalins and Endorphins: Stress and the Immune System* Plenum Press, New York (1986a), pp. 417–424.

Plotnikoff NP, Miller GC, Solomon S, Faith RE, Edwards L, and Murgo AJ: Methionine enkephalin: enhancement of T-cells in patients with Kaposi's sarcoma (AIDS). *Psychopharmacol Bull* 1986b; 22:695.

Riley V: Psychoneuroendocrine influences on immunocompetence and neoplasia. *Science* 1981; 212:1100.

Rossier J, French ED, Rivier C, Ling N, Guillemin R, and Bloom FE: Foot-shock induced stress increases β-endorphin levels in blood but not brain. *Nature (London)* 1977; 270:618.

Sapolsky R, Rivier C, Yamamoto G, Plotsky P, and Vale W: Interleukin-1 stimulates the secretion of hypothalamic corticotropin-releasing factor. *Science* 1987; 238:522.

Sardelli S, Petraglia F, Massolo F, Messori A, Santoro V, Facchinetti F, and Genazzani AR: Changes in immunoreactive β-endorphin, met-enkephalin and ACTH in bone marrow cells and fluid from leukemic children. *Clin Immunol Immunopathol* 1986; 41:247.

Schweigerer L, Schmidt W, Teschemacher H, and Gramsch C: β-Endorphin: surface binding and internalization in thymoma cells. *Proc Natl Acad Sci USA* 1985; 82:5751.

Sharp BM, Keane WF, Suh HJ, Gekker G, Tsukayama D, and Peterson PK: Opioid peptides rapidly stimulate superoxide production by human polymorphonuclear leukocytes and macrophages. *Endocrinology* 1985; 117:793.

Shavit Y, Lewis JW, Terman GW, Gale RP, and Liebeskind JC: Opioid peptides mediate the suppressive effect of stress on natural killer cell cytotoxocity. *Science* 1984; 223:188.

Shavit Y, Terman GW, Martin FC, Lewis JW, Liebeskind JC, and Gale RP: Stress, opioid peptides, the immune system, and cancer. *J Immunol* 1985; 135 (Suppl):834.

Shavit Y, Depaulis A, Martin FC, Terman GW, Pechnick RN, Zane CJ, Gale RP, and Liebeskind JC: Involvement of brain opiate receptors in the immuno-suppressive effect of morphine. *Proc Natl Acad Sci USA* 1986; 83:7114.

Shivers BD, Harlan RE, Romano GJ, Howells RD, and Pfaff DW: Cellular localization of proenkephalin mRNA in rat brain: gene expression in the caudate-putamen and cerebellar cortex. *Proc Natl Acad Sci USA* 1986; 83:6221.

Sibinga NES and Goldstein A: Opioid peptides and opioid receptors in cells of the immune system. *Annu Rev Immunol* 1988; 6:219.

Smith EM, Meyer WJ, and Blalock JE: Virus-induced corticosterone in hypophysectomized mice: a possible lymphoid-adrenal axis. *Science* 1982; 218:1311.

Smith EM, Morrill AC, Meyer WJ III, and Blalock JE: Corticotropin releasing factor induction of leukocyte-derived immunoreactive ACTH and endorphins. *Nature (London)* 1986; 321:881.

Smith EM, Brosnan P, Meyer WJ, and Blalock JE: An ACTH receptor on human mononuclear leukocytes: relation to adrenal ACTH-receptor activity. *N Engl J Med* 1987; 317:1266.

Smith AI and Funder JW: Proopiomelanocortin processing in the pituitary, central nervous system, and peripheral tissues. *Endocr Rev* 1988; 9:159.

Stefano GB, Leung MK, Zhao X, and Scharrer B: Evidence for the involvement of opioid neuropeptides in the adherence and migration of immunocompetent invertebrate hemocytes. *Proc Natl Acad Sci USA* 1989; 86:626.

Swaab DF, Pool CW, and Van Leeuwen FW: Can specificity ever be proved in immunocytochemical staining? *J Histochem Cytochem* 1977; 25:388.

Tatro JB and Reichlin S: Specific receptors for α-melanocyte-stimulating hormone are widely distributed in tissues of rodents. *Endocrinology* 1987; 121:1900.

Tsong SD, Phillips D, Halmi N, Liotta AS, Margioris A, Bardin CW, and Krieger DT: ACTH and β-endorphin-related peptides are present in multiple sites in the reproductive tract of the male rat. *Endocrinology* 1982; 110:2204.

Tubaro E, Borelli G, Croce C, Cavallo G, and Santiangeli C: Effect of morphine on resistance to infection. *J Infect Dis* 1983; 148:656.

Van Epps DE and Kutvirt SL: Modulation of human neutrophil adherence by β-endorphin and met-enkephalin. *J Neuroimmunol* 1987; 15:219.

Webster EL and De Souza EB: Corticotropin-releasing factor receptors in mouse spleen: identification, autoradiographic localization, and regulation by divalent cations and guanine nucleotides. *Endocrinology* 1988; 122:609.

Westly HJ, Kleiss AJ, Kelley KW, Wong PKY, and Yuen P-H: Newcastle disease virus-infected splenocytes express the proopiomelanocortin gene. *J Exp Med* 1986; 163:1589.

Whitcomb RW, Linehan WM, Wahl LM, and Knazek RA: Monocytes stimulate cortisol production by cultured human adrenocorticol cells. *J Clin Endocrinol Metab* 1988; 66:33.

Woloski BMRNJ, Smith EM, Meyer WJ III, Fuller GM, and Blalock JE: Corticotropin-releasing activity of monokines. *Science* 1985; 230:1035.

Wybran J: Enkephalins and endorphins as modifiers of the immune system: present and future. *Fed Proc* 1985; 44:92.

Wybran J, Appelboom T, Famaey J-P, and Govaerts A: Suggestive evidence for receptors for morphine and methionine-enkephalin on normal human blood T lymphocytes. *J Immunol* 1979; 123:1068.

Yamasaki Y, Shimamura O, Kizu A, Nakagawa N, and Ijichi H: Interactions of morphine with PGE_1, isoproteronol, dopamine and aminophylline in rat mast cells; their effect on IgE-mediated ^{14}C-serotonin release. *Agents Actions* 1983; 13:21.

Zagon IS, Rhodes RE, and McLaughlin PJ: Localization of enkephalin immunoreactivity in diverse tissues and cells of the developing and adult rat. *Cell Tissue Res* 1986; 246:561.

Zakarian S, Eleazar MS, and Silvers WK: Regulation of pro-opiomelanocortin biosynthesis and processing by transplantation immunity. *Nature (London)* 1989; 339:553.

Zurawski G, Benedik M, Kamb BJ, Abrams JS, Zurawski SM, and Lee FD: Activation of mouse T-helper cells induces abundant preproenkephalin mRNA synthesis. *Science* 1986; 232:772.

20

Opioid Systems and Immune Functions

Hemendra N. Bhargava
Department of Pharmacodynamics (m/c 865)
The University of Illinois at Chicago
College of Pharmacy
Chicago, Illinois

INTRODUCTION

Studies on the neurochemical control of immune function are still in their infancy. Much knowledge has been gained on the possible role of several neurotransmitter systems in centrally mediated behaviors and in the regulation of endocrine functions. For instance, dopamine, believed to be a pathogenetic factor in schizophrenia and movement disorders like Parkinsonism, and drug-induced dyskinetic behaviors (Bhargava, 1986), is also important in the control of the secretion of prolactin from the anterior pituitary. The hypothalamo-pituitary-adrenal axis is well established. The questions that then arise are (1) whether a nervous-endocrine-immune axis exists and (2) whether there are neurochemicals of brain and pituitary which influence the immune function. Attempts have been made recently to answer both these questions. In the first place, steroidal molecules like corticosterone and progesterone, which exhibit anti-inflammatory activity, inhibit the binding of ^{3}H-SKF 10,047, a specific ligand of σ-receptors to homogenates of brain and spleen. Since steroids induce mental disturbances and alter immune function, a link between endocrine, nervous, and immune function was suggested (Su et al., 1988). However, it must be noted that the inhibition constant (K_i) for steroid displacing the binding of ^{3}H-SKF 10,047 was in the micromolar range, and thus is far above the physiological concentrations. However, it is possible that at the target site, *in vivo,* the concentration of steroids may be high enough to observe the above phenomenon.

Neurotransmitters are the obvious candidates for examination in their role in immune function. Several neurotransmitters, including serotoninergic, catecholaminergic, and cholinergic, have been implicated in modulating immune function (Hall and Goldstein, 1981). The sum of this work suggests that catecholamines and acetylcholine stimulate immune function, whereas, serotonin has an inhibitory effect on the immune system. The details of the involvement of biogenic amines and acetylcholine will not be covered in this review.

In this paper, the possible role of opioid systems in modulating immune function will be discussed. The evidence for such an involvement will be based on the fact that opiate-addicted humans or animals have altered immune function, endogenous and exogenous opiates modify the functions of cells or markers of immune function, interferons and humoral factors which stimulate antibody production are known to interact with endogenous opiates, and, finally, opiate binding sites exist on lymphocytes or can be expressed after stimulation with mitogens. Each one of these areas will be elaborated in detail.

OPIATE ADDICTION AND IMMUNE FUNCTION

Human Studies

Because of the spread of AIDS, particularly among drug addicts, considerable attention has been focused on modification of the immune function by drugs commonly abused. Central nervous system (CNS) depressant agents like morphine or heroin, alcohol, and marijuana depress immune function (Watson et al., 1985; Lundy et al., 1975; Patel et al., 1985; Bhargava, 1990), which then leads to increased risk of infection. The possible mechanisms by which the immune function is compromised is still unclear. However, it should be emphasized that many opiates like morphine and heroin are self administered by addicts using intravenous injections. The sharing of unsterilized needles can lead to the entry of microorganisms into the bloodstream to produce infections. It is also possible that abused drugs like heroin may have direct action on various parameters of immune systems, which may lead to the diminished (impaired) immune function of the host. For almost half a century, clinical evidence has been gathered which shows that heroin addicts have an increased incidence of bacterial, protozoal, and viral infections. Bacterial endocarditis (Luttgens, 1949; Hussey et al., 1944; Olsson and Romansky, 1962), septicemia (Briggs et al., 1967; Hussey et al., 1944; Cherubin and Brown, 1968), pulmonary infections, tetanus, hepatitis, malaria, thrombophlebitis, and skin sepsis (Hussey and Katz, 1950; Louria et al., 1967) are some of the commonly encountered problems in heroin addicts.

Abnormalities in cellular and/or humoral immunity in heroin addicts also could be due to drug contaminants, needle contamination, and concomitant abuse of other drugs like alcohol and marijuana (Lundy et al., 1975; Patel et al., 1985).

In a recent study, Lazzarin et al. (1984) summarized various types of infections in 82 opiate addicts. The major infections included viral hepatitis, recurrent dental abscesses, subcutaneous abscesses, phlebitis, lues, and respiratory infections. The infections were also associated with compromised cellular immunity, as evidenced by functional deficits of polymorphonuclear leukocytes and T-lymphocytes. In another study of 38 heroin addicts, Brown et al. (1974) reported immunological abnormality, manifested as hypergammaglobulinemia with higher than normal levels of IgM and IgG, and a false positive test for syphilis. Cellular immunity was also found to be impaired, as evidenced by decreased responsiveness of lymphocytes to mitogen-induced blastogenesis. A decrease in the absolute number of total T-lymphocytes in the peripheral blood of opioid addicts, as measured by the ability of lymphocytes to rosette sheep red blood cells, was reported; however, B-lymphocytes or total white blood cell count was found to be unchanged (McDonough et al., 1980). The narcotic antagonist, naloxone, was found to reverse the above changes. Naloxone not only increased T-cell percentage, it also improved the appearance of E-rosettes. Another indicator of compromised immune function of addicted patients was the decreased ability of phytohemagglutinin (PHA)-induced stimulation of ^{3}H-thymidine incorporation into the DNA of lymphocytes. Tubaro et al. (1985) showed that morphine addicts exhibited a severe depression of phagocytosis and killing properties of polymorphonuclear leukocytes and monocytes and their ability to generate superoxide anion.

Animal Studies

In an effort to understand more precisely the mechanisms by which opioids, particularly morphine, modulate the immune function, several studies have been carried out in mice. Chronic administration of morphine to mice was shown to decrease the responsiveness of lymphocytes to stimulation by concanavalin A (ConA) (a T-lymphocyte mitogen) when compared to lymphocytes of nonaddicted mice. This suppressive effect was partially reversed by concurrent administration of naloxone (Ho and Leung, 1979). In mice addicted to morphine by multiple injection technique, the primary immune response was inhibited, as evidenced by decreases in the spleen-to-body weight ratio and serum hemolysin production against sheep red blood cells. These

effects were also reversed by naloxone (Gungor et al., 1980). Chronic treatment of mice for 3 d with morphine (75 mg/kg/d) produced immunosuppression, as shown by using a plaque-forming cell (PFC) assay to evaluate antibody-forming efficiency (Lefkowitz and Chiang, 1975) and a rosette-forming
cell test (Lefkowitz and Nemeth, 1976). Chronic administration of morphine
to mice also decreases the production of interleukin-2 (Peritt et al., 1988).
In guinea pigs, chronic treatment with morphine altered the lymphocyte metabolism of cyclic nucleotides and lymphocytic responsiveness to ConA stimulation (Law et al., 1978).

A time course of morphine pellet implantation on the immune function
of mice has been studied recently (Bryant et al., 1988). Forty eight and 72
h (but not at earlier times) after implantation of a morphine pellet, T-lymphocyte proliferation in response to ConA was reduced. B-lymphocyte proliferation in response to lipopolysaccharide (LPS) was reduced at 24, 48, and
72 h after implantation. However, at 96 h after implantation, T- and B-
lymphocyte proliferation was unaffected. The decrease in T- and B-lymphocytes was associated with atrophy of spleen and thymus. It is not clear why
at 24 and 96 h after the implantation of morphine pellets, a time at which
tolerance to morphine was evident, there was no change in mitogen-induced
proliferation of T- and B-lymphocytes.

Is there indeed a relationship between morphine tolerance-dependence
and the immune function? Manipulations which suppress the immune system
have been shown to inhibit the development of tolerance to and physical
dependence on morphine (Meisheri and Isom, 1978; Dougherty et al., 1986).

Is immunosuppression by morphine centrally or peripherally mediated?

Administration of morphine into the periaqueductal gray matter has been
shown to suppress NK cell activity and mitogen-induced proliferation of T-
lymphocytes in the rat, suggesting a central site of action of morphine in
immunomodulation (Weber and Pert, 1987). However, a peripheral site cannot
be ruled out.

From the above studies, however, it cannot be concluded whether morphine-induced altered immune function was related to the tolerant-dependent
state or to the abstinent state of animals.

In addition to evaluation of the lymphocyte function of morphine-addicted
animals, studies have also been carried out to determine their susceptibility
to a variety of microorganisms. Chronic treatment of mice with morphine
was found to result in decreased resistance to bacterial and fungal infections.
In an elegant study, Tubaro et al. (1983) demonstrated that in mice treated
chronically with morphine, the reticuloendothelial system activity was decreased and so were the lymphoid organ weight, phagocyte count, natural
killer (NK) cell activity, and superoxide anion formation in polymorphonuclear leukocytes and macrophages. These effects were associated with greater
susceptibility to infections due to *Klebsiella pneumoniae* and *Candida albicans,* as evidenced by decreases in the LD_{50} of these organisms in morphine-
treated mice.

In Vitro Effects of Morphine

Inconsistent results have been obtained on the *in vitro* effects of morphine on immune cell functions. Bocchini et al. (1983) showed that at 10^{-7} M concentration, morphine increased T-cell percentage, decreased null cells, did not affect B-cells, and enhanced PHA-stimulated lymphocyte response. On the other hand, Donahoe et al. (1985) reported that *in vitro* morphine inhibits T- and E-rosetting. It is possible that these effects are concentration dependent since morphine at high concentration (10^{-3} M) inhibits the lymphocyte response to PHA.

Evidence for the Presence of Endogenous Opiates in the Peripheral Blood and Its Compartments

With the discovery of opioid receptors in mammalian tissue, a search to isolate the endogenous ligands for the receptors resulted in the isolation of a family of peptides having opiate-like activity. Three major classes of compounds are the enkephalins (methionine and leucine), dynorphin-(1-13), and β-endorphin. These peptides have differential distribution in the CNS, pituitary, and peripheral tissues (Bhargava et al., 1988, 1989) and have been implicated in a number of physiological and pathophysiological states involving neural and hormonal actions (Morley et al., 1987). It is thus possible that the endogenous opioids are also involved in the modulation of immune function via the autonomic nervous system, the endocrine system, and the CNS. Many of the endogenous peptides are present in blood in intact form, as determined by radioimmunoassay. β-Endorphin-like immunoreactivity is present in rat serum, and under stress it is apparently released from the pituitary into the blood (Guillemin et al., 1977). Although the concentration of β-endorphin in human serum is low, appreciable concentrations have been found in the plasma of patients with certain endocrine disorders (Suda et al., 1978). Human leukocytes contain interferon (hIFN-α), which is a group of proteins with antiviral activity, and recognize β-endorphin and adrenocorticotrophic hormone (ACTH)-like activities (Smith and Blalock, 1981). Methionine-enkephalin is also present in human plasma in intact form in the amount of 55 pg/ml and is possibly secreted by the adrenal medulla (Clement-Jones et al., 1980). The plasma levels of methionine-enkephalin are independent of endogenous ACTH, β-lipotropin (β-LPH), and β-endorphin, and thus suggest that methionine-enkephalin is derived from its own precursor distinct from ACTH, β-LPH, and β-endorphin (Clement-Jones et al., 1980).

Methionine-enkephalin is a pentapeptide that has been found in a variety of tissues, including the brain, spinal cord, and gastrointestinal tract of several species (Simantov et al., 1977; Yang et al., 1977; Wesche et al., 1977; Gros et al., 1977; Hughes et al., 1977; Miller et al., 1978). It has also been detected in human gut, brain, and cerebrospinal fluid (Polak et al., 1977; Gramsch et al., 1979; Akil et al., 1978).

It has been indicated earlier that methionine-enkephalin, an endogenous opioid peptide, circulates as intact pentapeptide in human plasma (Clement-Jones et al., 1980). Although methionine-enkephalin is degraded rapidly by tissue enkephalinases and aminopeptideases, making its half-life extremely short (Roda et al., 1986), the presence of intact peptides in the blood raises questions concerning protective mechanisms present in the peripheral blood, its distribution patterns, and its physiological role. Picogram quantities of immunoreactive methionine-enkephalin were detected in human, rat, and rabbit platelets. The platelet methionine-enkephalin concentration in Sprague-Dawley rats was not affected by either adrenalectomy or hypophysectomy (DiGiulio et al., 1982). However, plasma concentrations of methionine-enkephalin were increased after adrenalectomy both in normal and hypophysectomized rats (Panerai, 1988). Therefore, the origin of methionine-enkephalin in blood is still not certain. The distribution and uptake of methionine-enkephalin into human blood cells has also been studied. Blood obtained from normal volunteers was separated into RBCs, WBCs, and platelets, and the methionine-enkephalin contents of cells was determined by radioimmunoassay. On a per cell basis, WBCs were found to contain about 100-fold greater amounts of methionine-enkephalin than either RBCs or platelets. Similarly, the uptake of ^{3}H-methionine-enkephalin was far greater in WBCs than in RBCs or platelets. These studies suggest that WBCs may act as a compartment of distribution for methionine-enkephalin in blood (Valentine et al., 1988).

Effects of Opioid Peptides on Immune Function

Wybran et al. (1979) provided suggestive evidence for the presence of methionine-enkephalin receptors on human blood T-lymphocytes. Human T-lymphocytes are easily recognized by their specific ability to form rosettes with sheep red blood cells (SRBCs). *In vitro,* methionine-enkephalin increased the percentage of active T-rosettes, an effect which was inhibited by naloxone (Wybran et al., 1979). Subsequently, the presence of opioid receptors on human phagocytic leukocytes was reported (Lopker et al., 1980). The distribution and presence of methionine-enkephalin receptors on cells involved in immune function prompted further studies on the possible role of methionine-enkephalin in the host defense mechanisms. Plotnikoff's group has shown that the enkephalins increase PHA-induced lymphocyte blastogenesis (Plotnikoff and Miller, 1983) and prolong survival of BDF$_1$ mice inoculated with an attenuated L1210 strain of tumor cells (Plotnikoff and Miller, 1983). Methionine-enkephalin significantly increases the active T-cell rosette-forming cells in peripheral blood lymphocytes from lymphoma patients (Miller et al., 1983). Enkephalins also stimulate at low doses and inhibit at high doses T-dependent antibody responses *in vitro* (Johnson et al., 1982). Both methionine- and leucine-enkephalin significantly increased NK cell activity in isolated human peripheral blood lymphocytes (Faith et al., 1984). NK cells belong to the subpopulation of lymphocytes which play an important role in host defense mechanisms against neoplastic diseases.

Further evidence for the possible role of methionine-enkephalin in immune function was provided by the studies of Zurawski et al. (1986), who demonstrated that mitogenic activation of mouse T-helper cells induces preproenkephalin mRNA synthesis. A complementary DNA library prepared from a cloned ConA-activated mouse T-helper cell line was found to encode preproenkephalin mRNA. The supernatants from induced T-helper cell cultures were found to have methionine-enkephalin immunoreactivity. These studies suggest that enkephalins like methionine-enkephalin serve a function as neuroimmunomodulators via T-dependent immune functions.

Several studies have been carried out with opioid peptides, particularly β-endorphin and methionine-enkephalin in animals and humans and also *in vitro* to understand their possible role in immune function. Although the concentration of circulating β-endorphin is very low in the rat, it is increased several fold following acute stress, producing plasma β-endorphin concentrations to almost 10 ng/ml (Guillemin et al., 1977). The possible relationship between stress, immune function, and endorphins has been reviewed (Amir et al., 1980). The effect of α-endorphin, β-endorphin, and D-Ala^2-Met^5-enkephalin to modulate the proliferative responses of splenic lymphocytes to mitogenic stimulation was measured. The results indicated that of the three peptides, only β-endorphin potentiated ConA and PHA-induced proliferation of T-lymphocytes, but had no effect on the response to the B-cell mitogen LPS/dextran sulfate (Gilman et al., 1982). The potentiating effect of β-endorphin was not reversed by naloxone, which suggests that the effect may be mediated by a nonopioid but β-endorphin-specific mechanism. On the other hand, McCain et al. (1982) reported that β-endorphin is a potent and efficacious suppressor of PHA-induced blastogenesis in cultured human T-lymphocytes which could not be antagonized by naloxone. The reduction in lymphocyte reactivity induced by β-endorphin did not appear to be due to cytotoxicity since the lactic dehydrogenase activity of the supernatant fluid, an indicator of cell lysis, was not affected. The differences in the studies of Gilman et al. (1982) and McCain et al. (1982) were that in the former splenocytes were used, whereas in the latter cultured human leukocytes were used. The influence of β-endorphin on lymphocyte function has been demonstrated to be dependent on the donor used. The β-endorphin-induced inhibition of lymphocyte proliferation appeared to be due to the fragment β-endorphin$_{10-16}$ amino acid sequence, and the effect is probably mediated by interference in the mobilization of intracellular calcium. β-Endorphin and methionine-enkephalin stimulate chemotaxis of human blood mononuclear cells, an effect which is antagonized by the opiate antagonist naloxone (van Epps and Saland, 1984), indicating that such an effect is mediated via endogenous opioids. A similar response has also been shown for neutrophils. β-endorphin at very low concentration (10^{-14} *M*) and methionine-enkephalin (10^{-9} *M*) have been shown to enhance the activity of NK cells from peripheral human blood, and this effect was blocked by naloxone (Matthews et al., 1983). Thus, endogenous opioids modify immune function via both opioid and nonopioid receptors. The opioid receptor-mediated effects include increased NK cell activity, increased α-interferon and interleukin-2 production, release of histamine from mast cells, enhancement of chemotaxis, and enhancement of T-cell subsets. The effects which do not appear to involve opioid receptors include modification of PHA-stimulated proliferation, superoxide production, and binding to terminal complexes of complement (SCSB-9 and CSB-9).

Evidence for the Presence of Opioid Recognition Sites (Receptors) on Cells Regulating Immune Function

Since morphine causes immunosuppression in both animals and humans which are at least partially reversed by naloxone, it is suggested that opiate receptors may be involved in immunomodulation. Since the discovery of opiate binding sites or receptors in mammalian tissue in 1975, at least five major types of opiate receptors have been postulated. They include μ- (preferring morphine), δ- (preferring enkephalins), κ- (preferring dynorphins or ethylketazocine), σ- (preferring *N*-allylnormetazocine, SKF 10,047), and ε- (preferring β-endorphin). In reality, σ-sites are nonopioid in nature. The endogenous opioids present in the circulation, CNS, pituitary, spleen and thymus (Bhargava et al., 1988, 1989b) interact with opiate receptors to different degrees. Much work has been done to characterize opiate receptors on T-lymphocytes, which are the major cells in immunoregulation. The first indirect evidence for the presence of opioid receptors on human T-lymphocytes was provided by the studies of Wybran et al. (1979), who showed that morphine inhibited and methionine-enkephalin increased the percentage of active T-rosettes. This effect was antagonized by naloxone but not by the inactive levomoramide, suggesting the presence of specific opioid receptors on T-lymphocytes. Binding sites for ^{3}H-leucine-enkephalin on cultured human T-lymphocytes were present, but the binding of the ligand could not be displaced or inhibited by naloxone (Ausiello and Roda, 1984). The binding sites for ^{3}H-naloxone were detected on lymphocytes and platelets from peripheral blood of healthy human volunteers. The binding was displaced by unlabeled naloxone and morphine (Mehrishi and Mills, 1983). In another study, ^{3}H-naloxone binding sites on rat lymphocytes have been demonstrated. Cultured human lymphocytes were shown to have specific binding sites for ^{125}I-h-[D-Ala^2]-β-endorphin. The binding was not inhibited by opiate agonists and antagonists or by enkephalin analogs, but was inhibited by β-endorphin or its analogs (Hazum et al., 1979). These studies demonstrated the presence of binding sites for β-endorphin on lymphocytes which were specific for β-endorphin and were nonopioid in nature. Similar binding sites have been found on the surface of mouse thymoma cells (Schweigerer et al., 1985). *In vitro* studies using PHA-stimulated human peripheral blood lymphocytes demonstrated the binding of ^{3}H-methionine-enkephalin, and this could be displaced by unlabeled methionine-enkephalin but not with 200 μM naloxone (Plotnikoff et al., personal communication). The δ-opiate receptor ligand, *cis*-(±)-3-methylfentanylisothiocynate (SUPERFIT), was found to label a protein from both B- and T-cell-enriched murine splenocytes, peripheral blood lymphocytes, and human peripheral blood lymphocytes (Carr et al., 1988).

SUMMARY AND CONCLUSIONS

Although not very convincing, several studies have demonstrated that binding sites for naloxone, opioid peptides, β-endorphin, and methionine-enkephalin exist on T-lymphocytes. β-Endorphin appears to be immunodepressant, whereas methionine-enkephalin is immunostimulant. Both *in vitro* and *in vivo* studies have shown that methionine-enkephalin can influence some immune functions. Since *in vitro* modifications of immune function require very low concentrations, it is reasonable to believe that methionine-enkephalin plays a physiological role in the immune system. Although not well established, methionine-enkephalin appears to activate T-lymphocytes via opioid receptors and triggers a series of intracellular signals leading to the activation of receptors for interleukin-2 (IL-2), OKT10, and active sheep T-red blood cell receptors. Methionine-enkephalin enhances the activity of NK cells and induces the production of IL-2, which in turn may recruit and activate other T-cell subsets like CD3 and CD4. Methionine-enkephalin also enhances mitogen-induced proliferation of lymphocytes.

Acute as well as chronic administration of morphine appears to suppress the immune function. However, it is not clear whether such an effect is direct or indirect. Chronic administration of opiates like morphine and U-50,488H (a κ-opiate agonist) are known to down-regulate central opiate receptors (Bhargava et al., 1989a; Bhargava and Gulati, 1990a) and affect other neurotransmitter receptors like dopamine and serotonin (Bhargava and Gulati, 1990b; Gulati and Bhargava, 1988, 1989, 1990). Evidence has been presented for the presence of dopamine receptors on rat lymphocytes (Ovadia and Abramsky, 1987) and sympathetic innervation of murine thymus and spleen (Felten et al., 1985; Williams et al., 1981). Chronic administration of morphine also alters the levels of opioid peptides in spleen and thymus (Bhargava et al., 1989b). Thus, the immunomodulation by morphine and other opiates may be both centrally and peripherally mediated, involving opioid peptides as well as neurotransmitter systems. Much more work is obviously required to understand the role of the opiate-opioid peptide-neurotransmitter chain in the CNS and periphery in immunomodulation.

REFERENCES

Akil H, Watson SJ, Sullivan S, and Barchas JD: Enkephalin-like material in normal human CSF: measurement and levels. *Life Sci* 1978; 23:121.

Amir S, Brown ZQ, and Amit Z: The role of endorphins in stress: evidence and speculations. *Neurosci Biobehav Rev* 1980; 4:77.

Ausiello CM and Roda LG: Leu-enkephalin binding to cultured human T lymphocytes. *Cell Biol Int Rep* 1984; 8:353.

Bhargava HN: Brain peptides, neuroleptic-induced tolerance and dopamine receptor supersensitivity: implications in tardive dyskinesia. In *Movement Disorders*. Shah NS and Donald AG, Eds. Plenum Press, New York, 1986, p. 159.

Bhargava HN: Opioid peptides, receptors and immune function. *NIDA Res Monogr* 1990; 96:220.

Bhargava HN and Gulati A: Down-regulation of μ-opiate receptors in spinal cord and discrete brain regions of non-abstinent morphine tolerant-dependent rats. *Eur J Pharmacol* 1990a; 190:305.

Bhargava HN and Gulati A: Modification of brain and spinal cord dopamine D_1 receptors labeled with ^{3}H-SCH 23390 following morphine withdrawal from tolerant and physically dependent rats. *J Pharmacol Exp Ther* 1990b; 252:901.

Bhargava HN, Gulati A, and Ramarao P: Effect of chronic administration of U-50,488H on tolerance to its pharmacological actions and on multiple opioid receptors in rat brain regions and spinal cord. *J Pharmacol Exp Ther* 1989a; 251:21.

Bhargava HN, Matwyshyn G, Hanissian S, and Tejwani GA: Opioid peptides in pituitary gland, brain regions and peripheral tissues of spontaneously hypertensive and Wistar-Kyoto normotensive rats. *Brain Res* 1988; 440:333.

Bhargava HN, Ramarao P, Gulati A, Gudehithlu KP, and Tejwani GA: Methionine-enkephalin and β-endorphin levels in spleen and thymus gland of morphine tolerant-dependent and abstinent rats. *Life Sci* 1989b; 45:2529.

Bocchini G, Bonanno G, and Canevari A: Influence of morphine and naloxone on human peripheral blood T-lymphocytes. *Drug Alcohol Depend* 1983; 11:233.

Briggs JH, McKerron CG, Souhami RL, Taylor DJE, and Andrews H: Severe systemic infections complicating "mainline" heroin addiction. *Lancet* 1967; 2:1227.

Brown SM, Stimmell B, Taub RN, Kochwa S, and Rosenfield RE: Immunologic dysfunction in heroin addicts. *Arch Intern Med* 1974; 134:1001.

Bryant HV, Berton EW, and Holaday JW: Morphine pellet induced immunomodulation in mice: temporal relationships. *J Pharmacol Exp Ther* 1988; 245:913.

Carr DJ, Kim CH, DeCosta B, Jacobson AE, Rice KC, and Blalock JE: Evidence for a δ-class opioid receptor on cells of the immune function. *Cell Immunol* 1988; 116:44.

Cherubin CE and Brown J: Systemic infections in heroin addicts. *Lancet* 1968; 1:298.

Clement-Jones V, Lowry PJ, Rees LH, and Besser GM: Met-enkephalin circulates in human plasma. *Nature* 1980; 283:295.

DiGiulio AM, Picotti GB, Cesura AM, Panerai AE, and Mantegazza P: Met-enkephalin immunoreactivity in blood platelets. *Life Sci* 1982; 30:1605.

Donahoe RM, Madden JJ, Hollingworth F, Schafer D, and Falek A: Morphine depression of T cell E-rosetting: definition of the process. *Fed Am Soc Exp Biol* 1985; 44:95.

Dougherty PM, Harper C, and Dafny N: The effect of alpha-interferon, cyclosporin A and radiation-induced immune suppression on morphine-induced hypothermia and tolerance. *Life Sci* 1986; 39:2197.

Faith RE, Liang HJ, Murgo AJ, and Plotnikoff NP: Neuroimmunomodulation with enkephalins: enhancement of human natural killer (NK) cell activity *in vitro*. *Clin Immunol Immunopathol* 1984; 31:412.

Felten DL, Felten SY, Carlson SL, Olschowska JA, and Livnat S: Noradrenergic and peptidergic innervation of lymphoid tissue. *J Immunol* 1985; 135(Suppl):755S.

Gilman SC, Schwartz JM, Milner RJ, Bloom FE, and Feldman JD: β-Endorphin enhances lymphocyte proliferative responses. *Natl Proc Acad Sci U.S.A.* 1982; 79:4226.

Gramsch C, Hollt V, Mehraien P, Pasi A, and Herz A: Regional distribution of methionine-enkephalin and beta endorphin-like immunoreactivity in human brain and pituitary. *Brain Res* 1979; 171:261.

Gros C, Pradelles P, Rouget C, Bepoldin O, Dray F, Fournie-Zaluski MC, Roques BP, Pollard H, Llorens-Cortes C, and Schwartz JC: Radioimmunoassay of methionine- and leucine-enkephalins in regions of rat brain and comparison with endorphins estimated by radioreceptor assay. *J Neurochem* 1977; 31:29.

Guillemin R, Vargo TM, Rossier J, Minick S, Ling N, Rivier C, Vale W, and Bloom F: β-Endorphin and adrenocorticotropin are secreted concomitantly by the pituitary gland. *Science* 1977; 197:1367.

Gulati A and Bhargava HN: Cerebral cortical 5-HT$_1$ and 5-HT$_2$ receptors of morphine tolerant-dependent and abstinent rats. *Neuropharmacology* 1988; 27:1231.

Gulati A and Bhargava HN: Brain and spinal cord 5-HT$_2$ receptors of morphine tolerant-dependent rats. *Eur J Pharmacol* 1989; 167:185.

Gulati A and Bhargava HN: Down-regulation of hypothalamic 5-HT$_{1A}$ receptors in morphine-abstinent rats. *Eur J Pharmacol* 1990; 182:253.

Gungor M, Genc E, Sagduyu H, Eroglu L, and Koyuncuoglu H: Effect of chronic administration of morphine on primary immune response in mice. *Experientia* 1980; 36:1309.

Hall NR and Goldstein AL: Neurotransmitters and the immune system. In *Psychoneuroimmunology*. Ader R, Ed. Academic Press, New York (1981).

Hazum E, Chang KJ, and Cuatrecasas P: Specific nonopiate receptors for β-endorphin. *Science* 1979; 205:1033.

Ho WKK and Leung A: The effect of morphine addiction on concanavalin A-mediated blastogenesis. *Pharmacol Res Commun* 1979; 11:413.

Hughes J, Kosterlitz HW, and Smith TW: The distribution of methionine-enkephalin and leucine enkephalin in the brain and peripheral tissues. *Br J Pharmacol* 1977; 61:639.

Hussey HH and Katz S: Infections resulting from narcotic addiction: report of 102 cases. *Am J Med* 1950; 9:186.

Hussey HH, Keliher TF, Schaffer BF, and Walsh BJ: Septicemia and bacterial endocarditis from heroin addiction. *JAMA* 1944; 126:535.

Johnson HM, Smith EM, Torres BA, and Blalock JE: Regulation of the in vitro antibody response by neuroendocrine hormones. *Proc Natl Acad Sci U.S.A.* 1982; 79:4171.

Law JS, Watanabe K, and West WL: Morphine effects on the responsiveness of lymphocytes to concanavalin A. *Pharmacologist* 1978; 20:231.

Lazzarin A, Mella L, Trombini M, Uberti-Foppa C, Franzetti F, Mazzoni G, and Galli M: Immunological status in heroin addicts: effects of methadone maintenance treatment. *Drug Alcohol Depend* 1984; 13:117.

Lefkowitz SS and Chiang CY: Effects of certain abused drugs on hemolysin forming cells. *Life Sci* 1975; 17:1763.

Lefkowitz SS and Nemeth D: Immuno-suppression of rosette-forming cells. *Adv Exp Med Biol* 1976; 73:269.

Lopker A, Abood LG, Hoss W, and Lionetti FJ: Stereoselective human phagocytic leukocytes. *Biochem Pharmacol* 1980; 29:1361.

Louria DB, Hensle T, and Rose J: The major medical complications of heroin addiction. *Ann Intern Med* 1967; 67:1.

Lundy J, Raaf JH, Deakins S, Wanebo HJ, Jacobs DA, Lee TD, Jacobwitz D, Spear C, and Oettgen HF: The acute and chronic effects of alcohol on the human immune function. *Surg Gynecol Obstet* 1975; 141:212.

Luttgens WF: Endocarditis in "mainline" opium addicts. *Arch Intern Med* 1949; 83:653.

Matthews PM, Froelich CJ, Sibbitt WL, and Bankhurst AD: Enhancement of natural cytotoxicity by β-endorphin. *J Immunol* 1983; 130:1658.

McCain HW, Lamster IB, Bozzone JM, and Grbic JT: β-Endorphin modulates human immune activity via non-opiate receptor mechanisms. *Life Sci* 1982; 31:1619.

McDonough RJ, Madden JJ, Falek A, Shafer DA, Pline M, Gordon D, Bokon, P, Kuehnle JC, and Mendelson J: Alteration of T and null lymphocyte frequencies in the peripheral blood of human opiate addicts: *in vivo* evidence for opiate receptor sites on T lymphocytes. *J Immunol* 1980; 125:2539.

Mehrishi JN and Mills IH: Opiate receptors on lymphocytes and platelets in man. *Clin Immunol Immunopathol* 1983; 27:240.

Meisheri KD and Isom GE: Influence of immune stimulation and suppression on morphine physical dependence and tolerance. *Res Commun Chem Pathol Pharmacol* 1978; 19:85.

Miller GC, Murgo AJ, and Plotnikoff NP: Enkephalin enhancement of active T-cell rosettes from lymphoma patients. *Clin Immunol Immunopathol* 1983; 26:446.

Miller RJ, Chang KJ, Cooper B, and Cuatrecasas P: Radioimmunoassay and characterization of enkephalins in rat tissues. *J Biol Chem* 1978; 253:531.

Morley JE, Kay NE, Solomon GF, and Plotnikoff NP: Neuropeptides: conductors of the immune orchestra. *Life Sci* 1987; 41:527.

Olsson RA and Romansky MJ: Staphylococcus tricuspid endocarditis in heroin addicts. *Ann Intern Med* 1962; 57:755.

Ovadia H and Abramsky O: Dopamine receptor on isolated membranes of rat lymphocytes. *J Neurosci Res* 1987; 18:70.

Panerai AE: Plasma [met]enkephalin concentrations after endocrine and pharmacological modifications. *Pharmacol Res Commun* 1988; 20:195.

Patel V, Borysenko M, Kumar MSA, and Millard WJ: Effects of acute and subchronic delta-9-tetrahydrocannabinol administration on the plasma catecholamine, β-endorphin, and corticosterone levels and splenic natural killer cell activity in rats. *Proc Soc Exp Biol Med* 1985; 180:400.

Peritt DJ, Holaday JW, and Bryant HU: Suppression of interleukin-2 production with chronic morphine treatment. *FASEB J* 1988; 2:A485.

Plotnikoff NP and Miller GC: Enkephalins as immunomodulators. *Int J Immunopharmacol* 1983; 5:437.

Polak JM, Bloom SR, Sullivan SN, Facer P, and Pearse AGE: Enkephalin-like immunoreactivity in the human gastrointestinal tract. *Lancet* 1977; 1:972.

Roda LG, Venturelli F, and Roscetti G: Hydrolysis and protection from hydrolysis of circulating enkephalins. *Comp Biochem Physiol* 1986; 85:449.

Schweigerer L, Schmidt W, Teschemacher H, and Gramsch C: β-Endorphin: surface binding and internalization in thymoma cells. *Proc Natl Acad Sci USA* 1985; 82:5751.

Simantov R, Childers SR, and Snyder SH: Opioid peptides: differentiation, radioimmunoassay and radioreceptor assay. *Brain Res* 1977; 135:358.

Smith EM and Blalock JE: Human lymphocyte production of corticotropin and endorphin-like substances: association with leucocyte interferon. *Proc Natl Acad Sci USA* 1981; 78:7530.

Su TP, London ED, and Jaffe JH: Steroid binding at σ-receptors suggests a link between endocrine, nervous and immune systems. *Science* 1988; 240:219.

Suda T, Liotta AS, and Krieger DT: β-Endorphin is not detectable in plasma from normal human subjects. *Science* 1978; 202:221.

Tubaro E, Borelli G, Croce C, Cavallo G, and Santiangeli C: Effect of morphine on resistance to infection. *J Infect Dis* 1983; 148:656.

Tubaro E, Avico U, Santiangeli C, Zuccaro P, Cavallo G, Pacifici R, Croce C, and Birelli G: Morphine and methadone impact on human phagocytic physiology. *Int J Immunopharmacol* 1985; 7:865.

Valentine JL, Plotnikoff NP, and Mayer RL: Distribution and uptake of methionine enkephalin into human blood cells. *Fed Proc* 1988; 46:A1073.

van Epps DE and Saland L: β-Endorphin and met-enkephalin stimulate human peripheral blood mononuclear cell chemotaxis. *J Immunol* 1984; 132:3046.

Watson RS, Jackson JC, Hartmann B, Sampliner R, Mobley D, and Eskelson C: Cellular immune functions, enkephalin, and alcohol consumption in males. *Alcohol Clin Exp Res* 1985; 9:248.

Weber RJ and Pert A: Opiate action in the periaqueductal gray matter causes suppression of immune function. *J Cell Biochem Suppl* 1987; 12D:317.

Wesche D, Hollt V, and Herz A: Radio-immunoassay of enkephalins. Regional distribution in rat brain after morphine treatment and hypophysectomy. *Naunyn Schmiedebergs Arch Pharmakol* 1977; 301:79.

Williams JM, Peterson RG, Shea PA, Schmedtjie JF, Bauer DC, and Felten DL: Sympathetic innervation of murine thymus and spleen. Evidence for a functional link between the nervous and immune systems. *Brain Res Bull* 1981; 6:83.

Wybran J, Appelboom T, Famey JP, and Govaerts A: Suggestive evidence for receptors for morphine and methionine enkephalin on normal human blood T lymphocytes. *J Immunol* 1979; 123:1068.

Yang HY, Hong JS, and Costa E: Regional distribution of leu- and met-enkephalin in rat brain. *Neuropharmacology* 1977; 16:303.

Zurawski G, Benedik M, Kamb BJ, Abraens JS, Zurawski SM, and Lee FD: Activation of mouse T-helper cells induces abundant proenkephalin mRNA synthesis. *Science* 1986; 232:772.

Chapter 21

The Role of Endogenous Opioids and Opioid Receptors in Human and Animal Cancer

Ian S. Zagon and Patricia J. McLaughlin
Neuroscience and Anatomy
The Pennsylvania State University
The M.S. Hershey Medical Center
Hershey, Pennsylvania

INTRODUCTION

The discovery of opioid receptors (Pert and Snyder, 1973; Simon et al., 1973; Terenius, 1973) and endogenous opioids (Hughes et al., 1975), which comprise the endogenous opioid systems, has led to considerable research regarding the function(s) of these elements (Akil et al., 1984; Beaumont and Hughes, 1979). A fascinating area of interest that has developed since the early 1980s has been concerned with the role of endogenous opioid systems in the growth of normal and abnormal tissues and cells. The early literature on opioids and cancer has been reviewed elsewhere (Zagon and McLaughlin, 1986) and will be summarized in this chapter. A comprehensive discussion of this field is precluded by limitations in space placed on this chapter. Thus, we have elected to direct our efforts to studies with model systems that have revealed the function and mechanisms underlying the influence of endogenous opioid systems on neoplasia, as well as the identification of the opioid peptide and opioid receptor involved with tumorigenic processes. We conclude with some exciting observations suggesting that endogenous opioids and opioid receptors also interact in human neoplasia, implying that endogenous opioid systems may be involved in the etiology and pathogenesis of human cancer.

ENDOGENOUS OPIOID SYSTEMS REGULATE CANCER: INITIAL OBSERVATIONS

For some time, it has been known that exogenous opioids such as methadone and morphine alter cell function, particularly of the developing nervous system (see bibliographies of Zagon et al., 1982, 1984, 1989). Intrigued by these findings, we conducted preliminary studies showing that mice injected with S20Y murine neuroblastoma cells, which results in a measurable — and ultimately lethal — tumor, had a prolonged survival if the animals received daily injections of heroin, an opioid agonist (Zagon and McLaughlin, 1981). This antitumor effect was blocked by concomitant administration of naloxone, an opioid antagonist, suggesting that opioid action resided at the level of the opioid receptor. Although it was known that neuroblastoma cells had opioid receptors (Klee and Nirenberg, 1974), the location of opioid-receptor interaction was unknown and could have been a direct action on the tumor cells or one that was mediated by other opioid functions (e.g., endocrine, immunity). Concurrently, we discovered that naloxone, at certain concentrations, could produce an antitumor action (Zagon and McLaughlin, 1981). After intensive study with an opioid antagonist paradigm using naltrexone, an extremely potent opioid antagonist, we concluded that endogenous opioids are involved with carcinogenesis (Zagon and McLaughlin, 1983a, 1984). Our strategy for many of these early studies was to use a low dosage of naltrexone to block the opioid receptor for either a short time each day (4 to 8 h/d) or a dosage and/ or schedule that blocked the opioid receptor for the entire period each day. The duration of opioid receptor blockade in these mice was determined in experiments challenging the animals with an opioid agonist and monitoring nociception. The premise of these experiments was that opioid agonists should diminish nociceptive capabilities unless opioid receptors are occupied by an opioid antagonist. We discovered that a daily intermittent receptor blockade significantly reduced the incidence of cancer, and dramatically prolonged the survival of tumor-bearing animals. Complete receptor blockade accelerated tumorigenesis and shortened the life span of the animals. Explanation of these results was revealed in subsequent experiments (Zagon and McLaughlin, 1989a). Autoradiographic and receptor binding assays of tumor tissue from mice subjected to opioid antagonists revealed an up-regulation of [D-Pen$^{2, 5}$]-enkephalin and [Met^5]-enkephalin binding sites, as well as an increase in β-endorphin and [Met^5]-enkephalin levels (determined by radioimmunoassay) relative to control specimens. Treatment of mice with naltrexone also produced a twofold increase in sensitivity to opioids. Thus, opioid receptor blockade (intermittent or complete) appears to produce an increase in opioid peptide levels and opioid receptors, and a supersensitivity to opioids. In the case of intermittent blockade, the increased levels of opioids are able to act on an increased number of receptors (presumably associated with tumor cells) and an exaggerated tumor inhibition is evoked. Thus, endogenous opioids serve as natural trophic inhibitory factors. Complete opioid receptor blockade prohibits the increased opioids from interacting with the increased number of receptors; hence, the endogenous opioids have no chance to interface and inhibit growth. The experiments with complete opioid receptor blockade also indicate that opioid-receptor interaction in regard to carcinogenic events must be quite active and under tonic regulation, since removal of opioid-receptor interfacing stimulates neoplasia. In essence, the opioids serve to repress certain tumorigenic events, and deprivation of opioids removes these controlling influences on neoplasia. A corollary to these observations was that the duration of opioid receptor blockade determines tumorigenic response (Zagon and McLaughlin, 1984). This conclusion came from experiments showing that administration of a low dosage of naltrexone at intervals over a 24-h period resulted in an acceleration of tumor growth. Administration of the cumulative amount of drug given once daily served to inhibit growth. Thus, the extent of opioid receptor blockade, rather than drug dosage, is the major factor involved in endogenous opioid control of tumorigenesis.

A number of other observations have been instrumental in arriving at the hypothesis that endogenous opioids modulate cancer. Opioids act in a stereospecific manner, and the demonstration of the enantiomeric specificity of opioids has been suggested by many investigators as a criterion for exclusion of nonopioid receptor-mediated pharmacological effects. The results from administration of naloxone stereoisomers to mice with transplanted neuroblastoma clearly showed that the (−) isomer of naloxone, but not the (+) isomer, decreased tumor incidence and prolonged survival time (Zagon and McLaughlin, 1985). Another aspect of these studies on endogenous opioids and their relationship to carcinogenesis was whether the effect of opioids seen earlier on a primary tumor model of neuroblastoma also was of importance in metastatic cancer; over 50% of the cases of human neuroblastoma are associated with metastatic tumors. To address the question of whether endogenous opioid systems function in metastatic tumors, the effects of opioids on a metastatic neuroblastoma in mice were examined (Zagon and McLaughlin, 1983b). Our results showed that metastatic tumors, just like primary tumors, are responsive to the action of opioids. Finally, the important question of whether endogenous opioids or opioid antagonists that alter growth produce identifiable qualitative alterations in the fine structure of cancer cells was investigated using transmission and scanning electron microscopy (Zagon, 1988). Utilizing cultures of neuroblastoma cells exposed to (1) [Met^5]-enkephalin, a naturally occurring opioid pentapeptide, at a concentration (10^{-6}

M) that inhibits cell replication by 66% of control levels, (2) [Met⁵]-enkephalin (10^{-6} *M*) and the opioid antagonist naloxone (10^{-6} *M*) which blocks opioid action, or (3) naltrexone (10^{-6} *M*), a potent opioid antagonist that disrupts endogenous opioid-opioid receptor interaction and increases cell number 76% above control values, morphological studies were performed. The ultrastructural profile of the cells exposed to these agents for 2 to 4 d was similar to controls (i.e., exposed to sterile water). These results support the hypothesis that endogenous opioid systems act as trophic factors as they regulate growth; their effects on cell growth and survival, however, do not alter the basic fine structural anatomy of the cells. Thus, the effects of opioids must be exerted through normal channels of growth and are not dependent on toxicity.

WHICH OPIOID PEPTIDE(S) IS(ARE) INVOLVED IN GROWTH?

An important question arising at this juncture was which opioid(s) is(are) selective for the growth regulation of animal tumors. To answer this question, we decided to employ a tissue culture system of murine S20Y neuroblastoma (the same tumor cell line used in earlier transplantation studies mentioned above) (Zagon and McLaughlin, 1989b). We devised an assay system whereby cells grown for 24 h were subjected to a drug and the number of cells determined 48 h later (72 h after seeding); preliminary studies in our laboratory indicated this to be the optimal time for detecting changes in cell proliferation. Using this assay system and drug concentrations ranging from 10^{-6} to 10^{-10} *M,* the effects of a wide range of opioid (synthetic and natural, exogenous and endogenous) and nonopioid compounds were examined (see Tables I and II). The results showed that [Met⁵]-enkephalin had the most potent action on cell proliferation; peptide concentrations as low as 10^{-10} *M* inhibited growth by 62% of control values. Closely related peptides such as [Met⁵, Arg⁶, Phe⁷]-enkephalin (heptapeptide), [Met⁵, Arg⁶, Gly⁷, Leu⁸]-enkephalin (octapeptide, proenkephalin), and [Leu⁵]-enkephalin also exhibited some inhibitory properties, but not to the extent of [Met⁵]-enkephalin. Experiments using analogs of [Met⁵]-enkephalin revealed the selectivity of this peptide; for example, no changes in growth occurred when the amino acids Tyr¹ or Met⁵ were deleted, smaller fragments of the [Met⁵]-enkephalin molecule such as L-tyrosylglycine or Tyr-Gly-Gly were used, or when alterations in the basic structure of [Met⁵]-enkephalin (e.g., [Met⁵]-enkephalinamide, [Met⁵]-enkephalin sulfoxide) were made. Interestingly, compounds selective for other opioid receptor types such as [D-Pen²,⁵]-enkephalin (DPDPE) and ICI 174,864 (δ-receptor ligands), ethylketocyclazocine (EKC) and U50,488 (κ-receptor ligands), D-Ala², MePhe⁴, [Glyol⁵]-enkephalin (DAGO) and β-funaltrexamine (β-FNA) (μ-receptor ligands), β-endorphin (ε-receptor ligand), and SKF-10,047 and haloperidol (σ-

TABLE I.

Effect of Opioid Peptides and Analogs, Related to Proenkephalin A, Prodynorphin, and POMC, on Proliferation of S20Y Neuroblastoma Cells in Culture

Compound	Structure	Peptide concentration (M)		
		10^{-6}	10^{-8}	10^{-10}
L-Tyrosylglycine	Tyr-Gly			
Tyr-Gly-Gly	Tyr-Gly-Gly			
[Des-Met⁵]-enkephalin	Tyr-Gly-Gly-Phe			
[Des-Tyr¹,Met⁵]-enkephalin/β-lipotropin₆₂₋₆₅	Gly-Gly-Phe-Met			
[Met⁵]-enkephalin	Tyr-Gly-Gly-Phe-Met	47**	59**	62**
[Met⁵]enkephalinamide	Tyr-Gly-Gly-Phe-Met-NH₂			
[Met⁵(O)]-enkephalin (sulfoxide)	Tyr-Gly-Gly-Phe-Met[O]			
[Met⁵,Lys⁶]-enkephalin	Tyr-Gly-Gly-Phe-Met-Lys			
[Met⁵,Arg⁶,Phe⁷]-enkephalin/heptapeptide	Tyr-Gly-Gly-Phe-Met-Arg-Phe	71**	77**	69**
[Met⁵,Arg⁶,Gly⁷,Leu⁸]-enkephalin/octapeptide/ proenkephalin	Tyr-Gly-Gly-Phe-Met-Arg-Gly-Leu	70**	76**	
Metorphinamide/adrenorphin	Tyr-Gly-Gly-Phe-Met-Arg-Arg-Val-NH₂			
BAM-12P (bovine adrenal medulla dodecapeptide)	Tyr-Gly-Gly-Phe-Met-Arg-Arg-Val-Gly-Arg-Pro-Glu			
β-Endorphin/β-lipotropin₆₁₋₉₁	Tyr-Gly-Gly-Phe-Met-Thr-Ser-Glu-Lys-Ser-Gln-Thr-Pro-Leu-Val-Thr-Leu-Phe-Lys-Asn-Ala-Ile-Ile-Lys-Asn-Ala-Tyr-Lys-Lys-Gly-Glu			
Peptide F	Tyr-Gly-Gly-Phe-Met-Lys-Lys-Met-Asp-Glu-Leu-Tyr-Pro-Leu-Glu-Val-Glu-Glu-Glu-Ala-Asn-Gly-Gly-Glu-Val-Leu-Gly-Lys-Arg-Tyr-Gly-Gly-Phe-Met			
[Leu⁵]-enkephalin	Tyr-Gly-Gly-Phe-Leu	62**	71**	
Dynorphin A₁₋₆	Tyr-Gly-Gly-Phe-Leu-Arg			
Dynorphin A₁₋₇	Tyr-Gly-Gly-Phe-Leu-Arg-Arg			
Dynorphin A₁₋₁₃	Tyr-Gly-Gly-Phe-Leu-Arg-Arg-Ile-Arg-Pro-Lys-Leu-Lys			
α-Neo-endorphin₁₋₈	Tyr-Gly-Gly-Phe-Leu-Arg-Lys-Tyr			
Dynorphin B/rimorphin	Tyr-Gly-Gly-Phe-Leu-Arg-Arg-Gln-Phe-Lys-Val-Val-Thr			

*Note:*Values represent mean cell number as percentage of controls.

**Significantly different from controls at $p < 0.01$.

TABLE II.
Opioid and Nonopioid Compounds
Having No Effect on Cell Proliferation of
S20Y Neuroblastoma Cells in Culture

DPDPE	Heroin*
DPLPE	Codeine
DADLE	LAAM
DADME	Methadone
[D-Ala^7,Met^5]-	Haloperidol
enkephalinamide	
DAGO	β-FNA
Kyotorphin	ICI 174,864
β-Casomorphin$_{1-5}$	EKC
(+)-Naloxone	U50,488
(−)-Naloxone	SKF-10,047
Levorphanol	Somatostatin
Dextrorphan	[Arg^8]-vasopressin
Levallorphan tartrate	α-MSH
Morphine	PHe-Leu-Glu-Glu-Val

Note: Each compound was tested at concentration of 10^{-6}, 10^{-8}, and $10^{-10}M$.

*Heroin, at a concentration of 10^{-6} M, inhibited cell growth (see text).

receptor ligands) had no effect on growth at concentrations of 10^{-6} to 10^{-10} M (Figures 1 and 2). Full growth curves (Figure 1) using [Met^5]-enkephalin showed a dose-dependent effect at concentrations of 10^{-4} to 10^{-12} M; the median effective concentration (EC$_{50}$) was 10^{-10} M. [Met^5]-enkephalin's effect on growth was blocked by concomitant administration of (−)-naloxone, but not (+)-naloxone, indicating stereospecificity and the involvement of opioid receptors. Cell proliferation appeared to be the target of [Met^5]-enkephalin, with [^{3}H]-thymidine autoradiography showing a 48% decrease from control values in cells synthesizing DNA in cultures subjected to 10^{-6} M [Met^5]-enkephalin for 48 h. The labeling index of cultures exposed to both [Met^5]-enkephalin and (−)-naloxone was comparable to controls (Figure 2). Evaluation of the mitotic index showed 62.5% fewer mitotic profiles in cultures exposed to [Met^5]-enkephalin than in controls; once again, this decrease was blocked by concomitant exposure to naloxone (Figure 2). Immunocytochemical studies revealed [Met^5]-enkephalin-like immunoreactivity in the cytoplasm and cell processes of S20Y neuroblastoma cells, but not in the cell nucleus. Immunoelectron microscopic investigations confirmed these results at the light microscopic level of resolution, and revealed that [Met^5]-enkephalin immunoreactivity was associated with the plasma membrane, outer nuclear envelope, and a variety of organelles (Zagon, 1989). Radioimmunoassays indicated that neuroblastoma cells in culture contained a [Met^5]-

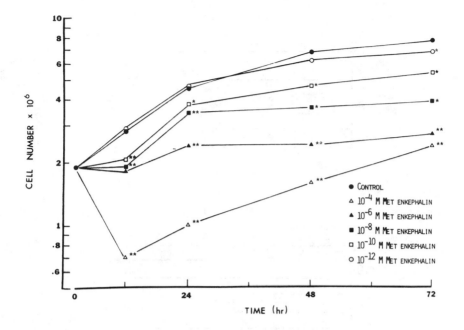

Figure 1. The growth of S20Y neuroblastoma cells subjected to various concentrations of [Met⁵]-enkaphalin (Met enkephalin). Twenty-four h after seeding, [Met⁵]-enkephalin was added to cultures containing a comparable number of cells (time of drug addition − 0 h); fresh media and drug were changed every 24 h thereafter. Control cultures were given an equivalent volume of vehicle (sterile water) only. Significantly different from control at $*p < 0.05$ and $**p < 0.01$.

enkephalin-like substance and that this peptide was secreted and accumulated in the media. Receptor binding assays with [³H]-[Met⁵]-enkephalin revealed specific and saturable binding that fit a single homogeneous binding site, with a binding affinity of 1.2 nM and a binding capacity of 50.2 fmol/mg protein; we estimated 15,000 receptors per cell (Figure 3). These results suggest that (1) the naturally occurring pentapeptide, [Met⁵]-enkephalin, derived from proenkephalin A, is the opioid peptide involved with carcinogenesis, (2) opioid action, as mediated by opioid receptors, is targeted to cell replication, (3) opioids act as inhibitory trophic factors, (4) tumor cells produce [Met⁵]-enkephalin, and (5) the median effective concentration of [Met⁵]-enkephalin is comparable to the dissociation constant (i.e., the $EC_{50} = K_d$).

To confirm that [Met⁵]-enkephalin can influence the growth of a tumor, S20Y neuroblastoma cells were transplanted into mice and the animals received daily injections of peptides (Zagon and McLaughlin, 1988; Zagon et al., 1985). Dosages of 0.5 to 30 mg/kg [Met⁵]-enkephalin (but not 0.1 mg/kg) delayed tumor appearance and prolonged survival; antitumor effects were blocked by concomitant injections of naloxone. Daily administration of 10 mg/kg [Leu⁵]-enkephalin, a closely related pentapeptide, had no effect on

MITOTIC INDEX

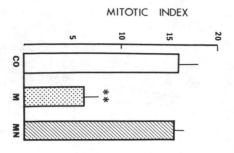

LABELING INDEX

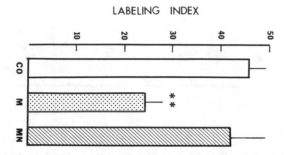

Figure 2. The mitotic and labeling indices of S20Y neuroblastoma cells subjected to 10^{-6} *M* [Met⁵]-enkephalin (M), 10^{-6} *M* [Met⁵]-enkephalin, and 10^{-6} (−)-naloxone (MN), or sterile water (vehicle) (CO) and assessed 48 h after drug exposure. Cells were seeded and allowed to grow for 24 h prior to addition of drug, and fresh media and drug were changed every 24 h. All cultures contained a comparable number of cells prior to addition of drug. (−)-naloxone (10^{-6} *M*) had no effect on growth. Bars − SEM. Significantly different from control at **$p < 0.01$.

[³H]-[MET⁵]-ENKEPHALIN

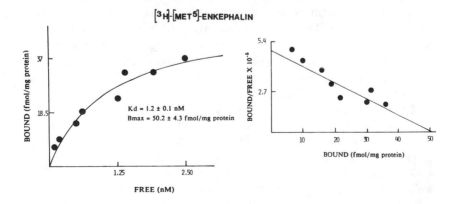

Figure 3. Representative saturation binding isotherm and Scatchard plot (inset) of the specific binding of [³H]-[Met⁵]-enkephalin to S20Y neuroblastoma cells in culture for 72 h.

neurotumor growth. [D-Ala², D-Leu⁵]-enkephalin (DADLE), EKC, and β-FNA, ligands selective for δ, κ, and μ receptors, respectively, also did not influence neural oncogenesis. These results demonstrate (1) the potent inhibitory effects on tumor growth of the naturally occurring opioid pentapeptide, [Met⁵]-enkephalin, (2) [Met⁵]-enkephalin acts at the level of the opioid receptor since its action is reversed by naloxone, (3) neither δ, κ, nor μ receptors are involved with modulating the growth of neural neoplasia, and (4) [Met⁵]-enkephalin acts in a receptor-mediated fashion at concentrations (nM) in the range of the K_d to alter neural tumor growth.

WHICH OPIOID RECEPTOR(S) IS(ARE) INVOLVED IN CARCINOGENESIS?

Although the endogenous opioid related to neural cancer growth was identified, the nature of the opioid receptor related to this action was unclear. [Met⁵]-enkephalin is known to interact with a number of opioid receptors, at least in adult neural tissues, and further work is needed to characterize the opioid receptor subtype involved in neoplasia. Using tumor tissue harvested from mice with transplanted S20Y neuroblastoma (Zagon et al., 1989) and in subsequent studies with S20Y neuroblastoma cells grown in culture (Zagon et al., 1990), we performed detailed receptor binding experiments with radiolabeled [Met⁵]-enkephalin using homogenates of tumor tissue or cells grown in culture. In both cases, our results showed specific and saturable binding, with the data most consistent for a single binding site. Scatchard analysis yielded a K_d of 0.49 and 1.6 nM in tumor tissues and cell cultures, respectively, and a binding capacity of 5.3 and 48.1 fmol/mg protein, respectively; the results with tumor cells in culture were consistent with the preliminary data obtained earlier (Zagon and McLaughlin, 1989b). Binding of [Met⁵]-enkephalin was dependent on protein concentration, time, temperature, and pH. Optimal binding required protease inhibitors, and pretreatment of the homogenates with trypsin markedly reduced binding, indicating the proteinaceous character of the binding site. Displacement experiments revealed that [Met⁵]-enkephalin was the most potent competitor of [³H]-[Met⁵]-enkephalin. Given the functional significance of [Met⁵]-enkephalin as a potent regulator of normal and abnormal growth, and that the receptor recognized by [Met⁵]-enkephalin did not resemble any previously described receptor, these studies demonstrated the presence of a new opioid receptor termed zeta (ζ) (from the Greek word "zoe", life). The function of this receptor is related to cell proliferation. The increased binding capacity in cell cultures with respect to tumor tissue probably reflected the heterogenous nature of the tumor tissue and the presence of varying proportions of necrotic and viable areas, which were eliminated by homogenous cell cultures.

Human Studies

The impact of endogenous opioid systems on the growth of neural tumors in animals stimulated our interest in obtaining information about the relationship of opioids and human cancer. Initially, our studies focused on determining whether endogenous opioids and/or opioid receptors were present in human tumors. Using a wide variety of human tumors obtained at biopsy or autopsy, we discovered that endogenous opioids and opioid receptors are ubiquitous in human tumor tissue (Zagon et al., 1987). Receptor binding assays demonstrated specific, high-affinity, and saturable binding of a number of opioid ligands. Radioimmunoassays revealed the presence of β-endorphin and [Met^5]-enkephalin in these tumors. Both [Met^5]- and [Leu^5]-enkephalin were detected in tumor tissue by immunocytochemistry, with immunoreactivity related to the cortical cytoplasm of tumor cells, but not to cell nuclei. Endogenous opioids and receptors were found in benign and malignant tumors representative of ectodermal, mesodermal, and endodermal origin. These results suggested that endogenous opioids and opioid receptors are fundamental features of human cancer.

In order to examine whether human neuroblastoma was influenced by endogenous opioid systems, experiments were undertaken with the opioid antagonist paradigm (i.e., using naltrexone) and human neuroblastoma (SK-N-MC) transplanted into nude mice (McLaughlin and Zagon, 1987). The latency for appearance of a measurable tumor (5 mm diameter) in the intermittent receptor blockade group (0.1 mg/kg naltrexone) was 27% longer than controls (11 d), and the first death in this group occurred 33% later than controls (day 27). Mice inoculated with human neuroblastoma cells in the 10 mg/kg naltrexone group, a dosage which rendered a complete opioid receptor blockade for each 24-h injection period, had an acceleration (18%) in the latency of tumor appearance. Two weeks after cell inoculation, 70% of the mice in the 10 mg/kg naltrexone group had tumors, in contrast to 10% of the controls. At the termination of the experiment (day 45), only 33% of the mice in the 10 mg/kg naltrexone group were alive, in contrast to 90% of the controls. These results were similar to those obtained earlier with opioid antagonists and murine S20Y neuroblastoma, and indicate that endogenous opioid systems regulate human neural oncogenesis, with opioids being active inhibitors of growth.

Experiments in tissue culture cells using human neuroblastoma (SK-N-MC) and human fibrosarcoma (HT-1080) reveal that 10^{-6} M [Met^5]-enkephalin depresses cell growth in a naloxone-reversible fashion (Zagon and McLaughlin, 1989b). Moreover, exposure to the potent opioid antagonist naltrexone (10^{-6} M) accelerates tumor cell proliferation (Zagon and McLaughlin, 1990). These results are consistent with those described earlier for murine S20Y neuroblastoma and indicate that endogenous opioid systems operate in human neural and nonneural tumor cells in culture.

If, indeed, endogenous opioid systems are involved in neural neoplasia, it is important to know whether the ζ-receptor related to tumor growth exists in human brain tumors. During the course of a study on the ζ-receptor in developing and adult human cerebellum (Gibo et al., 1989; Zagon et al., 1990b), we received brain tissue from an individual with a primary adenocarcinoma of the stomach and a metastatic adenocarcinoma of the cerebellum. Using receptor binding assays, we found the growth-related opioid receptor, ζ, was present and in abundance in the subject with metastatic adenocarcinoma of the cerebellum, but not in normal cerebellar tissue (Zagon et al., 1990a). Since the ζ-receptor is related to cell proliferation, these results suggest that endogenous opioid systems are present and function as trophic growth regulators in neoplasia of the human nervous system.

SUMMARY

Considerable evidence has been accumulated from both *in vivo* and *in vitro* studies indicating that endogenous opioid systems play a substantial role in regulating the growth of neural and nonneural cancers. The endogenous opioids function as inhibitory growth factors, with their action targeted to cell proliferation and mediated by opioid receptors. [Met^5]-enkephalin has now been identified as the most potent opioid peptide associated with growth, and the ζ-receptor as the opioid receptor involved with carcinogenesis. It appears that human neoplasia is also governed by endogenous opioid systems with respect to growth. Further studies of endogenous opioid systems and oncogenesis should provide valuable information about the etiology, pathogenesis, and therapeutic intervention of human cancer.

ACKNOWLEDGMENTS

This work was supported by NIH Grants NS-20500 and NS-20623.

REFERENCES

Akil H, Watson WJ, Young E, Lewis ME, Khachaturian H, and Walker JM: Endogenous opioids: biology and function. *Annu Rev Neurosci* 1984; 7:223.

Beaumont A and Hughes J: Biology of opioid peptides. *Annu Rev Pharmacol* 1979; 19:245.

Gibo DM, McLaughlin PJ, and Zagon IS: Presence of zeta and other opioid binding sites in cerebellum of adult and developing humans. *Soc Neurosci Abstr* 1989; 15:566.

Hughes JA, Smith TW, Kosterlitz HW, Fothergill LA, Morgan BA, and Morris HR: Identification of two pentapeptides from the brain with potent opiate agonist activity. *Nature* 1975; 258:577.

Klee WA and Nirenberg M: A neuroblastoma × glioma hybrid cell line with morphine receptors. *Proc Natl Acad Sci U.S.A.* 1974; 71:3474.

McLaughlin PJ and Zagon IS: Modulation of human neuroblastoma transplanted into nude mice by endogenous opioid systems. *Life Sci* 1987; 41:1465.

McLaughlin PJ and Zagon IS: Zeta (ζ), a growth-related opioid receptor, is present in metastatic adenocarcinoma of human cerebellum. *FASEB J* 1990; 4:A1001.

Pert CB and Snyder SH: Opiate receptor: demonstration in nervous tissue. *Science* 1973; 179:1011.

Simon EJ, Miller JM, and Edelman I: Stereospecific binding of the potent narcotic analgesic (³H)etorphine to rat brain homogenate. *Proc Natl Acad Sci U.S.A.* 1973; 70:1947.

Terenius L: Stereospecific interaction between narcotic analgesics and a synaptic plasma membrane fraction of rat cerebral cortex. *Acta Pharmacol Toxicol* 1973; 32:317.

Zagon IS: Endogenous opioid systems and neural cancer: transmission and scanning electron microscopic studies of murine neuroblastoma in tissue culture. *Brain Res Bull* 1988; 21:775.

Zagon IS: Endogenous opioids and neural cancer: an immunoelectron microscopic study. *Brain Res Bull* 1989; 22:1023.

Zagon IS, Goodman SR, and McLaughlin PJ: Characterization of zeta (ζ): a new opioid receptor involved in growth. *Brain Res* 1989; 482:297.

Zagon IS, Goodman SR, and McLaughlin PJ: Demonstration and characterization of zeta (ζ), a growth-related opioid receptor, in a neuroblastoma cell line. *Brain Res* 1990; 511:181.

Zagon IS and McLaughlin PJ: Heroin prolongs survival time and retards tumor growth in mice with neuroblastoma. *Brain Res Bull* 1981; 7:25.

Zagon IS and McLaughlin PJ: Naltrexone modulates tumor response in mice with neuroblastoma. *Science* 1983a; 221:671.

Zagon IS and McLaughlin PJ: Opioid antagonists inhibit the growth of metastatic murine neuroblastoma. *Cancer Lett* 1983b; 21:89.

Zagon IS and McLaughlin PJ: Duration of opiate receptor blockade determines tumorigenic response in mice with neuroblastoma: a role for endogenous opioid systems in cancer. *Life Sci* 1984; 35:409.

Zagon IS and McLaughlin PJ: Stereospecific modulation of tumorigenicity by opioid antagonists. *Eur J Pharmacol* 1985; 113:115.

Zagon IS and McLaughlin PJ: Endogenous opioid systems, stress, and cancer. In *Enkephalins-Endorphins: Stress and the Immune System.* Plotnikoff N, Murgo AJ, Faith RE, and Good RA, Eds. Plenum Press, New York, 1986, pp. 81–100.

Zagon IS and McLaughlin PJ: Modulation of murine neuroblastoma in nude mice by opioid antagonists. *J Natl Cancer Inst* 1987; 78:141.

Zagon IS and McLaughlin PJ: Endogenous opioids and the growth regulation of a neural tumor. *Life Sci* 1988; 43:1313.

Zagon IS and McLaughlin PJ: Opioid antagonist modulation of murine neuroblastoma: a profile of cell proliferation and opioid peptides and receptors. *Brain Res* 1989a; 480:16.

Zagon IS and McLaughlin PJ: Endogenous opioid systems regulate growth of neural tumor cells in culture. *Brain Res* 1989b; 490:14.

Zagon IS and McLaughlin PJ: Opioid antagonist (naltrexone) stimulation of cell proliferation in human and animal neuroblastoma and human fibrosarcoma cells in culture. *Neuroscience* 1990; 37:223.

Zagon IS, Gibo DM, and McLaughlin PJ: Expression of zeta (ζ), a growth-related opioid receptor, in metastatic adenocarcinoma of the human cerebellum. *J Natl Cancer Inst* 1990a; 82:325.

Zagon IS, Gibo DM, and McLaughlin PJ: Adult and developing human cerebella exhibit different profiles of opioid binding sites. *Brain Res* 1990b; 523:62.

Zagon IS, McLaughlin PJ, Goodman SR, and Rhodes RE: Opioid receptors and endogenous opioids in diverse human and animal cancers. *J Natl Cancer Inst* 1987; 79:1059.

Zagon IS, McLaughlin PJ, Takemori AE, and Portoghese PS: β-funaltrexamine (β-FNA) and neural tumor response in mice. *Eur J Pharmacol* 1985; 116:165.

Zagon IS, McLaughlin PJ, Weaver DJ, and Zagon E: Opiates, endorphins, and the developing organism: a comprehensive bibliography. *Neurosci Biobehav Rev* 1982; 6:439.

Zagon IS, McLaughlin PJ, and Zagon E: Opiates, endorphins, and the developing organism: a comprehensive bibliography, 1982-1983. *Neurosci Biobehav Rev* 1984; 8;387.

Zagon IS, Zagon E, and McLaughlin PJ: Opioids and the developing organism: a comprehensive bibliography, 1984-1988. *Neurosci Biobehav Rev* 1989; 13:207.

Enhancement of Tumor Resistance in Mice by Enkephalins

Anthony J. Murgo
Section of Hematology-Oncology
Department of Medicine
West Virginia University School of Medicine
Morgantown, West Virginia

Robert E. Faith
Department of Biology
University of Houston
Houston, Texas

Nicholas P. Plotnikoff
Pharmacodynamics Department
College of Pharmacy and School of Medicine
The University of Illinois at Chicago
Chicago, Illinois

SUMMARY

There is mounting evidence that the endogenous opioids have significant effects on the immune response. Presently, we show that the administration of [Met]enkephalin and [Leu]enkephalin into mice inhibits the growth and metastasis of B16 melanoma and that enkephalin administration enhances the natural killer (NK) cell activity of splenic lymphocytes. These results suggest that the antitumor effect of the enkephalins is related, at least in part, to the stimulation of host immunological defense. We propose that the enkephalins are biological response modifiers and that these neuropeptides may play a protective role in maintaining homeostasis in the immune system during periods of stress.

It is well known that psychological as well as physical stress can influence immune response and tumor growth (Riley, 1981). Although most investigations have focused on the adrenal corticosteroids as the mediators of these changes (Monjon and Collector, 1977; Riley, 1981), there is mounting evidence that other substances play a role. First, corticosteroids are generally considered to be immunosuppressive. However, under experimental conditions, certain stressful stimuli can result in immunoenhancement and tumor growth inhibition (Greenberg et al., 1984; Monjon and Collector, 1977; Steplewski et al., 1985). Furthermore, stress-induced suppression of the immune response can occur in adrenalectomized animals (Keller et al., 1983), and hypothalamic lesioning can cause alterations in the immune system that are not related to changes in corticosteroids (Brooks et al., 1982). Finally, stress brings about a variety of biochemical changes, including the release of neurotransmitters and hormones other than corticosteroids, that have direct effects on the elements of the immune system and can alter host defense mechanisms (Evans et al., 1986).

Among the potential mediators of stress-induced immunomodulation and tumor growth regulation are the endogenous opioids, including β-endorphin, dynorphin, methionine-enkephalin, and leucine-enkephalin. These peptides are found within the central nervous system, pituitary gland, adrenal glands, sympathetic neurons, and other tissues and can be released in response to stressful stimuli (Evans et al., 1986; Olson et al., 1987). The endogenous opioids may be responsible for a variety of physiological effects which are mediated through specific opioid receptors (Olson et al., 1987). There has been recent interest in studying the effects of the endogenous opioids on the immune system, and substantial evidence from numerous *in vitro* experiments indicates that these substances can influence immune function. Various elements of the immune system, including lymphocytes, phagocytic leukocytes, and terminal complexes of complement, possess receptors or binding sites for opioid peptides (Murgo et al., 1986). β-endorphin and the enkephalins can increase the formation of active T-cell rosettes by human peripheral blood lymphocytes (Miller et al., 1984; Murgo et al., 1985; Wybran et al., 1979). Also, the opioid peptides can regulate mitogen-induced lymphocyte proliferation (Plotnikoff and Miller, 1983) and the *in vitro* antibody response to sheep erythrocytes (Johnson et al., 1982). Furthermore, several investigators have shown that the incubation of human peripheral blood lymphocytes with β-endorphin and the enkephalins enhances the activity of natural killer cells (Faith et al., 1984, 1987; Kay et al., 1984; Mandler et al., 1986; Mathews et al., 1983). The stimulation of natural killer cells *in vivo* may enhance host defenses against viral infections, tumor growth, and tumor metastasis. However, the role of the endogenous opioid peptides in the modulation of the immune system and tumor growth *in vivo* remains unclear. Several studies suggest that the enkephalins stimulate the immune response and inhibit tumor growth *in vivo* (Murgo et al., 1986; Zagon and McLaughlin, 1986). The administration of methionine-enkephalin and leucine-enkephalin into mice can improve the survival of animals bearing L1210 tumors (Plotnikoff and Miller, 1983). In addition, enkephalin treatment increases the weight of the thymus in both mice (Murgo, 1986; Plotnikoff et al., 1985) and rats (Plotnikoff et al., 1985). It has also been shown that the administration of enkephalin to mice inhibits the growth and metastases of B16 melanoma (Faith and Murgo, 1988; Murgo, 1985; Scholar et al., 1987), and we have found that methionine-enkephalin stimulates splenic natural killer cell activity *in vivo* (Faith and Murgo, 1988). These studies which support the role of the endogenous opioid system in the modulation of the immune response and tumor growth will be reviewed in this paper.

MATERIALS AND METHODS

Mice

Four-week-old male C57Bl/6 mice were obtained from either Jackson Laboratories (Bar Harbor, ME) or Harlan Sprague Dawley, Inc (Indianapolis, IN). The mice were housed in plastic bottom cages in groups of five and were permitted free access to food and water. The mice were allowed to adjust to their environment for 1 week prior to experimentation.

Drugs

Methione-enkephalin ([Met]enk) and leucine-enkephalin ([Leu]enk) were purchased from Peninsula Laboratories (Belmont, CA) or Sigma Chemical Co. (St. Louis, MO). [D-Ala^2,D-Leu^5]enkephalin (DADLE) was purchased from Sigma. Naloxone was kindly provided by DuPont® Pharmaceuticals (Wilmington, DE). The drugs were diluted in sterile water, phosphate-buffered saline (PBS), or Hank's balanced saline solution (HBSS). Injections of drug were administered subcutaneously (s.c.) except for the spleen cell cytotoxicity studies in which case the intraperitoneal (i.p.) route was utilized. Control mice received injections of diluent.

Tumor cells

B16-BL6 and B16-F10 melanoma cells were maintained in monolayer culture in minimum essential media (MEM) supplemented with 10% fetal bovine serum. Single cell suspensions were prepared by brief exposure to trypsin-EDTA. These cells were suspended in PBS without Ca^{+2} or Mg^{+2} for injection or with medium for the cytotoxicity assay. The YAK-1 tumor cells were maintained in suspension culture in RPMI 1640 medium containing 10% fetal calf serum.

Monitoring of Tumor Growth and Metastasis

In the studies involving local tumor growth, B16-BL6 melanoma cells were injected in a volume of 0.1 ml s.c. into the right flank region. Tumor diameters were measured with the use of a vernier calipers and the geometric means of the two largest perpendicular diameters (mm) were recorded. In the studies of experimental metastasis, B16 melanoma cells were inoculated intravenously (i.v.) into the lateral tail vein. The mice were sacrificed by cervical dislocation 12 to 14 d later; the lungs were removed and placed in formalin and the number of metastatic pulmonary lesions were counted with a dissecting microscope.

Natural Killer (NK) Cell Cytotoxicity Assay

All cytotoxicity assays were performed using freshly isolated splenic lymphocytes as effector cells. The mice were injected i.p. with various doses of [Met]enk, and 18 h later the mice were sacrificed by cervical dislocation. The spleens were removed aseptically and pooled into groups of two. Single cell suspensions were prepared from these spleens and used as effector cells in the cytotoxicity assays. Both YAC-1 and B16-F10 melanoma tumor cells were used as targets.

A ^{51}Cr release cytotoxicity assay was utilized. Aliquots containing 2×10^6 cells per ml were labeled with 150 μCi of $Na^{51}CrO_4$ (^{51}Cr) solution per milliliter of cells by incubation at 37°C for 45 min. After washing the cells three times, 5×10^3 viable cells in 0.1 ml of RPMI 1640 medium was pipetted into 96-well Linbro plates (Linbro Scientific, Hamden, CT). Various effector cell concentrations in 0.1 ml of medium were added to triplicate wells to give effector:target cell ratios of 200:1, 100:1, and 50:1. After incubation at 37°C in 5% CO_2 in air for 4 h, 100 μl of supernatant from each well was collected and counted for 2 min in a γ-counter. The percentage of isotope released was used as a measure of cytotoxicity and was calculated by the formula:

$$\% \text{ specific release} = \frac{\text{cpm experimental release} - \text{cpm from medium control}}{\text{cpm maximum release} - \text{cpm from medium control}} \times 100$$

where cpm experimental release = counts released after incubation of target cells with effector cells, cpm from medium control = counts spontaneously released by target cells incubated in medium alone, and cpm maximum release = counts released by lysis of target cells with 1% Triton® X-100.

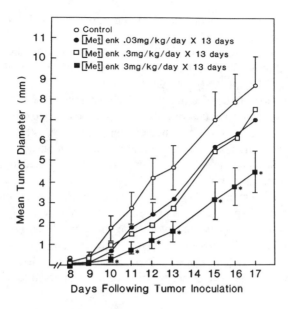

Figure 1. The effect of various doses of [Met]enk on local tumor growth is shown. All mice were inoculated with 10^5 B16-BL6 melanoma cells s.c. on day 0. Injections of [Met]enk were begun the day following tumor cell inoculation. Control mice received injections of diluent (H_2O). The results represent the means ± S.E. of ten mice per group and the asterisk sign indicates statistically significant ($p < 0.05$) differences from the control group.

Statistical Analysis

Student's T-test was used to determine differences in mean tumor diameters and in cytotoxic activity between treatment groups. The Mann Whitney test was used to determine differences in the number of metastases.

RESULTS

Effects on Local Tumor Growth

In order to assess the effect of enkephalin on tumor growth, mice were inoculated with B16-BL6 melanoma tumor cells s.c. into the flank region. The day following tumor cell inoculation, the mice received daily s.c. injections of various doses of enkephalin. Control mice received injections of diluent. The mice were examined daily or every other day for the appearance of palpable tumors. The effect of [Met]enk at doses of .03, 0.3, and 3 mg/kg/d for 13 d on local tumor growth is shown in Figure 1. Tumor growth was significantly inhibited with the 3 mg/kg dose. Although the mean time to tumor appearance was slightly prolonged in the treated mice, [Met]enk did not significantly reduce the incidence of tumors by the time the experiment was terminated (day 17). Local tumor growth was similarly inhibited by the administration of [Leu]enk (Figure 2).

The antitumor effect of enkephalin is most marked during the first 2 weeks following tumor inoculation, after which time the rate of tumor growth in the treated groups approaches that of controls. Also, we found that enkephalin treatment did not result in the regression of established tumors. Thus far, similar studies with the enkephalin analog, DADLE, failed to demonstrate a significant antitumor effect.

In order to determine if the effect of enkephalin on local tumor growth is mediated through specific opioid receptors, [Met]enk was administered in combination with the opioid receptor antagonist, naloxone. Beginning the day following the s.c. inoculation of B16-BL6 tumor cells, mice were injected daily for 7 d with [Met]enk alone, naloxone just prior to [Met]enk, naloxone alone, or diluent alone. The effect of this treatment on local tumor growth is

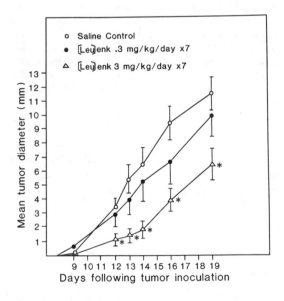

Figure 2. The effect of [Leu]enk on the local tumor growth of B16-BL6 melanoma is shown. 10^5 tumor cells were inoculated s.c. on day 0 and treatment was begun on the following day. The results represent the means ± S.E. of ten mice per group. The asterisk sign indicates statistically significant differences ($p < 0.05$) from the control group.

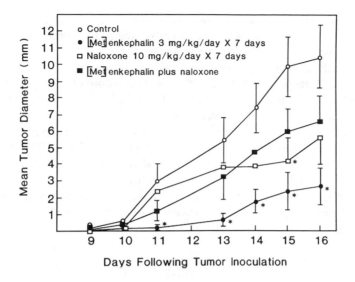

Figure 3. The effect of [Met]enk and/or naloxone on the local tumor growth of B16-BL6 melanoma is shown. 10^5 tumor cells were inoculated s.c. on day 0 and treatment was begun on day 1. Control mice received injections of diluent (H$_2$O). In the group which received the combination, naloxone was administered 5 to 10 min prior to [Met]enk. The results represent the means ± S.E. of eight mice per group and the asterisk sign indicates statistically significant differences ($p < 0.05$) from the control group.

shown in Figure 3. The antitumor effect of [Met]enk was inhibited by the concomitant administration of naloxone. Although naloxone inhibited the antitumor effect of enkephalin, naloxone alone also tended to reduce tumor growth. This antitumor effect of naloxone was seen in repeated experiments.

Effects on Experimental Metastasis

The following experiments were performed to determine the effect of enkephalin on the development of pulmonary metastasis. Groups of mice were injected with enkephalin 1 d prior to the i.v. administration of B16-BL6 melanoma cells. Twelve to 14 d later, the mice were sacrificed and the number of metastases counted. The median number of metastatic lesions in control groups in these experiments was about 3 to 4. The relatively low number of metastases observed in these experiments probably results from a variety of factors, including the early time of sacrifice, tumor dose, and, possibly, because the tumor cells used in these experiments had been maintained in culture for approximately 2 years and may have lost some of their *in vivo* virulence. In any event, both [Met]enk and [Leu]enk caused a reduction in metastasis. The results with various doses of [Met]enk is shown in Table I. The number of metastases was significantly reduced by a dose of 30 mg/kg. Table II shows the results of various doses of [Leu]enk on metastasis. Significant reduction in pulmonary metastasis with [Leu]enk occurred with 0.3 mg/kg and 30 mg/kg, but not with an intermediate dose of 12 mg/kg. Similar experiments with various doses of DADLE have thus far failed to demonstrate a significant effect on tumor metastasis.

In order to determine if the inhibitory effect of enkephalin on experimental pulmonary metastasis is mediated through opioid receptors, [Met]enk was administered in combination with the opioid receptor antagonist, naloxone. The results of this study are shown in Table III. The antimetastatic effect of [Met]enk was inhibited when this substance was administered in combination with naloxone. Again, naloxone by itself had an antitumor effect, causing a reduction in the number of metastases.

TABLE I.
Effect of [Met]Enk on Experimental Pulmonary Metastasis

Dose (mg/kg)	Incidence (%)	Number of Metastases		p
		Median	(Range)	
0	16/20 (80)	3.0	(0–16)	
3	8/10 (80)	4.0	(0–10)	NS
12	9/10 (90)	3.0	(0–18)	NS
30	11/20 (55)	1.0	(0–6)	0.005

Note: [Met]enk was administred s.c. on day − 1. 5×10^4 B16-BL6 melanoma cells were given i.v. on day 0. The mice were sacrificed on day 14. The p-values indicate differences in the number of lesions from the control group, using the Mann-Whitney test. NS = not significant. (From Faith and Murgo, 1988. With permission.)

TABLE II.
Effect of [Leu]Enk on Experimental Pulmonary Metastasis

Dose (mg/kg)	Incidence (%)	Number of Metastases		p
		Median	(Range)	
0	14/15 (93)	3.5	(0–18)	
3	4/15 (27)	0	(0–5)	0.0002
12	8/10 (80)	2.5	(0–11)	NS
30	5/10 (50)	0.5	(0–6)	0.015

Note: [Leu]enk was administered s.c. on day − 1. 5×10^4 B16-BL6 melanoma cells were given i.v. on day 0. The mice were sacrificed on day 14. The p-values indicate differences in the number of lesions from the control group, using the Mann-Whitney test. NS = not significant.

TABLE III.
Effect of [MET]Enk and Naloxone on Experimental
Pulmonary Metastasis

Group	Incidence (%)	Number of Metastases Median	(Range)	p
Control	8/10 (80)	4.5	(0–24)	
[Met]Enk alone	3/10 (30)	0	(0–1)	0.007
Nal + [Met]Enk	7/10 (70)	1.5	(0–10)	NS
Nal alone	4/10 (40)	0	(0–8)	0.049

Note: Naloxone (60 mg/kg) and [Met]enk (30 mg/kg) were administered on day −1. Control mice received diluent (PBS). 10^5 B16-BL6 melanoma cells were given i.v. on day 0. Half of the mice from each group were sacrificed on days 12 and 14 and the number of pulmonary metastases determined. The *p*-values indicate differences in the number of lesions from the control group, using the Mann-Whitney test. NS = not significant. (From Faith and Murgo, 1988. With permission.)

Effect on Splenic NK Cell Activity

In these experiments, mice were injected with various doses of [Met]enk i.p. The day following enkephalin administration, the mice were sacrificed and the spleens were removed and tested for NK activity against YAC-1 and B16 melanoma targets in a 4-h ^{51}Cr release assay. The results of these studies are shown in Figure 4. [Met]enk significantly enhanced NK cell activity against both of these tumor cell targets. The degree of enhancement varied with the dose of [Met]enk administered. The optimal dose of [Met]enk was 1 to 3 mg/kg and 3 to 10 mg/kg against YAC-1 and B16 tumor cell targets, respectively.

DISCUSSION

The results of the studies presented herein support the role of the endogenous opioid system in the modulation of the immune response and tumor growth. We have found that the administration of the natural opioid peptides [Met]enk and [Leu]enk in mice inhibits the growth and metastasis of B16 melanoma. Similar results with [Met]enk and [Leu]enk against B16 melanoma have recently been published by Scholar et al. (1987), and it has previously been shown that these enkephalins can also improve the survival of mice inoculated with L1210 leukemia (Plotnikoff and Miller, 1983).

The mechanism by which the enkephalins inhibit tumor growth is not clear. We have shown that the antitumor effects of the enkephalins can be inhibited by the concomitant administration of the opioid receptor antagonist naloxone, suggesting that the effects are mediated through opioid receptors.

It was interesting to find that naloxone, by itself, also tended to inhibit B16 melanoma growth and metastasis. The antitumor effect of naloxone against B16 melanoma has been confirmed by additional *in vivo* and *in vitro* studies (Murgo, 1989). These results with naloxone are consistent with those of previously reported investigations which have shown that the opioid receptor antagonists can inhibit the growth of neuroblastoma in mice (Zagon and

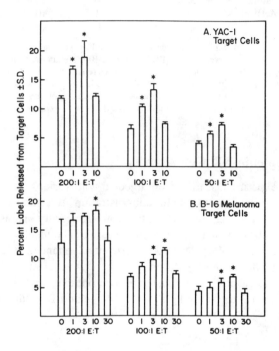

Figure 4. The effect of [Met]enk administration on splenic NK cell activity is shown. Mice were injected with various doses of [Met]enk i.p. The doses used (0, 1, 3, 10, or 30 mg/kg) are indicated in the figure under the bars. Eighteen h after the treatment, the mice were sacrificed and the spleens were removed. A 4-h ^{51}Cr release assay for cytotoxicity was performed as indicated in the methods section. Both YAC-1 (A) and B16-F10 (B) tumor cells were used as targets. Assays were performed at effector:target (E:T) cell ratios of 200:1, 100:1, and 50:1. The results are reported as the mean percent specific release from target cells for each of the treatment groups. The data shown represent pooled data from two experiments, with six animals in each dosage group. The vertical lines indicate the S.E. The asterisk sign indicates statistically significant ($p < 0.05$) differences from the group receiving no [Met]enk. (From Faith and Murgo, 1988. With permission.)

McLaughlin, 1986) and mammary carcinoma in rats (Alysworth et al., 1979). It is somewhat difficult to explain how naloxone could possess both antagonistic and agonistic effects in regards to the growth of B16 melanoma. However, similar phenomena have previously been described with other systems (Bocchini et al., 1983; Carr and Klimpel, 1986; Kraut and Greenberg, 1986). It is possible that the endogenous opioids and the opioid receptor antagonists inhibit tumor growth by changing the hormonal milieu of the host in a manner that is unfavorable to tumor cell proliferation. Alternately, the opioids and the opioid receptor antagonists may affect tumor cells directly. Zagon et al. (1987) have recently identified specific opioid receptors on a variety of human and animal tumors, including B16 melanoma. Since the opioids and their antagonists can bind to tumor cells, a direct cytotoxic effect may be possible. Zagon (1988) has recently reported that treatment with [Met]enk inhibits the proliferation of S20Y neuroblastoma cells *in vitro*. Preliminary results thus far have failed to demonstrate a direct effect of [Met]enk on the proliferation of B16 melanoma *in vitro* (Murgo, unpublished data). However, naloxone does inhibit the proliferation of B16 melanoma cells *in vitro,* but relatively high concentrations are required for this effect, i.e., higher than that which is capable of inhibiting tumor growth *in vivo* (Murgo, 1989). Other possible mechanisms by which the endogenous opioids or their antagonists inhibit tumor growth include altering the characteristics of the tumor cells, making them more vulnerable to the host's defenses, and stimulating immunological responses.

In this chapter, we provide evidence that the antitumor effect of the enkephalins may be related, at least in part, to the stimulation of the immune response. NK cells are a population of lymphocytes which can recognize and kill a variety of tumor cells, and represent a host function believed to play an important role in the inhibition of tumor development and metastasis (Reynolds and Ortaldo, 1987). These lymphocytes are also capable of killing virus-infected cells and, thereby, may be important in the defense against viral illness. The activation of NK cells by the enkephalins may be an important mechanism by which the enkephalins inhibit tumor growth and metastasis. Homeostasis during periods of stress may rely on the protective properties of the endogenous opioids such as [Met]enk and [Leu]enk.

Certainly, there is mounting evidence that the opioids, including the enkephalins, have significant effects on the immune response. Much of the data supporting the immunomodulatory role of the endogenous opioids are based upon *in vitro* experiments with murine and human cells. Since many of these investigations have been reviewed elsewhere (Murgo et al., 1986), this discussion will focus mainly on those properties of the opioids that are likely to effect tumor growth and metastasis.

As noted earlier in this chapter, several groups of investigators have shown that the endorphins and the enkephalins can enhance the NK cell activity of human peripheral blood lymphocytes. Stimulation of NK cell activity occurs *in vitro* with what may be considered physiological concentrations of the opioid peptides, or that which can occur during periods of stress (10^{-14} to 10^{-10} M). We have found that both [Met]enk and [Leu]enk can enhance the NK cell activity of peripheral blood lymphocytes obtained from cancer patients (Faith et al., 1984) as well as healthy volunteers (Faith et al., 1987). In addition, Mandler et al. (1986) have shown that the endogenous opioid peptide β-endorphin enhances both the cytotoxicity and interferon production of purified large granular lymphocytes (NK cells). Since these effects were inhibited by naloxone, they concluded that β-endorphin enhances NK cell activity by binding directly to opioid receptors on large granular lymphocytes. Brown and Van Epps (1986) found that both β-endorphin and [Met]enk enhanced interferon production by concanavalin-stimulated peripheral blood mononuclear cells from the majority of subjects they studied. The endogenous opioids have also been shown to enhance the antitumor cytotoxicity of macrophages. Foster and Moore (1987) found that dynorphin, an opioid peptide that binds to κ-opioid receptors, and [Leu]enk, which binds to δ-receptors, can enhance the tumoricidal function of activated mouse peritoneal macrophages. The enhancement of tumoricidal activity by both of these opioid peptides could be inhibited by naloxone, indicating that opioid receptors are involved.

As previously noted, stress can have significant effects on the resistance to tumor growth. Greenberg et al. (1984) found that the natural resistance of DBA/2 mice to SL2-5 lymphoma is suppressed by tail electroshock (TES) early after the stress, but enhanced with continued stress. In addition, these investigators found that 30 to 60 min after TES, there is a significant suppression of splenic NK cell activity which could be prevented by the administration of naloxone or naltrexone (Kraut and Greenberg, 1986). They also found that the administration of morphine or [D-Ala^2-Met^5]-β-endorphin, an analog of β-endorphin, enhanced splenic NK activity. These investigators proposed that the endogenous opioids may participate in a homeostatic rebound from the suppression mediated by other neurohormonal mechanisms activated during TES. Steplewski et al. (1985), using a model of forced restraint in rats, found that splenic NK cell activity was unaffected by the stress, but was actually increased after the recovery period. Whether the release of endogenous opioids occurred during this recovery period was not determined. Our results that [Met]enk and [Leu]enk can inhibit tumor growth and metastasis and stimulate NK cell activity are consistent with a protective role for these neuropeptides.

The effect of stress on NK cell activity has been observed clinically (Irwin et al., 1987; Locke et al., 1984). NK cell activity has been found to be decreased in patients with depression (Irwin et al., 1987) and significantly lower in individuals who are considered "poor copers" compared to those who are "good copers" (Locke et al., 1984). Levy et al. (1987) found that the level of NK cell activity in a group of patients who had undergone treatment for clinically localized breast cancer was reduced in those with certain emotional distress indicators such as fatigue-depression and lack of social support. The role of neurohormones, including the endogenous opioids, in the modulation of host resistance in various clinical disorders certainly warrants further investigation.

There are increasing data to suggest that the endogenous opioid peptides, including the enkephalins, represent a new class of biological response modifiers that may have potential clinical usefulness. [Met]enk has been safely administered to normal volunteers (Plotnikoff et al., 1986), and the results of preliminary clinical trials in patients with cancer and acquired immunodeficiency disorders have been encouraging (Plotnikoff et al., 1987; Wybran et al., 1987; Zunich and Kirkpatrick, 1988).

As biological response modifiers, the enkephalins should be grouped with the cytokines such as γ-interferon, the interleukins, and tumor necrosis factor. Support for this contention is based upon recent data which show that both lymphocytes (Smith et al., 1985; Zurawski et al., 1986) and macrophages (Lolait et al., 1986) can produce significant quantities of opioid peptide. Zurawski et al. (1986), utilizing complementary DNA techniques, have shown that concanavalin-stimulated murine helper T-lymphocytes can produce quantities of [Met]enk that are equivalent to that of other lymphokines, such as interferon, colony stimulating factor, and interleukin-2. These results are supportive of the important role of the endogenous opioids and opioid receptors in a regulatory circuit between the immune and neuroendocrine systems (Smith et al., 1985). Since the administration of interferon, and possibly other biological response modifiers presently in clinical use, can result in significant pertubations of the endocrine system (Goldstein et al., 1987), it is conceivable that some of the immunomodulatory effects of these agents are mediated by changes in the levels of various neuropeptides, including the endogenous opioids. Certainly, this is an area that deserves further investigation. We propose that the endogenous opioid system is an important modulator of the immune response and tumor growth, and that the enkephalins may play a protective role in maintaining homeostasis during periods of stress.

ACKNOWLEDGMENTS

This work was supported in part by intramural funds from the University of Houston and from WVU Medical Corporation and NIH Biomedical Research Grants 2 S07RR05433-24 and 2 S07 RR05433-25.

REFERENCES

Alysworth CF, Hodson CA, and Meites J: Opiate antagonists can inhibit mammary tumor growth in rats. *Proc Natl Soc Exp Biol Med* 1979; 161:18.

Bocchini G, Bonanno G, and Canevari A: Influence of morphine and naloxone on human peripheral blood T-lymphocytes. *Drug Alcohol Abuse* 1983; 11:233.

Brown SL and VanEpps DE: Opioid peptides modulate production of interferon-gamma by human mononuclear cells. *Cell Immunol* 1986; 103:19.

Carr DJJ and Klimpel GR: Enhancement of the generation of cytotoxic T cells by endogenous opiates. *J Neuroimmunol* 1986; 12:75.

Cross RJ, Markesbery WR, Brooks WH, and Roszman TL: Hypothalamic-immune interactions: neuromodulation of natural killer activity by lesioning of the anterior hypothalamus. *Immunology* 1984; 51:399.

Evans CJ, Erdely E, and Barchas JD: Candidate opioid peptides for interaction with the immune system. In *Enkephalins and Endorphins: Stress and the Immune System*. Plotnikoff NP, Faith RE, Murgo AJ, and Good RA, Eds. Plenum Press, New York, 1986.

Faith RE, Liang HJ, Murgo AJ, and Plotnikoff NP: Neuroimmunomodulation with enkephalins: enhancement of human natural killer (NK) cell activity in vitro. *Clin Immunol Immunopathol* 1984; 31:412.

Faith RE, Liang HJ, Plotnikoff NP, Murgo AJ, and Nimeh NF: Neuroimmunomodulation with enkephalins: in vitro enhancement of natural killer cell activity in peripheral blood lymphocytes from cancer patients. *Nat Immun Cell Growth Regul* 1987; 6:88.

Faith RE and Murgo AJ: Inhibition of pulmonary metastases and enhancement of natural killer cell activity by methionine-enkephalin. *Brain Behav Immun* 1988; 2:114.

Foster JS and Moore RN: Dynorphin and related opioid peptides enhance tumoricidal activity mediated by murine peritoneal macrophages. *J Leuk Biol* 1987; 42:171.

Goldstein D, Gockerman J, Krishnan R, Richie J, Tso CY, Hood LE, Ellinwood E, and Laszlo J: Effects of gamma-interferon on the endocrine system: results from a phase I study. *Cancer Res* 1987; 47:6397.

Greenberg AJ, Dyck DG, Sandler LS, Pohajdak B, Dresel KM, and Grant D: Neurohormonal modulation of natural resistance to a murine lymphoma *JNCI* 1984; 72:653.

Irwin M, Smith TL, and Gillin JC: Low natural killer cytotoxicity in major depression. *Life Sci* 1987; 41:2127.

Johnson HM, Smith EM, Torres BA, and Blalock JE: Neuroendocrine hormone regulation of in vitro antibody production. *Proc Natl Acad Sci U.S.A.* 1982; 79:4171.

Kay N, Allen J, and Morley JE: Endorphins stimulate normal human peripheral blood lymphocyte natural killer activity. *Life Sci* 1984; 35:53.

Keller SE, Weiss JM, Schleifer SJ, Miller NE, and Stein M: Stress-induced suppression of immunity in adrenalectomized rats. *Science* 1983; 221:1301.

Kraut RP and Greenberg AH: Effects of endogenous and exogenous opioids on splenic natural killer cell activity. *Nat Immun Cell Growth Regul* 1986; 5:28.

Levy S, Herberman R, Lippman M, and d'Angelo T: Correlation of stress factors with sustained depression of natural killer cell activity and predicted prognosis in patients with breast cancer. *J Clin Oncol* 1987; 5:348.

Locke SE, Kraus L, Leserman J, Hurst MW, Heisel JS, and Williams RM: Life change stress, psychiatric symptoms, and natural killer cell activity. *Pschosom Med* 1984; 46:441.

Lolait SJ, Clements JA, Markwick AJ, Cheng C, McNally M, Smith AI, and Funder JW: Pro-opiomelanocortin messenger ribonucleic acid and posttranslational processing of beta endorphin in spleen macrophages. *J Clin Invest* 1986; 77:1776.

Mandler RN, Biddison WE, Mandler R, and Serrate SA: Beta-endorphin augments the cytolytic activity and interferon production of natural killer cells. *J Immunol* 1986; 136:934.

Mathews PM, Froelich CJ, Sibbitt WL, and Bankhurst AD: Enhancement of natural cytotoxicity by beta-endorphin. *J Immunol* 1983; 130:1658.

Miller GC, Murgo AJ, and Plotnikoff NP: Enkephalins: enhancement of active T-cell rosettes from normal volunteers. *Clin Immunol Immunopathol* 1984; 31:132.

Monjon AA and Collector MI: Stress-induced modulation of the immune response. *Science* 1977; 196:307.

Murgo AJ: Inhibition of B16-BL6 melanoma growth in mice by methionine-enkephalin. *JNCI* 1985; 75:341.

Murgo AJ: Effects of [Met]enkephalin and corticosterone on thymus weight and tumor growth. *Neuroendocrinol Lett* 1986; 8:79.

Murgo AJ: Modulation of murine melanoma growth by naloxone. *Cancer Lett* 1989; 44:137.

Murgo AJ, Plotnikoff NP, and Faith RE: Effect of methionine-enkephalin plus $ZnCl_2$ on active T cell rosettes. *Neuropeptides* 1985; 5:367.

Murgo AJ, Faith RE, and Plotnikoff NP: Enkephalins: mediators of stress-induced immunomodulation. In *Enkephalins and Endorphins: Stress and the Immune System*. Plotnikoff NP, Faith RE, Murgo AJ, and Good RA, Eds. Plenum Press, New York, 1986.

Olson GA, Olson RD, and Kastin AJ: Endogenous opiates: 1986. *Peptides* 1987; 8:1135.

Plotnikoff NP and Miller GC: Enkephalins as immunomodulators. *Int J Immunopharmacol* 1983; 5:437.

Plotnikoff NP, Murgo AJ, Miller GC, Corder CN, and Faith RE: Enkephalins: immunomodulators. *Fed Proc* 1985; 44:118.

Plotnikoff NP, Miller GC, Solomon S, Faith RE, Edwards L, and Murgo AJ: Methionine enkephalin: immunomodulator in normal volunteers (in vivo). In *Enkephalins and Endorphins: Stress and the Immune System*. Plotnikoff NP, Faith RE, Murgo AJ, and Good RA, Eds. Plenum Press, New York, 1986.

Plotnikoff NP, Miller GC, Nimeh N, Faith RE, Murgo AJ, and Wybran J: Enkephalins and T-cell enhancement in normal volunteers and cancer patients. *Ann NY Acad Sci* 1987; 496:608.

Reynolds CW and Ortaldo JR: Natural killer activity: the definition of a function rather than a cell type. *Immunol Today* 1987; 8:172.

Riley V: Psychoneuroendocrine influences on immunocompetence and neoplasia. *Science* 1981; 212:1100.

Scholar EM, Violi L, and Hexum TD: The antimetastatic activity of enkephalin-like peptides. *Cancer Lett* 1987; 35:133.

Smith EM, Harbour-McMenamin D, and Blalock JE: Lymphocyte production of endorphins and endorphin-mediated immunoregulatory activity. *J Immunol* 1985; 135:779s.

Steplewski Z, Vogel WH, Ehya H, Poropatich C, and Smith JMcD: Effects of restraint stress on inoculated tumor growth and immune response in rats. *Cancer Res* 1985; 45:5128.

Wybran J, Appelboom T, Famaey J-P, and Govaerts A: Suggestive evidence for receptors for morphine and methionine-enkephalin on normal human blood T lymphocytes. *J Immunol* 1979; 123:1068.

Wybran J, Schandene L, Van Vooren J-P, Vandermoten G, Latinne D, Sonnet J, De Bruyere M, Taelman H, and Plotnikoff NP: Immunologic properties of methionine-enkephalin, and therapeutic implications in AIDS, ARC, and cancer. *Ann NY Acad Sci* 1987; 496:108.

Zagon IS and McLaughlin PJ: Endogenous opioid systems, stress, and cancer. In *Enkephalins and Endorphins: Stress and the Immune System*. Plotnikoff NP, Faith RE, Murgo AJ, and Good RA, Eds. Plenum Press, New York, 1986.

Zagon IS, McLaughlin PJ, Goodman SR, and Rhodes RE: Opioid receptors and endogenous opioids in diverse human and animal cancers. *JNCI* 1987; 79:1059.

Zagon IS: Endogenous opioid systems and neural cancer: transmission and scanning electron microscopic studies of murine neuroblastoma in tissue culture. *Brain Res Bull* 1988; 21:777.

Zunich KM and Kirkpatrick CH: Methionine-enkephalin as immunomodulator therapy in human immunodeficiency virus infections: clinical and immunological effects. *J Clin Immunol* 1988; 8:95.

Zurawski G, Benedik M, Kamb BJ, Abrams JS, Zurawski SM, and Lee FD: Activation of mouse T-helper cells induces abundant preproenkephalin mRNA synthesis. *Science* 1986; 232:772.

Interaction of Immune Cytokines and CNS Opioids: A Possible Interface for Stress-Induced Immune Suppression?

P.M. Dougherty
Department of Anatomy and Neurosciences
Marine Biomedical Institute
University of Texas Medical Branch
Galveston, Texas

Nachum Dafny
Department of Neurobiology and Anatomy
University of Texas Medical School at Houston
Houston, Texas

INTRODUCTION

Stress-induced immune suppression is one phenomenon that highlights the emerging significance of reciprocity between the nervous, endocrine, and immune systems (Locke et al., 1985). For example, the CNS areas activated by stress exposure to produce an endocrinologic response are also activated upon stimulation of the immune system and again produce an identical endocrinologic response (Besedovsky et al., 1986; Spector and Korneva, 1981).

Lymphoid tissues produce a large number of products upon mitogenic stimulation, including ACTH and endorphins (Smith et al., 1985) as well as interleukins (ILs), interferons (IFNs), and muramyl-peptides (MDPs) which may possess neuromodulatory activities in addition to their immunoregulatory actions (Besedovsky et al., 1986; Dafny et al., 1985; Dinarello and Krueger, 1986; Smith et al., 1985). Thus, stimulation of the immune system itself can be considered as a "stressor". However, the "stress" response of hormone and peptide release associated with immune stimulation must be carefully regulated to ensure an effective defense to pathogenic invasion (Besedovsky et al., 1986). It has been proposed that stress-induced immune suppression results from an inappropriate and deleterious level of various hormones which result in a disregulation of shared neuroendocrine pathways (Plotnikoff et al., 1985).

One neuroendocrine pathway shared by the CNS and the immune system involves the endogenous opioids (Faith et al., 1987; Plotnikoff et al., 1985). The neuroanatomical distribution of opioid-receptor and opioid peptide-containing neurons overlaps the hypothalamus and limbic brain areas shown to possess immunomodulatory function (Akil et al., 1984; Locke et al., 1985). CNS opioid systems are implicated in many of the deleterious effects of severe emotions, such as stress and depression, upon immune system function (Shavit et al., 1985). Stress mobilizes various opioid components evidenced by naloxone blockade of stress-induced analgesia (Akil et al., 1984), and increased levels of enkephalin and endorphin messenger RNA detectable in the hypothalamus immediately following exposure to stress in rats (Lightman and Young, 1987). Moreover, the suppressive effect of restraint and footshock stress upon antibody formation and natural killer (NK) cell activity is reversed or attenuated by the opiate antagonist naloxone (Shavit et al., 1985).

Hypothalamic opioids regulate sympathetic and parasympathetic outflow (Jaffe and Martin, 1985), which, in turn, provides important immune regulatory functions (Felten et al., 1985). In addition, opioids regulate the secretion of several hormones (Jaffe and Martin, 1985) which have potent immune regulatory activity (Locke et al., 1985). Finally, opioid and opioid-related peptides are produced by peripheral blood leukocytes of humans and rats when stimulated with mitogens (Smith et al., 1985). Indeed, the specific opioid peptides produced are dependent upon the type of mitogen which is used (Smith et al., 1985). Moreover, opiate alkaloids as well as endogenous opioid peptides modify the reactions of all lymphoid cell types when administered systemically, intracranially, or *in vitro* (Jankovic and Maric, 1986; Wybran, 1985).

Over the past several years, immune cytokines such as IFN-α and MDP were demonstrated to alter opioid-related properties. For example, the naloxone-precipitated withdrawal syndrome of morphine-dependent rats is attenuated following either systemic or intracranial administration of IFN or

MDP (Dafny, 1983a; Dafny et al., 1985; Dougherty et al., 1987). In addition, IFN and MDP alter the EEG, evoked potential, and single unit electrical activity of brain nuclei involved in the manifestation of this behavioral syndrome when given alone or in combination with opiates (Dafny, 1983b; Dougherty and Dafny, 1988a; Krueger et al., 1986). These studies are summarized and discussed in terms of the potential that cytokines such as IFN and MDP may exert direct effects upon the CNS by modulation of central opioid activity.

METHODS

Behavioral Experiments

Morphine dependence was induced in male Sprague-Dawley rats (180 to 220 g, TIMCO, Houston, TX) by subcutaneous implantation of 75 mg morphine base pellets as described previously (Dafny, 1983a; Dafny et al., 1983; Dougherty and Dafny, 1988b). On the third day after pellet implantation, naloxone (1.0 mg/kg) was injected to assess the degree of opiate dependence using the index of precipitated withdrawal behavior (Dafny, 1983a; Dougherty et al., 1987b). Two experiments were conducted. The first experiment tested the effect of systemically (i.p.) administered IFN and MDP on morphine withdrawal. The second experiment tested the effect of intracerebroventricular (i.c.v.) administration of these agents on morphine withdrawal. In both cases, the MDP or IFN was given 2 h before naloxone injection and withdrawal scoring.

Electrophysiology Experiments

Male Sprague-Dawley rats (180 to 240 g) were used in two electrophysiology experiments: sensory-evoked potential recording from awake animals and single unit recording from anesthetized animals. Rats in both studies were housed with food and water freely available, lights on 6 a.m. to 6 p.m., and room temperature maintained at 22 to 24°C.

Surgical Procedure

Animals prepared with permanent electrodes (evoked potential recordings) were anesthetized with pentobarbital (50.0 mg/kg, i.p.), and those prepared for the acute experiments (microiontophoresis) were anesthetized with urethane (1.25 g/kg, i.p.). Electrode locations were based on the atlas of Paxinos and Watson (1982). Stainless steel electrodes (120 μm, Medwire) insulated with teflon, were used for the awake experiments (Dafny et al.,

1988; Dougherty and Dafny, 1988a). A multibarrel electrode assembly was composed of a low-impedance (5 to 10 MΩ) six-barreled glass micropipette, and a seventh high-impedance (20 to 30 MΩ) recording electrode (Dafny et al., 1985; Reyes-Vazquez et al., 1984a) was used for the acute experiments.

Experimental Protocol (Awake Experiments)

On the experimental day, each animal was placed within a soundproofed Faraday cage and the electrodes were connected via a counterbalanced swivel commutator arm to Grass P511 amplifiers. Electrical activity was monitored on Tektonix storage oscilloscopes and simultaneously fed to a signal averager (evoked-potential experiments, NIC 1070; Dafny et al., 1988; Dougherty and Dafny, 1988a). Following establishment of baseline activity, the animals were injected i.p. first with saline and subsequently with IFN or MDP. Following the cytokine trial, the animals were injected with either 1.0 mg/kg naloxone or 10.0 mg/kg morphine sulfate and recording resumed. All injections were i.p. in 1 ml total volume.

Experimental Protocol (Acute Experiments)

Experiments and recording began after obtaining a 3-min baseline. The cell was then tested for drug responses to glutamate (GLUT, 0.1 M, pH 8.0), then to MDP (N-acetyl-muramyl-L-alanyl-D-isoglutamine, 0.1 mM, pH 6.0), ISO-MDP (N-acetyl-muramyl-D-alanyl-D-isoglutamine), morphine (MS, 0.5 M, pH 4.5), IFN (Hoffman LaRoche recombinant human α-A, pH 7.0), IFN-γ (purified human, pH 7.0), and naloxone (NAL, 0.15 M, pH 5.0) presented in random orders. In some cases, the effect of the cytokines was evaluated in the presence of morphine and/or naloxone to investigate the possible localized interactions with central opioid systems.

Histological Verification

At the conclusion of each experiment, the animal was sacrificed by pentobarbital overdose and perfused with a 10% formalin solution containing 3% potassium ferrocyanide and the electrode recording sites were marked (Dafny et al., 1985; Dougherty and Dafny, 1988a). Data are reported only for those electrodes confirmed to have been within the target locations.

Drug Administration

Systemic administration of IFN was done by injection of 1.50×10^5 IU/kg suspended in 1 ml saline. The bioactivity of IFN was verified prior to use as described by Langford et al. (1981). The dosage of IFN used in the i.c.v.

experiments was chosen based on preliminary radioimmunoassay measurements of IFN in the cerebrospinal fluid of rats 2 h following injection of IFN as described above. Total dosage volume was 10 μl. Time of administration was always at 2 h prior to naloxone-precipitated withdrawal. Finally, IFN and partially purified human γ-interferon were used in the microiontophoresis experiments.

MDP was suspended in normal saline and administered i.p. in 1 ml at a dosage of 200.0 μg/kg. This dosage comprises one pyrogenic unit. MDP was injected i.c.v. in 10 μl total volume at a dosage of 10.0 μg to morphine-dependent rats. The dosage range was chosen to be equivalent in pyrogenic activity to 200.0 μg/kg injected systemically (Dougherty et al., 1987a). Finally, for microiontophoretic application, MDP as well as an inactive stereoisomer (ISO-MDP) were used.

RESULTS

Behavioral Experiments

The effects of systemic administration of IFN and MDP on naloxone-precipitated morphine withdrawal are summarized in Figure 1. Each agent attenuated all seven signs observed, although IFN reduced the severity of

EFFECT OF SYSTEMIC MDP AND IFN ON
MORPHINE WITHDRAWAL IN RATS

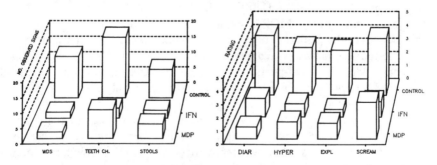

Figure 1. Bars summarizing the group mean for the observed (left) and rated (right) signs of naloxone (1.0 mg/kg, i.p.) precipitated morphine withdrawal behaviors. WDS = wet dog shakes; Teeth Ch. = teeth chatters; STOOLS = formed fecal boli; DIAR = diarrhea; HYPER = hyperactivity; EXPL = exploratory behavior; SCREAM = scream to touch. Those animals treated with MDP (N = 12), IFN (N = 12), or saline controls (N = 12) received the agents by i.p. injection. The figure demonstrates that IFN and MDP attenuate all signs of morphine withdrawal measured.

EFFECT OF INTRACRANIAL MDP AND IFN ON MORPHINE WITHDRAWAL IN RATS

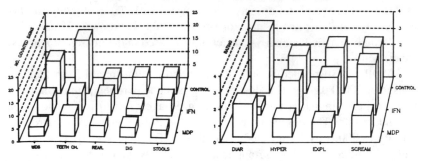

Figure 2. Bars summarizing the group mean for the observed (left) and rated (right) signs of naloxone (1.0 mg/kg, i.p.) precipitated morphine withdrawal behaviors. The animals treated with MDP (N = 8), IFN (N = 8), or saline carrier (N = 12) received a 10-μl injection 2 h before naloxone. Abbreviations as in Figure 1, except for REAR, which represents rearing behavior, and DIG, which represents digging behaviors. The figure demonstrates that IFN and MDP attenuate the severity of morphine withdrawal upon direct intracranial administration.

withdrawal to a slightly greater extent than MDP, as evidenced by the difference between the reduction in teeth chatters and scream to touch.

The effect of IFN on withdrawal is known to be specific to IFN-α vs. IFN-γ (Dafny, 1983a; Dafny et al., 1983). The effect of IFN is not affected by longer periods of morphine exposure (Dafny and Reyes-Vazquez, 1987; Dafny et al., 1985) or by dosages of the antagonist naloxone as high as 5.0 mg/kg. Finally, IFN attenuates withdrawal when administered prior to initiation of chronic morphine treatment as well as when administered just prior to naloxone (Dafny, 1983a; Dafny et al., 1983, 1985).

In contrast to IFN, MDP does not alter withdrawal severity when administered prior to initiation of chronic morphine treatment, consistent with the time course for other *in vivo* pharmacologic effects of muramyl-dipeptides (Chedid, 1986). Muramyl-peptides are cleared from the blood within a matter of hours after systemic administration and thus result in only a transient period of effects upon various biological targets.

The main finding of the i.c.v. administration studies was that IFN and MDP retained an effect upon withdrawal severity when administered directly into the brain ventricles. MDP was more effective than IFN through this route of administration, as evidenced by the reduction of all signs by MDP vs. only four of nine by IFN (Figure 2).

Electrophysiology Experiments

Representative observations from the averaged visual (sensory)-evoked response (AVER) studies are shown in Figure 3. In both cases, IFN and MDP induced an alteration in the electrical activity of brain regions important for opioid phenomena when given alone and in the presence of morphine and naloxone. The cytokines were most frequently excitatory upon AVER amplitude and not mediated at an opioid receptor type, as in neither case could naloxone block the activity. Yet IFN and MDP induced a modification of opioid activity as the effect of morphine within the hypothalamus was reversed from predominantly inhibitory to predominantly excitatory (Figure 3). In summary, these experiments have demonstrated that IFN and MDP induce an effect upon brain activity and also modify opiate-induced effects.

Representative results of the single unit microiontophoresis studies are shown in Figures 4 and 5, and further suggest that the observed evoked potential responses of brain nuclei following IFN and MDP administration are due to an effect on the single neurons of some of these brain sites. Similar

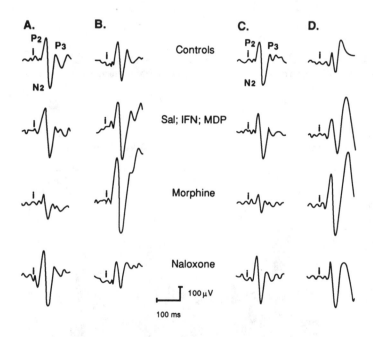

Figure 3. Representative averaged visual (sensory)-evoked reponses (AVERs) obtained from the ventromedial hypothalamus (VMH) of four animals. The control recordings appear in the columns labeled "A" and "C". The responses of the animals treated with IFN are in column "B", and those for animals treated with MDP are in column "D". Saline in control animals had no effect, morphine in these animals suppressed the AVERs, and naloxone reversed the morphine-induced changes. IFN and MDP potentiated the AVERs, morphine in these animals paradoxically induced further potentiation, and naloxone reversed the morphine effect.

EFFECT OF IONTOPHORETIC APPLIED IFN WITHIN VMH

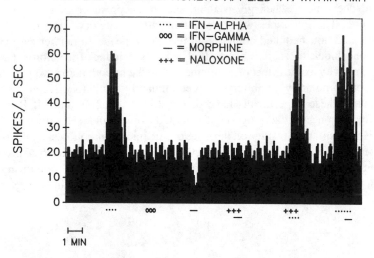

Figure 4. Representative frequency histograms for a VMH cell illustrating the effect of IFN upon the single unit discharge rate and the interaction with morphine and naloxone.

EFFECT OF IONTOPHORETIC APPLICATION OF MDP WITHIN VMH

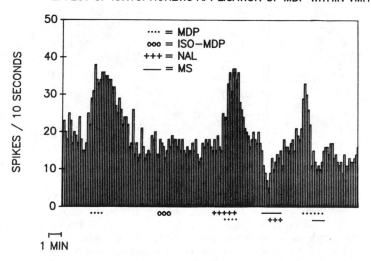

Figure 5. Representative frequency histograms for a VMH cell illustrating the effect of MDP on the single unit discharge rate and the interaction with morphine and naloxone.

to the AVER studies, both agents are most frequently observed to induce an excitation in single-unit firing of all the brain sites studied. This effect was not naloxone sensitive, and thus again appears to be nonopioid. Finally, similar to the AVER studies, the responses to morphine were altered by IFN or MDP pretreatment, as a much lower frequency of the neuronal populations responded to morphine treatment than expected from controls.

DISCUSSION

Human IFN-α is a 22-kDa molecule with a variety of immune regulatory actions upon both human and rat tissues. These activities include modification of lymphoproliferative responses, alteration of lymphocyte trafficking, induction of viral resistance, and stimulation of NK cell activities (Herberman, 1984). IFN has receptors on brain tissue (Aguet, 1980), and possesses several neuropharmacological properties (Herberman, 1984; Reite et al., 1987). These activities include the production of malaise, anorexia, and fever as well as the promotion of slow-wave sleep (Dafny, 1983b; Reite et al., 1987). In addition, IFN stimulates the neuroendocrine axis to induce secretion of anterior pituitary hormones (Roosth et al., 1986).

MDP is formed by reticuloendothelial cell digestion of Gram-negative bacterial cell walls (endotoxin), and can be isolated from all biological fluids (Chedid, 1986). MDP is an activator of macrophages within the immune compartment, and thus promotes a nonspecific heightened state of immunity. MDP also acts within the CNS, where it promotes slow-wave sleep and acts to increase body temperature (Chedid, 1986; Krueger et al., 1986). These activities, although not blockable by naloxone, possess opioid-mediated components (Ahmed et al., 1985; Ahokas et al., 1985; Bernton et al., 1987). The pyrogenic and sleep-promoting effects of MDPs are suggested as due to the induction or mimicry of the biologic effects of interleukin-1 (IL-1; Dinarello and Krueger, 1986). The demonstration that IL-1 modifies opiate receptor binding (Ahmed et al., 1985), as well as induces the release of corticotropin-releasing factor, which activates various endogenous opioid pathways, may underlie at least part of the observed effects upon withdrawal (Bernton et al., 1987). On the other hand, prostaglandins (PGs) provide yet another possible intermediary for the expression of MDPs neuromodulatory activity. PGs are responsible for the induction of MDP and IL-1-induced fever within the hypothalamus (Dinarello and Krueger, 1986). In addition, these substances modify morphine-induced analgesia and the development of morphine dependence (Leslie and Watkins, 1985).

The goal of the present study was to determine whether IFN and/or MDP modify opiate-mediated phenomena by a direct action within the CNS, thus supporting the contention that immune-derived peptides convey information from the immune system into the brain. Each agent modified naloxone-precipitated morphine withdrawal, which suggests that central opioid systems are very sensitive to immunomodulator agents in general and/or immunologic alterations. The prolonged time course of the effects induced by IFN suggests that either this agent induces a very long-acting suppressive effect on withdrawal expression, or IFN alters the development of dependence. In addition, lack of competition with naloxone in the withdrawal model and with morphine in the guinea pig ileum preparation (Reyes-Vazquez et al., 1984b) and on neuronal activity (Dafny et al., 1985; Reyes-Vazquez et al., 1984a) suggests a nonopioid site of action. Since both the development of physical dependence upon morphine as well as the expression of withdrawal are dependent upon the activity of several discrete brain structures which border the brain ventricles, it appears that IFN and MDP have direct neuromodulatory activity. The extent to which these signs were attenuated by each agent varied between agents as well as with the dosage of a given agent. These observations suggest that each agent has an effect upon more than one site of withdrawal regulation, and that these sites of regulation are differentially sensitive to each agent. Nevertheless, the alternate possibilities that a metabolite of the full protein or perhaps an intermediary product induced by IFN or MDP within the CNS remain as important issues to address.

The effect of IFN on the single neuron discharge rate is observable upon addition of the agent to cultured neuronal elements (Calvet and Gresser, 1979), and is specific to IFN-α vs. IFN-γ (Reyes-Vazquez et al., 1984a). IFN and MDP effects on single unit discharge frequency are also observed following systemic administration of the agents to awake, freely behaving animals prepared with permanent semimicroelectrodes (Dafny et al., 1985; Dougherty et al., 1988b). The effects induced by both agents are identical to that following microiontophoretic application, save for a prolonged latency for onset. In addition, IFN and MDP each modified baseline hypothalamic sensory-evoked potential activity as well the effects of morphine in this same region (Dafny, 1983b; Dafny et al., 1988; Dougherty and Dafny, 1988). The hypothalamus is one of those sites essential for various opioid activities (Kerr and Pozuelo, 1971). Lesioning of this area prevents withdrawal, reverses morphine tolerance, and prevents the onset of morphine-induced changes in feeding, nociception, and temperature regulation (Akil et al., 1984). The hypothalamus is also an important immune-regulatory area (Locke et al., 1985). Thus, the hypothalamus may provide a common neuroanatomical site of opioid-modulatory activity for the specific immune modulators studied. The observation that restraint stress attenuates the unit response of neurons within the hypothalamus and several limbic-related areas (Figure 6) underscores this possibility.

In summary, these studies demonstrate that the immune cytokines IFN and MDP have differential neuromodulatory actions. Systemic and intracranial administration of IFN and MDP result in the modification of opioid activity.

% RESPONDING UNITS TO S—MDP IN NAIVE VS STRESSED RATS

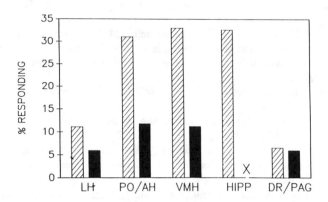

Figure 6. Bars represent the percentage of the population (N = 48) studied which exhibited a significant change in discharge frequency following systemic administration of MDP in freely behaving animals implanted with permanent electrodes. LH = lateral hypothalamus, PO/AH = preoptic/anterior hypothalamus, HIPP = dorsal hippocampus, and DR/PAG = dorsal raphe/periaqueductal gray. The "X" in the hippocampus results following stress represents a zero percentage. Recordings were obtained from naive unstressed animals (stripe bars) and from stressed animals (filled bars). Stress exposure consisted of overnight (8 h) restraint of the rats.

Therefore, the first conclusion which may be drawn is that both cytokines possess modulatory activity upon the CNS in addition to their peripheral effects upon the immune and endocrine systems. Second, opioids are potent modifiers of behavior, hormone secretion, temperature balance, and integration of emotions (Akil et al., 1984). Considering that all of these indices are also modified during infection as well as following administration of IFN and MDP, the finding of multiple immune products which affect opioid functions suggests this neuropharmacologic system as one of the pathways by which the immune system communicates with the central nervous system.

REFERENCES

Aguet M: High affinity binding of I^{125}-labelled mouse interferon to specific cell surface receptors. *Nature* 1980; 284:459.

Ahmed MS, Llanos-QJ, Dinarello CA, and Blatteis CM: Interleukin-1 reduces opioid binding in guinea pig brain. *Peptides* 1985; 6:1149.

Ahokas RA, Seydoux J, Llanos-QJ, Mashbrun TA Jr, and Blatteis CM: Hypothalamic opioids and the acute phase glycoprotein response in guinea pigs. *Brain Res Bull* 1985; 15:603.

Akil H, Watson SJ, Young E, Lewis ME, Khachaturian H, and Walker JM: Endogenous opioids: biology and function. *Annu Rev Neurosci* 1984; 7:223.

Berton EW, Beach JE, Holaday JW, Smallridge RC, and Fein HG: Release of multiple hormones by a direct action of interleukin-1 on pituitary cells. *Science* 1987; 238:519.

Bresedovsky H, DelRey A, Sorkin E, and Dinarello CA: Immunoregulatory feedback between interleukin-1 and glucocorticoid hormones. *Science* 1986; 233:652.

Calvet MC and Gresser I: Interferon enhances the excitability of cultured neurons. *Nature* 1979; 278:558.

Chedid L: Neuropharmacological activities of MDP. Methods and findings. *Exp Clin Pharmacol* 1986; 8:101.

Dafny N: Interferon modifies morphine withdrawal phenomena in rodents. *Neuropharmacology* 1983a; 22:647.

Dafny N: Interferon modifies EEG and EEG-like activity recorded from sensory, motor, and limbic system structures in freely behaving rats. *Neurotoxicology* 1983b; 4:235.

Dafny N and Reyes-Vazquez C: Single injection of three different preparations of alpha-interferon modifies morphine abstinence signs for a prolonged period. *Int J Neurosci* 1987; 32:953.

Dafny N, Lee JR, and Dougherty PM: Immune response products alter CNS activity: interferon modulates central opioid functions. *J Neurosci Res* 1988; 19:140.

Dafny N, Pietro-Gomez B, and Reyes-Vazquez C: Does the immune system communicate with the central nervous system? Interferon modifies central nervous system activity. *J Neuroimmunol* 1985; 9:1.

Dafny N, Zielinski M, and Reyes-Vazquez C: Alteration of morphine withdrawal to naloxone by interferon. *Neuropeptides* 1983; 3:453.

Dinarello CA and Krueger JM: Induction of interleukin-1 by synthetic and naturally occurring muramyl peptides. *Fed Proc* 1986; 45:2545.

Dougherty PM and Dafny N: Neuroimmune intercommunication, central opioids and the immune response to bacterial endotoxin. *J Neurosci Res* 1988a; 19:140.

Dougherty PM, Drath DB, and Dafny N: Evidence of an immune system to brain communication axis that affects central opioid functions: muramyl peptides attenuate opiate withdrawal. *Eur J Pharmacol* 1987a; 141:253.

Dougherty PM and Dafny N: Muramyl-dipeptides alter the neuronal firing rate of the hypothalamus and hippocampus but not the dorsal raphe. *Proc Soc Neurosci* 1988b; 14:1282.

Dougherty PM, Pearl J, Krajewski KJ, Pellis NR, and Dafny N: Differential modification of morphine and methadone dependence by interferon alpha. *Neuropharmacology* 1987b; 26:1595.

Faith RE, Liang HJ, Plotnikoff NR, Murgo AJ, and Nimeh NF: Enkephalins: immunomodulators. *Nat Immun Cell Growth Regul* 1987; 6:88.

Felton DL, Felten SY, Carlson SL, Olschowka JA, and Livnat S: Noradrenergic and peptidergic innervation of lymphoid tissues. *J Immunol* 1985; 135:755s.

Herberman RB: Interferon and cytotoxic effector cells. In *Interferon, Volume 2: Interferons and the Immune System*. Vilcek J and DeMaeyer E, Eds. Elsevier, 1984, pp. 61–84.

Jaffe JH and Martin WR: Opioid analgesics and antagonists. In *The Pharmacologic Basis of Therapeutics*. 7th ed. Goodman LS, Gilman A, Rall TW, and Murad F, Eds. MacMillan, New York, 1985, pp. 497–534.

Jankovic BD and Maric D: Modulation of in vivo immune responses by enkephalins. *Clin Neuropharmacol* 1986; 9:476.

Kerr FWL and Pozuelo J: Suppression of physical dependence and induction of tolerance to morphine by stereotaxic hypothalamic lesions in addicted rats. *Mayo Clin Proc* 1971; 46:653.

Krueger JM, Karaszewski JW, Davenne D, and Shoham S: Somnogenic muramyl peptides. *Fed Proc* 1986; 45:2552.

Langford MP, Weigert DA, Stanton GJ, and Baron S: Virus plaque-reduction assay for interferon: microplaque and regular macroplaque reduction assays. In *Methods in Enzymology, Vol. 78A*. Pestka S, Ed. Academic Press, New York, 1981, pp. 339–345.

Leslie JB and Watkins WD: Eicosanoids in the central nervous system. *J Neurosurg* 1985; 63:659.

Lightman SL and Young WS III: Changes in hypothalamic preproenkephalin A mRNA following stress and opiate withdrawal. *Nature* 1987; 328:643.

Locke S, Ader R, Besedovsky HO, Hall N, Solomon G, Strom T, and Spector NH, Eds. *Foundations of Psychoneuroimmunology*. Aldine, New York, 1985.

Paxinos G and Watson C: *The Rat Brain in Stereotaxic Coordinates*. Academic Press, New York, 1982.

Plotnikoff NR, Murgo AJ, Miller GC, Corder CC, and Faith RE: Enkephalins: immunomodulators. *FASEB* 1985; 44:118.

Reite M, Laudenslager M, Jones J, Crnic L, and Kaemingk K: Interferon decreases REM latency. *Biol Psychiatry* 1987; 22:104.

Reyes-Vazquez C, Prieto-Gomez B, Georgiades JA, and Dafny N: Alpha and gamma interferon effects upon cortical and hippocampal neurons: microionotophoretic application and single cell recording. *Int J Neurosci* 1984a; 25:113.

Reyes-Vazquez C: Weisbrodt N, and Dafny N: Does interferon exert its action through opiate receptors? *Life Sci* 1984b; 35:1015.

Roosth J, Polland RB, Brown SL, and Meyer WJ III: Cortisol stimulation by recombinant interferon-alpha$_2$. *J Neuroimmunol* 1986; 12:311.

Shavit Y, Terman GW, Martin FC, Lewis JW, Liebeskind JC, and Gale RP: Stress, opioid peptides, the immune system and cancer. *J Immunol* 1985; 135:834s.

Smith EM, Harbour-McMenamin D, and Blalock JE: Lymphocyte production of endorphins and endorphin-mediated immunoregulatory activity. *J Immunol* 1985; 135:779s.

Spector NH and Korneva EA: Neurophysiology, immunophysiology and neuroimmunomodulation. In *Psychoneuroimmunology*. Ader R, Ed. Academic Press, New York, 1981, pp. 449–473.

Wybran J: Enkephalins and endorphins as modifiers of the immune system: present and future. *Fed Proc* 1985; 44:92.

Erythrocyte-Opioid Peptide Interactions

Cuthbert O. Simpkins
*Department of Surgery
Division of Trauma
University of Maryland
Baltimore, Maryland*

INTRODUCTION

The area of opioid peptide-erythrocyte interactions is largely unexplored. In contrast, there has been intense experimental activity with regard to opioids, and other circulating cells, namely, lymphocytes (Wybran et al., 1979; Hazum et al., 1979), monocytes (Van Epps et al., 1983; Ruff et al., 1985), and neutrophils (Simpkins et al., 1984; Falke and Fisher, 1985). The reason for this inequity is not readily apparent. Perhaps it is because the red cell is not considered a part of the immune system, as are the other cells. It is also possible that the report of an absence of *opiate* receptors on erythrocytes led many investigators to conclude that significant *opioid* binding would not be present (Pert and Snyder, 1973). The erythrocyte may appear to be a less interesting cell to some researchers, since it lacks a nucleus, ribosomes, mitochondria, or active motility. Moreover, the erythrocyte is not known to secrete multifaceted substances such as interleukins, proopiomelanocortin fragments, or prostaglandins. Nonetheless, a careful examination of erythrocyte physiology reveals a potential role for this cell in stress and immunity.

It is widely known that the erythrocyte transports oxygen from the alveolar space of the lung to the tissues, and carbon dioxide from the tissues to the alveolar space. A drop in the blood oxygen concentration causes an increase in erythropoietin, a hormone which stimulates the proliferation and differentiation of medullary red cells, hemoglobin synthesis, and the release of immature erythrocytes from the bone marrow. Erythropoietin also binds to erythrocytes and increases the uptake of ribose (Baciu and Invanof, 1983).

Thus, there is a possible connection between the stress of hypoxia, blood loss, and erythrocytes. Under these same conditions, opioid peptide release into the bloodstream increases.

The erythrocyte may transport opioid peptides, just as it transports O_2 and CO_2. As older or damaged erythrocytes are sequestered by the spleen, erythrocyte-associated opioid peptides may be deposited into this organ and go on to modulate splenic function. β-endorphin (β-EP) has been shown to increase the proliferation response of rat spleen cells to phytohemagglutinin and concanavalin A (Gilman et al., 1982).

There is evidence that the erythrocyte may be involved in an integral way in the functioning of the immune system. T-lymphocytes and leukemic B-cells are known to possess erythrocyte receptors (Zalewski et al., 1984). Early work, which underscored the still evolving concept of a relationship between stress and immunity, utilized T-cell rosettes (Wybran et al., 1979; Plotnikoff and Miller, 1983). The erythrocyte has binding sites for complement fragments (Kirschfink and Borsos, 1988). The C5b-9 complement complex lyses erythrocytes (Hu et al., 1987). The C5b-9 complex has also been shown to bind to β-EP (Schweigerer et al., 1982). Other experiments have revealed that erythrocytes can process immune complex so that the binding of complex to Raji cells is enhanced and to neutrophils is decreased (Rasmussen et al., 1987). Finally, Cornacoff et al. (1983) showed that erythrocytes may serve as a clearing mechanism for immune complex.

Erythrocytes have also been shown to process immune complexes so that their binding to B-cell lines and guinea pig spleen cells is enhanced (Medoff et al., 1983, 1982). When sickle cells are induced to sickle by lowering the partial pressure of oxygen, they bind more IgG. Normal cells do not bind IgG (Green and Kalra, 1988). The work of Simpkins et al. (1989), which shows that β-EP specifically binds to human erythrocytes, further raises the possibility that opioid peptides modulate erythrocyte function. The finding by this same group that some erythrocytes bind β-EP better than others raises possibilities that have yet to be pursued.

In this discussion, work has been cited which suggests that the areas of opioid peptides, stress, immunity, and erythrocyte physiology may be highly congruent. The binding and sequestering capabilities of the erythrocyte, its metabolic machinery, its movement, albeit passive, throughout the body, and its propensity for lysis make this cell a potential transporter, processor, and release mechanism for many substances, including opioid peptides. In this chapter, we will review information which pertains to this premise.

NONSPECIFIC BINDING TO ERYTHROCYTES

At concentrations from 10^{-7} to 10^{-4} *M,* morphine uptake by human erythrocytes was shown to be independent of time, temperature, quabain, dinitrophenol, saponin, or ATP. The erythrocyte membrane/buffer partition coefficient was also shown to decrease with increasing NaCl concentration (Seeman et al., 1972). Other reports of measured erythrocyte membrane/ buffer partition coefficients for opiates were made by Garrett and Gurkan (1979) and Garrett and Jackson (1979). In 1984, Owen and Nakatsu showed that the Km and Vmax of morphine diester hydrolysis by erythrocyte membrane esterases decreased as the alkyl chain length of the ester moiety increased.

Later work was done with peptides. β-EP like immunoreactivity was found in the plasma as well as the erythrocytes in blood of humans and other animals (Fisher et al., 1984). Addition of ^{125}I-β-EP (I-β-EP) to blood was followed after 10 min by detection in the plasma of only about 40% of the original amount. Analysis by high-pressure liquid chromatography (HPLC) showed that there was no loss due to plasma enzymatic factors. The "lost" 60% of I-β-EP was found to be associated with the cell fraction. Only 3% was associated with leukocytes. The remainder was associated with the erythrocytes. HPLC also showed that the erythrocyte-associated I-β-EP was not degraded. In humans, the erythrocyte pool of I-β-EP was found to comprise 72% of the total blood I-β-EP. In the rabbit, this figure was 68%. Rat and mouse were nearly equal, at 53 and 54%, respectively. The authors concluded that previous measurements of circulating erythrocyte pool were not assessed. They also suggested that the addition of bacitracin to blood samples did not yield higher β-EP levels because of inhibition of β-EP degradation as was previously thought. Instead, bacitracin caused the lysis of red cells, which thereby resulted in the release of β-EP into the plasma.

In a subsequent study, erythrocyte and plasma β-EP were determined in pregnant women who had diabetes, hypertension, or other medical problems (Evans et al., 1985). Both plasma and erythrocyte β-EP increased during gestation. Diabetic patients had lower levels of plasma β-EP and higher levels of erythrocyte β-EP. Total β-EP was unchanged. In hypertensive women and women with other medical problems, there was no difference from those with normal pregnancies.

Also in 1985, Vanderberg et al. reported results of studying the rapid degradation of leucine-enkephalin (TyrGlyGlyPheLeu) by erythrocyte cytosolic peptidases, with nuclear magnetic resonance. The pathway of degradation was deduced to be initiated by cleavage of the Tyr-Gly bond, followed by cleavage of the Gly-Phe bond, thus resulting in the following fragments: Tyr, Gly-Gly, and Phe-Leu. The Phe-Leu bond is next degraded, followed by the final and slowest step, hydrolysis of the Gly-Gly link. However, leucine-enkephalin was not degraded when incubated with intact erythrocytes for as long as 2 h.

SPECIFIC BINDING TO ERYTHROCYTES

No specific binding of ^{3}H-naloxone to intact erythrocytes was found by two groups: Pert and Snyder (1973) and Mehrishi and Mills (1983). In 1976, using human erythrocyte membranes and ^{3}H-dihydromorphine, Abood et al. published the first report of an erythrocyte opiate receptor. The Kd was $9 \times 10^{-9} M$. Specific binding was completely inhibited by $10^{-7} M$ hydromorphine. $10^{-7} M$ morphine inhibited specific binding by 85%. This receptor was similar to the brain opiate receptor in some ways and different in others. As in brain, binding to the opiate receptor was completely inhibited by $10^{-3} M$ CaCl$_2$, 0.05 M NaCl, phospholipase A, and trypsin. Differences between the erythrocyte and brain receptors consisted of phosphatidylserine inhibition of binding by 58% in erythrocytes and enhancement of binding by 35% in brain, phospholipase C inhibition in erythrocytes by 100% and only 50% in brain, codeine inhibition of 25% in erythrocytes and 45% in brain, and naloxone inhibition of only 18% (Abood, personal communication, 1989) in erythrocytes and 95% in brain. Also, erythrocytes demonstrated only one receptor, while in brain there were two with Kd values of 5×10^{-10} and $8 \times 10^{-9} M$. The number of erythrocyte receptors was small, with maximum specific counts of 243 cpm/mg of tissue. These investigators also found that the erythrocyte membranes of heroin addicts exhibited 43% more specific binding than controls.

The disparity between the findings of Pert and Snyder (1973) and Mehrishi and Mills (1973), who found no erythrocyte opiate receptor, and Abood et al. (1976), who did detect the receptor, may be due to the presence of free hemoglobin in the preparation of the first two groups. Hemoglobin was found to inhibit opiate binding (Abood, personal communication, 1989). Another factor may be the use of ^{3}H-naloxone by the first two groups, while Abood et al. used ^{3}H-dihydromorphine. It may be that ^{3}H-dihydromorphine has a greater affinity for erythrocytes than ^{3}H-naloxone. An inhibitor of opiate binding to rat brain was found in human erythrocytes (Marzullo and Friedhoff, 1977). The inhibitor was shown to be glutathione-bound copper. Therefore, this inhibitor might also contribute to the inability to detect opiate receptors.

Fisher et al., in 1984, detected no specific binding of β-EP to human erythrocytes. However, in our experiments, we observed specific binding of β-EP to human erythrocytes in ten consecutive and different individuals (Simpkins et al., 1989). The techniques employed by these two groups were markedly different. Fisher et al. incubated I-β-EP with a mixture of 5.6×10^8 erythrocytes and 1.6×10^5 leukocytes for 45 min at 40°C. This was followed by the addition of 1 ml of phosphate-buffered saline and centrifugation for 5 min. White cells were separated from the erythrocytes by discarding the supernatant. The washing procedure was repeated twice, after which erythrocyte radioactivity was counted. This procedure might have washed

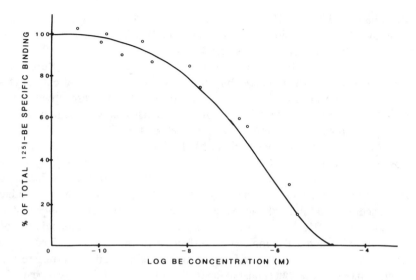

Figure 1. Displacement of 0.5 nM monoiodinated ^{125}I-labeled β-endorphin 61–91 (IBE) to human erythrocytes by unlabeled BE. Each data point is the average of ten different individuals. The assay was done in duplicate, with each sample being within 10% of the mean value.

away any membrane-bound and displaceable β-EP. Incubation with leukocytes may have degraded the I-β-EP.

In our experiments, we first separated the erythrocytes from other cellular components by centrifugation through hypaque-ficoll and washing in HEPES-TRIS buffer. Next, we added I-β-EP to 2.04×10^9 erythrocytes per ml and concentrations of unlabeled β-EP up to 3×10^{-5} M. This mixture was incubated at 15°C for 3.5 h. Preliminary studies showed these to be equilibrium conditions and that the erythrocyte concentration was in the linear portion of a curve relating specific counts to cell concentration. After incubation, 200 μl aliquots of the incubated suspension was centrifuged at 4°C for 5 min. The cell pellets were then counted in a γ-counter. We found that nonspecific binding was 50% of the total bound ligand. Our technique involved a pure preparation of erythrocytes, equilibrium conditions, and a minimum of washing steps which could wash the ligand off the receptor. Another significant difference in our techniques may have been that we used monoiodinated β-EP, while Fisher et al. used what probably was diiodinated β-EP.

Figure 1, from Simpkins et al. (1989), shows the competition between various concentrations of unlabeled β-EP and 5×10^{-10} M I-β-EP. The Kd ± SE for this interaction was $3.76 \pm 0.09 \times 10^{-7}$ M, with an apparent receptor number ± SE of 1418 ± 27.3 per cell. The low affinity of this binding site is unlike that of the opiate receptor discovered by Abood et al., which had a Kd of $9 \times 10^{-9} M$. The Kd we obtained does agree with values found by others for opioid receptors on other cells, from outside of the central nervous system. In lymphocytes and fibroblasts (Hazum et al., 1979), Kd values between 1×10^{-7} and $1 \times 10^{-6} M$ were found. Lopez-Ruiz et al. (1985) detected two leu-enkephalin binding sites on guinea pig enterocytes which had Kd values of 7×10^{-7} and $5.6 \times 10^{-5} M$, respectively. The low number of binding sites which we found is consistent with the low amount of specific opiate binding found by Abood et al. (1976).

We also studied the competition of I-β-EP with a variety of other related substances, as shown in Table I. Unlike opiate binding sites in the central nervous system, binding to the erythrocyte β-EP receptor was not inhibited by leu-enkephalin, met-enkephalin or (D-Ala²-D-Leu⁵)-enkephalin. Another difference was that in erythrocytes, β-endorphin 66–91 was just as potent as β-endorphin 61–91. The absence of the five N-terminal amino acids 61–66 would have rendered the molecule ineffective in brain tissue. Finally, the inability of naloxone to compete for binding is strikingly different from results obtained in CNS tissue, but similar to the finding of Abood et al. in erythrocytes.

Immunocytochemical techniques for light and electron microscopy were used as an alternative means of detecting the erythrocyte β-EP binding site. Human erythrocytes were incubated with or without β-EP at 10^{-4} or 10^{-9} M in HEPES-TRIS buffer. After incubation, the cells were reacted with anti-β-endorphin antibody. This primary antibody was stained by a biotinylated

TABLE I.

Percentage Decrease in Specific ¹²⁵-I-β-Endorphin Binding Obtained with 10^{-6} and $10^{-5} M$ Concentrations of Various Unlabeled Ligands

Opioid or Opiate	Concentration (M)	% Inhibition of Specific Binding
β-Endorphin	10^{-5}	100
61–91	10^{-6}	83
β-Endorphin	10^{-5}	94
66–91	10^{-6}	90
(−)-Naloxone	10^{-5}	22
	10^{-6}	0
Met-enkephalin	10^{-5}	15
	10^{-6}	0
Leu-enkephalin	10^{-5}	11
	10^{-6}	0
(D-Ala²-D-Leu⁵	10^{-5}	10
enkephalin	10^{-6}	0

Note: Each data point is the result of experiments performed with red cells from two different individuals.

secondary antibody and avidin-biotin-complexed horseradish peroxidase. Control experiments done (Figure 2A) without β-EP showed no staining. At 10^{-9} M β-EP and a magnification of 16,640×, staining is clearly seen (Figure 2B). At a β-EP concentration of 10^{-4} M and 400×, intense staining of the cells is seen. Some cells showed no stain at all, while others (about 20%) stained intensely (Figure 3B). Examination of the field at 16,640× and 10^{-4} M β-endorphin shows that all cells are stained, except that some show a patchy distribution on the surface and others are completely blackened. We did not expect to see this differential staining and do not presently have an explanation for it.

FUNCTIONAL EFFECTS OF OPIATES AND OPIOIDS

To date, there has been no systematic study of the effect of opiates and opioids on erythrocyte function. In 1972, Roth and Seeman showed that morphine protected human erythrocytes from hypotonic lysis. Lysis was reduced by 50% with a morphine concentration of 5.2×10^{-3} M. Among the compounds tested in this study, the most effective was chlorpromazine, which had an EC_{50} of 8.1×10^{-6} M. The least effective was butanol, which had an EC_{50} of 4.2×10^{-2} M. In 1978, Vadas and Hosein published their observation of a small (2 to 7%) increase in mean cell volume and a lessening of the cellular concavity caused by the i.v. injection of rabbits with varying doses of morphine. In 1980, Au found no effects of morphine on erythrocyte $(Ca^{2+} + Mg^{2+})$-ATPase.

In 1983, Yamaski and Way showed that ATP-dependent $^{45}Ca^{2+}$ efflux from rat erythrocyte ghosts was inhibited by opioids and opiates. The order of potency was dynorphin>ethylketocyclazocine>β-EP>morphine, with respective ID_{50} values of 1.07, 1.40, 12.7, and 18.7 nM. Naloxone blocked the action of these agonists at concentrations of 25 to 30 nM. In contrast, levorphanol and leu-enkephalin had no effect at concentrations less than 10^{-6} M. None of the agonists significantly affected the influx of $^{45}Ca^{2+}$. Naloxone at 100 nM also had no effect on influx. The antagonist effect of naloxone observed in this experiment appears incompatible with the findings of Pert and Snyder (1983), Mehrishi and Mills (1983), and Simpkins et al. (1989), in which naloxone was at most minimally effective. Further work must be done to resolve this contradiction.

The experimental evidence of the investigators reviewed in this chapter strongly supports the association of opioids and opiates with erythrocytes. Future work should consist of a comprehensive mapping of specific erythrocyte binding with a number of radioactive opioid and opiate ligands. The binding of opioids and opiates to free hemoglobin should be determined. Since the experiments of Simpkins et al. show that some erythrocytes associated

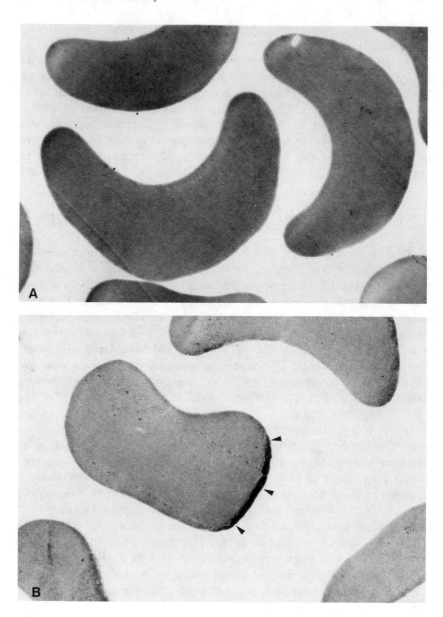

Figure 2. Immunocytochemical localization of β-endorphin binding sites on human erythro-cytes. (Magnification × 16,640.) (A) No β-endorphin added. No staining is seen; (B) β-endorphin at $10^{-9}M$ added. Patchy staining of the cell surface is observed.

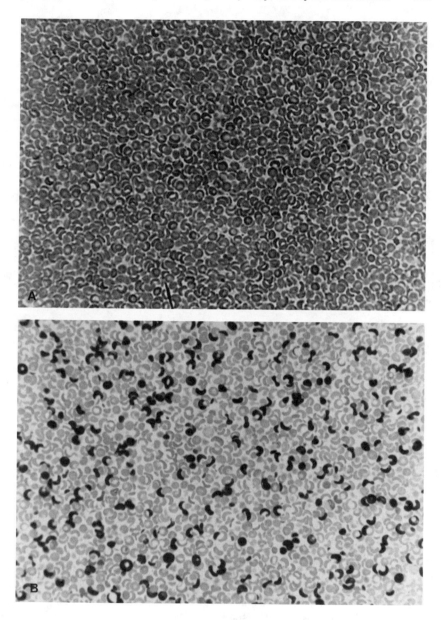

Figure 3. Immunocytochemical localization of β-endorphin binding sites on human erythrocytes. (Magnification × 400.) (A) No β-endorphin added; (B) β-endorphin added at $10^{-4}M$. Some cells are seen to stain heavily, while others do not, at this magnification. At higher magnification, (× 16,640), all cells are seen to be stained, although some are stained heavily, while others are stained lightly in a patchy configuration.

more strongly than others with β-EP, the various populations of erythrocytes should be separated and studied. One may find that the distinguishing feature between the erythrocytes which strongly bind β-EP and those which do not is age or degree of cell damage.

Once the opioid binding properties of the erythrocyte is worked out, the effects of these ligands on erythrocyte function will require further investigation. There is a need to look at a broad variety of operational properties of this cell, for example, O_2 dissociation and association, Cl^- and HCO_3 exchange, glucose uptake, erythropoietin-stimulated ribose uptake, deformability, and erythrocyte lifespan. If opioids modulate erythrocyte immune system interactions, then one should see effects on the C5b-9 lysis of erythrocytes and the processing of immune complex.

Another phase of experimentation might examine the hypothesis of a role of the erythrocyte as a transporter of opioids to multiple sites of action in various organs of the body, in particular, the spleen and liver where erythrocyte sequestion occurs. Considering the evidence that has been accumulated to date, the erythrocyte should provide a rich field of research for many years to come.

ACKNOWLEDGMENT

Appreciation is expressed to Mrs. Carolyn McCoy for preparation of this manuscript.

REFERENCES

Abood LG, Atkinson HG, and McNeil M: Stereospecific opiate binding in human erythrocyte membranes, and changes in heroin addicts. *J Neurosci Res* 1976; 2:427.
Abood LG: There is an error in Table 1 of Dr. Abood's paper above in which naloxone administration yields 713 counts. According to Dr. Abood, the bound counts should be 800, which would be equivalent to naloxone causing only an 18% decrease in specific binding. Personal communication, 1989.

> Leo G. Abood, Ph.D.
> Center for Brain Research
> Box 605
> University of Rochester Medical Center
> Rochester, N.Y. 14642
> 716-275-4024

Au KS: $(Ca^{2+}Mg^{2+})$-ATPase of chlorpromazine containing rabbit erythrocyte membrane. *Gen Pharmacol* 1980; 12:285.
Baciu I and Ivanof L: Erythropoietin interaction with the mature red cell membrane. *Ann NY Acad Sci* 1983; 414:66–72.

Cornacoff JB, Herbert LA, Smead WL, Vanaman ME, Birmingham DJ, and Waxman FJ: Primate erythrocyte-immune complex — clearing mechanism. *J Clin Invest* 1983; 71:236.

Evans MI, Fisher AM, Robishaux AG, Staton RC, Rodbard D, Larsen JW, and Murherjee AB: Plasma and red blood cell beta-endorphin immunoreactivity in normal and complicated pregnancies: gestational age variation. *Am J Obstet Gynecol* 1985; 151:433.

Falke NE and Fisher EG: Cell shape of polymorphonuclear leukocytes is influenced by opioids. *Immunobiology* 1985; 169:532.

Fisher AM, Comly RD, Tamarkin L, Ghazanfari AF, and Mukherjee AB: Two pools of beta endorphin-like immunoreactivity in blood: plasma and erythrocytes. *Life Sci* 1984; 34:1839.

Garrett ER and Gurkan T: Pharmacokinetics of morphine and its surrogates. II. Methods of separation of stabilized heroin and its metabolites from hydrolyzing biological fluids and applications to protein binding and red cell partition studies. *J Pharm Sci* 1979; 68:26.

Garrett ER and Jackson AJ: Pharmacokinetics of morphine and its surrogates. III. Morphine and morphine 3 — monoglucuronide pharmacokinetics in the dog as a function of dose. *J Pharm Sci* 1979; 68:753.

Gilman SC, Schwartz JM, Milner RJ, Bloom FE, and Feldman JD: Beta-endorphin enhances lymphocyte proliferative responses. *Proc Natl Acad Sci USA* 1982; 79:422.

Green GA and Kalra VK: Sickling induced binding of immunoglobulin to sickle erythrocytes. *Blood* 1988; 71:636.

Hazum E, Chang KJ, and Cuatrecasas P: Specific nonopiate receptors for beta-endorphin. *Science* 1979; 205:1033.

Hu VW, Mazorow DL, Nicholson-Weller A, and Shin ML: Enhancement of complement-mediated lysis of dithiothreitol treated erythrocytes involves increased C9 insertion and polymerization. *Mol Immunol* 1987; 24:887.

Kirschfink M and Borsos T: Binding and activation of C4 and C3 on the red cell surface by non-complement enzymes. *Mol Immunol* 1988; 25:505.

Lopez-Ruiz MP, Arilla E, Gomez-Pan A, and Prieto JC: Interactions of leu-enkephalin with isolated enterocytes from guinea pig. Binding to specific receptors and stimulation of cAMP accumulation. *Biochem Biophys Res Commun* 1985; 126:404.

Marzullo G and Frieldhoff AJ: An inhibitor of opiate receptor binding from human erythrocytes identified as a glutathione-copper complex. *Life Sci* 1977; 21:1559.

Medoff ME, Lam T, Prince GM, and Mold C: Requirements for human red blood cells in inactivation of C3b in immune complexes and enhancement of binding to spleen cells. *J Immunol* 1983; 130:1336.

Medoff ME, Prince GM and Mold C: Release of soluble immune complexes from immune adherence receptors on human erythrocytes is mediated by C3b inactivators independently of beta/H and is accompanied by generation of C3c. *Proc Natl Acad Sci USA* 1982; 79:5047.

Mehrishi JN and Mills IH: Opiate receptors on lymphocytes and platelets in man. *Clin Immunol Immunopathol* 1983; 27:240.

Owens JA and Nakatsu K: Morphine diesters. II. Blood metabolism and analgesic activity in the rat. *Can J Physiol Pharmacol* 1984; 62:452.

Pert CB and Snyder SH: Opiate receptor: demonstration in nervous tissue. *Science* 1973; 179:1011.

Plotnikoff NP and Miller GC: Enkephalins as immunomodulators. *Int J Immunopharmacol* 1983; 5:437.

Rasmussen JM, Hepsen HH, and Svehay SE: Influence of processing by erythrocyte C3b/C4b receptors (CRI) on binding of immune complexes to Raji cells and polymorphonuclear granulocytes. *Scand J Immunol* 1987; 26:437.

Roth S and Seeman P: The membrane concentrations of neutral and positive anesthetics (alcohols, chlorpromazine, morphine) fit the Meyer-Overton rule of anesthesia: negative narcotics do not. *Biochim Biophys Acta* 1972; 255:207.

Ruff MR, Wahl SM, Mergenhagen S, and Pert CB: Opiate receptor mediated chemotaxis of human monocytes. *Neuropeptides* 1985; 5:363.

Schweigerer L, Bhakdi S, and Teschemacher H: Specific non-opiate binding sites for beta-endorphin on the terminal complex of human complement. *Nature* 1982; 296:572.

Seeman P, Chau-Wong M, and Moyyen S: The membrane binding of morphine, diphenylhydantoin, and tetrahydrocannibinol. *Can J Physiol Pharmacol* 1972; 50:1193.

Simpkins CO, Chenet B, Kang Y, and Hollis V: Beta-endorphin receptors on human erythrocytes. *J Natl Med Assoc* 1989; 81:1199.

Simpkins CO, Dickey CA, and Fink MP: Human neutrophil migration is enhanced by beta-endorphin. *Life Sci* 1984; 34:2251.

Vadas EB and Hosein EA: Alteration of the erythrocyte ultrastructure and blood viscosity by morphine. *Can J Physiol Pharmacol* 1978; 56:245.

Vanderberg JI, King GF, and Kuchel PW: Enkephalin degradation by human erythrocytes and hemolysates studied using ^{1}H NMR spectroscopy. *Arch Biochem Biophys* 1985; 242:515.

Van Epps DE, Saland L, Taylor C, and Williams R: In-vitro and in-vivo effects of beta-endorphin and met-enkephalin on leukocyte locomotion. *Prog Brain Res* 1983; 59:361.

Wybran J, Appelbloom T, Famaey JP, and Govaerts A: Suggestive evidence for receptors for morphine and methionine — enkephalin on normal and human blood T lymphocytes. *J Immunol* 1979; 123:1068.

Yamasaki Y and Way EL: Possible inhibition of Ca^{++} pump of rat erythrocyte ghosts by opioid K agonists. *Life Sci* 1983; 33(1):723.

Zalewski PD, Forbes IJ, Valente L, and Comacchio R: Mechanism of induction of mouse erythrocyte receptor switch in human B cells. *J Immunol* 1984; 133:1278.

Chapter 25

Physiological Stress and Immune Response: Myelopeptides

R.V. Petrov and L.A. Zakharova
Shemyakin Institute of Bioorganic Chemistry,
U.S.S.R. Academy of Sciences,
Moscow, U.S.S.R.

Today, biomedical sciences have accumulated a wealth of information that evidences a crucial role of the mechanisms of neuroimmune interactions in stress and adaptation reactions. The list of human diseases accompanied or induced by different immunodeficient states continues to expand. Various forms of stress have been shown to bring on many immunological defects. Immunologic status determination and immunocorrection confirm their value in the case of many pathological disorders (i.e., traumas, starvation, extreme physical and psychic exercises, and side effects of chemotherapy).

Prevention and correction of stress-induced immunodeficiency requires a comprehensive investigation into the mechanisms of interaction between the nervous and immune systems. The study of endogenic opioid peptides and mediators of the immune system unraveled novel earlier, unknown aspects of the neuroimmune interaction. Stress-induced changes in the metabolism of opioid peptides might be a mechanism of development of functional disorders in the immune system. The functional significance of extraimmune opioids was established (Plotnikoff et al., 1985; Shavit et al., 1985; Wybran, 1985; Fisher, 1988) and their synthesis by the immune system cells was demonstrated (Petrov et al., 1982, 1986; Lolait et al., 1984; Zozulya et al., 1985).

In the central immunity organ, bone marrow, we discovered biologically active myelopeptides (MPs) with diverse functions that overstep the immune system borders. This group of mediators was found in the 1970s by their ability to increase antibody production at the peak of the immune response (Petrov et al., 1972, 1975; Zakharova et al., 1973). MPs are accumulated in the supernatant of the animal or human cell cultures upon their 15 to 20-h incubation. Later, MPs were isolated from the supernatant of porcine bone marrow cell cultures as highly purified fractions by gel chromatography on Sephadex G-25®, followed by reverse-phase high-pressure liquid chromatography (RP-HPLC). Thorough investigations into the physicochemical and functional properties of these molecules showed their peptide nature (Petrov et al., 1986) and revealed a wide spectrum of immunoregulatory properties. MPs stimulated a three- to tenfold increase in antibody production not only at the inductive, but also at the productive phase of the immune response, affected the functional activity of T-cells, increased the phagocytic activity of macrophages and neutrophils, and influenced the proliferation of blood-forming stem cells and their differentiation (Petrov et al., 1980, 1987). The MP immunostimulating properties are most pronounced at the decreased level of the immune response, i.e., in the case of immunodeficiency development (Petrov et al., 1987).

We succeeded in the HPLC separation of MP with immunostimulating and differentiation properties. The former were the basis for designing a new immunocorrecting preparation, Myelopidum. It was successfully tested and approved by the Pharmacological Committee for application as an immuno-stimulating drug to cure some clinical forms of secondary immunodeficient states (Stepanenko, 1989).

Immunodeficient states, which require application of immunocorrecting means, develop upon intense physical and psychoemotional exercises typical of sports activities. Some immunologic reactivity properties of leading athletes at the peak of their physical abilities undergo changes typical of the gerontal involution of the immune system: the number of macrophages decreases, their activity falls, the quantity of T-cells diminishes, their proliferative activity on mitogens and synthesis of immunoglobulins are inhibited, titers of specific antibodies decrease, and the amount of autoantibodies rises. Such immuno-deficient states can last 3 to 4 weeks after competition is finished (Pershin et al., 1981).

Previous investigations showed that Myelopidum is a promising remedy for the prevention and correction of immunodeficiency induced by stress. Myelopidum influence on the humoral immune response was studied on a model of stress induced by hypobaric hypoxia. It was elicited in mice immunized by sheep red blood cells (SRBCs) during a 3-d stay in a pressure chamber initiating a height of 8000 m. Antibody production in the mice on the 3rd day in the pressure chamber diminished by 50 to 60%. Administration

TABLE I.
MP-Induced Cancellation of Stress Immunosuppressor Action

Stress Model and Experimental Conditions	Number of Animals	AFC Number (10^6) of Nucleated Cells, $M \pm m$	K_1	K_2
Stress-Swimming				
Control N1 immunized lymph nodes	92	72.6 ± 2.2		
Control N2 swimming (immunized lymph nodes)	92	52.7 ± 2.2^a	0.72	
MP + swimming (immunized lymph nodes)	77	93.1 ± 4.1^c	1.29	1
Swimming (immunized lymph nodes) + MP	39	74.2 ± 3.9^b	1.02	1
Stress-Hypoxia				
Control N1 (immunized lymph nodes)	66	177 ± 15.1		
Control N2 (immunized lymph nodes)	61	96 ± 10.1^a	0.54	
MP + hypoxia (immunized lymph nodes)	48	188 ± 23.1^b	1.0	2
Hypoxia (immunized lymph nodes) + MP	48	326 ± 39^c	1.84	3

[a] Differences as compared to control N1 ($p < 0.01$).
[b] Differences as compared to control N2.
[c] Differences as compared to control N1 + N2.
Note: K_1 and K_2 on the coefficients of stimulation (suppression) of antibody production relative to control N1 and N2, respectively; they are calculated as the ratio of experimental to control AFC numbers.

of Myelopidum to animals at a dose of 50 mg per mouse immediately after the stress completely restored the immune response (Table I) (Sarybaeva et al., 1988). In 1 d, the MP level in the experimental animals decreased by two- to threefold. Deficiency of the MP production was retained on the 2nd and 3rd days. It is proposed that immune response can fall during pressure chamber hypoxia due to the depression of MP production. Restoration of the MP level in the organism achieved by exogenous administration prevents the development of hypoxia-induced immunodeficiency.

Besides the immunocorrecting action, Myelopidum exhibits a clearly expressed preventative effect. No decrease in antibody production is observed when the drug is injected before hypobaric hypoxia.

The stress model also revealed immunocorrecting and preventative effects developing in mice due to swimming. Mice were to swim once a day at the same time at a water temperature of 30°C. Each swim lasted 60 min and was repeated every 2 or 4 d. Parameters of the stress action used in the experiment led to a reliable decrease in antibody production, by 30 to 40%, in the cell population of immunized spleen and lymph nodes. Administration of Myelopidum before swimming effectively prevented development of the stress-induced immunodeficiency. In animals injected immediately after the stress action or at the peak of the immune response to SRBCs, the number of antibody-producing cells achieved a virtually normal level (Kirilina et al., 1989) (Table I).

The antistress action of Myelopidum is probably linked with its immunoprotective effect in rats with severe cranial injury. The most pronounced effect of the drug was observed on the 1st day after the experimental trauma. Injection of Myelopidum prevented, to a great extent, cellular devastation of bone marrow and thymus, and posttraumatic redistribution of lymph cell subpopulations. It resulted in high resistance in animals infected with *Staphylococcus aureus* and averted their death (Lisyany et al., 1988).

The changing dynamics of early stress reactions of the immune system, i.e., alterations of spleen and peripheral blood, provides evidence for the preventative effect of Myelopidum. Injections before a 6-h immobilization increased the quantity of neutrophils in murine peripheral blood immediately after the stress action and somewhat inhibited this reaction during the next 2 d (Vasilenko et al., 1985). The characteristic property of Myelopidum is considerable retardation of the cell migration from spleen and rapid restoration of their normal level.

The Myelopidum protective effect not only increases the immunocompetence level of the organism upon stress. Daily 14-fold injections of physiological solution (of a volume that induced stress in rats) retarded development of typical stress features, such as behavioral disorders, body-mass decrease, and change in the number of eosinophils and neutrophil leukocytes.

Experimental evidence in favor of the immunocorrecting and protective action of Myelopidum allows its wide application in different forms of stress-induced immunodeficiency.

Investigation into the mechanisms of immunological disorders induced by hypobaric hypoxia and stress-inducing swimming unraveled the increasing activity of nonspecific T-cell suppressors which interacted with Myelopidum (Peterov et al., 1975). The stress-provoked suppression of the immune response mediated by T-cell suppressors might be caused by triggering the opiatergic mechanisms. Naloxone administered to mice before or after swimming prevented the immune response decrease, as in the case of Myelopidum (Figure 1). Their combined application initiated an analogous effect. Taking into account that MPs competitively replace radioactively labeled opiates at their specific binding sites on the brain cells, we proposed that MP immunomodulating action depended on the μ- and δ-opioid receptor ligands discovered among MPs.

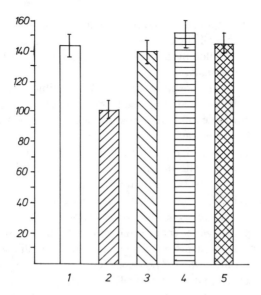

Figure 1. Abolishment of stress-induced suppression of immune response with naloxone. X: 1 = control, 2 = swimming-induced stress, 3 = naloxone injection before stress paradigm, 4 = Myelopidum injection before stress paradigm, 5 = combined injection of naloxone and Myelopidum before stress paradigm. Y: AFC number (10^6) nucleated cells.

The Myelopidum immunocorrecting effect was also observed in patients with developing immunodeficiency provoked by various stress factors (e.g., traumas, operation stress, burns, etc.) Myelopidum treatment of post-surgical patients (prothesis of cardiac valves) diminished the number of post-operative complications (pneumonia, mediastinitis, etc.) by two- to 2.5-fold on average. Their decrease was accompanied by positive changes in immune status properties and selective activation of B-cell immunity. The drug also provided correction of the post-traumatic immunodeficiency and prevented osteomyelitis development in patients with injured facial bones (Stepanenko, 1989). The frequency of these complications fell from 27.5 to 6.8%. The general state of the persons with cranial injury was markedly improved after Myelopidum injection. In addition, Myelopidum abolished a trauma-induced epileptic attack that apparently was associated with the MP affinity not only to the immune system, but to the central nervous system as well.

MP activities are not confined to immunoregulatory functions. In the early 1980s, we investigated the hypoalgesic naloxone-dependent MP action on animals and men (Petrove et al., 1982, 1986). The dynamics of the analgesic MP effect in men was analogous to that in animals.

MPs lower the evoked potentials in the cortical somato-sensory region caused by nociceptive stimulation and increase the summation-threshold index and latent period of the tail-flick and hot-plate reactions (Petrov et al., 1986, 1987). Hypoalgesia developing after MP injection did not influence the behavioral reactions in animals.

Along with the antinociceptive action, MPs exhibit a pronounced cardiotropic effect on the isolated frog heart. Addition of MP (5.5×10^{-8} to 10^{-5} g/l) to a perfusate exhibited a positive inotropic effect on the heart. Increasing the MP concentration up to 5.5×10^{-3} g/l led to a negative inotropic effect accompanied by bradycardia of the contracture type, with subsequent cardiac arrest. The preliminary addition of naloxone (1×10^{-6} M) to perfusate completely blocked the MP inotropic effect on the heart (Mikhailova et al., 1987). The cardiotropic effect can also be considered as a component of the antistress and protective action of MPs.

The opioid peptides were recently shown to play an important role in the central and peripheral mechanisms of regulation of the cardiovascular system activities (Laurent et al., 1985). The dependence of antinociceptive and cardiotropic MP effects on naloxone as well as electrophysiological characteristics of the MP action demonstrate the involvement of opioid receptors. Hence, MPs are able to bind the opiate receptors of neurons and lymphocytes (Petrov et al., 1983). Radioimmunoassay revealed β-lypotropin, β-, γ-, and α-endorphins, and Leu- and Met-enkephalins in MPs and bone marrow cell culture supernatant (Zozulya et al., 1985). Proopiomelanocortin, a precursor of endorphins, was found in bone marrow. These data demonstrate that bone marrow cells are a previously unknown source of endogenic opioid peptides.

According to radioreceptor assay, the amount of substances bound to opiate receptors is larger than the total amount of opioids determined by radioimmunoassay. Along with the already discovered opioids, MPs probably are composed of other ligands of opioid receptors. This is confirmed by the MP influence on pain reactions.

The nociceptive action of MP showed a dose-dependent pattern. Two h after MP injections in milligram concentrations, hypoalgesia developed in mice (Figure 2B). The effect is naloxone dependent. Nanogram amounts of MP caused hyperalgesia in 15 min that lasted about 2 h (Figure 2A). Naloxone decreased the latent period of the nociceptive reaction, i.e., enhanced the MP-induced pain reaction.

There is a strong correlation between MP influence on pain sensitivity and the immune response. MP hyperalgesia is always accompanied by a clearly expressed antibody-stimulating effect, whereas upon hypoalgesia, the immune response to SRBCs does not change (Vasilenko et al., 1989; Zakharova et al., in press).

Hence, the close interrelationship between such vitally important systems of the organism as those for pain and immune control is clearly traced. However, the interrelationship between MP immunostimulating activity and that influencing the pain sensitivity threshold is still obscure. Moreover, the question arises as to what concrete molecular structures perform this interaction. The comparative estimation of the antibody stimulation of intact MP and the artificial opioid mixture composed in proportions close to their content in MPs showed that they provoke the same enhancement of antibody production (Table II). The antibody-stimulating effect of the synthetic opioid mixture (α-, γ-, and β-endorphins and β-lipotropin) is dose dependent and maximal in compound concentrations corresponding to the MP active dose (13 to 16 fmol/ml). If injected separately, opioids showed no antibody-stimulating activity similar to that of MP, except for β-endorphin in a concentration 1000-fold lower than its content in MP. β-Endorphin exhibited a stimulating effect both in culture *in vitro* and upon administration to animals. Synthetic α- and γ-endorphins as well as Leu- and Met-enkephalins used in a wide range of doses elicited no antibody production. Naloxone, which itself produced no immune response, prevented the antibody-stimulating effect of all three tested substances (Zakharova et al., 1988). Analogous immunostimulating effects of synthetic opioid peptides, MPs, and their similar dependence on naloxone imply the significance of opiate mechanisms in immune response regulation.

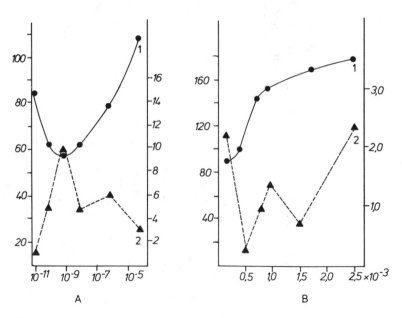

Figure 2. Myelopeptide influence on pain sensitivity (1) and antibody production (2) in mice. X: myelopeptide concentration (grams per mouse); * = $p < 0.05$, ** = $p < 0.01$, *** = $p < 0.001$., Y: (A) changes in the latent period of nociceptive reaction; (B) coefficient of antibody production stimulation, calculated as the ratio of experimental to control content.

TABLE II.

Naloxone Influence on MP Antibody-Stimulating Activity, Mixture of Synthetic Opioid Peptides (OP) and β-Endorphin

Substance	AFC Number (10^6) of Nucleated Cells, M±m		Coefficient of Stimulation
	Control	Experimental	
Immunized lymph nodes + MP	183± 5.06	366±16.94*	2.0
Immunized lymph nodes + OP mixture (13 fmol/ml)	189± 4.53	350±23.58*	1.9
Immunized lymph nodes + β-endorphin (2.4×10^{-2} fmol/ml)	171±14.74	386±21.98*	2.1
Immunized lymph nodes + naloxone + MP	200± 8.88	206± 6.34	1.0
Immunized lymph nodes + naloxone + OP mixture (13 fmol/ml)	198± 4.70	222±17.55	1.1
Immunized lymph nodes + naloxone + β-endorphin (2.4×10^{-2} fmol/ml)	209±19.37	196±18.41	0.9

* Statistically significant difference from the control ($p < 0.01$)

According to HPLC results, the retention times differ for antibody-stimulating MP and synthetic β-endorphin. Apparently, different peptides are responsible for the immunostimulating and opioid activities. It is not excluded that bone marrow opioid peptides can effect the humoral immune response through the chain of signals of cell differentiation processes.

The ability of bone marrow peptides to cause immune stimulation and to bind to the opioid receptors of neurons testifies to their involvement in the mechanisms of neuroimmune interaction. Due to the aforementioned properties, MPs can be considered as mediators regulating the immunocompetence of the organism following stress.

The stress-limiting MP action experimentally discovered and confirmed by clinical trials can be effectively applied to prevent various widespread stress-induced immunodeficient states.

REFERENCES

Fisher EG: Opioid peptides modulate immune functions. A review. *Immunopharmacol Immunotoxicol* 1988; 10:265.

Laurent S, Marsh JD, and Smith TW: Enkephalins have a direct positive inotropic effect on cultured cardiac myocytes. *Proc Natl Acad Sci U.S.A* 1985; 82:5930.

Lisyany MI, Radzievsky AA, and Zakharova LA: Immunomodulating effect of myelopeptides in severe closed experimental cranial trauma in rats. *Bull Exp Biol Med* 1988; 3:310 (in Russian).

Lolait S, Lim A, Toh BH, and Funder JW: Immunoreactive β-endorphin in a subpopulation of mouse spleen macrophages. *J Clin Invest* 1984; 73:277.

Kirilina EA, Zakharova LA, Vasilenko AM, and Mikhailova AM: Myelopide influence on early manifestation of immunosuppressive action of stress. *Immunology* 1989; 1:41 (in Russian).

Mikhailova AA, Zakharova LA, and Sorokin SV: Myelopeptides — a new class of endogenic immunoregulators. *Med Genet Immunol* 1987; 1:1 (in Russian).

Petrov RV and Mikhailova AA: Cell interactions in the immune response: collaboration at the level of mature antibody producers. *Cell Immunol* 1972; 5:392.

Petrov RV, Mikhailova AA, Stepanenko RN, and Zakharova LA: Cell interaction in the immune response: effect of humoral factor, related from the bone marrow cells on the quantity of mature antibody producers in culture of immune lymph node cells. *Cell Immunol* 1975; 17:342.

Petrov RV, Mikhailova AA, and Zakharova LA: Cell interactions at the level of mature antibody producers: the properties of the bone marrow humoral factor stimulating antibody production. *Ann Immunol (Paris)* 1980; 131D:161.

Petrov RV, Durinyan RA, and Vasilenko AM: Endorphin-like properties of the bone marrow factor stimulating antibody production. *Proc Acad Sci USSR* 1982; 265:501 (in Russian).

Petrov RV, Vartanyan ME, and Zozulya AA: Opiate activity of humoral factor in the bone marrow stimulating antibody production. *Bull Exp Biol Med* 1983; 5:46 (in Russian).

Petrov RV, Durinyan RA, and Vasilenko AM: Analgesic effect of myelopeptides. *Pathol Physiol Exp Ther* 1986a; 1:13 (in Russian).

Petrov RV, Mikhailova AA, Zakharova LA, Vasilenko AM, and Katlinsky AV: Myelopeptides — bone marrow mediators with immunostimulating and endorphin-like activity. *Scand J Immunol* 1986b; 24:237.

Petrov RV, Mikhailova AA, Sergeev JO, and Sorokin SV: Regulator bone marrow peptides and immunocorrection. *EOS* 1987a; 2:88.

Petrov RV, Mikhailova AA, and Zakharova LA: Myelopeptides: mediators of interaction between the immune system and the nervous system. *Ann NY Acad Sci* 1987b; 496:271.

Pershin BB, Kuzmin CN, and Levando VA: Immunologic responsiveness in athletes. *Immunology* 1981; 3:13 (in Russian).

Plotnikoff NP, Murgo AJ, Miller GC, Corder CN, and Faith RE: Enkephalins: immunomodulators. *Fed Proc* 1985; 44:118.

Sarybaeva DV, Zakharova LA, and Vasilenko AM: Immunostimulating effect of myelopeptides in hypoxic hypoxia in animals. *Immunology* 1988; 12:691 (in Russian).

Stepanenko RN: Clinical use of myelopidum. Advances in science and engineering. *Immunology* 1989; 26:192 (in Russian).

Shavit Y, Terman GW, and Martin FC: Stress, opioid peptides, the immune system and cancer. *J Immunol* 1985; 135:834S.

Vasilenko AM, Zakharova LA, and Belousova OI: Effect of auricular electric stimulation on myelopeptide production and early reactions of blood system cell populations in immobilization stress. *Pathol Physiol Exp Ther* 1985; 5:26 (in Russian).

Vasilenko AM, Yanovsky OG, and Zakharova LA: Hyperalgesic action of myelopeptides in low dose. *Proc Acad Sci USSR* 1989; 306:999 (in Russian).

Wybran Y: Enkephalins and endorphins: activation molecules for the immune system and natural killer activity? *Neuropeptides* 1985; 5:371.

Zakharova LA and Galkina NS: Interaction *(in vitro)* of cells of immune lymph nodes and of intact bone marrow separated by millipore membrane. *Bull Exp Biol Med* 1974; 9:67 (in Russian).

Zakharova LA, Belyovskaya RG, and Mikhailova AA: The effect of opioid bone marrow peptides on antibody formation during the productive phase of immune response. *Bull Exp Biol Med* 1988; 1:50 (in Russian).

Zakharova LA, Belyovskaya RG, and Yanovsky OG: Opioids involved into the myelopeptide antibody stimulating activity. *Biomed Sci* In press.

Zozulya AA, Pshenichkin SP, and Shchurin MR: Thymus peptides interacting with opiate receptors. *Acta Endocrinol* 1985; 110:284.

Zozulya AA, Patsakava E, Mikhailova AA, and Zakharova LA: Radioimmunoassay of α-, β-, γ-endorphines and β-lipotropin in the bone marrow mediator stimulating antibody production. *Immunology* 1986; 5:37 (in Russian).

Opioids and the Physiological Regulation of Natural Killer Cell Activity and Flushing

John E. Morley
St. Louis VA Medical Center
Geriatrics Research Education and Clinical Center,
St. Louis, Missouri
and
Division of Geriatrics, Department of Medicine,
St. Louis University Medical School,
St. Louis, Missouri

George F. Solomon
Department of Psychiatry,
Sepulveda VA Medical Center,
Sepulveda, California

Donna Benton
Geriatric Research Education and Clinical Center,
Sepulveda VA Medical Center,
Sepulveda, California

INTRODUCTION

It is now well accepted that opioid peptides can modulate a variety of immune system functions *in vitro* (Morley et al., 1989). However, there is a paucity of evidence that endogenous opioids play a physiological role *in vivo* in the modulation of the immune system. Recently, the use of infusions of opiate antagonists *in vivo* in humans has provided some preliminary evidence that natural killer cell activity and flushing are, at least under some conditions, physiologically under the regulation of endogenous opioids.

OPIOIDS AND NATURAL KILLER CELL ACTIVITY *IN VITRO*

A number of endogenous opioids have been reported to enhance natural killer (NK) cell activity *in vitro* (Matthews et al., 1983; Faith et al., 1984; Kay et al., 1984). β-endorphin stimulates NK cell activity at concentrations of 10^{-16} to 10^{-18} M. The dose response curve showed an inverted U shape. However, in studies in our laboratory, less than 50% of subjects showed an increase in NK activity in response to β-endorphin (Kay et al., 1984). Once a subject was demonstrated to be a β-endorphin responder, his or her peripheral blood lymphocytes were shown to respond to β-endorphin in a reproducible manner. This effect is naloxone reversible, suggesting that it may involve the activation of an opioid receptor. However, data showing a lack of effect of D-naloxone are not published, thus failing to establish stereospecificity for the effect.

In our early studies, we noted that γ-endorphin, but not α-endorphin, enhanced NK activity (Kay et al., 1984). This led us to more fully characterize the role of nonopioid fragments of β-endorphin in the stimulation of NK activity. We found that certain nonopioid fragments of β-endorphin (12–16, 2–7, and 6–17) enhanced NK activity, with peak dose responses between 10^{-12} to 10^{-15} M concentrations (Kay et al., 1987). The effect of these Des-Tyr endorphins was reversed by naloxone. In addition, the 2–9 fragment was active, but at a lower molarity. Both the 10–13 and 10–16 fragments were inactive. This suggested that the ability of β-endorphin to enhance NK activity rests, at least in part, in the α-helical portion (amino acids 6–9) of the molecule. However, the ability of naloxone to reduce the effect of des-Tyr-γ-endorphin suggested to us that the receptor was of the "double-lock" or "address-message" type, with the α-helical portion representing the address portion and the opioid moiety representing the message (Morley and Kay, 1986). This type of opioid receptor conformation has been previously suggested for the dynorphin molecule (Chavkin and Goldstein, 1981; Morley and Levine, 1983).

Oleson and Johnson (1988) noticed a bidirectional effect of opioids on NK cell activity. In low NK-responder populations, they found NK activity to be enhanced by endogenous opioids, while endogenous opioids suppressed NK activity in high-responder populations.

NK cell activity is stimulated by both interferon and interleukin-2. We have found that stimulation of NK cell activity by interferon or by interleukin-2 can be suppressed by naloxone (Morley and Kay, 1986). In ongoing studies using PHA-stimulated lymphocytes, we have found that labeled interleukin-2 is displaced by naloxone and β-endorphin and that tritiated naloxone is displaced by interleukin-2 (Kay and Morley, unpublished studies). In addition, naloxone administration modulates the TAC antigen which is related to the low-affinity interleukin-2 receptor. These data suggest that either endogenous opioids and interleukin-2 share similar receptors on the surface of human lymphocytes or that activation of one receptor modulates the configuration of the other receptor.

NK CELL ACTIVITY AND EXERCISE

Acute exercise in humans results in an increase in total leukocyte count (Busse et al., 1980; Martin, 1932), plasma interferon (Viti et al., 1985), and interleukin-1 (Cannon et al., 1986) levels, alterations in lymphocyte subset numbers and function (Kanonchoff et al., 1984; Robertson et al., 1981), and NK cell activity (Brahmi et al., 1985; Targen et al., 1981). Fiatarone et al. (1989) showed that in response to maximal bicycle ergometry exercise, there was a marked increase in NK activity that declined to baseline values within 15 min of completing the exercise. In addition to the increase in NK activity, there was an increase in Leu-11a and Leu-19 lymphocyte markers. The pre-exercise *in vitro* stimulation of NK activity by recombinant DNA interleukin-2 was markedly attenuated following exercise. Old individuals (over the age of 65 years) had a similar NK response to exercise compared to that seen in younger subjects.

β-endorphin is released rapidly during physical exercise (Fraioli et al., 1980; Carr et al., 1981). This suggested to us that β-endorphin may be the link between exercise and enhanced NK cell activity. To determine if this was the case, we studied eight women ranging in age from 24 to 35 years (Fiatarone et al., 1988). All underwent a maximal bicycle ergometer test on two occasions. On one occasion they received naloxone (100 mg/kg) before exercise, and on the second occasion they received an equal volume of normal saline placebo. Naloxone did not significantly alter any of the parameters of exercise performance.

Naloxone reduced the increase in NK activity seen with exercise (Fiatarone et al., 1988). Naloxone did not prevent the increase in Leu 11a and

Leu 19 cell markers seen with exercise. We also studied the ability of β-endorphin to stimulate NK activity *in vitro* before and after exercise. While before exercise β-endorphin stimulated NK activity, after exercise β-endorphin no longer stimulated NK activity *in vitro*. Administration of naloxone before exercise significantly blunted the fall in β-endorphin stimulation which was present after exercise. The ability of β-endorphin to stimulate NK activity after exercise is not a nonspecific phenomenon, as exercise-stimulated NK cells can be further stimulated by interferon *in vitro* (Brahmi et al., 1985; Targan et al., 1981). It should be noted that the two other acute stress hormones, catecholamines and cortisol, that are released during exercise suppress NK activity *in vitro,* making it unlikely that they are involved in the increase in NK activity seen with acute exercise (Hellstand et al., 1985; Katz et al., 1984).

Our data strongly support a role of β-endorphin in the increase in NK activity during acute exercise. To summarize this evidence: (1) naloxone, an opioid antagonist, attenuated the increase in NK activity that occurred with exercise, (2) *in vitro* β-endorphin stimulation was reduced after exercise, suggesting receptor down-regulation, and (3) naloxone attenuated the reduced β-endorphin stimulation that occurred after exercise.

Epidemiologic data in humans have suggested that regular moderate exercise produces a decrease in cancer of the colon (Gerhardsson et al., 1986) and cancer of the breast (Frosch et al., 1985). The discovery that opioids stimulate NK activity *in vivo* now provides a pathophysiological explanation for this finding. Preliminary studies by our group have now shown that mild mental stress can also lead to an increase in NK activity in young subjects. It is likely that this effect is also mediated by endogenous opioid release.

MAST CELLS AND FLUSHING

Up to 15% of patients receiving morphine either flush or have pruritus associated with histamine release from mast cells. *In vitro* β-endorphin has been shown to antagonize prostaglandin E_1-induced inhibition of IgE-mediated serotonin release from rat mast cells (Yamasaki et al., 1982). This effect was reversed by naloxone. Administration *in vivo* of the enkephalin analog, [D-Ala^2, MePhe^4, Met *(0)*-01]-enkephalin (DAMME) results in facial flushing in normal humans (Stubbs et al., 1978). Naloxone has attenuated the flushing seen with ethanol-induced flushing in association with chlorpropamide ingestion (Baraniuk et al., 1987). The post-menopausal flush has been blunted by naloxone in some cases (Lightman et al., 1980). Naloxone blocked flushing in a child with hyperendorphin syndrome associated with neurotizing encephalomyelopathy (Brandt et al., 1980). In a patient with flushing associated with cyclic psychosis, naloxone was reported to attenuate her symptoms (Goldstein and Keiser, 1983).

For these reasons, we decided to study in detail the effects of opioid blockade, using nalmefene, on subjects who exhibit spontaneous ethanol-induced flushing. Ethanol-induced flushing occurs in approximately 80% of Asians and 6 to 13% of Caucasians (Wolf, 1972). It is associated with elevated concentrations of plasma acetaldehyde due to the absence of the high-affinity isoenzyme necessary for normal acetaldehyde metabolism (Goedde et al., 1983).

In flushers, ethanol induced an increase in skin temperature which was markedly attenuated by prior administration of nalmefene (Ho et al., 1989). Ethanol had no effect on skin temperature in nonflushers and nalmefene, likewise, had no effects. Nalmefene had no effect on ethanol levels. Flushers, but no nonflushers, showed a marked increase in acetaldehyde levels following ethanol administration. Nalmefene did not alter the rise in acetaldehyde levels. This suggests that opioids modulate alcohol-induced flushing at a site distal to the increase in acetaldehyde.

In flushers, as opposed to nonflushers, alcohol induced a marked tachycardia which was attenuated by both nalmefene and indomethacin pre-treatment (Ho et al., 1989). Indomethacin had no effect on flushing. Alcohol-induced flushing resulted in an increase in serum cortisol levels, which increased further with the concomitant administration of nalmefene. A single dose of 100 mg methylprednisolone intravenously had no effect on ethanol-induced flushing or tachycardia, suggesting that the flushing inhibition by nalmefene was not due to mast cell stabilization secondary to cortisol release. Ethanol-induced flushing had no effects on substance P, vasoactive intestinal peptide, and pancreatic polypeptide. Addition of nalmefene further failed to alter the values of these circulating peptides.

To summarize, our studies showed that ethanol-induced flushing in Orientals can be inhibited by a single intravenous dose of the opioid antagonist, nalmefene (Ho et al., 1989). Opioid blockade was more effective than prostaglandin inhibition at decreasing flushing. The opioid antagonist effects were independent of acetaldehyde release and did not appear to involve substance P or vasoactive intestinal peptide.

SUMMARY

There is increasing evidence that β-endorphin plays a physiological role in the enhancement of NK cell activity during exposure to acute stressors. The β-endorphin-mediated increase in NK activity during acute exercise may play a role in the decrease in the development of cancer in subjects who exercise moderately. Alcohol appears to produce flushing in susceptible subjects by releasing endogenous opioids which may then release vasodilatory substances from mast cells.

REFERENCES

Baraniuk JN, Murray RB, and Mabbee WG: Naloxone, ethanol and the chlorpropamide alcohol flush. *Alcohol Clin Exp Res* 1987; 11:518.

Brahmi Z, Thomas JE, Park M, and Dowdeswell JRG: The effect of acute exercise on natural killer cell activity of trained and sedentary human subjects. *J Clin Immunol* 1985; 5:32.

Brandt NJ, Terenius L, Jacobsen BB, Klinken L, Norduis A, Brandt S, Blegvad K, and Yssing M: Hyperendorphin syndrome in a child with neurotizing encephalo-myelopathy. *N Engl J Med* 1980; 303:914.

Busse WN, Wilson CL, Hanson DA, and Folts J: The effect of exercise on the granulocyte response to isoproterenol in the trained athlete and unconditioned individual. *J Allergy Clin Immunol* 1980; 65:358.

Cannon JG, Evans WJ, Hugh VA, Meredith CN, and Dinarello CA: Physiological mechanisms contributing to increased interleukin-1 secretion. *J Appl Physiol* 1986; 61:1869.

Carr DB, Ballen BA, Skroner GS, et al: Physical conditioning facilitates the exercise induced secretion of beta-endorphin and beta-lypotropin in women. *N Engl J Med* 1981; 305.

Chavkin C and Goldstein A: Specific receptor for the opioid peptide dynorphin: structure-activity relationships. *Proc Natl Acad Sci USA* 1981; 78:6534.

Faith RE, Liang HJ, Murgo AJ, et al: Neuroimmunomodulation with enkephalins: enhancement of natural killer (NK) cell activity in vitro. *Clin Immunol Immuno-pathol* 1984; 31:412.

Fiatarone MA, Morley JE, Bloom ET, Benton D, Makinodan T, and Solomon GF: Endogenous opioids and the *exercise* induced augmentation of natural killer cell activity. *J Lab Clin Med* 1988; 112:566.

Fiatarone MA, Morley JE, Bloom ET, Benton D, Solomon GF, and Makinodan T: The effect of exercise on natural killer cell activity in young and old subjects. *J Gerontol Med Sci* 1989; 44:M37.

Fraioli F, Moretti C, Paolucci D, Alicicco E, Crescenzi F, and Fortunio G: Physical exercise stimulates marked concomitant release of beta-endorphin and adrenocor-ticotropic hormone (ACTH) in peripheral blood in man. *Experientia* 1980; 36:987.

Frosch RE, Wyshak G, Albright NL, Albright TE, Schiff I, Jones KP, Witschi J, Shiang E, Koff E, and Marguglio M: Lower prevalence of breast cancer and cancer of the reproductive system among former college athletes compared to non-athletes. *Br J Cancer* 1985; 52:885.

Gerhardsson M, Norell SE, Kiviranta H, Pedenen NL, and Ahlbom A: Sedentary jobs and colon cancer. *Am J Epidemiol* 1986; 123:775.

Goedde HW, Agarwal DP, and Harada S: The role of alcohol dehydrogenase and aldehyde dehydrogenase isoenzymes in alcohol metabolism, alcohol sensitivity and alcoholism. *Isozymes Curr Top Biol Med Res* 1983; 8:175.

Goldstein DJ and Keiser HR: A case of episodic flushing and organic psychosis: reversal by opiate antagonists. *Ann Intern Med* 1983; 98:30.

Hellstand K, Hesmodsson D, and Strannegard O: Evidence for a beta-adreno receptor-mediated regulation of human natural killer cells. *J Immunol* 1985; 134:4095.

Ho SB, DeMaster EG, Shafer RB, Levine AS, Morley JE, Go VLW, and Allen JI: Opiate antagonist nalmefene inhibits ethanol-induced flushing in Asians: a preliminary study. *Alcohol Clin Exp Res* 1989; 12:705.

Kanonchoff AD, Cavanaugh DJ, Mehl VL, Bartel RC, Penn GM, and Budd JA: Changes in lymphocyte subpopulations during acute exercise. *Med Sci Sports* 1984; 16:175.

Katz P, Zuytoun AM, and Lee HJ: The effects of in vivo hydrocortisone on lymphocyte-mediated cytotoxicity. *Arthritis Rheum* 1984; 27:72.

Kay N, Allen J, and Morley JE: Endorphins stimulate normal peripheral blood lymphocyte natural killer activity. *Life Sci* 1984; 35:53.

Kay N, Morley JE, and Van Ree JM: Enhancement of human lymphocyte natural killing function by non-opioid fragments of beta-endorphin. *Life Sci* 1987; 40:1083.

Lightman S, Maguire A, Jacobs H: Evidence of opioid control of menopausal flushing and luteinizing hormone pulses. *Clin Sci* 1980; 59:19P.

Martin HE: Physiological leukocytosis: the variation in leukocyte count during rest and exercise and after hypodermic injection of adrenaline. *J Physiol (London)* 1932; 75:113–129.

Matthews PM, Froelich CJ, Sidbit WL, et al: Enhancement of natural cytotoxicity by beta-endorphin. *J Immunol* 1983; 130:1658.

Morley JE and Kay N: Neuropeptides as modulators of immune function. *Psychopharmacol Bull* 1986; 22:1089.

Morley JE, Kay N, and Solomon GF: Opioid peptides, stress and immune function. In *Neuropeptides and Stress.* Tachey, Morley JE, and Brown MR, Eds. Springer-Verlag, New York, 1989, p. 222.

Morley JE, Levine AS: Involvement of dynorphin and the kappa opioid receptor in feeding. *Peptides* 1983; 6:797.

Oleson DR and Johnson DR: Regulation of human natural cytoxicity by enkephalins and selective opiate agonists. *Brain Behav Immun* 1988; 2:171.

Robertson AJ, Ramescar KCR, Potts RC, Gibbs JH, Browning MCK, Brown RA, Hayes AC, and Beck JC: The effect of strenuous physical exercise on circulating blood lymphocytes and serum cortisol levels. *J Clin Lab Immunol* 1981; 5:53.

Stubbs WA, Delitala G, Jones A, Jeffcoate WI, Edwards CRW, Rattes SJ, Beser GM, Bloom SR, Alberti KGMM: Hormonal and metabolic responses to an enkephalin analogue in normal man. *Lancet* 1978; 2:1225.

Targan S, Britvan L, and Dorey F: Activation of human NKCC by moderate exercise: increased frequency of NK cells with enhanced capability of effector-target lytic interactions. *Clin Exp Immunol* 1981; 45:352.

Viti A, Muscettola M, Paulsu C, Bocci V, and Almi A: Effect of exercise on plasma interferon levels. *J Appl Physiol* 1985; 59:426.

Wolf PM: Ethnic differences in alcohol sensitivity. *Science* 1972; 175:449.

Yamasaki Y, Shimamura O, Kizu H, et al: IgE mediated ^{14}C-serotonin release from rat mast cells modulated by morphine and endorphins. *Life Sci* 1982; 31:671.

Methionine Enkephalin, A New Lymphokine for the Treatment of ARC Patients

Joseph Wybran
Hôpital Erasme
Université Libre de Bruxelles
Belgium

Nicholas P. Plotnikoff
College of Pharmacy and College of Medicine
University of Illinois at Chicago
Chicago, Illinois

ABSTRACT

Methionine enkephalin (MEK), a new lymphokine derived from T-helper cells, has been found to elevate T-cell subsets, natural killer (NK) activity, mitogen blastogenesis, and reduce constitutional symptoms in 8/12 ARC patients. We are proposing that MEK is an essential lymphokine of the immune system and may be of therapeutic value in immunodeficiency states.

INTRODUCTION

MEK is an endogenous opioid peptide endowed with immunomodulatory properties (Wybran et al., 1979; Plotnikoff and Miller, 1983). Numerous *in vitro* studies have shown that MEK has direct immunomodulatory effects (Wybran et al., 1985; Van Epps and Saland, 1984). Most important, MEK has been shown to be derived from T-helper cells (Zurawski et al., 1986).

TABLE I.
Description of Patients on MEK Treatment

Patient/ Symptoms Before Treatment	MEK Doses	MEK Treatment	p24 ELISA Absorbance Units	Symptoms During Mek Treament
7 27-yr male homosexual Weight loss IPT Lymph nodes Thrombocytopenia (100,000) III PGL IV E	20μ/kg 3×/week 50 μ/kg 1×/week 3 months	MEK 6 months	0.00 0.00	weight gain: 2 kg Stable ITP No changes in lymph nodes or platelet count
8 25-yr male homosexual Weight loss (3 kg) Lymph nodes III PGL	20 μ/kg 3×/week 50 μ/kg 1×/week 5 months	MEK 7 months	0.00 0.00	weight gain: 2 kg Slight decrease in nodes
9 20-yr female Caucasian Lymph nodes Fatigue Weight loss (3 kg) Thrush IV A	20 μ/kg 3×/week	MEK 3 months	0.00 0/00	Slight node regression No fatigue 2 kg weight No thrush
10 37-yr male homosexual Weight loss (6 kg) Night sweats IV A	20 μ/kg 3×/week 100 μ/kg 3×/week	MEK 7 months	4.04 0.00	Interstitial pneumonia responding to anti-tuberculosis treatment (month 6)
11 57-yr male Caucasian Weight loss (5 kg) Night sweats Fatigue IV A	20 μ/kg 3×/week	MEK 4 months +	7.40 7.10	Weight gain: 3 kg No night sweats No fatigue Excellent mood

Patient	Dose	Treatment	Values	Outcome
12 36-yr male homosexual Weight loss (11 kg) Night sweats Lymph nodes Scrotal infections IV A	20 µg/kg 3×/week 100 µg/kg 1×/week (6m)	MEK 19 months	0.00 0.00	In 1 to 4 months, complete clinical recovery: weight gain 11 kg, node regression, no night sweats, no infection
13 36-yr male homosexual Interstitial pneumonia Weight loss Fatigue Recurrent oral herpes IV E	20 µg/kg 3×/week 100 µg/kg 1×/week	MEK 11 months +	1.73 0.00	Weight gain: 2 kg Decreased fatiguability Decreased oral herpes Increase mood
14 25-yr female African Tetraplegia IV B CSF-high HIV titer	20 µg/kg 3×/week	MEK 1 month	0.00 0.00	Recovery of tetraplegia in 3 weeks
15 57-yr male Caucasian Polyneuritis Tuberculosis Malnutrition	20 µg/kg 3×/week 100 µg/kg 3×/week	MEK 3 months	—	Presented malnutrition and gastrointestinal bleeding of unknown origin Death after 3 months
16 48-yr African Weight loss Diarrhea Confusion IV A, B	20 µg/kg 3×/week	MEK 1 month	1.4 0.0	Weight gain: 3 kg Treatment stopped for ITP (steroid treatment) Death in dementia after 6 months (off treatment)

(continued)

TABLE I (Cont.).
Description of Patients on MEK Treatment

Patient/ Symptoms Before Treatment	MEK Doses	MEK Treatment	p24 ELISA Absorbance Units	Symptoms During Mek Treatment
17 62-yr male Caucasian Weight loss Night sweats Confusion IV A, B	20μ/kg 3 ×/week 50 μ/kg 3 ×/week 1 month	MEK 2 months plus Suramin	—	No clinical improvement Death in dementia after 7 months (off treatment)
18 Weight loss CMV infection IV ?	20 μ/kg 3 ×/week	MEK 1 month	—	Weight gain: 2 kg Death from cerebral hemorrhage (Arterial hypertension)

TABLE II. Summary-Immunology

	Responders to MEK Treatment		(patients 7 to 14)
	Day 0	1 month	4 months
Lymphocytes/mm³	1142	1399 NS	1330 NS
T₃/mm³	916	1047 NS	1029 NS
T₄/mm³	243	350 p <0.05	285 NS
T4/T8	0.37	0.54 p <0.05	0.41 NS
PHA (10³ CPM)	198	291 p <0.02	404 p <0.05
PWM (10³ CPM)	43	63 p <0.05	77 p <0.05
NK (%)	18	27 p <0.05	19 NS
(1:40)			

Early clinical studies have shown that MEK can reduce symptomatology and improve immunological functions in ARC-AIDS patients (Wybran et al., 1987; Plotnikoff et al., 1987). The present clinical study expands on these earlier clinical reports, showing that MEK may also reduce p 24 serum levels and reduce symptomatology in ARC patients when administered over prolonged treatment periods (1 to 19 months).

METHODS

All the patients included in this study were HIV seropositive, diagnosed by ELISA and confirmed by immunofluorescence of Western blot analysis. They were classified in four stages, according to Centers for Disease Control (CDC) criteria.

All the patients (except patient 14) received, at least for 3 months, MEK injections. The patients are described in Table I and include two patients with persistent generalized lymphadenopathy, (PGL) (Stage III), four patients with ARC (Stage IVA), and three other patients with miscellaneous manifestations of the HIV disease (patient 13 with interstitial pneumonia, patient 14 with tetraplegia, and patient 15 with polyneuritis, tuberculosis, and malnutrition). None of these patients had been previously included in a therapeutic study for HIV infection. All of the patients were fully informed about the therapeutic protocol, which had been approved by the Hospital Ethical Committee.

This was an open study in which the patients were fully cooperative. This study included patients who were in treatment for at least 3 months. They were followed both clinically and immunologically during various periods of time. Tables I and II summarize all their clinical data as well as the immunological follow-up.

METHIONINE ENKEPHALIN (MEK)

MEK was purchased from UCB (Belgium). It was constituted in sterile vials containing 750 μg of pure synthetic compound. MEK was further dissolved in a 500-ml normal saline solution. It was injected intravenously in a period of 60 to 120 min. MEK was injected in the morning. The patients received MEK at a dose of 20 μg/kg three times weekly (Monday, Wednesday, and Friday) for a period of at least 4 months in order to be included in the study (patient 14 received only 1 month of treatment). No adverse reactions were observed.

The treatment was, however, longer in most of the patients, as reported in Table I. The treatment was as follows for the ARC patients. Patients 7 and 8 (PGL) received the initial treatment for 3 and 4 months, respectively, and then received a weekly injection of MEK at a dose of 50 μg/kg body weight for another 3 months. Patient 9 (ARC) received 3 months of treatment. Patient 10 (ARC) received, after the initial 3 months, 100μg/kg body weight three times weekly. Patient 12 received the initial treatment and then received the treatment for another 10 months at 100 μg/kg once a week. Patient 13 (interstitial pneumonia), after receiving the initial treatment, was continued at 100 μg/kg once weekly for another 6 months.

IMMUNOLOGY

All the patients were immunologically monitored at the entry of the study and at 1 and 4 months during treatment. Venous blood was always drawn in the morning before MEK injection. The percentage and the absolute number of lymphocytes was determined using the OKT3 monoclonal antibody (Ortho, Raritan, NJ), and the subpopulations of CD4 and CD8 cells were measured by the OKT4 and OKT8 monoclonal antisera using flow cytometry (FACS, Becton Dickinson). The response to mitogens was assessed using phytohem-agglutinin (PHA, Wellcome) at an optional concentration of 1 μg/ml and pokeweed mitogen (PWM) at an optimal dilution of 1/50 (GIBCO). The Ficoll-Hypague peripheral blood mononuclear isolated cells were cultured for 3 days in a 96-well flat-bottomed microtiter plate at a concentration of 2 × 10^8 cells pulsed with labeled thymidine and harvested in glass filter papers.

The NK assay used K562 cells labeled with CR^{51} as target cells in a classical 4-h cytotoxicity assay. The results were expressed by calculating the percentage of CR^{51} release.

STATISTICAL ANALYSIS

Immunological variables were compared before and during treatment (day 0, 1 month, and 4 months) using both the student *t* test and the Wilcoxon rank test for paired data.

ARC PATIENTS

Clinical Results

Seven out of eight ARC patients (7 to 14) showed a reduction of constitutional symptoms with MEK treatment (Table I). These symptoms included body weight changes, lymphadenopathy, fatigue, night sweats, scrotal infections, thrush, oral herpes, and tetraplegia.

One patient (16) showed a weight gain of 3 kg, but was taken off MEK treatment after 1 month for steroid treatment of ITP. Three advanced ARC patients (15, 17, and 18) showed no clinical improvement during 3 months (15), 2 months (17), and 1 month (18) of MEK treatment. These four patients (15 to 18) expired 3, 6, 7, and 1 months, respectively, *off* MEK treatment in follow-up observation.

p 24 Serum Levels (Table I)

ARC Patients. Patients 10, 11, 13, and 16, while on MEK treatment, had a decrease in p 24 levels (Table I). Patients 7, 8, 9, 12, and 14 had no detectable antigen levels before or during MEK treatment.

Immunological Parameters (Table II)

ARC Patients (7 to 14) — Responders. Significant increases in T4, T4/T8, PHA, PWM, and NK function were seen in eight ARC patients the first month of MEK treatment (Table II). Significant increases in PHA and PWM responses were also observed at 4 months of treatment.

Lymphocytes (Table III)

MEK Responders. Five of eight patients had increases in lymphocyte numbers at 1 month and four patients at 4 months.

T3 (Table IV)

Five patients had increases in T3 numbers at 1 month and four patients at 4 months. Two patients had increases at 6 months (7) and 9 months (13).

T4 (Table V)

Seven patients had increases of T4 cells at 1 month and five patients at 4 months.

T8 (Table VI)

Four patients had increased T8 counts at 1 and 4 months; conversely, the other four patients had decreases at 1 and 4 months.

T4/T8 (Table VII)

Seven patients had increased T4/T8 ratios at 1 month and four patients at 4 months. Two patients had increased ratios at 7 months (8) and 19 months (12).

PHA (Table VIII)

Seven patients had increased blastogenesis at 1 month and five patients at 4 months. Three patients had increased activity at 6 months (7), 7 months (8), and 19 months (12).

PWM (Table IX)

Six patients had increased blastogenesis at both 1 and 4 months. Two patients had increased activity at 7 months (8) and 19 months (12).

NK (Table X)

Six patients had increased NK cell activity at 1 month and three patients at 4 months. Two patients had increased functional activity at 6 and 7 months (7 and 8, respectively).

IL2 (Table XI)

Two patients had increased levels at 1 and 4 months. Two patients had increased levels at 6 and 19 months (7 and 12, respectively).

ARC Patients (15 to 18) (Nonresponders)

Lymphocytes, T4, T3, T8, PHA, PWM, and IL-2 decreased in numbers. Slight increases were seen in patient 17 (T3, T8, PHA, and NK).

TABLE III. Lymphocytes (/mm³)

Patient	Day 0	1 Month	4 Months		Treatment Duration (months)
			Responders to MEK Treatment		
7	1550	1315	1258	1500 (6 M)	6
8	1702	1560	1194	1517 (7 M)	7
9	966	864	1066*	—	3
10	1222	1305*	864	—	7
11	1066	1470*	896	—	4 +
12	1681	2418*	1920*	1369 (19 M)	19
13	946	1596*	1755*	920 (9 M)	11 +
14	560	660*	1092*	—	1
			Nonresponders		
15	1700	1140	1080 (2 M)	—	3
16	1560	532	—	—	1
17	352	322	312 (2 M)	—	2
18	—	—	—	—	1

TABLE IV. T3 Cells (/mm³)

Patient	Day 0	1 Month	4 Months		Treatment Duration (months)
			Responders to MEK Treatment		
7	1271	1105	855	1305* (6 M)	6
8	1361	1263	1166	1137 (9 M)	7
9	676	640	810*	—	3
10	880	887*	674	—	7
11	853	1029*	627	—	4 +
12	1177	1958*	1613	917 (19 M)	19
13	738	1037*	1421*	745* (9 M)	11 +
14	375	462*	666*	—	1
			Nonresponders		
15	1326	889	820 (2 M)	—	3
16	1185	345	—	—	1
17	204	241*	262* (2 M)	—	2
18	—	—	—	—	1

TABLE V. T4 Cells (/mm³)

Patient	Day 0	1 Month	4 Months		Treatment Duration (months)
Responders to MEK Treatment					
7	387	320	201	375 (6 M)	6
8	340	405*	394*	303 (7 M)	7
9	290	307*	341*	—	3
10	256	261*	104	—	7
11	85	118*	63	—	4+
12	336	991*	730*	397 (19 M)	19
13	85	255*	280*	83 (9 M)	11+
14	95	165*	164	—	1
Nonresponders					
15	510	262	345 (2 M)	—	3
16	109	37	—	—	1
17	28	22	25 (2 M)	—	2
18	—	—	—	—	1

TABLE VI. T8 Cells (/mm³)

Patient	Day 0	1 Month	4 Months		Treatment Duration (months)
Responders to MEK Treatment					
7	837	829	604	885* (6 M)	6
8	1021	842	843	789 (7 M)	7
9	367	346	469*	—	3
10	708	626	510	—	7
11	757	882*	547	—	4+
12	840	967*	864*	657 (19 M)	19
13	643	686*	1123*	662* (9 M)	11+
14	269	290*	491*	—	2
Nonresponders					
15	816	604	488 (2 M)	—	3
16	1045	287	—	—	1
17	172	225*	225* (2 M)	—	2
18	—	—	—	—	1

TABLE VII. T4/T8 Ratios

Patient	Day 0	1 Month	4 Months		Treatment Duration (months)
			Responders to MEK Treatment		
7	0.46	0.36	0.33	0.42 (6 M)	6
8	0.33	0.48*	0.47*	0.38* (7 M)	7
9	0.79	0.87*	0.77	—	3
10	0.36	0.42*	0.20	—	7
11	0.11	0.14*	0.12*	—	4 +
12	0.40	1.05*	0.85*	0.60* (19 M)	19
13	0.13	0.37*	0.25*	0.13 (9 M)	11 +
14	0.35	0.57*	0.33	—	1
			Nonresponders		
15	0.62	0.44	0.71* (2 M)	—	3
16	0.10	0.13*	—	—	1
17	0.16	0.10	0.11 (2 M)	—	2
18	—	—	—	—	1

TABLE VIII. PHA (10^3 CPM)

Patient	Day 0	1 Month	4 Months		Treatment Duration (months)
			Responders to MEK Treatment		
7	235	370*	653*	388* (6 M)	6
8	270	425*	588*	632* (7 M)	7
9	250	304*	468*	—	3
10	239	256*	182	—	7
11	81	138*	—	—	4 +
12	147	338*	414*	421* (19 M)	19
13	143	123	127	162 (9 M)	11 +
14	224	378*	398*	—	1
			Nonresponders		
15	228	215	280* (2 M)	—	3
16	60	50	—	—	1
17	176	195*	76 (2 M)	—	2
18	—	—	—	—	1

TABLE IX. PWM (10³ CPM)

Patient	Day 0	1 Month	4 Months		Treatment Duration (months)
			Responders to MEK Treatment		
7	64	54	88*	38 (6 M)	6
8	67	123*	178*	188* (7 M)	7
9	38	76*	66*	—	3
10	74	82*	90*	—	7
11	15	31*	—	—	4 +
12	38	76*	56*	59* (19 M)	19
13	24	16	10	21 (9 M)	11 +
14	27	45*	52*	—	1
			Nonresponders		
15	82	51	70 (2 M)	—	3
16	26	29*	—	—	1
17	82	—	54 (2 M)	—	2
18	—	—	—	—	1

TABLE X. NK (%) (T:E, 1:40)

Patient	Day 0	1 Month	4 Months		Treatment Duration (months)
			Responders to MEK Treatment		
7	19	11	11	21* (6 M)	6
8	14	20*	12	16* (7 M)	7
9	11	21*	16*	—	3
10	17	12	13	—	7
11	18	29*	18	—	4 +
12	22	55*	43*	16 (19 M)	19
13	20	32*	22*	12 (9 M)	11 +
14	21	32*	18	—	1
			Nonresponders		
15	9	6	8 (2 M)	—	3
16	16	18*	—	—	1
17	16	36*	20* (2 M)	—	2
18	—	—	—	—	1

TABLE XI. IL-2 (Units)

Patient	Day 0	1 Month	4 Months		Treatment Duration (months)
			Responders to MEK Treatment		
7	1.2	1.5*	0.6	1.7 (6 M)	6
8	1.4	0.5	0.5	1.2 (7 M)	7
9	1.1	1.1	1.8*	—	3
10	0.9	0.3	0.3	—	7
11	0.2	0	—	—	4+
12	0.6	0.6	2.1*	1.3* (19 M)	19
13	0.5	0.3	0.1	0.3 (9 M)	11+
14	0.2	0.4*	—	—	1
			Nonresponders		
15	2.0	1.8	1.0 (2 M)	—	3
16	0	0.3*	—	—	1
17	—	0.34	0.29 (2 M)	—	2
18	—	—	—	—	1

DISCUSSION

Recent findings indicate that cytotoxic T-cells destroy HIV (Walker et al., 1988). These cells bear CD3, CD8 monoclonal markers and may also cross-react with Leu 7, Leu 11, and Leu 19 monoclonals. In the present study, increases were observed in NK function while on MEK treatment. Similar increases in NK function were reported earlier against K562 and Molt 4 target cells in patients on MEK treatment (Wybran et al., 1987). In addition, HIV-positive patients on MEK treatment were also reported earlier to have increases in Leu 11- and Leu 19-labeled cells (Plotnikoff et al., 1989). Finally, increases in CD3 and CD8 cells were also observed (Plotnikoff et al., 1989). These increases support our hypothesis that MEK is activating cytotoxic cells that destroy HIV. In further support of this interpretation is the present study showing that p 24 serum levels may be reduced during MEK treatment. Most importantly, none of the patients exhibited any increase in antigen levels, thus negating possible activation of HIV (Plotnikoff et al., 1988).

Sustained increases in T4 numbers were observed in patients 8, 9, 12, 13, and 14, suggesting that tolerance to MEK did not develop. However, changes of MEK dosage during treatment may have accounted for the reduction of T4 counts in patients 7 and 10.

It is challenging to consider the role of MEK in the immune system. MEK has been shown to be derived from its prohormone, proenkephalin A, found in T-helper cells (Zurawski et al., 1986). MEK has been found to stimulate expression of interleukin 1 and 2 (IL-1, IL-2) as well as γ-interferon (Wybran et al., 1987; Wybran and Schandene, 1986; Plotnikoff et al, 1987; Brown and Van Epps, 1985; Youkilis et al., 1985). MEK can now be considered to be a lymphokine, derived from T-helper cells, that activates NK-K-LAK cells. Recently, MEK has been found to activate LAK cells against Daudi target cells and also potentiate IL-2 (Wybran and Plotnikoff, 1989). In addition, Melder et al. (1989) reported that LAK cells destroy HIV-infected human monocytes.

We are proposing that AIDS patients have a deficiency of MEK, in addition to other lymphokines such as IL-2 (Lane et al., 1985). Replacement therapy with MEK may retard the progression of the disease by activating and increasing NK-K-LAK cells that destroy HIV. Cytotoxic cell activity has been found to be markedly depressed in HIV-positive patients (Plata et al., 1988). It is possible that treatment of asymptomatic HIV-positive patients with MEK may prevent conversion to ARC and AIDS status by activating NK-K-LAK cells. In addition, MEK may be found useful as an adjuvant to vaccine development for the treatment of HIV-positive patients (Koenig et al., 1988).

We believe the present clinical study, together with earlier clinical reports, supports the further clinical development of MEK in the treatment of HIV-positive patients in the early stages of the disease (ARC status). The nonresponders in the present study may have been more advanced in their disease states. Furthermore, combination therapy with antiviral agents such as zidovudine may be appropriate since MEK has been reported to have bone marrow stimulatory properties, in addition to its immunostimulant effects on NK-K-LAK cells (Plotnikoff et al., 1986; Jankovic et al., 1987).

REFERENCES

Brown SL and Van Epps DE: Beta endorphin (BE), metenkephalin (ME), and corticotrophin (ACTH) modulate the production of gamma interferon (IFN) in vitro. *Fed Proc* 1985; 44(4):949.

Carr DJJ and Klimpel GR: Enhancement of the generation of cytotoxic T cells by endogenous opiates. *J Neuroimmunol* 1986; 12:75–87.

Foris G, Medgyesi GA, Gyimesi E, and Hauck M: Metenkephalin induced alterations of macrophage functions. *Mol Immunol* 1984; 21(8):242–250.

Jankovic BD, Markovic BM, and Spector NH: 4 Neuroimmune interactions. *Ann NY Acad Sci* 1987; 496.

Koenig S, Eral P, Powell D, Lane HC, Merli SL, and Fauci AS: Cell mediated cytotoxicity against target cells expressing HIV-I proteins. In 4th Int Conf AIDS. Stockholm, June 1988.

Lane HC, Depper JM, Greene WC, Whalen G, Waldman TA, and Fauci AS: Qual-ititative analysis of immune function in patients with the acquired immunodefi-ciency syndrome. *N Engl J Med* 1985; 313(2):79–84.

Mathews PM, Froelich CJ, Sibbett WL Jr, and Bankhurst AD: Enhancement of natural cytotoxicity by endorphin. *J Immunol* 1983; 130(4):1658–1662.

Melder RJ, Balachandra R, Gupta P, Rinaldo CR, Whiteside TL, and Herberman RB: Lymphokine-activated killer (LAK) cell cytotoxicity against HIV-infected human monocytes. *FASEB J* 1989; 3:4.

Morley JE, Kay NE, Solomon GF, and Plotnikoff NP: Neuropeptides; conductors of the immune orchestra. *Life Sci* 1987; 41:527–544.

Plata, Hoffenbach FA, Langlade-Demoyen P, Dadaglio G, Vilmer E, and Sansonetti P: Quantitative analysis of HIV specific cytotoxic T lymphocytes in humans. In 4th Int Conf AIDS. Stockholm, June 1988.

Plotnikoff NP and Miller GC: Enkephalins as immunomodulators. *Int J Immuno-pharmacol* 1983; 5:437–441.

Plotnikoff NP, Murgo AJ, Faith RE, and Good RA: Enkephalins-Endorphins: Stress and the Immune System. Plenum Press, New York, 1986.

Plotnikoff NP, Miller GC, Nimeh N, Faith RE, Murgo AJ, and Wybran J: Enkephalins and T-cell enhancement in normal volunteers and cancer patients. *Ann NY Acad Sci* 1987; 496:608–619.

Plotnikoff NP, Miller GC, Nimeh N, and Wybran J: Methionine enkephalin: antiviral effects against herpes and AIDS. In Symp Stress and Immunity. AAAS, Boston, February 1988.

Plotnikoff NP, Miller GC, Nimeh N, and Wybran J: Methionine-enkephalin (MEK): enhancement of cytotoxic T cells in ARC patients. In 4th Int Conf AIDS. Stock-holm, June 1988.

Plotnikoff NP, Miller GC, and Wybran J: Activation by methionine-enkephalin (MEK): enhancement of cytotoxic T cells in HIV + patients. In 5th Int Conf AIDS. Mon-treal, 1989, p. 400.

Van Epps DE and Saland L: Endorphin and metenkephalin stimulate human peripheral blood mononuclear cell chemotaxis. *J Immunol* 1984; 132:3046–3053.

Walker BD, Flexner C, Paradis TJ, Fuller TC, Hirsch MJ, Schooley RT, and Moss B: HIV-I reverse transcriptase is a target for cytotoxic T lymphocytes in infected individuals. *Science* 1988; 240:64–65.

Wybran J, Appleboom T, Famaey JP, and Govaerts A: Suggestive evidence for morphine and methionine enkephalin receptors on normal blood T lymphocytes. *J Immunol* 1979; 123:108–114.

Wybran J: Enkephalins and endorphins as modifiers of the immune system. *Fed Proc* 1985; 44:92–94.

Wybran J and Schandene: Some immunological effects of methionine enkephalin in man; potential therapeutic use. In *Roles of Leucocytes in Host Defense.* Oppenheim J, Ed. Alan R. Liss, New York, 1986, pp. 205–212.

Wybran JL, Schandene, Van Vooren J-P, Vandermoten G, Lattine D, Sonnect J, DeBruyere M, Taelman H, and Plotnikoff NP: Immunologic properties of methi-onine enkephalin, and therapeutic implications in AIDS, ARC, and cancer. *Ann NY Acad Sci* 1987; 496:108–114.

Wybran J and Plotnikoff NP: Enhancement of immunological mechanisms, including LAK induction, by methionine enkephalin. In 7th Int Cong Immunology. Berlin, 1989.

Youkilis E, Chapman J, Woods E, and Plotnikoff NP: In vivo immunostimulation and increased in vitro production of interleukin 1 (IL-1) activity by met-enkephalin. *Int J Immunopharmacol* 1985; 7(3):79.

Zurawski G, Benedik M, Kamb BJ, Abram JS, Zurawski SM, and Lee FD: Activation of T-helper cells induces abundant preproenkephalin in RNA synthesis. *Science* 1986; 232:772–774.

Growth Hormone and Prolactin as Natural Antagonists of Glucocorticoids in Immunoregulation

Keith W. Kelley
Professor of Immunophysiology
University of Illinois
Department of Animal Sciences
207 Plant and Animal Biotechnology Laboratory
Urbana, Illinois

Robert Dantzer
Directeur de Recherches
INRA-INSERM
Unité de Recherches de Neubiologie des Comportements
Bordeaux Cedex (France)

INTRODUCTION

The field of immunophysiology has virtually exploded during the past 10 years. It is now known that (1) lymphoid tissue is innervated with autonomic sympathetic noradrenergic neurons, (2) the brain, which has long been considered to be an immunologically privileged site, contains functionally active macrophage-like cells of bone marrow origin (microglial cells) and possesses Thy-1 and CD4 surface-like molecules, (3) lymphocytes and macrophages have receptors for a variety of pituitary hormones and neuropeptides, (4) these cells synthesize and appear to secrete several classic pituitary hormones, and (5) lymphoid and myeloid cells secrete other hormone-like molecules (cytokines) that act both locally (autocrine and paracrine effects) and at distant targets such as the brain (endocrine effects) to affect the neuroendocrine system. Findings such as these have led to the growing appreciation that neuropeptides and hormones not only affect cells of the immune system, but that soluble products from lymphoid and myeloid cells affect the central nervous system. This concept of bidirectional communication between the immune and neuroendocrine systems has recently been reviewed (Blalock, 1989), and the implications of this concept in the maintenance of homeostasis during stress have been discussed (Dantzer and Kelley, 1989; Griffin, 1989).

The role of stress in health and disease was reviewed a decade ago (Kelley, 1980). Although many kinds of adverse stimuli increase the susceptibility of animals to a variety of infectious diseases and suppress different types of immune events, it is noteworthy that a number of reports have shown that some stressors can enhance disease resistance and augment certain immune responses. The classic example was reported 20 years ago by Gross and Colmano (1969). Psychosocial stress (the mixing of unfamiliar chickens) reduced resistance to Newcastle disease virus and *Mycoplasma gallisepticum,* and much of this reduction in host resistance was caused by the stress-induced release of adrenal glucocorticoids (Gross, 1989). However, Gross and Colmano (1969) also showed that psychosocial stress actually increased the bird's resistance to *Staphylococcus aureus* and *Escherichia coli* infections. It was subsequently demonstrated that social stress increased resistance to Eimeria infections and northern fowl mites (Gross, 1976; Hall and Gross, 1975), but reduced host resistance to Marek's disease (Gross, 1972; Gross and Colmano, 1971).

The mechanisms that are responsible for these differential effects are virtually unexplored. The problem with stressors is that they change peripheral concentrations of a number of hormones so that finding out which one is preferentially involved is a difficult task. It is somewhat analogous to a fishing expedition.

Five years ago, it was speculated that hormonal changes were likely to be responsible for stress-induced alterations in disease susceptibility (Kelley, 1985). The major hormones that are sensitive to stressors, and which were known at that time to affect cells of the immune system, are glucocorticoids, catecholamines, and endogenous opiates. Of these, glucocorticoids are the most widely recognized group of hormones that are known to suppress the synthesis of a variety of cytokines such as interleukin 2 (IL-2), inteferon-γ (IFN-γ), interleukin 1 (IL-1), and tumor necrosis factor-α (TNF-α). This results in a reduction in a number of activities of lymphocytes and macrophages. It is therefore widely believed that stress-induced increases in plasma glucocorticoids are responsible for most of the immunosuppressive effects of stress, although it is now known that other as yet undefined stress-induced immunosuppressive mechanisms exist (Keller et al., 1983, 1988).

AN HYPOTHESIS: STRESS-INDUCED PROTECTIVE HORMONES

A number of years ago, Denckla (1978) suggested that the pituitary gland secretes substances which antagonize the effects of other pituitary hormones. Since adrenocorticotropic hormone (ACTH) is responsible for inducing the synthesis and release of glucocorticoids from the adrenal cortex, it is possible that stress-responsive pituitary hormones exist that might augment rather than suppress functional activities of cells of the immune system. Physical and psychological stress increases the release of both growth hormone and prolactin in most animal species, the exception being the rat. In this species, stress augments the release of prolactin and inhibits growth hormone. Certain types of infections also increase the release of growth hormone and prolactin, and these neuroendocrine effects are probably mediated by microbial and viral agents inducing the release of proteins from macrophages (i.e., IL-1 and TNF-α; see Kelley, 1989 for discussion).

The global statement that stress causes immunosuppression is no longer tenable. Ample evidence has now accumulated that certain stressors actually increase host resistance to some pathogenic organisms and also augment certain immune responses. Of the variety of hormones that affect lymphoid cells and macrophages, we have specifically chosen to discuss growth hormone and prolactin. This chapter will highlight data which show that growth hormone and prolactin augment many activities of lymphoid and myeloid cells in both *in vitro* and *in vivo* systems. These data are then extended by hypothesizing that the stress-induced, immunosuppressive properties of adrenal glucocorticoids are counterbalanced by the stress-induced increase in prolactin and growth hormone. This idea is entirely consistent with recent results which showed that a protein product of T-lymphocytes, IFN-γ, reverses the suppressive effects of glucocorticoids on the secretion of reactive oxygen intermediates by human mononuclear cells (Szefler et al., 1989; *vide infra*).

In the case of the rat, it is suggested that stress-induced increases in prolactin mimic the effects of growth hormone on the immune system of other species, therefore overcoming the problem of stress reducing the release of growth hormone in this species. Furthermore, an imbalance in the ratio of glucocorticoids to growth hormone/prolactin may lead to either immunosuppression or immunoenhancement and therefore explain the paradoxical

TABLE I.

Restraint Stress Suppresses Evanescent Delayed Hypersensitivity Responses to Sheep Erythrocytes but Augments Contact Sensitivity Reactions to DNFB

Treatment	Sheep Erythrocytes (%)	DNFB (%)
Control	100	100
Restraint	38*	143*
+ Adrenalectomy	100	124*
+ Metyrapone	85	136*

* Indicates statistical difference from control values. (From Blecha et al., 1982. With permission.)

effects of stress on immunity. Although these ideas are clearly speculative, the idea of stress-induced release of protective hormones from the pituitary gland is appealing because it suggests that recovery from immunosuppressive treatments (e.g., glucocorticoids, immunosuppressive viruses) is an active rather than a passive process that is simply associated with healing. This concept also forms a unified theory for explaining the network of communication signals between the immune and neuroendocrine systems that are activated during stress.

STRESS AND AUGMENTATION OF THE IMMUNE RESPONSE

The broad effects of psychological factors on immune responses of both man and animals have recently been summarized (Dantzer and Kelley, 1989; Griffin, 1989), so only specific examples will be used to illustrate the concept that certain stressors can augment immune responses. When mice that have previously been sensitized to an immunizing agent are closely restrained for 2 h and then challenged with this same agent, cell-mediated immune responses to these immunogens can be either suppressed or augmented (Table I). Specific, *in vivo* cellular immune responses to sheep erythrocytes (SRBC) are suppressed, while contact sensitivity responses to dinitrofluorobenzene (DNFB) are significantly augmented. It is therefore clear that effector cells for one type of immune response are differentially affected by immobilization-induced stress. Furthermore, adrenalectomy totally abrogates the immunosuppressive effects of restraint on SRBC responses, whereas there is no significant effect on the restraint-induced augmentation in DNFB reactions. Neither of these effects is mediated by catecholamines because metyrapone, which is an 11-β-hydroxylase inhibitor of corticosterone biosynthesis that does not affect catecholamine synthesis, also abrogates the immunosuppressive effects of restraint on the SRBC response without affecting the potentiation in DNFB contact sensitivity reactions. These data confirm that a stressor such as restraint can suppress one type of cellular immune response and that this suppressive effect is mediated by adrenal glucocorticoids. However, the results also show that even in the presence of high levels of corticosterone, a different type of cellular immune response is enhanced.

A number of recent experiments from other laboratories have also shown that stress can augment certain immune responses. Pain stimuli increase the number of plaque-forming cells that secrete antibodies against sheep erythrocytes (Fujiwara and Orita, 1987). Similarly, handling and exploration of a new cage augments lectin-induced proliferative responses of splenocytes and increases the number of antibody-forming cells in rats, and this enhancement is reversed by passive avoidance conditioning (Croiset et al., 1987; Croiset, 1989). The stress-induced enhancement of plaque-forming cells that was observed by these authors is probably mediated by catecholamines. Chronic exposure to noise and chronic isolation augments lectin-induced proliferative responses of lymphocytes (Monjan and Collector, 1977; Jessop et al., 1987). Separation of mother and infant squirrel monkeys augments the chemiluminescence response of peripheral blood monocytes (Coe et al., 1988). Since chemiluminescence measures the production of reactive oxygen intermediates, and these molecules are very important for killing intracellular pathogens, these observations on neonatal separation are particularly important.

As emphasized above, data such as these indicate that (1) resistance to infectious diseases is not always reduced by stress and in some cases is actually increased and (2) stress can augment a number of immune responses. Since stress-induced immunoenhancement is often observed under chronic stress, this change may be a natural physiologic response that maintains homeostasis and resistance to disease during long-term, adverse situations. Unfortunately, absolutely nothing is known about the mechanisms that may mediate these changes in host resistance. A few years ago, it was speculated that β-endorphin might be an important mediator because it is elevated by certain stressors and augments immune events such as lectin-induced proliferation of lymphocytes and natural killer (NK) cell activity (Kelley, 1985). This speculation remains a possibility, but the effects of opioid peptides on many types of immune responses are often contradictory (reviewed by Sibinga and Goldstein, 1988). A number of other mechanisms are probably involved, such as direct secretion of catecholamines by noradrenergic neurons in lymphoid tissue. We believe that another likely possibility for stress-induced immunoenhancement is that elevations in growth hormone and prolactin augment certain immune events, or at least counteract the immunosuppressive effects of glucocorticoids on cell-mediated immune functions. It is therefore important to discuss the immunomodulatory role of these two hormones in the normal functioning of the immune system.

GROWTH HORMONE, PROLACTIN, AND IMMUNE FUNCTION

The role of growth hormone and prolactin in modulating immune events has recently been reviewed (Kelley, 1991; Berczi and Nagy, 1986, 1987). These reviews specifically address the immunological state of growth hormone-deficient or prolactin-deprived animals and the role of these hormones in thymic development, lymphocyte proliferation, hemopoiesis, and the function of phagocytic cells. These results will not be further discussed here. Instead, specific examples will be used to illustrate the contrasting effects of these hormones and glucocorticoids on a number of immune events.

THYMIC INVOLUTION

The cardinal sign of acute stress is thymic involution. This change is caused by the stress-induced rise in glucocorticoids which leads to lysis of cortical thymocytes. Half a century ago, Hans Selye showed that acute stress caused thymic atrophy and that this effect was mediated by the release of glucocorticoids from the adrenal gland (Selye, 1936a, 1936b). It was subsequently shown that cortical thymocytes of species such as the mouse, rat, and rabbit are very susceptible to the lytic effects of glucocorticoids (Claman, 1972). It is now believed that glucocorticoids cause the death of thymocytes by activating an endogenous pathway within the cell (a calcium-activated endonuclease) that leads to suicide (Ucker, 1987; McConkey et al., 1989).

When ACTH is used to induce thymic involution, regeneration of the thymus gland occurs more rapidly in normal than in hypophysectomized rats (Brolin and Hellman, 1955). This finding could be interpreted to indicate that the pituitary gland produces a hormone that leads to rapid restoration of thymus growth following an acute stress. This interpretation has been directly supported using a different type of endpoint; namely, cortisol-induced leukopenia (Chatterton et al., 1973), which is characterized by a reduction in circulating lymphocytes. In these experiments, it was noted that the leukopenia disappeared within 6 h following cortisol injection into normal rats. However, the cortisol-induced leukopenia remained in hypophysectomized rats, with no return to normal values. Anterior pituitary extracts, as well as partially purified growth hormone, reversed the cortisol-induced leukopenia. These workers concluded that the stress-induced release of growth hormone opposed the leukopenic effects of the stress-induced rise in corticosterone.

One of the earliest reported immunological effects of growth hormone was to increase size of the thymus gland. Hypophysectomy leads to thymic involution (Smith, 1930), and both growth hormone (Shrewsbury and Reinhardt, 1959; Pandian and Talwar, 1971; Li and Evans, 1948) and prolactin

(Berczi and Nagy, 1986) partially reverse this effect of hypophysectomy. Indeed, purified growth hormone and growth-hormone secreting cells can even induce normal growth of thymus glands that are atrophied in old animals (Kelley et al., 1986; Roth et al., 1984; Goff et al., 1987; Monroe et al., 1987). Since growth hormone declines with age, it could be that this decline is causally related to involution of the thymus gland.

These data clearly support the idea that glucocorticoids lead to thymic atrophy while growth hormone and probably prolactin promote thymic growth. The classic sign of acute stress is thymic involution, and the thymus often returns to normal size soon after cessation of the stress. It is possible that the stress-induced release of both growth hormone and prolactin antagonize the thymolytic effects of glucocorticoids, although this experiment has not yet been reported. Similarly, both growth hormone and prolactin probably participate in stress-induced recovery by causing a repopulation of cells within the cortical region of the thymus gland that occurs after the stressful episode ceases.

ANTIBODY SYNTHESIS

A number of different kinds of stressors have been shown to suppress antibody synthesis (reviewed by Kelley, 1980), and the use of antibody production to a specific ligand to measure the immunosuppressive properties of stress has recently been emphasized (Laudenslager et al., 1988). The classic experiment that tested potential antagonisms between pituitary hormones on antibody synthesis was reported in 1971 by Gisler and Schenkel-Hulliger (Table II). These workers demonstrated that either acute stress, ACTH injections, or hypophysectomy caused a reduction in the capability of murine spleen cells to synthesize and secrete antibodies to a defined antigen *in vitro*. Growth hormone restored this immunodeficiency in hypophysectomized mice, and a significant growth hormone-induced recovery occurred even when hypophysectomized animals were injected with ACTH. Similar results were observed *in vivo* by Hayashida and Li (1957), who showed that growth hormone could reverse the defect in both growth rate and antibody synthesis to a Pasteurella antigen that was caused by injecting ACTH into normal rats (Table III). These experiments offer direct proof for antagonism between two pituitary hormones that are responsive to acute stress: ACTH, acting via adrenal glucocorticoids, suppresses antibody synthesis whereas growth hormone reverses this effect.

Since growth hormone declines in the blood of rats following acute stress, it can be argued that elevated levels of this hormone do not promote recovery from the immunosuppressive effects of glucocorticoids in this species. However, two other explanations can be offered to explain the case of the rat. (1)

TABLE II.

Growth Hormone Reverses Suppression in Antibody Synthesis *In Vitro* Caused by Hypophysectomy, Even After Injection of ACTH

Treatment	Plaque-Forming Cells/10^6 Cells
Normal mice	750
Hypophysectomized mice + saline	35
Hypophysectomized mice + bovine growth hormone	500
Hypophysectomized mice + bovine growth hormone + ACTH	250

Note: Hypophysectomy significantly reduced the number of plaque-forming cells, and growth hormone augmented this response in both the presence and absence of ACTH. (From Gisler and Schenkel-Hulliger, 1971. With permission.)

TABLE III.

Antagonistic Effects of Growth Hormone and ACTH on Antibody Synthesis to *Pasteurella pestis* in Normal Rats

Treatment	Change in Body Weight (g)	Antibody Titer (base$_{10}$)
Control	20.3	2.2
Growth Hormone	60.4	2.6
ACTH	−2.1	1.3
Growth Hormone + ACTH	34.6	1.9

Note: ACTH significantly suppressed growth rate and antibody synthesis, and this suppression was significantly reveresed by growth hormone. (From Hayashida and Li, 1957. With permission.)

It is likely that the closely-related hormone, prolactin, may serve the role of growth hormone on immune events following stress. Growth hormone (191 amino acids) and prolactin (199 amino acids) share substantial homology at the amino acid level, and they arose by gene duplication nearly 400 million years ago. Receptors for both of these hormones also appear to have been derived from a common ancestral gene. It is suggested that the stress-induced rise in prolactin is responsible for reversing the immunosuppressive effects of ACTH treatment in the rat *(vide infra)*. (2) A more speculative possibility is that the reduction in growth hormone following acute stress in rats is short-lived, as suggested by the rapid compensatory growth response shown by rats following stress. It could be that rats, as other species, show a heightened compensatory growth hormone response that follows the stress-induced reduction in growth hormone.

The original experiments by Istvan Berczi and colleagues have clearly shown that prolactin shares many of the immunological effects of growth hormone. An early report from his group (Nagy and Berczi, 1978) showed that completely hypophysectomized rats display a generalized immuno-deficiency, such as prolonged skin graft survival, suppressed contact sensitivity reactions, and reduced primary and secondary antibody responses to T-dependent antigens (sheep erythrocytes). These suppressed immune responses in hypophysectomized rats can be totally reversed by syngeneic pituitary grafts (which primarily secrete prolactin and some growth hormone) or pituitary-derived prolactin or growth hormone of rat, human or bovine origin (Nagy et al., 1981, 1983a; Berczi et al., 1981). Similarly, when prolactin release is inhibited by the dopamine type 2 agonist, bromocryptine, antibody synthesis, contact sensitivity reactions, and the development of adjuvant-induced arthritis are inhibited (Nagy et al., 1983b; Berczi and Nagy, 1982; Berczi et al., 1984). Others have also shown that complete hypophysectomy suppresses antibody synthesis (Cross et al., 1987) and that growth hormone can reverse this defect (Pandian and Talwar, 1971).

These data show that a reduction in plasma levels of pituitary hormones by hypophysectomy, or in plasma prolactin by bromocryptine, suppresses antibody synthesis, contact sensitivity reactions, and adjuvant-induced arthritis. All of these responses in rats can be reversed by injections of either growth hormone or prolactin. However, the studies by Berczi and colleagues also revealed that the immunopotentiating properties of both growth hormone and prolactin can be inhibited by injections of ACTH, while other experiments (Tables II and III) suggest that growth hormone can effectively counteract the effects of ACTH. One might therefore speculate that the immunosuppressive properties of glucocorticoids are more potent than the enhancing effects of growth hormone and prolactin. This would be consistent with the finding that the immunoenhancing properties of exogenous growth hormone and prolactin are easier to demonstrate in hypophysectomized (with low levels of glucocorticoids) than in normal animals. It is more likely to postulate that growth hormone aids in the recovery of immunological tissues after an insult caused by a stress-induced rise in glucocorticoids. In the rat, prolactin mimics this property of growth hormone. Therefore, even though growth hormone and prolactin may not directly antagonize the immunosuppressive effects of glucocorticoids, they certainly may act to restore the damage to lymphoid and myeloid cells that is caused by glucocorticoids.

NATURAL KILLER CELLS

Glucocorticoids suppress the activity of NK cells (Hochman and Cudkowicz, 1979; Holbrook et al., 1983; Onsrud and Thorsby, 1981), an effect which may be mediated by glucocorticoid inhibition of the synthesis of IL-2. Similarly, certain stressors inhibit the activity of splenic NK cells in rodents (Shavit et al., 1984; Pollock et al., 1987; Cunnick et al., 1988; Keller et al., 1988), and this suppression is mediated by the stress-induced release of corticosterone (Keller et al., 1988). Hypophysectomy reduces the activity of NK cells (Cross et al., 1984; Keller et al., 1988), and this defect is significantly reversed by treatment with growth hormone (Saxena et al., 1982). Similarly, activity of NK cells and plasma concentrations of growth hormone decline with age. Injection of growth hormone augments NK cell activity in both aged rats (Davila et al., 1987) and humans (Crist et al., 1987). Growth hormone may be essential for normal development of NK cells as well as for augmenting cytolytic activity. Kiess et al. (1988) recently demonstrated that the activity of NK cells is suppressed in growth hormone-deficient children. However, these cells did not respond to *in vivo* treatments with growth hormone, growth hormone-releasing hormone, and IFN-α, which suggests that there is a defect in the development or activation of NK cells in growth hormone-deficient patients.

These experiments demonstrate that both stress and glucocorticoids inhibit the activity of NK cells, that the pituitary is needed for optimal development of NK cells and NK cell activity, and that growth hormone augments NK cell activity in both hypophysectomized and aged animals. It is as yet unknown whether prolactin shares this property of growth hormone, and whether growth hormone or prolactin can reverse the suppressive effect of glucocorticoids on the activity of NK cells.

ACTIVATED MACROPHAGES

Macrophages are essential for almost all types of immune responses. They not only participate in host defense against a variety of microorganisms, such as obligate intracellular bacteria, but they are essential for the bidirectional cellular interactions with T-and B-lymphocytes that control humoral and cellular immune functions. An important concept in macrophage immunology is that these cells can be specifically activated to nonspecifically kill intracellular bacteria. Macrophages from animals that are infected with a gram positive bacterium, such as *Listeria monocytogenes,* will kill other bacteria as well (e.g., Salmonella, Chlamydia) and even protozoa (e.g., Trypanosomes) and fungi (e.g., Candida). Activated macrophages also nonspecifically kill tumor cells. Therefore, it is important to learn whether stress and neuropeptides affect functional activities of activated macrophages.

The mechanisms by which macrophages become activated to nonspecifically kill intracellular bacteria and cancer cells are still being elucidated. Although other cytokines are now known to prime macrophages (e.g., IL-4,

TNF-α), it is generally recognized that a protein secreted by antigen-stimulated T-lymphocytes, known as interferon-γ, is the prototype molecule for inducing activation of macrophages. Glucocorticoids suppress the production of IFN-γ (Kelso and Munck, 1984; Arya et al., 1984). It is also known that glucocorticoids inhibit the synthesis of proteins by macrophages, such as IL-1, TNF-α, and the expression of class II genes of the major histocompatibility complex (Snyder and Unanue, 1982; Beutler et al., 1986; Szefler et al., 1989). Glucocorticoids also inhibit phagocytosis and intracellular killing of some microorganisms (Masur et al., 1982; Rinehart et al., 1974, 1975). In both human monocytes and polymorphonuclear granulocytes, the inhibition of intracellular killing may be mediated by a reduction in the respiratory burst and the subsequent production of reactive oxygen intermediates (Chretien and Garagusi, 1972; Szefler et al., 1989; Dunham et al., 1990).

Macrophages and granulocytes can be triggered by a number of agents to produce a respiratory burst (Johnston, 1988), which is characterized by the consumption of oxygen and the generation of toxic metabolites, including superoxide anion (O_2^-) and hydrogen peroxide (H_2O_2). Phagocytic cells can be primed by agents such as IFN-γ to produce enhanced amounts of these microbicidal oxygen metabolites. We recently demonstrated that growth hormone can prime phagocytes *in vitro* and when injected into hypophysectomized rats *in vivo* produces heightened amounts of (Edwards et al., 1988a; Fu et al., 1991). Preliminary data indicate that prolactin may share this same property (Edwards et al., 1988b). Since growth hormone and prolactin appear to be synthesized by leukocytes (Hiestand et al., 1986; Montgomery et al., 1987; Weigent et al., 1988), it is interesting to speculate that these hormones have the potential of counteracting the suppressive effects of glucocorticoids on the production of reactive oxygen intermediates by phagocytic cells. If so, both growth hormone and prolactin would share with IFN-γ (Szefler et al., 1989; Dunham et al., 1990) the capability of overcoming the glucocorticoid-induced inhibition of priming for H_2O_2 release from human monocytes.

Macrophages can also be primed by IFN-γ to produce increased quantities of TNF-α. New data from our laboratory show that growth hormone shares this property with IFN-γ when injected into hypophysectomized rats (Edwards et al., 1991). However, in contrast to IFN-γ, growth hormone does not prime rat peritoneal macrophages when incubated with these cells *in vitro*. The potential role of prolactin in regulating the synthesis of TNF-α *in vivo,* and the possibility that growth hormone and/or prolactin can antagonize the suppressive effects of glucocorticoids *in vivo,* are unknown.

When serum concentrations of prolactin are continuously suppressed by treatment with bromocryptine, peritoneal cells do not develop into effective tumoricidal macrophages (Bernton et al., 1988). However, if bromocryptine-treated mice are given an exogenous source of prolactin, tumoricidal activity of peritoneal macrophages is completely restored. A conditioned supernatant

made from splenocytes of BCG-infected mice and then stimulated with purified protein derivative reverses the defect in tumoricidal macrophages from
bromocryptine-treated mice. This finding suggests that the defect is not in the
macrophage, but, rather, in the development of T-cell-derived macrophage
activating factors. Since IFN-γ is well-known to prime macrophages for
enhanced production of reactive oxygen intermediates, Bernton et al. (1988)
speculated that the synthesis of this protein is affected by bromocryptine.
They found that IFN-γ synthesis by appropriately stimulated splenocytes was
dramatically reduced in mice that were treated with this D-2 agonist, and that
this suppression was reversed by injections of prolactin. These results demonstrate that the synthesis of a very important macrophage priming agent,
IFN-γ, is suppressed in hypoprolactinemic mice, and that prolactin can amel-
iorate this suppression. Since psychosocial stress (examinations) suppresses
IFN-γ synthesis in medical students (Glaser et al., 1987), and this suppression
returns to normal after the examinations, it could be that prolactin is involved
in the recovery of IFN-γ synthesis.

LYMPHOCYTE PROLIFERATION

Using the drug bromocryptine, Bernton et al. (1988) demonstrated that
splenocytes from hypoprolactinemic mice had reduced proliferative responses
to concanavalin A, phytohemagglutinin, and lipopolysaccharide. This
suppression could be significantly (although only partially) reversed by the
in vivo administration of either ovine or murine prolactin. Neither bromocryptine nor prolactin affected the percentage of B-, T-helper, or T-suppressor
lymphocytes.

The role of growth hormone in lymphocyte proliferation is equivocal,
with some investigators reporting increases, decreases, and no change (reviewed by Kelley, 1989). However, synthetic glucocorticoids are well known
to suppress almost all cell-mediated immune events. For example, glucocorticoids inhibit the synthesis of IL-2 (Gillis et al., 1979; Kelso and Munck,
1984), expression of IL-2 receptors (Reed et al., 1986), and synthesis of IFN-
γ and colony stimulating factor (Kelso and Munck, 1984), and these effects
are mediated by inhibiting the accumulation of messenger RNA for these
cytokines (Arya et al., 1984). Natural glucocorticoids, at physiological concentrations, also inhibit lectin-induced proliferation of lymphoid cells in domestic animals (Blecha and Baker, 1986; Westly and Kelley, 1984; Franklin
et al., 1987).

It is as yet unknown whether the suppressive effects of glucocorticoids
on lymphoid cell proliferation are affected by either growth hormone or
prolactin. However, Keller et al. (1988) provided direct proof that the pituitary

gland produces a factor that antagonizes the suppressive effect of shock on the lectin-induced proliferation of peripheral blood lymphocytes from rats (Table IV). In these experiments, shock significantly suppressed lymphocyte proliferation in both groups of animals with pituitary glands. The magnitude of this suppression in the sham hypophysectomized animals was 44%, but the suppression was nearly doubled in hypophysectomized rats (79%). As the authors suggested, these data indicate that the pituitary gland produces something that counteracts the immunosuppressive effects of shock. We suggest that this pituitary product is either growth hormone or prolactin.

HEMOPOIESIS

All cells in the blood are derived from common multipotential progenitor stem cells in the bone marrow. Specific precursor cells proliferate and differentiate along defined pathways to each of the eight lineages of blood cells. This process is known as differentiation-commitment, and it occurs only in the presence of specific glycoproteins known as hemopoietic growth factors (Metcalf, 1989). Hypophysectomized rats develop a reduction in the number of peripheral blood leukocytes, erythrocytes, and platelets. Nagy and Berczi (1989) recently demonstrated that both growth hormone and prolactin can reverse the leukopenia, anemia, and thrombocytopenia that occur in hypophysectomized rats. Similar results have also been reported for growth hormone in human hypopituitary dwarfs (Jepson and McGarry, 1972). These data led Nagy and Berczi (1989) to speculate that both growth hormone and prolactin can act as competence signals for bone marrow cells. In this model, these hormones would have no effect on inducing the differentiation of hemato-

TABLE IV.

The Pituitary Gland Produces a Factor That Protects Rats Against Stress-Induced Suppression in Peripheral Blood Lymphocytes Stimulated with Phytohemagglutinin

Treatment	^{3}H-Thymidine Incorporation (cpm)		% Change
	No Shock	Shock	
Nonoperated	100,000	40,000	60
Sham hypophysectomy	100,000	56,000	44
Hypophysectomy	14,000*	3,000*	79

* Significantly lower incorporation of ^{3}-thymidine when compared to rats with pituitary glands.
The concentration of phytohemagglutinin was 3.2 μg per culture. (From Keller et al., 1988. With permission.)

poietic colonies from myeloid progenitors. Consistent with current ideas (Metcalf, 1989), this event is controlled by growth factors such as colony-stimulating factor-1 and granulocyte/macrophage colony-stimulating factor (GM-CSF). However, even though pituitary hormones have no effect on the differentiation-commitment process which is caused by specific hemopoietic growth factors, they are able to act as competence factors to enhance the effect of these commitment factors. Therefore, growth hormone and prolactin would act as permissive competence hormones with significant synergizing activity with hemopoietic growth factors.

These ideas are in accord with recent findings that recombinant human growth hormone significantly augments the maturation of cells of the granulocyte and erythroid series in human marrow mononuclear cells (Merchav et al., 1988a, 1988b; Claustres et al., 1987). Growth hormone does not affect colony formation in the absence of GM-CSF or erythropoietin. It is unknown whether growth hormone or prolactin can antagonize any potential direct effect of glucocorticoids on stem cells or any indirect effects on the synthesis of specific differentiating factors.

CONCLUSION

Certain stressors increase the resistance of animals to infectious diseases and also augment a number of immune responses. Although glucocorticoids mediate many of the immunosuppressive effects of stress, little is known about the physiologic mechanisms that mediate stress-induced immunoenhancement. Stress increases the circulating concentrations of both growth hormone and prolactin in most animal species. In this chapter, it is hypothesized that both of these hormones can counteract the immunosuppressive effects of glucocorticoids, and therefore participate in stress-induced recovery of the immune system. Direct proof has been obtained which shows that growth hormone can reverse the immunosuppressive effects of glucocorticoids on antibody synthesis. Similar results suggest that growth hormone and/or prolactin accelerate repopulation of the cortical thymocytes following stress-induced thymic involution. A number of other immunological events are augmented by growth hormone and/or prolactin and are suppressed by glucocorticoids (Table V), but it is not yet known whether these pituitary hormones can block the immunosuppressive effects of glucocorticoids. It is concluded that the neuroendocrine system is a major participant in maintaining homeostasis of the immune system following infectious episodes, and these effects are mediated by the pituitary gland secreting hormones that have dual activities of augmenting and suppressing a variety of immune events. The concept of the pituitary gland secreting hormones that promote the recovery of cells of the immune system after a pathological insult provides fascinating

TABLE V.
Counteracting Effects of the Immunosuppressive Properties of Glucocorticoids and the Immunoenhancing Effects of Growth Hormone and Prolactin on Activities of Lymphocytes and Macrophages

Immune Event
Thymic Size
Antibody Synthesis
NK Activity
Activated Macrophages
Superoxide anion
Tumoricidal macrophages
IFN-γ synthesis
TNF-α synthesis
Lymphocyte proliferation
Hemopoiesis

Note: See text for discussion.

insights into the complex mechanisms which animals and humans use to maintain homeostasis.

ACKNOWLEDGMENTS

Partially supported by Grants from the National Institutes of Health (National Institute on Aging AG06246), Office of Naval Research (N00014-89-J-1956), and the U.S. Department of Agriculture (86-CRCR-1-2003).

REFERENCES

Arya SK, Wong-Staal F, and Gallo RC: Dexamethasone-mediated inhibition of human T cell growth factor and γ-interferon messenger RNA. *J Immunol* 1984; 133:273.

Berczi I and Nagy E: A possible role of prolactin in adjuvant arthritis. *Arthritis Rheum* 1982; 25:591.

Berczi I, Nagy E, Asa SL, and Kovacs K: The influence of pituitary hormones on adjuvant arthritis. *Arthritis Rheum* 1984; 27:682.

Berczi I and Nagy E: Prolactin and other lactogenic hormones. In *Pituitary Function and Immunity*. Berczi I, Ed. CRC Press, Boca Raton, FL, 1986, pp. 161–183.

Berczi I and Nagy E: The effect of prolactin and growth hormone on hemolymphopoietic tissue and immune function. In *Hormones and Immunity*. Berczi I and Kovacs K, Eds. MTP Press, Lancaster, 1987, pp. 145–171.

Berczi I, Nagy E, Kovacs K, and Horvath E: Regulation of humoral immunity in rats by pituitary hormones. *Acta Endocrinol* 1981; 98:506.

Bernton EW, Meltzer MS, and Holaday JW: Suppression of macrophage activation and T-lymphocyte function in hypoprolactinemic mice. *Science* 1988; 239:401.

Beutler B, Krochin N, Milsark IW, Luedke C, and Cerami A: Control of cachectin (tumor necrosis factor) synthesis: mechanisms of endotoxin resistance. *Science* 1986; 232:977.

Blalock JE: A molecular basis for bidirectional communication between the immune and neuroendocrine systems. *Physiol Rev* 1989; 69:1.

Blecha F and Baker PE: Effect of cortisol *in vitro* and *in vivo* on production of bovine interleukin 2. *Am J Vet Res* 1986; 47:841.

Blecha F, Kelley KW, and Satterlee DG: Adrenal involvement in the expression of delayed-type hypersensitivity to SRBC and contact sensitivity to DNFB in mice. *Proc Soc Exp Biol Med* 1982; 169:239.

Brolin SE and Hellman B: An experimental procedure applied to test the reaction of the thymus after hypophysectomy. *Acta Pathol Microbiol Scand* 1955; 37:414.

Chatterton RT Jr, Murray CL, and Hellman L: Endocrine effects of leukocytopoiesis in the rat. I. Evidence for growth hormone secretion as the leukocytopoietic stimulus following acute cortisol-induced lymphopenia. *Endocrinology* 1973; 92:775.

Chretien JH and Garagusi VF: Corticosteroid effect on phagocytosis and NBT reduction by human polymorphonuclear neutrophils. *J Reticuloendothel Soc* 1972; 11:358.

Claman HN: Corticosteroids and lymphoid cells. *New Engl J Med* 1972; 287:388.

Claustres M, Chatelain P, and Sultan C: Insulin-like growth factor I stimulates human erythroid colony formation *in vitro*. *J Clin Endocrinol Metab* 1987; 65:78.

Coe CL, Rosenberg LT, and Levine S: Prolonged effect of psychological disturbance on macrophage chemiluminescence in the squirrel monkey. *Brain Behav Immun* 1988; 2:151.

Crist DM, Peake GT, MacKinnon LT, Sibbit WL Jr, and Kraner JC: Exogenous growth hormone treatment alters body composition and increases natural killer cell activity in women with impaired endogenous growth hormone secretion. *Metabolism* 1987; 36:1115.

Croiset G: *The Impact of Emotional Stimuli on the Immune System*. Rudolf Magnus Institute, Het Wilhelmina Kinderziekenhuis, Utrecht (Proefschrift), 1989, pp. 1–111.

Croiset G, Heijnen CJ, Dick Veldhuis H, de Wied D, and Ballieux RE: Modulation of the immune response by emotional stress. *Life Sci* 1987; 40:775.

Cross RJ, Brooks WH, and Roszman TL: Modulation of T-suppressor cell activity by central nervous system catecholamine depletion. *J Neurosci Res* 1987; 18:75.

Cross RJ, Markesbery WR, Brooks WH, and Roszman TL: Hypothalamic-immune interactions. Neuromodulation of natural killer activity by lesioning of the anterior hypothalamus. *Immunology* 1984; 51:399.

Cunnick JE, Lysle DT, Armfield A, and Rabin BS: Shock-induced modulation of lymphocyte responsiveness and natural killer activity: differential mechanisms of induction. *Brain Behav Immun* 1988; 2:102.

Dantzer R and Kelley KW: Stress and immunity: an integrated view of relationships between the brain and the immune system. *Life Sci* 1989; 44:1995.

Davila DR, Brief S, Simon J, Hammer RE, Brinster RL, and Kelley KW: Role of growth hormone in regulating T-dependent immune events in aged, nude, and transgenic rodents. *J Neurosci Res* 1987; 18:108.

Denckla WD: Interactions between age and the neuroendocrine and immune systems. *Fed Proc* 1978; 37:1263.

Dunham DM, Arkins S, Edwards CK III, Dantzer R, and Kelley KW: Role of interferon-γ in counteracting the suppressive effects of transforming growth factor-B2 and glucorticoids on the production of tumor necrosis factor-α. *J Leukocyte Biology* 1990, 48:473.

Edwards CK III, Ghiasuddin SM, Schepper JM, Yunger LM, and Kelley KW: A newly defined property of somatotropin: priming of macrophages for production of superoxide anion. *Science* 1988a; 239:769.

Edwards CK III, Lorence RM, Dunham DM, Arkins S, Yunger LM, Greager JA, Walter RJ, Dantzer R, and Kelley KW: Hypophysectomy inhibits the synthesis of tumor necrosis factor-α by rat macrophages: partial restoration by exogenous growth hormone or interferon-γ. *Endocrinology* 1991, 128:989.

Edwards CK III, Schepper JM, Yunger LM, and Kelley KW: Somatotropin and prolactin enhance respiratory burst activity of macrophages. *Ann NY Acad Sci* 1988b; 540:698.

Franklin RA, Davila DR, and Kelley KW: Chicken serum inhibits lectin-induced proliferation of autologous splenic mononuclear cells. *Proc Soc Exp Biol Med* 1987; 184:225.

Fu YK, Arkins S, Wang BS, and Kelley KW: A novel role of growth hormone and insulin-like growth factor-I: Priming neutrophils for superoxide anion secretion. *J Immunol* 1991, 146:1602.

Gillis S, Crabtree GR, and Smith KA: Glucocorticoid-induced inhibition of T cell growth factor production. II. The effect on the *in vitro* generation of cytolytic T cells. *J Immunol* 1979; 123:1632.

Gisler RH and Schenkel-Hulliger L: Hormonal regulation of the immune response. II. Influence of pituitary and adrenal activity on immune responsiveness in vitro. *Cell Immunol* 1971; 2:646.

Glaser R, Rice J, Sheridan J, Fertel R, Stout J, Speicher C, Pinsky D, Kotur M, Post A, Beck M, and Kiecolt-Glaser KK: Stress-related immune suppression: health implications. *Brain Behav Immun* 1987; 1:7.

Goff BL, Roth JA, Arp LH, and Incefy GS: Growth hormone treatment stimulates thymulin production in aged dogs. *Clin Exp Immunol* 1987; 68:580.

Griffin JFT: Stress and immunity: a unifying concept. *Vet Immunol Immunopathol* 1989; 20:263.

Gross WB: Effect of social stress on occurrence of Marek's disease in chickens. *Am J Vet Res* 1972; 33:2275.

Gross WB: Plasma steroid tendency, social isolation and *Eimeria necatrix* infection. *Poult Sci* 1976; 55:1508.

Gross WB: Effect of adrenal blocking chemicals on viral and respiratory infections of chickens. *Can J Vet Res* 1989; 53:48.

Gross WB and Colmano G: The effect of social isolation on resistance to some infectious diseases. *Poult Sci* 1969; 48:514.

Gross WB and Colmano G: Effect of infectious agents on chickens selected for plasma corticosterone response to social stress. *Poult Sci* 1971; 50:1213.

Hall RD and Gross WB: Effect of social stress and inherited plasma corticosterone levels in chickens on populations of northern fowl mites, *Ornithonyssus sylviarum*. *J Parasitol* 1975; 61:1096.

Hayashida T and Li CH: The influence of adrenocorticotropic and growth hormones on antibody formation. *J Exp Med* 1957; 105:93.

Hiestand PC, Mekler P, Nordmann R, Grieder A, and Permmongkol C: Prolactin as a modulator of lymphocyte responsiveness provides a possible mechanism of action for cyclosporine. *Proc Natl Acad Sci USA* 1986; 83:2599.

Hochman PS and Cudkowicz G: Suppression of natural cytotoxicity by spleen cells of hydrocortisone-treated mice. *J Immunol* 1979; 123:968.

Holbrook NJ, Cox WI, and Horner HC: Direct suppression of natural killer activity in human peripheral blood leukocyte cultures by glucocorticoids and its modulation by interferon. *Cancer Res* 1983; 43:4019.

Jepson JH and McGarry EE: Hemopoiesis in pituitary dwarfs treated with human growth hormone and testosterone. *Blood* 1972; 39:238.

Jessop JJ, Gale K, and Bayer BM: Enhancement of rat lymphocyte proliferation after prolonged exposure to stress. *J Neuroimmunol* 1987; 16:261.

Johnston RB Jr: Current concepts: immunology—monocytes and macrophages. *N Engl J Med* 1988; 318:747.

Keller SE, Schleifer SJ, Liotta AS, Bond RN, Farhoody N, and Stein M: Stress-induced alterations of immunity in hypophysectomized rats. *Proc Natl Acad Sci USA* 1988; 85:9297.

Keller SE, Weiss JM, Miller NE, and Stein M: Stress-induced suppression of immunity in adrenalectomized rats. *Science* 1983; 221:1301.

Kelley KW: Stress and immune function. A bibliographic review. *Ann Rech Vet* 1980; 11:445.

Kelley KW: Immunological consequences of changing environmental stimuli. In *Animal Stress*. Moberg GP, Ed. American Physiological Society, Bethesda, 1985, pp. 193–223.

Kelley KW: Growth hormone, lymphocytes and macrophages. *Biochem Pharmacol* 1989; 38:705.

Kelley KW: Growth hormone in immunobiology. In *Psychoneuroimmunology II*. 2nd ed. Ader R, Felten D, and Cohen N, Eds. Academic Press Inc., New York, 1991, pp. 377–402.

Kelley KW, Brief S, Westly HJ, Novakofski J, Bechtel PJ, Simon J, and Walker EB: GH$_3$ pituitary adenoma cells can reverse thymic aging in rats. *Proc Natl Acad Sci U.S.A.* 1986; 83:5663.

Kelso A and Munck A: Glucocorticoid inhibition of lymphokine secretion by alloreactive T lymphocyte clones. *J Immunol* 1984; 133:784.

Kiess W, Malozowski S, Gelato M, Butenand O, Doerr H, Crisp B, Eisl E, Maluish A, and Belohradsky BH: Lymphocyte subset distribution and natural killer activity in growth hormone deficiency before and during short-term treatment with growth hormone releasing hormone. *Clin Immunol Immunopathol* 1988; 48:85.

Laudenslager ML, Fleshner M, Hofstadter P, Held PE, Simons L, and Maier SF: Suppression of specific antibody production by inescapable shock: Stability under varying conditions. *Brain Behav Immun* 1988; 2:92.

Li CH and Evans HM: The biochemistry of pituitary growth hormone. *Recent Prog Horm Res* 1948; 3:3.

McConkey DJ, Hartzell P, Nicotera P, and Orrenius S: Calcium-activated DNA fragmentation kills immature thymocytes. *FASEB J* 1989; 3:1843.

Merchav S, Tatarsky I, and Hochberg Z: Enhancement of human granulopoiesis *in vitro* by biosynthetic insulin-like growth factor I/somatomedin C and human growth hormone. *J Clin Invest* 1988a; 81:791.

Merchav S, Tatarsky I, and Hochberg Z: Enhancement of erythropoiesis *in vitro* by human growth hormone is mediated by insulin-like growth factor I. *Br J Haematol* 1988b; 70:267.

Masur H, Murray HW, and Jones TC: Effect of hydrocortisone on macrophage response to lymphokine. *Infect Immun* 1982; 35:709.

Metcalf D: The molecular control of cell division, differentiation commitment and maturation in haemopoietic cells. *Nature* 1989; 339:27.

Monjan AA and Collector MJ: Stress induced modulation of immune response. *Science* 1977; 196:307.

Monroe WE, Roth JA, Grier RL, Arp LH, and Naylor PH: Effects of growth hormone on the adult canine thymus. *Thymus* 1987; 9:173.

Montgomery DW, Zukoski CF, Shah GN, Buckley AR, Pacholczyk T, and Haddock Russell D: Concanavalin A-stimulated murine splenocytes produce a factor with prolactin-like bioactivity and immunoreactivity. *Biochem Biophys Res Commun* 1987; 145:692.

Nagy E and Berczi I: Prolactin and contact sensitivity. *Allergy* 1981; 36:429.

Nagy E and Berczi I: Immunodeficiency in hypophysectomized rats. *Acta Endocrinol* 1978; 89:530.

Nagy E and Berczi I: Pituitary dependence of bone marrow function. *Br J Haematol* 1989, 71:457.

Nagy E, Berczi I, and Friesen HG: Regulation of immunity in rats by lactogenic and growth hormones. *Acta Endocrinol* 1983a; 102:351.

Nagy E, Berczi I, Wren GE, Asa SL, and Kovacs K: Immunomodulation by bromocriptine. *Immunopharmacology* 1983b; 6:231.

Onsrud M and Thorsby E: Influences of *in vivo* hydrocortisone on some human blood lymphocyte subpopulations. I. Effect on natural killer cell activity. *Scand J Immunol* 1981; 13:573.

Pandian MR and Talwar GP: Effect of growth hormone on the metabolism of thymus and on the immune response against sheep erythrocytes. *J Exp Med* 1971; 134:1095.

Pollock RE, Lotzova E, Stanford SD, and Romsdahl MM: Effect of surgical stress on murine natural killer cell cytotoxicity. *J Immunol* 1987; 138:171.

Reed JC, Abidi AH, Alpers JD, Hoover RG, Robb RJ, and Nowell PC: Effect of cyclosporin A and dexamethasone on interleukin 2 receptor gene expression. *J Immunol* 1986; 137:150.

Rinehart JJ, Balcerzak SP, Sagone AL, and LoBuglio AF: Effects of corticosteroids on human monocyte function. *J Clin Invest* 1974; 54:1337.

Rinehart JJ, Sagone AL, Balcerzak SP, Ackerman GA, and LoBuglio AF: Effects of corticosteroid therapy in human monocyte function. *N Engl J Med* 1975; 292:236.

Roth JA, Kaeberle ML, Grier RL, Hopper JG, Spiegel HE, and McAllister HA: Improvement in clinical condition and thymus morphologic features associated with growth hormone treatment of immunodeficient dwarf dogs. *Am J Vet Res* 1984; 45:1151.

Saxena QB, Saxena RK, and Adler WH: Regulation of natural killer activity *in vivo*. III. Effect of hypophysectomy and growth hormone treatment on the natural killer activity of the mouse spleen cell population. *Int Arch Allergy Appl Immunol* 1982; 67:169.

Selye H: A syndrome produced by diverse nocuous agents. *Nature* 1936a; 138:32.

Selye H: Thymus and adrenals in the response of the organism to injuries and intoxications. *Br J Exp Pathol* 1936b; 17:234.

Shavit Y, Lewis JW, Terman GW, Gale RP, and Liebeskind JC: Opioid peptides mediate the suppressive effect of stress on natural killer cell cytotoxicity. *Science* 1984; 223:188.

Shrewsbury MM and Reinhardt WO: Effect of pituitary growth hormone on lymphatic tissues, thoracic duct lymph flow, lymph protein and lymphocyte output in the rat. *Endocrinology* 1959; 65:858.

Snyder DS and Unanue ER: Corticosteroids inhibit murine macrophage Ia expression and interleukin 1 production. *J Immunol* 1982; 129:1803.

Sibinga, NES and Goldstein A: Opioid peptides and opioid receptors in cells of the immune system. *Annu Rev Immunol 1988; 6:219.*

Szefler SJ, Norton CE, Ball B, Gross JM, Aida Y, and Pabst MJ: IFN-γ and LPS overcome glucocorticoid inhibition of priming for superoxide release in human monocytes: evidence that secretion of IL-1 and tumor necrosis factor-α is not essential for monocyte priming. *J Immunol* 1989; 142:3985.

Ucker DS: Cytotoxic T lymphocytes and glucocorticoids activate an endogenous suicide process in target cells. *Nature* 1987; 327:62.

Westly HJ and Kelley KW: Physiologic concentrations of cortisol suppress cell-mediated immune events in the domestic pig. *Proc Soc Exp Biol Med* 1984; 177:156.

Chapter
29

Neurohormones, Serotonin, and Their Receptors in the Immune System

E.M. Smith, D.V. Harbour, T.K. Hughes, T. Kent,
M.J. Ebaugh, A. Jazayeri, and W.J. Meyer, III
Departments of Psychiatry and Behavioral Sciences, Microbiology,
Neurology, and Human Biological Chemistry and Genetics
University of Texas Medical Branch
Galveston, Texas

INTRODUCTION

The endocrine, nervous, and immune systems communicate intrasystemically through a variety of signal molecules, generally referred to as neurotransmitters and lymphokines, respectively. It appears these same signal molecules may be used for communication between the two systems as well. Other chapters in this book have discussed the best-characterized molecules, the endogenous opiates and interleukin-1 (IL-1). This chapter will attempt to broaden this perspective by reviewing the evidence that many other pituitary and hypothalamic hormones, plus serotonin, play a role in neural-immune communication.

The relevance of these less-characterized peptides is beginning to become evident. For instance, the hypothalamic peptide, thyrotropin-releasing hormone (TRH), will stimulate lymphocytes *in vitro* to produce thyrotropin (TSH) (Harbour et al., 1988, 1989). TSH has been found previously to enhance the *in vitro* antibody response (Blalock et al., 1984). At that time, significant concentrations of TRH were thought to be only in the portal circulation. This made it questionable whether there was sufficient TRH in the periphery to

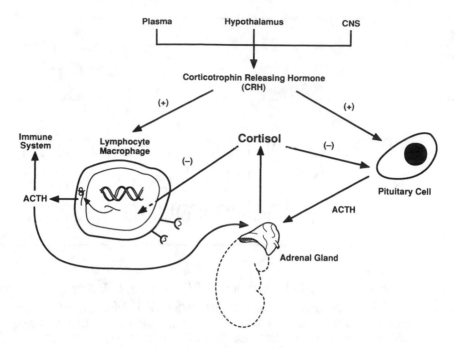

Figure 1. A putative scheme of interactions between the hypothalamic-pituitary-adrenal axis and the immune system.

have a significant impact on immune function *in vivo*. With more extensive investigation, TRH and its precursor have been found in many peripheral organs, but especially pertinent is its location in the spleen and thymus (Simard et al., 1989). One of the main concepts to be emphasized in this chapter is that lymphocytes produce neuroendocrine hormones and they may serve to modulate immune function.

PITUITARY PEPTIDES

Corticotropin (ACTH)

ACTH Production by Leukocytes

In 1980, Blalock and Smith discovered ACTH production by peripheral mononuclear leukocytes of the mouse and human. Since that time, this finding has been expanded to include the full schemata outlined in Figure 1. The pituitary and mononuclear leukocyte share pathways in the stimulation and release of ACTH. Both corticotropin-releasing hormone (CRH) and interferon-inducing agents, *in vitro* and *in vivo*, stimulate the immune system to make ACTH (Blalock and Smith, 1980; Smith and Blalock, 1981; Smith et al., 1982, 1986; Meyer et al., 1987). The ACTH from the mononuclear leukocyte has the ability to stimulate cultured Y-1 adrenal cells to make corticosterone (Smith and Blalock, 1981). Recently, Smith et al. showed that ACTH from the immune system has an identical sequence to pituitary ACTH (Smith et al., 1990). In 1986, Lolait et al. confirmed ACTH production in spleen macrophages. Messenger RNA work has confirmed the protein findings; the messenger RNA for proopiomelanocortin (POMC) as well as ACTH protein was identified in immunocytes. Westly et al. (1986) found messenger RNA for POMC in splenocytes. These findings were supported by those of Oates et al. (1988), who extended these findings to virus-infected human leukocytes. *In vivo* ACTH production by the immune system was supported by the identification of ectopic ACTH in patients with lymphoid malignancy (Pfluger et al., 1981) and in a patient with lymphoma (Buzzetti et al., 1989). DuPont et al. (1984) were the first to show *in vivo* ACTH production by lymphoid cells in a nonmalignant granuloma. In this case, the leukocytes produced enough ACTH to cause the subject to become "Cushingoid". In another nonmalignant situation, Reder et al. (1988) have identified ACTH production in mononuclear leukocytes from patients with multiple sclerosis.

Glucocorticoids block ACTH production by the immune system in a way similar to its negative feedback blocking pituitary ACTH secretion (Smith et al., 1982; Blalock and Smith, 1982). In one series of experiments with hypophysectomized mice, enough ACTH was produced by the immune system of Newcastle disease virus-infected mice to give measurable stimulation of the adrenal gland (Smith et al., 1982). We also have demonstrated in normal individuals as well as patients with hypopituitarism that stimuli such as insulin-induced hypoglycemia and/or typhoid vaccination will cause an increase in ACTH production by peripheral mononuclear leukocytes (Meyer et al., 1987). Mouse spleen cells produce POMC in response to Erlich ascites tumor cells (Larsson et al., 1988). The form of ACTH is determined by the stimulus. Full-length ACTH (1–39) production is stimulated by CRH, but a truncated form, ACTH (1–24) production, is stimulated by bacterial lipopolysaccharide (LPS) interferon-inducing protein (Harbour et al., 1987; Smith et al., 1990).

Further support for CRH induction of ACTH in lymphocytes has come from expanded studies into CRH action. Heijnen et al. (1989) found that CRH indirectly induced lymphocytes to produce POMC-related peptides through induction of IL-1 by macrophages. This agrees with the results of Webster and De Souza (1988), who demonstrated specific CRH binding to splenic areas known to contain high concentrations of macrophages. This same group (Webster et al., 1989) and ours (Smith and Johnson, 1988) have shown that CRH stimulates adenylase cyclase activity in mouse spleen cells. CRH activities are not limited to monocytic cells. McGillis et al. (1989) have shown CRH induction of B-lymphocyte proliferation. Modulation of natural killer cell activity, directly (Pawlikowski et al., 1988) and centrally (Irwin et al., 1987), plus T-cell function (Singh 1989) have also been shown with CRH.

ACTH Action in the Immune System

Based on the findings discussed above, it is clear that both ACTH from the pituitary gland and ir-ACTH from the lymphocyte or macrophage-derived ACTH may act on the immune system. Johnson et al. (1982) showed that both T-cell-dependent and -independent antibody responses by murine spleen cells can be inhibited by ACTH. The T-cell response appeared to be more sensitive than the B-cell response. Later, they showed that ACTH was a potent inhibitor of interferon (IFN) production by murine spleen cell cultures (Johnson et al., 1984). In 1985, Koff and Dunegan demonstrated that ACTH would block IFN-γ activation of murine peritoneal macrophages to a tumoricidal state and suggested that stress-induced rises of ACTH would thereby enhance neoplastic disease. A few months later, Alvarez-Mon et al. (1985) showed that ACTH was also active in regulating human B-cell function.

In 1987, Heijnen et al. demonstrated that ACTH as well as β-endorphin modulate the proliferative response of human lymphocytes. That response seems to be donor specific as well as neuropeptide specific. For instance, they found ACTH (1–39) to be inhibitory in 65% of the donors tested, but stimulatory in 23% of those tested; 12% did not react.

Recently, Hughes and Smith (1990) have found that ACTH (1–39) will induce TNF-α from the adherent fraction of peripheral blood leukocytes and potentiate IFN-γ induction of TNF-α from these cells. ACTH also acts independently of steroid production to restore the Bmax of splenic adrenoreceptors to their normal pre-shock levels (Sandrini et al., 1988).

ACTH Stimulation of Second Messengers in Lymphocytes

Recently, Johnson et al. (1988) have demonstrated that cyclic AMP increases are associated with ACTH binding in the nanomolar range in mononuclear leukocytes. Spleen cells treated with ACTH respond by elevating cyclic AMP production. There is no ACTH stimulation of cyclic AMP release in Molt 4 cells, a human T-cell lymphoblast cell line which is ACTH receptor negative, but there is a very marked stimulation in the S49A T-cells, a human T-cell lymphoma cell line which has a very high percentage of ACTH receptor-positive cells. However, forskolin will stimulate the rise of cyclic AMP levels in other cell lines. Therefore, the ACTH production by the immune system seems to be identical to the ACTH produced by the pituitary. Kavelaars et al. (1989) have demonstrated another possible second messenger, intracellular calcium. They noted that ACTH ($10^{-10}\,M$) enhanced the cytosolic free calcium concentration in T-cells being activated by concanavalin A (ConA) stimulation or RIV9 induction. ACTH did not affect the baseline free Ca^{2+} concentration.

This suggests that ACTH might act through interference with the phosphorylation state of G proteins.

ACTH Binding

If ACTH has direct action on mononuclear leukocytes as described above, then there should be ACTH receptors on lymphocytes and macrophages. In order to characterize cellular binding of ACTH on isolated mononuclear cells (Boyum, 1968), an adrenal ACTH receptor assay (McIlhenney and Schuester, 1975) was adapted (Smith et al., 1987). A Scatchard plot of the binding with ^{125}I-ACTH is curvilinear, indicating at least two sites: a high-affinity, low-number site with a Kd of 0.04 nM and Bmax of 2000 sites per cell, and a lower-affinity, high-number receptor site with a Kd of 3.4 nM and a Bmax of 40,000 sites per cell.

The high-affinity receptor is very similar to that found on adrenal cells (McIlhenney and Schuester, 1975). Utilizing complementary peptide technology, Bost et al. (1985) were able to make an antibody against the ACTH receptor. With an affinity column prepared with anti-ACTH receptor antibody, they later were able to isolate the ACTH receptor and its components from murine adrenal (Y-1) cells as well as human mononuclear leukocytes (Bost and Blalock, 1986). Electrophoresis of affinity-purified ACTH receptor on a 7.5% SDS-polyacrylamide gel reveals four major bands: 83, 64, 52, and 22 kDa for receptors isolated from either tissue. ^{125}I-ACTH overlay of a washed gel revealed specific ACTH binding to only the 83-kDa band. A Scatchard plot of the specific binding of purified ACTH receptor to increasing concentrations of ^{125}I-ACTH looked like that for whole cells. Again, two ACTH binding sites were identified; they had a similar Kda and Bmax to those seen in the whole cells.

ACTH binding for the types of mononuclear leukocytes differs quantitatively (Johnson et al., 1990, in press). Using immunofluorescence with an antibody to the ACTH receptor, about 47% of murine spleen cells are ACTH receptor positive; similarly, 36% of lymph node cells are ACTH receptor positive, as are less than 1% of resting thymocytes. Among peripheral purified murine mononuclear leukocyte populations, 47% of the macrophages, 47% of the B-lymphocytes, and 24% of the T-lymphocytes have measurable ACTH receptor by immunofluorescence. After mitogen stimulation by ConA or phytohemagglutinin (PHA), there is a very striking up-regulation of ACTH receptors on thymocytes. Furthermore, 47% of unstimulated peritoneal macrophages express ACTH receptors.

Clarke and Bost (1989) have had similar findings using radioligand binding. Using rats, they found that B- and T-cells from the rat, but not thymocytes, bound ACTH. The affinity for ACTH of B- and T-cells was similar, but the T-cells had only 1000 high-affinity sites while the B-cells had 3500 sites per cell. In response to mitogenic stimulation, all populations increased their ACTH receptor number with no change in Kd. Working with a mouse B-lymphocyte cell line, Bost et al. (1987) demonstrated high- and low-affinity binding sites (Kd = 4.5×10^{-12}, 2.8×10^{-9}). The cell line also produced ACTH, so an autocrine function of ACTH is indicated.

Leukocyte ACTH Receptors and Disease

Because of the similarities between the immune and endocrine ACTH receptors, we decided to use the immune cells and their receptors to examine diseases involving ACTH action. The syndrome of ACTH insensitivity was first described in 1959 by Shepard et al. (1959). In a large number of patients, the inheritance is usually autosomal recessive (Kershnar et al., 1972). The patients have high circulating levels of ACTH with very low cortisol, but normal aldosterone and adrenal androgen concentrations. Their adrenals are unresponsive to exogenous ACTH, but will respond to lowering of salt intake with an aldosterone rise.

To examine the role of ACTH binding in the syndrome of ACTH insensitivity, a 5-year-old affected male child was examined (Smith et al., 1987). ACTH binding studies of his lymphocytes revealed no significant ACTH binding and the Scatchard plot was a horizontal line. Therefore, the cause of ACTH insensitivity is probably a deficiency in functional ACTH binding sites, not only on the peripheral mononuclear leukocyte, but probably in the adrenal, as well.

From the perspective of adrenal ACTH responsiveness, adrenoleukodystrophy (ALD) is very similar to ACTH insensitivity (Kershnarr et al., 1972; Moser et al., 1980). In both diseases, the adrenal continues to produce aldosterone appropriately after it no longer makes significant amounts of cortisol. The symptoms of ALD begin between 3 and 12 years, slightly later in life than that of ACTH insensitivity. ALD, an X-linked disease, is characterized by adrenal failure associated with progressive CNS deterioration (Moser et al., 1980, 1983).

The diagnostic biochemical characteristic is an increased amount of long-chain C26 fatty acids in the plasma and in most cell types (Singh et al., 1984; Menkes and Corbo, 1977; Rizzo et al., 1984). To date, the etiology of the adrenal failure is unknown. Theories, such as the cells filling up with so much lipid that they actually burst, have been suggested (Menkes and Corbo, 1977). On histologic examination, these patients often have atrophied adrenals, which suggests a lack of ACTH action in spite of high ACTH levels (Powers and Schaumburg, 1973). Therefore, we hypothesized that ACTH binding to the adrenal ACTH receptors is deficient, and we proposed to measure the binding characteristics of ACTH to mononuclear leukocytes (as a model of the ACTH receptor on adrenal cells).

ACTH binding to the mononuclear leukocytes showed that the total binding was equal to the nonspecific binding. The Scatchard plots were a straight line with no X-intercept; therefore, there was no measurable specific ACTH binding. Individuals with ALD have been reported to have very stiff cellular membranes (Knazek et al., 1983). Perhaps the ALD patients have a generalized defect of all mononuclear leukocyte membrane receptors. To test that possibility, we measured the binding characteristics of mononuclear leukocyte β-adrenergic receptors and found that the β-adrenergic receptors were normal in both Kd and Bmax. We have also showed *in vitro* that when normal leukocytes were exposed to 3 μg/ml C26 hexacosanoic acid, the C26 will block the ACTH receptors but not the β-adrenergic receptors.

Therefore, ALD has an ACTH receptor abnormality as the probable etiology for the adrenal atrophy and subsequent Addison's disease. C26 binding specifically to the ACTH receptor provides a possible mechanism for the decreased measurable ACTH receptor binding. We believe that ALD may be an example of nonantibody-related acquired polypeptide hormone receptor defect.

Both the immune system and the neuroendocrine system produce ACTH which binds to a specific high-affinity receptor. By studying the ACTH receptor on immune system cells such as mononuclear leukocytes, one can gain insight into, and draw conclusions about, the characteristics of the ACTH receptor on the adrenals of those patients. To date, this methodology has been used to identify an ACTH receptor abnormality in two hereditary diseases involving adrenal function: ACTH insensitivity and ALD.

Thyrotropin (TSH)

TSH Production by the Immune System

Another common signal mediator between the immune, neural, and endocrine systems appears to be TSH. A member of a family of glycoprotein hormones, TSH consists of two noncovalently joined subunits, α and β. Pituitary TSH is released after binding of hypothalamic TRH to the pituitary TRH receptors.

As seen in the ACTH system, TSH production is not limited to the pituitary. Peripheral blood mononuclear cells will synthesize ir-TSH when stimulated with the T-cell mitogen, Staphylococcus enterotoxin A (SEA) (Smith et al., 1983) or by the hypothalamic releasing hormone, TRH (Harbour et al., 1988, 1989).

The ir-TSH appears identical to pituitary TSH in all major characteristics, including antigenicity, molecular size, multiple chain composition, and elution on HPLC (Smith et al., 1983; Harbour et al., 1989). Harbour et al. (1989) found that the Molt 4, T-lymphoblastoid cell line produces ir-TSH in response to TRH and that mRNA for both the β- and α-chains of TSH can be detected by Northern blotting. Another continuous T-cell line, HUT 78, interestingly expresses TSH β-chain-related mRNA, but no β-chain protein appears to be translated.

Besides the similarity of pituitary and lymphocyte TSH induction by TRH, the two respond similarly to negative regulators. Triiodothyronine (T_3) pretreatment of lymphocytes produced reduced amounts of ir-TSH when stimulated by TRH (Harbour et al., 1989). This inhibition seemed to occur not only in the amount of TSH secretion, but also in the number of cells expressing this hormone. Therefore, the similarities between lymphocyte and pituitary TSH are not only in the structure of the molecule, but also in regulation of its production.

TSH Action in the Immune System

Pituitary TSH is released after binding of hypothalamic TRH to the pituitary TRH receptors. The TSH then causes release of thyroid hormones, T_3, and T_4, which function to increase the basal metabolic rate. This hypothalamic-pituitary-thyroid (HPT) axis functions to regulate metabolism and is also activated during times of stress (See Ingbar and Brauerman, 1986). In addition, TSH has been shown to turn on the expression of the c-fos and c-myc oncogenes in thyroid cells (Colletta et al., 1986; Tramontano et al., 1986), cause enhanced T-cell-dependent and -independent *in vitro* antibody responses (Blalock et al., 1984; Kruger et al., 1986, 1989), plus bind to neutrophils, monocytes, and some cultured cell lines, increase cAMP in some β-cells, PMN, and monocytes, and decrease iodine uptake and phagocytosis (Stolc, 1972a, 1972b; Chabaud and Lissitsky, 1977; Pehoxen and Weintraub, 1979; Harbour et al., 1989b) in phagocytes. The evidence indicates a direct interaction of TSH with B-cells and phagocytic cells since both cell types have been reported to express high-affinity receptors, approximately 1 nM, on both types of cells with varying degrees of receptor density (Stolc, 1972a, 1972b; Chabaud and Lissitsky, 1977; Pehoxen and Weintraub, 1979; Harbour et al., 1989b). Evidence seems to indicate that T-lymphocytes are the primary cell type producing TSH in response to various *in vitro* stimuli, including SEA and TRH (Smith et al., 1983; Harbour et al., 1989). The possibility that the T-cell-derived TSH is functioning *in vivo* is suggested by the reports that athymic mice (those without functioning T-cells and, therefore, no source of T-cell-derived TSH) are hypothyroid (Pierpaoli and Sorkin, 1972). We have postulated that there exists a hypothalamic-lymphoid-thyroid (HLT) axis (Figure 2) which proposes that the immune cells respond to similar stimuli and produce TSH in much the same manner as do the pituitary cells (Harbour et al., 1988, 1990a, in press).

TRH and TRH Receptors

Currently, the major action of TRH on cells of the immune system appears to be to effect the release and to induce the synthesis of leukocyte-derived

TSH (Harbour et al., 1988, 1989). TRH also enhances antibody responses *in vitro*. Kruger et al. (1989) reported that the TRH-induced antibody enhancement occurs through a TSH intermediate since the enhancement kinetics paralleled an increase in mRNA for TSH-β and the effect could be abrogated by the addition of antibody to TSH-β. Taken together, these data suggest that TRH may be interacting with TRH receptors in the immune system. We have identified specific TRH binding sites on Molt 4 cells as well as on mouse spleen cells which express TSH genes after treatment with TRH (Harbour et al., 1989; Kruger et al., 1989). The binding of TRH to these Molt 4 cells is specifically compatable with cold TRH and two binding sites are detectable. One site has a Kd in the nanomolar range with a Bmax ranging from approximately 30 to 70 fmol/mg of protein. The receptor parameters are similar to what has been reported for TRH binding sites in brain and pituitary, suggesting that these cells of the immune system are expressing classical TRH receptors. Our data suggests that these receptors are coupled to the inositol triphosphate pathway, which is further evidence for a classical TRH receptor.

In addition, we have also identified a unique, higher-affinity receptor which has not been reported in brain or pituitary (Harbour et al., 1990b). The receptor parameters include a Kd of approximately 40 p*M* with a Bmax of 1 to 5 fmoles/mg of protein. Our characterization of this higher-affinity

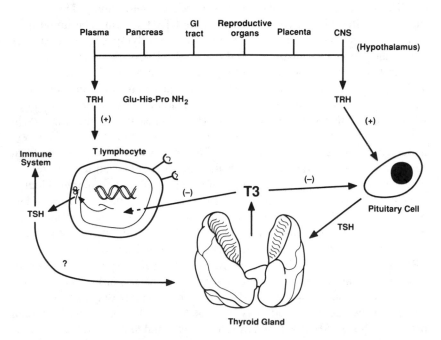

Figure 2. A putative scheme of interactions between the hypothalamic-pituitary-thyroid axis and the immune system.

receptor suggests that it is not coupled to the inositol phosphate pathway, and its binding characteristics strongly suggest that it is not a classical TRH receptor. However, our evidence suggests that this receptor is functional since concentrations of TRH equivalent to this receptors' Kd elicit a release of TSH from immune cells (Harbour et al., 1989; Kruger et al., 1989).

The evidence of TRH on leukocytes becomes even more intriguing when one considers the many extrahypothalamic sources of TRH, including a recent report describing pathways for TRH expression in the spleen (Simard et al., 1989). Our data strongly suggest the existence of an HLT axis functioning both *in vivo* and *in vitro*. In testing this hypothesis, we have found strong evidence that abnormalities in the HPT axis are manifested as defects in the HLT axis (Harbour et al., 1990a). Since the HPT axis is altered and activated in stress, most notably through the central input and activation of TRH neurons, one might expect that the HLT axis is also activated. The pituitary-thyroid axis is regulated by environmental changes such as those associated with stress, environmental temperature, and circadian rhythms, and our evidence is beginning to suggest that these same mechanisms may be operating in the HLT axis.

Leukocyte TSH and TRH Receptors in Disease

The previous section suggests that defects of the pituitary TSH system may be manifested as defects in the lymphoid TSH system. The initial publication demonstrated a blunted TSH response from lymphocytes of patients with major depressive disorder (Harbour et al., 1988). A subgroup of individuals with major depressive disorder have an impaired TSH response to TRH. The molecular relationship between the mechanism of this "blunted" TSH response and depression is unknown. Harbour et al. (1988) examined whether the lymphocyte response to TRH mimicked that of the pituitary in controls and subjects with major depressive disorder. As predicted, there was a significant decrease in the measured TSH response of lymphocytes from depressed subjects, even considering that this first study did not control for drug therapy of the subjects. Shortly after that, Halbreich reported blunted lymphocyte response in patients with premenstrual distress syndrome (Halbreich and Liu, 1989). In a separate series of patients with major depression, we have demonstrated that a significant number of individuals with an abnormal pituitary response to TRH have an abnormal leukocyte response to TRH (Harbour et al., 1990, in press). Most individuals with a normal pituitary cell response also had a normal leukocyte hormone response. These results suggest that while lymphocyte TSH production is no more diagnostic of major depressive disorder than is pituitary function testing, there is a high correlation between *in vitro* TSH production by lymphocytes and *in vivo* TSH production.

Thus, these various results suggest that the *in vitro* leukocyte TSH response may be a useful reflection of pituitary TSH responses. These data also have implications for other disease states, including autoimmune thyroiditis and hypothyroidism. Also, since TSH is a member of the HPT axis which is activated during times of stress, there may be activation of the HLT axis in stress as well.

Gonadoptropins

Chorionic Gonadotropin (CG)

Pregnancy has been referred to as a natural allotransplant. In fact, a great deal of evidence suggests that the greater the HLA disparity between the parental cells, the greater the likelihood of successful implantation and pregnancy (for a review, see Harbour and Blalock, 1990). Our finding that chorionic gonadotropin (CG) is produced in a mixed leukocyte culture (MLR) is very intriguing in this regard (Harbour and Blalock, 1990). It suggests that the immune system may play an active role in conception. This is in contrast to previous concepts that the immune response, in particular graft rejection processes, must be suppressed for a successful pregnancy.

Allogeneic stimulation in a mixed leukocyte reaction stimulated human lymphocytes to produce CG-like molecules (ir-cg) (Harbour and Blalock, 1990). Biochemical characterization of this material showed the lymphocyte CG to have a two-chain structure, molecular weight, glycosylation, and antigenicity similar to placental CG. The lymphocyte-derived CG is also luteotropic, stimulating mouse Leydig cells *in vitro* to produce testosterone. We hypothesized that since successful implantation requires CG and a recognition of the graft as foreign, then CG production by sensitized leukocytes in the preimplantation milieu may be tantamount to successful implantation and modulation of local immune response. The finding that the CG produced in a MLR possessed luteotropic activity suggests that this material may be important for promoting local progesterone production. Stress and the subsequent neurochemical and biologic changes may have implications on the local release of factors involved in luteotropic activity and immunotropism. In addition to promoting growth, CG has been reported to have numerous immunomodulatory activities, including suppression of NK and CTL activity, and inhibition of MLR and mitogen response (for a review, see Berczi, 1986). In an apparent controversy, others have found either no effects, or activity with a very high dose of CG.

However, besides being luteotropic, the ir-CG produced in an *in vitro* MLR has an immunomodulatory effect (Harbour-McMenamin et al., 1986). At very low concentrations, the ir-CG was shown to enhance the *in vitro* MLR in both humans and mice. Conversely, at very high concentrations, the MLR is inhibited. This bimodal effect suggests a mechanism whereby the ir-CG could promote an allogeneic response at very early times, and at later time points when the concentration of ir-CG is increased, the allogeneic response is turned off. Through such a mechanism, ir-CG may promote successful implantation and protection of the blastocyst.

Luteinizing Hormone

Recent studies indicate that human leukocytes produce immunoreactive luteinizing hormone (ir-LH). We have shown that ir-LH production and secretion can be consistently (Ebaugh and Smith, 1989a, 1989; Costa et al., 1990) and significantly enhanced by exposure to gonadotropin-releasing hormone (GnRH) at doses typically used to elicit maximal LH production in primary, pituitary cell cultures. Metabolic labeling studies indicate that the effect of GnRH upon β-chain synthesis appears to be specific for the production of ir-LH, as it has an insignificant effect upon total protein synthesis while increasing the production of ir-LH β-chain 2.08 ± 0.17 (p <0.005 vs. control). An examination of carrier-free sulfate incorporation (Horton et al., 1982) by GnRH-stimulated lymphocyte cultures reveals that secretion of sulfated ir-LH is greatly enhanced under the influence of GnRH (5.84 ± 2.07, p <0.01 vs. control), and this effect can be completely blocked with antiserum to GnRH. The report that GnRH could enhance the blastogenic response of thymocytes to ConA (Marchetti et al., 1989) may indicate a potential role for GnRH interaction with these immune cells. These observations are consistent with the presence of GnRH receptors on an, as of yet, unidentified population of lymphoid cells.

Structurally, ir-LH is closely related to, and perhaps identical with pituitary LH by a variety of criteria (Ebaugh and Smith, 1989, and submitted for publication). Analysis of ir-LH detected by gel electrophoresis, ConA affinity chromatography, reverse-phase HPLC, and western blotting was highly similar to LH. Polyacrylamide gel electrophoresis of ir-LH showed polypeptide species of the appropriate molecular weights and antigenicity consistent with the α- and β-chains of LH. By ConA chromatography, we demonstrated that the ir-LH could be eluted with 100 mM α-D-methylmannoside and thus was glycosylated; the observation that ir-LH will incorporate carrier free sulfate and bind ConA is consistent with the presence of terminal sulfated high-mannose oligosaccharides characterized for LH (Parsons and Pierce, 1980). The N-terminal amino acid sequence of the HPLC fraction corresponding to the β-chain of intrinsically labeled ir-LH was found to be identical to that of human LH-β for the first five residues examined. Fiddes and Talmadge (1984) have demonstrated that only a single human LH-β gene is present in the genome. Thus, taken in total, these characteristics indicate that the lymphocyte-derived molecule will be identical in amino acid sequence to pituitary LH and that, in addition to other recently characterized endocrine hormones, lymphocytes produce LH.

The exact physiological significance of lymphocytic production of LH is at present unclear. Because LH is a pH-labile hormone, we examined ConA chromatography as a method for concentrating ir-LH from PBL supernates, since the elution can be performed at physiologic pH, resulting in recovery of *bioactive* LH. ConA affinity column eluates (CAEs) from GnRH stimulated lymphocyte cultures stimulated testosterone production similar to that reported for LH in a primary mouse LC assay when incubated in the presence or absence of forskolin (LeFevre et al., 1985). The stimulatory effect of the CAE is most striking in the presence of forskolin and is inhibited by hLH-β antibody. Thus, at least one of the active components of the PBL-derived CAE appears to be LH. Preliminary evidence indicates that co-culture of lymphocytes and Leydig cells results in a dose-dependent modulation of testosterone production; this effect was not observed when control smooth muscle cells were mixed in culture. It will be of interest to determine what role ir-LH has in reproductive and immune regulation. It is tantalizing to postulate that the reversal of hypophysectomy-induced thymic atrophy seen by Marchetti et al. (1989) is due to ir-LH production.

LH Action in the Immune System

The production of LH by lymphocytes implies a potential role in immune and reproductive regulatory function. Thymic dysfunction correlated with reproductive anomalies has been documented by several groups (Michael et al., 1980; Rebar et al., 1981), as has lymphopenia (Alila and Hanson, 1984). Thymosin peptides have been shown to either stimulate LH or GnRH release, depending on the fraction assayed (Hall et al., 1988). While these investigators suggest that the target of thymosin factors is within the hypothalamic-pituitary axis, our study indicates that a localized function acting directly upon the immune system may also exist. Supporting this concept, GnRH receptors have been characterized within the thymic compartment (Marchetti et al., 1989) and on lymphocytes (Costa et al., 1990). Observations that LH in combination with thymosin fraction V will enhance NK activity *in vivo* and *in vitro* and modulate T-cell antigen expression (Rouabhia et al., 1988) indicate a direct role for LH modulation of immune function. Several lines of evidence obtained *in vivo* and *in vitro* suggest that the gonadotropins have an important intermediary role in immune modulation. These include alteration of gonadotropin levels in mice after inoculation with allogeneic cells (Pierpaoli et al., 1978), and castration studies that indicate a modulating function for both estrogens and androgens in the development of autoimmune disorders (Roubinian et al., 1979; Talal, 1981), antibody response, and stem cell differentiation (Eidinger and Garrett, 1972). Studies *in vitro* have shown that estrogenic steroids can influence NK activity (Seaman et al., 1979a, 1979b), and B-cell maturation (Paavonen et al., 1981). Thus, besides direct effects, another role of gonadotropin production by immune cells may be to elicit steroid production which then acts upon immune or reproductive tissues.

AVP: Effects of Arginine Vasopressin and Oxytocin on Immunity

Arginine vasopressin (AVP) is a nine-amino acid peptide hormone derived from the posterior pituitary gland. AVP plays important regulatory roles in homeostasis which include (1) antidiuretic effects (Sawyer, 1961), (2) vasopressor effects (Rossie and Schrier, 1986), (3) modulation of stress responses (Gibbs, 1986), (4) enhancement of learning and memory, and (5) neurotransmitter functions (Doris, 1984). Oxytocin is also a neurohormone that is structurally related to AVP, but with a different hormone action. These actions primarily include promotion of uterine contraction and milk ejection (Tepperman, 1980).

Several reports implicate AVP and oxytocin as also having an important role(s) in immune function and action. Early reports of AVP affecting the lymphoid system include those by Whitfield et al. in 1969. These authors demonstrated that AVP, in addition to other hormones, would promote a calcium-dependent mitotic activity in rat thymocyte populations maintained *in vitro*. However, the mitogenic activity was promoted at supraphysiologic concentrations of the hormone. Additional evidence of AVP affecting the lymphoid system was provided by Hunt et al. in 1977. This report demonstrated that 2 d after a severe hemorrhage in hypophysectomized rats, vasopressin was able to stimulate bone marrow mitotic activity, both *in vitro* and *in vivo*. The authors suggested that this novel hypophysial bone marrow system may assist in post-hemorrhagic recovery in blood cell numbers in the circulation.

Block et al., in 1981, reported on the specific binding of ^{125}I-8-L-AVP to mononuclear phagocytes. Binding was shown to be saturable (2.8 ± 0.4 fmol per 2×10^6 cells per ml), linear with cell number, and reversible. Scatchard analysis of the binding provided a dissociation constant of 25 ± 0.21 pM and an estimated 640 ± 80 sites per cell. The specificity of the binding was demonstrated with a series of vasopressin analogs and, in addition, showed that the cells responded to 40 pM AVP by demonstrating a rise in intracellular cyclic AMP levels.

In 1982, Johnson et al. provided evidence that AVP was capable of replacing the IL-2 requirement for IFN-γ production by Lyt-2$^+$ C57BL/6 mouse spleen cells. In addition, they showed that the structurally related oxytocin was also capable of replacing IL-2 in this system. Both AVP and oxytocin were shown to act at near-physiologic concentrations (8×10^{-9} M). Building on these observations of AVP receptors on mononuclear phagocytes, Locher et al., in 1983, studied the interactions of AVP and prostaglandin E_2 in these cells. 8-L-AVP was shown to increase prostaglandin E_2 synthesis. Oxytocin, however, was shown to have little effect.

Johnson and Torres, in 1985, showed that a structural basis for the helper signal provided by AVP and oxytocin during T-cell mitogen induction of IFN-γ exists. They provided evidence that the six N-terminal amino acids of

AVP provide the helper signal based on the relative ability of AVP, oxytocin, vasotocin, and pressinoic acid (AVP1–6, N-terminal amino acid peptide) to help in IFN-γ production. Since an AVP competitive antagonist of vasopressor activity blocked the helper activity, it was suggested that the AVP signal operated through an AVP vasopressor-type receptor on the lymphocyte. Thibonnier et al. (1985, 1986), in the next 2 years, reported on the presence of vasopressin receptors on human platelets and rat spleen cells. In both these studies, it was suggested that the receptors were of the V_1 vascular type. These reports were further confirmed in 1986 by Vittet et al.

In the same year, Marwick et al. (1986) described an ir-AVP in the rat thymus. In the mouse thymus, they have also shown the presence of these immunoreactive molecules (Greenen et al., 1986a, 1986b). It is, at present, uncertain as to whether their synthesis occurs in these tissues or if they have been sequestered there.

Oxytocin receptors in the rat thymic gland were described by Elands et al. in 1988. These receptors appeared to have a ligand specificity that was similar to that of the uterine receptors. Evidence for a novel AVP receptor on mouse lymphocytes was described by Torres and Johnson in 1988. As previously described, they found that AVP could provide a helper signal during IFN-γ production. They found that two V_1 vasopressor receptor antagonists that work identically on liver cells differed in their ability to block AVP help in the lymphocyte system. V_2 antidiuretic receptor antagonists had no effect. Torres and Johnson, in a separate communication in the same year, showed that a peptide communication could block AVP modulation of immune function. Since AVP requires conformational flexibility for signal transduction, they hypothesized that the complementary peptide was binding to AVP and converting it to an antagonist of its own action.

Smith et al. (1986) showed that AVP in conjunction with CRF induced lymphocytes to synthesize ACTH and endorphins. Kavelaars et al. (1989) expanded this finding and reported on the role of IL-1 in corticotropin-releasing factor (CRF) and AVP induction of immunoreactive β-endorphin in human lymphocytes. They found that the presence of monocytes was requisite for AVP and CRF to induce β-endorphin. It appeared that AVP and CRF induced the monocyte to secrete IL-1 which, in turn, caused the B-cell to secrete β-endorphin.

Serotonin

In addition to communication by neuropeptides, another facet of neuroimmunological research involves the effects of neurotransmitters on leukocyte function. Our laboratory has a recent focus on serotonin (5-HT). The pharmacology of 5-HT is particularly complex (Peroutka, 1988), with several receptor subtypes mediating responses at the different affinities identified. In peripheral blood, 5-HT is localized primarily in platelets and is released at sites of injury. In some species, mast cells can also take up and release serotonin. It is this presence of 5-HT in injury or inflammation (Henson, 1970) which suggests the opportunity for 5-HT to play a role in a local immune response.

Several studies have demonstrated 5-HT effects on immune function both *in vivo* and *in vitro*. The *in vivo* studies include complex effects of 5-HT on lymphocyte subpopulation numbers, suppression of immune response (decreased IgM and IgG plaque-forming response to sheep red blood cells in mice) (Jackson et al., 1985), and a permissive role in delayed-type hypersensitivity (Ameisen et al., 1989). There are also intriguing suggestions that lesioning central 5-HT neuronal systems affects peripheral leukocyte function (Devoino et al., 1987; Steplewski and Vogel, 1985).

In vitro, a 50% decrease in mitogen-induced lymphocyte proliferation (10^{-6} to 10^{-4} *M*) and nearly complete inhibition of the production of IFN-γ and other lymphokines (at 10^{-4} *M* 5-HT) (Khan et al., 1986; Arzt et al., 1988), suppression of IFN-γ-induced Ia expression by macrophages and phagocytes (10^{-7} to 10^{-6} *M*) (Sternberg et al., 1987), release of certain lymphokines and a PMN chemotactic factor (at 10^{-6} to 10^{-4} *M* 5-HT) (Paegelow et al., 1985), and up to 50% augmentation of NK cell cytotoxicity (at 10^{-6} to 10^{-4} *M* 5-HT) (Hellstrand and Hermodsson, 1987) have been reported. A recent report demonstrates, through the use of subtype-specific pharmacological probes, that the 5-HT$_{1a}$ receptor subtype mediates the effect of 5-HT (10^{-4} to 10^{-7} *M*) on the activation of NK cells by monocytes (Hellstrand and Hermodsson, 1990). With regard to the latter finding, it is noteworthy that the 5-HT$_{1a}$ receptor subtype also participates in the release of ACTH from the hypothalamus/pituitary (Calogero et al., 1990). Because the 5-HT$_{1a}$ subtype is a target for newly developed anxiolytic medications (Glennon, 1990), these drugs may have effects on immune function. In addition to these effects on immune function, 5-HT (10 μM) has been found to affect K$^+$ channels in a transformed lymphocyte cell line (Chouquet and Korn, 1988).

Presumably, an essential factor for 5-HT to directly affect leukocytes is the presence of functional receptors. However, controversy exists as to whether these receptors are present, as assessed by radioligand receptor techniques. Leukocyte receptors would not be necessary if the effects of 5-HT function were indirect, e.g., 5-HT released from platelets or mast cells could effect the release of immunologically active substances from other cells and affect the endothelial cell matrix or vascular permeability (Doukas et al., 1987; Walker and Codd, 1985; Meade et al., 1988). However, many, but not all, *in vitro* studies support a possible direct effect of 5-HT. Because of the complex pharmacology of serotonin, we suspect one possible reason for these discrepancies has been insufficient attention to details such as the concentrations of 5-HT required for a response. Some effects which require high 5-HT concentrations (i.e., 10^{-4} *M*) may reflect nonspecific effects. However, in several reports, effects on immune function occur at more reasonable concentrations, and studies to address the pharmacological specificity have been performed using appropriate receptor agonists or antagonists (e.g., Ameisen et al., 1989; Hellstrand and Hermodsson, 1987, 1990; Nordlind and Sundstrom, 1988, and others).

The presence of 5-HT binding sites on lymphocytes, eosinophiles, or macrophages has been reported (Bonnet et al., 1987; Martelletti et al., 1988; Silverman et al., 1986), although not consistently (Jackson et al., 1988). Many of these studies had methodological weaknesses, such as a limited range of 5-HT concentrations, lack of antioxidant protection for the ligand, and incomplete analysis of binding specificity by the use of pharmacological probes in displacement experiments.

With the availability of improved methodologies and ligands, we thought we could clarify the authenticity of this 5-HT binding site. Binding of ^{3}H-5-HT to a crude membrane preparation of human peripheral blood lymphocytes was studied using methods that minimize oxidation of the ligand (Jazayeri et al., 1989). We performed extensive heparin washes to eliminate platelet contamination and incubated the cells for 10 min at 37°C to eliminate residual 5-HT which may have been released during the isolation procedure and potentially could obscure binding sites.

By Scatchard analysis, we found >90% specific binding, and a curvilinear saturation curve, suggesting the presence of a very high affinity (K_d = 0.4 nM), low capacity (Bmax = 12 fmoles/mg protein) and low affinity (K_d = 3000 nM), high capacity binding site (Bmax = 30,000 fmoles/mg protein).

The high-affinity binding site was a consistent finding. However, the low-affinity site was less readily analyzed, as it was difficult to saturate and often was curvilinear itself, with a convex hump at submicromolar concentrations, resembling positive cooperativity. To further analyze these binding sites, we evaluated the kinetics of association and dissociation. We analyzed the kinetics based on a one- or two-exponential model of the rate of association and dissociation, using an iterative nonlinear least-squares fit (program written by Dr. J.M. Simard, Departments of Surgery and Physiology and Biophysics, University of Texas Medical Branch). Leukocytes were incubated with ^{3}H-5-HT (7 nM) from 30 s to 80 min. Parallel tubes contained 10^{-5} M unlabeled 5-HT to define specific binding. At equilibrium (based on the association experiments), an excess of unlabeled 5-HT was added to reaction tubes containing only ^{3}H-5-HT. We found that a two-exponential model described the association kinetics considerably better than the one-exponential model (fourfold lower residual sum of squares). We found a rapidly equilibrating compartment (ca. 4 min), consistent with a high-affinity site, and a slowly equilibrating compartment (ca. 60 min). However, only a small portion of the specific binding was readily reversible, with greater than 50% binding remaining at 80 min. This irreversible binding could explain the difficulty we encountered in saturating the low-affinity site, and could suggest that the site was not a classical biogenic amine receptor, whose effects are usually rapidly turned on and off.

Reports that human leukocytes take up serotonin (Read et al., 1985), and that murine splenic macrophages also take up serotonin with an affinity of 40 nM (Jackson et al., 1988) prompted us to examine 5-HT uptake in human lymphocytes. We found that three times as much ^{3}H-5-HT (at 0.1 μM) was taken up by lymphocytes at 37°C than at 4°C. Unlike Jackson et al. (1988), we could not block this uptake by the classic uptake blockers, imipramine or paroxetine, so this uptake could be either a novel mechanism or nonspecific diffusion.

Further studies using radioligands and oligonucleotide probes to 5-HT subtypes are in progress to assess the nature of the binding sites. However, the results of both the saturation and association/dissociation experiments suggest the presence of high- and low-affinity binding sites for ^{3}H-5-HT on lymphocytes. The high-affinity site could be occupied at circulating, nano-molar concentrations of 5-HT. The binding kinetic properties of the low-affinity site may not make analysis of this site amenable to classic equilibrium methods. Alternatively, the lower-affinity site may be an uptake channel and not a classic 5-HT receptor. In support of the latter concept, there are reports that leukocytes not only take up, but also metabolize 5-HT (Finocchiardo et al., 1988) (a process which was found to be regulated by IFN-γ). The effects of higher concentrations of 5-HT on immune function, reviewed above, may be due to uptake into leukocytes. The affinity of this site would be compatible with occupancy by 5-HT in concentrations attained after local release of 5-HT, such as in thrombosis.

Although the precise nature of the leukocyte binding sites for ^{3}H-5-HT has not been completely characterized, our results do lend support to findings of *in vitro* and *in vivo* immunomodulatory effects of 5-HT. The issue of whether 5-HT effects are receptor mediated, and which receptor mediates these effects remains unclear, with notable exceptions (e.g., Ameisen et al., 1989; Hellstrand and Hermodsson, 1987, 1990; Nordling and Sundstrom, 1988, and others). Nevertheless, these studies offer substantial evidence for the notion that 5-HT is a signal molecule common to the brain and immune system.

CONCLUSIONS AND IMPLICATIONS

One conclusion that is clear from the data reviewed above is that the neuropeptides, serotonin, and their receptors are present in the immune system. Other chapters in this book present the converse situation: lymphokines and their respective receptors present in the nervous and neuroendocrine systems.

There are many implications, but few known roles, for these common signal molecules. We have tried to present the specific possibilities when the molecules were discussed. The general implication is that these molecules and receptors are the basis of one type of immune-nervous system communication. The other major pathway is thought to be direct neural connections through the innervation of lymphoid organs.

A repeated question concerning the former pathway is whether the concentration of neuropeptides naturally attains the levels utilized for *in vitro* modulation of immune responses. This was especially worrisome with the hypothalamic-releasing hormones which are most concentrated in the portal circulation and, presumably, below functional levels in the periphery.

There are at least two reasons that argue against peripheral concentration being a problem. One: we and others are showing that these factors are synthesized and released in active forms in the periphery. This production can be from epithelial cells, peptidergic neurons, or the leukocytes themselves in lymphoid organs. This is well-documented throughout this book. TRH in particular is one neuropeptide in high concentrations in the periphery (Engler et al., 1981). The second reason is that, while some neuropeptide receptors on lymphocytes have binding characteristics similar to the neuroendocrine prototypes, Harbour et al. (1990a, 1990b) have found an exception where TRH binding differs. Contrary to its single type of pituitary binding site, TRH binds to lymphocytes at two sites. One has a neuroendocrine-like Kd of $\sim 1 \times 10^{-9} M$. The second site is a novel higher-affinity site with a Kd of approximately $4 \times 10^{-11} M$. Thus, the novel lymphoid site can be activated by much lower concentrations of ligand, possibly at levels such as found in the periphery.

The major difficulty in proving that a regulatory communication pathway exists has been the complexity of *in vivo* systems. In particular, many of these pituitary hormones are released during stress and rise with experimental manipulations. Another confounding factor is the redundancy of the immune and neuroendocrine systems. Some functions in both systems can be mediated by more than one hormone or lymphokine. Thus, it will be difficult to do the definitive experiment unless multiple factors can be controlled.

A basic knowledge of immune neuroendocrine interactions may be important to understanding certain disease processes. Other chapters have addressed the influence of stress and behavior on immune function. Aspects of this effect may be the result of, or influenced by, these common mediators. Production of hormones and their receptors may explain endocrinopathies and other systemic effects seen with immunologic diseases such as AIDS (Dlahy, 1990) or autoimmune disorders like Graves' disease.

A final implication is for clinical diagnosis and therapy. If the neuropeptides and receptors expressed by lymphocytes correlate with the pituitary, it should be possible to use leukocytes as indicators of central neuropeptide functioning. Evidence suggests that ACTH receptors (Smith et al., 1987) and TSH (Harbour et al., 1989) production by lymphocytes do correlate with the neuroendocrine state.

Last is the possibility of using hormonal treatment to manipulate immune responses. While not a new idea, the information in this chapter and book suggests new hormones to try and the possibility of enhancing beneficial immune responses. Thus, the potential for hormonal modulation of immune responses is much greater than the classical use to suppress the major responses by glucocorticoid treatment.

REFERENCES

Alvarez-Mon M, Kehrl JH, and Fauci AS: A potential role for adrenocorticotropin in regulating human B lymphocyte functions. *J Immunol* 1985; 135:3823.

Ameisen J-C, Meade R, and Askenase PW: A new interpretation of the involvement of serotonin in delayed-type of hypersensitivity. *J Immunol* 1989; 142:3171.

Arzt ES, Fernandez-Castello S, Finnocchiaro LM, Criscuolo ME, Diaz A, Finkielman S, and Nahmod VE: Immunomodulation by indoleamines: serotonin and melatonin action on DNA and interferon-γ synthesis by human peripheral blood mononuclear cells. *J Clin Immunol* 1988; 8:513.

Berczi I, Gonadotropins and sex hormones. In *Pituitary Function and Immunity*. Berczi I, Ed. CRC Press, Boca Raton, FL, 1986, pp. 184.

Blalock JE and Smith EM: Human leukocyte interferon: structure and biological relatedness to adrenocorticotropic hormone and endorphins. *Proc Natl Acad Sci USA* 1980; 77:5972.

Blalock JE and Smith EM: Human lymphocyte production of neuroendocrine hormone-related substances. In *Human Lymphocines*. Khan A, Hill NO, and Dumonds DC, Eds. Academic Press, New York, 1982, pp. 323-332.

Blalock JE, Smith HM, and Torres BA: Enhancement of the in vitro antibody response by thyrotropin. *Biochem Biophys Res Commun* 1984; 125:30.

Block L, Locher R, Tenschert W, Siegenthaler W, Hofman T, Mettler, R, and Vetter W: ^{125}I-8-L Arginine vasopressin binding to human mononuclear phagocytes. *J Clin Invest* 1981; 68:374.

Bonnet MG, Espinates L, and Burtin C: Evidence for serotonin (5HT) binding sites on murine lymphocytes. *Int J Immunopharmacol* 1987; 9:551.

Bost KL and Blalock JE: Molecular characterization of a corticotroph (ACTH) receptor. *Mol Cell Endocrinol* 1986; 44:1.

Bost KL, Smith EM, and Blalock JE: Similarity between the corticotropin (ACTH) receptor and a peptide encoded by an RNA that is complementary to ACTH mRNA. *Proc Natl Acad Sci USA* 1985; 82:1372.

Bost KL, Smith EM, Wear LB, and Blalock JE: Presence of ACTH and its receptor on a B-lymphocytic cell line: a possible autocrine function for a neurocrine hormone. *J Biol Regul Homeost Agents* 1987; 1:23.

Boyum A: Isolation of mononuclear cells and granulocytes from human blood. Isolation of mononuclear cells by centrifugation and of granulocytes by combining centrifugation and sedimentation at 1g. *Scand J Clin Lab Invest* 1968; 21(Suppl):31.

Buzzetti R, McLoughlin L, Lavender PM, Clark AJL, and Rees LH: Expression of pro-opiomelanocortin gene and quantification of adrenocorticotropin hormone-like immunoreactivity in human normal peripheral mononuclear cells and lymphoid and myeloid malignancies. *J Clin Invest* 1989; 83:733.

Calogero AE, Bagdy G, Szemeredi K, Tartaglia ME, Gold PW, and Chrousos GP: Mechanisms of serotonin receptor agonist-induced activation of the hypothalamic-pituitary-adrenal axis in the rat. *Endocrinology* 1990; 126:1888.

Chabaud O and Lissitsky S: Thyrotropin specific binding to human peripheral blood monocytes and polymorphonuclear leukocytes. *Mol Cell Endocrinol* 1977; 7:79.

Choquet D and Korn H: Dual effects of serotonin on a voltage-gated conductance in lymphocytes. *Proc Natl Acad Sci USA* 1988; 85:4557.

Clarke BJ and Bost KE: Differential expression of functional adrenocorticotropin hormone receptors by subpopulations of lymphocytes. *J Immunol* 1989; 143:464.

Colletta G, Cirafici AM, and Vecchio G: Induction of the c-fos oncogene by thyrotropic hormone in rat thyroid cells in culture. *Science* 1986; 233:458.

Costa O, Mulchahey JJ, and Blalock JE: Structure and function of luteinizing hormone releasing hormone (LHRH) receptors on lymphocytes. *Prog Neuro Endocrinol Immunol* 1990; 3(1):55.

Devoino L, Idova G, Alperina E, and Cheido M: Distribution of immunocompetent cells underlying psychoneuroimmunomodulation. *Ann NY Acad Sci* 1987; 496:292.

Doris PA: Vasopressin and central integrative processes. *Neuroendocrinology* 1984; 38:75.

Doukas J, Shepro D, and Hechtman HB: Vasoactive amines directly modify endothelial cells to affect polymorphonuclear leukocyte diapedis in vitro. *Blood* 1987; 69:1563.

Dupont AG, Somers G, Van Steirteghem AC, Warson F, and Vanhaelst L: Ectopic adrenocorticotropin production: disappearance after removal of inflammatory tissue. *J Clin Endocrinol Metab* 1984; 58:654.

Ebaugh MJ and Smith EM: Characterization of human lymphocyte immunoreactive luteinizing hormone. *FASEB J* 1989; 3:A1474.

Eidinger D and Garrett TJ: Studies of the regulatory effects of the sex hormones on antibody formation and stem cell differentiation. *J Exp Med* 1972; 136:1098.

Elands J, Annelies R, and DeKloet ER: Oxytocin receptors in the rat thymus gland. *Eur J Pharmacol* 1988; 151:345.

Engler D, Scanlon MF, and Jackson IMD: Thyrotropin releasing hormone receptors in the systemic circulation of the neonatal rat are derived from the pancreas and other extraneural tissues. *J Clin Invest* 1981; 67:800.

Fiddes JC and Talmadge K: Structure, expression and evolution of the genes for the human glycoprotein hormones. *Recent Prog Horm Res* 1984; 40:43.

Finnocchairo LME, Arzr ES, Fernandez-Castelo S, Criscuolo M, Finkielman S, and Nasmod VE: Serotonin and melatonin synthesis in peripheral immunomodulatory pathway. *J Interferon Res* 1988; 8:705.

Garssen J, Nijkamp FP, Wagenaar SS, Zwart A, Askenase PW, and van Loveren H: Regulation of delayed-type hypersensitivity-like responses in the mouse lung, determined with histological procedures: serotonin, T-cell suppressor-inducer factor and high antigen dose tolerance regulate the magnitude of T-cell dependent inflammatory reactions. *Immunology* 1989; 68:51.

Gibbs DM: Vasopressin and oxytocin: hypothalamic regulations of a stress response. *Psychoneuroendocrinology* 1986; 11:131.

Glennon RA: Serotonin receptors: clinical implications. *Neurosci Biobehav Rev* 1990; 14:35.

Greenen V, Legros JJ, Defresne MP, and Boniver J: The thymus as a neuroendocrine organ. In 1st Int Congr Neuroendocrinology. San Francisco, 1986a, p. 107.

Greenen V, Legros JJ, Franchimont P, Baudrihaye M, Defresne MP, and Boniver J: The endocrine thymus: coexistence of oxytocin and neurophysin in the human thymus. *Science* 1986b; 323:508.

Halbreich U and Liu X: *In vitro* ir-TSH response of mononuclear leukocytes to TRH in normal women and depressed patients — relationship to *in vivo* TRH test. In American College of Neuropsycholopharmacology Meeting Abstracts, 1989, p. 183.

Hall NRS, O'Grady MP, Stemer RC, Roth LC, and Goldstein AL: Regulation of reproductive and other neuroendocrine circuits by immune system peptides. In *Neural Control of Reproductive Functions*. Lakoski JM, Perez-Polo JR, and Rassin DK, Eds. Alan R. Liss, New York, 1988, p. 311.

Harbour DV, Anderson A, Farrington J, et al. Decreased mononuclear leukocyte TSH responsiveness in patients with major depression. *Biol Psychiatry* 1988; 23:797.

Harbour DV and Blalock JE: Lymphocytes and lymphocyte hormone in pregnancy. *Prog Neuroendocrinol Immunol* 1990; 2(2):55.

Harbour DV, Kruger T, Coppenhaver D, et al. Differential expression and regulation of thyrotropin (TSH) in T cell lines. *Mol Cell Endocrinol* 1989; 64:229.

Harbour DV, Kruger TE, Smith EM, and Meyer WJ: Thyrotropin releasing hormone receptors in the immune system. *FASEB Proc Abstr* 1990b; 4(7):2024.

Harbour DV, Smith EM, and Blalock JE: Novel pathway for pro-opiomelanocortin in lymphocytes: endotoxin induction of a new prohormone-cleaving enzyme. *J Neuro Res* 1987; 18:95.

Harbour-McMenamin DV, Smith EM, and Blalock JE: Production of immunoreactive gonadotropin in mixed leukocyte reactions: a possible mechanism for the generation of genetic diversity. *Proc Natl Acad Sci USA* 1986; 83:6834.

Harbour DV, Smith EM, and Meyer WJ: The thyrotropin releasing hormone induced leukocyte TSH response correlates with the TRH induced leukocyte TSH response. *Ann NY Acad Sci* 1990; 594:385.

Harbour DV and Wilhite SE: Expression of bioactive TSH receptors on cells of the immune system. *FASEB Proc Abstr.* 1989; 48:1475.

Heijnen CJ, Zulstra J, Kavelaars A, Croiset G, and Ballieux RE: Modulation of the immune response by POMC-derived peptides. *Brain Behav Immun* 1987; 1:284.

Hellstrand K and Hermodsson S: Enhancement of human natural killer cell cytotoxicity by serotonin: role of non-T/CD10$^+$ NK cells, accessory monocytes and 5-HT$_{1A}$ receptors. *Cell Immunol* 1990; 127:199.

Hellstrand K and Hermodsson S: Role of serotonin in the regulation of human natural killer cell cytotoxicity. *J Immunol* 1987; 139:869–875.

Henson PM: Mechanisms of release of constituents from rabbit platelets by antigen-antibody complexes and complement. *J Immunol* 1970; 105:476.

Hiestand PC, Mekler P, Nordmann R, et al. Prolactin as a modulator of lymphocyte responsiveness provides a possible mechanism of action for cyclosporin. *Proc Natl Acad Sci USA* 1976; 83:2599.

Hortin G, Natowicz M, Pierce J, Baenzinger J, Parsons T, and Boime I: Metabolic labeling of lupotropin with ^{35}S sulfate. *Proc Natl Acad Sci USA* 1982; 78:7468.

Hughes TK and Smith EM: Corticotropin (ACTH) induction of tumor necrosis factor α by monocytes. *J Biol Regul Homeo Agents* 1990; 3:163.

Hunt NN, Perris AD, and Sanford PA: Role of vasopressin in the mitotic response of rat bone marrow cells to hemorrhage. *J Endocrinol* 1977; 72:5.

Ingbar SH and Brauerman LE, Eds. *The Thyroid: A Fundamental and Clinical Text.* Lippincott, Philadelphia, 1986.

Irwin MR, Vale W, and Britton KT: Central corticotropin-releasing factor suppresses natural killer cytotoxicity. *Brain Behav Immun* 1987; 1:81.

Jackson JC, Cross RJ, Walker RF, Markesbery WR, Brooks WH, and Roszman TL: Influence of serotonin on the immune response. *Immunology* 1985; 54:505.

Jackson JC, Walker RF, Brooks WH, and Rozman TL: Specific uptake of serotonin by murine macrophages. *Life Sci* 1988; 42:1641.

Jazayeri A, Meyer WJ III, and Kent TA: 5-HT$_{1B}$ and 5-HT$_2$ serotonin binding in cultured Wistar-Kyoto rat aortic smooth muscle cells. *Eur J Pharmacol* 1989; 169:183.

Johnson EW, Blalock JE, and Smith EM: ACTH receptor induction of leukocyte cyclic AMP. *Biochem Biophys Res Commun* 1988; 157(3):1205.

Johnson EW, Bost KE, Blalock JE, and Smith EM: Distribution of ACTH receptors among murine mononuclear leukocyte populations. In press (1989).

Johnson HM, Farrar WL, and Torres B: Vasopressin replacement of interleukin-2 requirement in gamma interferon production: lymphokine activity of a neuroendocrine hormone. *J Immunol* 1982a; 129(3):983.

Johnson HM, Smith EM, Torres BA, and Blalock JE: Regulation of the *in vitro* antibody response by neuroendocrine hormones. *Proc Natl Acad Sci USA* 1982b; 79:4171.

Johnson HM and Torres BA: Regulation of lymphokine production by arginine, vasopressin and oxytocin: modulation of lymphocyte function by neurohypophyseal hormones. *J Immunol* 1985; 135(2):773s.

Johnson HM and Torres BA: A novel arginine vasopressin modulation of immune function. *J Immunol* 1988; 141(7):2420.

Johnson HW, Torres BA, Smith EM, Dion LD, and Blalock JE: Regulation of lymphokine (gamma-interferon) production by corticotropin. *J Immunol* 1984; 132:246.

Kao T-L, Keenan BS, and Meyer WJ: Characterization of human growth hormone secreted by lymphocytes. In Endocrine Society Annu. Meet. Abstr. (1990).

Kahn IA, Bhardwaj G, Wattal C, and Agarwal SC: Effect of serotonin on T-lymphocyte proliferation *in vitro* in healthy individual. *Int Arch Allergy Appl Immunol* 1986; 81:378.

Kavelaars A, Ballieux RE, and Heijnen C: Modulation of the immune response by pro-opiomelanocortin-derived peptides. *Brain Behav Immun* 1988; 2:57.

Kavelaars A, Ballieux RE, and Heijnen CJ: The role of interleukin-1 in the corticotropin-releasing factor and arginine vasopressin-induced secretion of immunoreactive β-endorphin by human peripheral blood mononuclear cells. *J Immunol* 1989; 142(7):2338.

Kershnar AK, Roe TF, and Kougat MD: Adrenocorticotropic hormone unresponsiveness: report of a girl with extensive growth and review of 16 reported cases. *J Pediatr* 1972; 80:610.

Knazek RA, Rizzo WB, Schulman JD, and Dave JR: Membrane microviscosity is increased in the erythrocytes of patients with adrenoleukodystrophy and adrenomyeloneuropathy. *J Clin Invest* 1983; 72:245.

Koff WC and Dunegan MA: Modulation of macrophage-mediated tumoricidal activity of neuropeptides and neurohormones. *J Immunol* 1985; 135:350.

Kruger TE and Blalock JE: Cellular requirements for thyrotropin enhancement of the in vitro antibody production. *J Immunol* 1986; 137:197.

Kruger T, Smith LR, Harbour DV, et al. Thyrotropin: an endogenous regulator of the *in vitro* immune response. *J Immunol* 1989; 142:744.

Larsson LI, Blume-Jensen P, Skovsgaard T, and Scopi L: Pro-opiomelanocortin producing cells of spleen: increase after transplantation with opioid-peptide producing Ehrlich ascites tumor cells. *Eur J Cell Biol* 1988; 47:373.

Lefevre A, Finaz C, Berthelon MC, and Saez JM: Modulation of cultured mouse Leydig cell adenylate cyclase by forskolin and hCG. *Mol Cell Endocrinol* 1985; 40:107.

Locher R, Vetter W, and Block L: Interactions between 8-L-arginine vasopressin and prostaglandin E2 in human mononuclear phagocytes. *J Clin Invest* 1983; 71:884.

Marchetti BV, Guarcello MC, Morale G, Bostoloni A, Farinella G, Cordaro S, and Scapagnini U: Characteristics and functions of thymic luteinizing hormone-releasing hormone (LHRH) receptors. *Endocrinology* 1989; 125:1025.

Martelletti MD, Alteri E, Pesce A, Rinaldi-Garaci C, and Giacovazzo M: Defect of serotonin binding to mononuclear cells from episodic cluster headache patients. *Headache* 1987; 27:23.

Martelletti MD, Alteri E, Pesce A, Rinaldi-Garaci C, and Giacovazzo M: In vitro interactions of serotonin (5-HT) with mononuclear cells from migraine patients: alterations related to the phase of the attack. *J Neuroimmunol* 1988; 18:17.

Marwick AJ, Lolait SJ, and Funder JW: Immunoreactive arginine vasopressin in the rat thymus. *Endocrinology* 1986; 119:960.

McGillis JP, Park A, Rubin-Fletter P, Turck C, Dallman MF, and Payan DG: Stimulation of rat B-lymphocyte proliferation by corticotropin-releasing factor. *J Neurosci Res* 1989; 23:346.

McIlhenney RAI and Schuester D: Studies on the binding of ^{125}I labeled corticotropin to isolated rat adrenocortical cells. *J Endocrinol* 1975; 64:175.

Meade R, van Lovern H, Parmentier H, Iverson GM, and Askenase PW: The antigen-binding T-cell factor PCI-F sensitizes mast cells for in vitro release of serotonin: comparison with monoclonal IgE antibody. *J Immunol* 1988; 141:2704.

Menkes J and Corbo L: Adrenoleukodystrophy: accumulation of cholesterol esters with very long fatty acids. *Neurology* 1977; 31:1241.

Meyer WJ, Harbour DV, Gardner R, Wassef A, and Smith EM: Correlation of TRH stimulation of *in vitro* production of TSH lymphocytes with *in vivo* TRH pituitary testing. Abstr. 291.8. In Society for Neuroscience Annu Meet (1989).

Meyer WJ, Smith EM, Richards GE, Cavallo A, Morrill AC, and Blalock JE: *In vivo* immunoreactive ACTH production by human lymphocytes from normal and ACTH-deficient individuals. *J Clin Endocrinol Metab* 1987; 64:331.

Meyer WJ, Smith EM, Richards GE, Greyer NG, Gauzier A, Brosnan PG, and Keenan BS: ACTH receptor defect in adrenoleukodystrophy (ALD). *Pediatr Res* 1987; 21:251A.

Michael SD, Taguchi O, and Nishizuka: Effect of thymectomy on ovarian development of plasma LH, FSH, GH and PRL in the mouse. *Biol Reprod Mar* 1980; 22(2):243.

Moser H, Moser A, Kawamura N, Migeon B, O'Neill B, Fenselau C, and Kishimoto Y: Adrenoleukodystrophy: studies of the phenotype, genetics and biochemistry. *Johns Hopkins Med J* 1980; 147:217.

Moser HW, Moser AE, Trojak JE, Supplee SW: Identification of female carriers of adrenoleukodystrophy. *J Pediatr* 1983; 103:54.

O'Dorisio MS and Panerai A, Eds. Neuropeptides and immunopeptides: messengers in a neuroimmune axis. *Abstr. NY Acad Sci,* 1989.

Oates EL, Allaway GP, Armstrong GR, Boyajian RA, Kehrl JH, and Prabhaker BS: Human lymphocytes produce pro-opiomelanocortin gene related transparencies. *J Biol Chem* 1988; 263:10041.

Paavonen T, Anderson LC, and Aldercreutz H: Sex hormone regulation of in vitro response. *J Exp Med* 1981; 154:1935–1945.

Paegelow I, Werner H, Hagen M, Wartner U, and Lange P: Influence of serotonin on lymphokine secretion *in vitro. Int J. Immunopharmacol* 1985; 7:889.

Parsons TF and Pierce JG: Oligosaccharide moieties of glycoprotein hormone bovine lupotropin acetylhex resists enzymatic deglycosylation because of terminal O-sulfated N-acetyhexosamines. *Proc Natl Acad Sci USA* 1980 77:7089.

Pekonen F and Weintraub BD: Thyrotropin receptors on bovine thyroid membranes: two types with different affinities and specifics. *Endocrinology.* 1979; 105:35.

Peroutka SJ: 5-Hydroxytryptamine receptor subtypes: molecular biochemical and psychological characterization. *TINS* 1988; 11:496.

Pfluger KH, Gramse M, Gropp C, and Havermann K: Ectopic ACTH production with autoantibody formation in a patient with acute myeloblastic leukemia. *N Engl J Med* 1981; 305:1632.

Pierpaoli W and Sorkin E: Role of the thymus in programming in mice with congenital absence of thymus. *Nature* 1972; 238:282.

Pierpaoli W and Maestroni GJM: Pharmacologic control of the hormonally mediated immune response. *Immunology* 1978; 34:419.

Read NG, Beesley JE, Blackett NM, and Trist DG: The accumulation of an aryloxylkylamide (501C) and 5-hydroxytryptamine in human polymorphonuclear leucocytes: a quantitative electron microscopy study. *J Pharm Pharmacol* 1985; 37:96.

Rebar RW, Morandini IC, Erickson GF, and Petze JE: The hormonal basis of reproductive defects in athymic mice: diminished gonadotropin concentrations in prepubertal females. *Endocrinology* 1981; 108(1):120.

Reder AT, Pinamaneni S, Smyka W, and Nutter D: ACTH production by human mononuclear cells. *Ann NY Acad Sci* 1988; 540:589.

Rizzo WB, Avigan J, Chemke J, and Schulman JD: Adrenoleukodystrophy: very long fatty acid metabolism in fibroblasts. *Neurology* 1984; 34:163.

Rossi NF and Schrier RW: Role of the arginine vasopressin in regulation of systemic arterial pressure. *Annu Rev Med* 1986; 37:13.

Roubinian J, Talal N, Siiteri PK, and Sadakian JA: Sex hormone modulation of autoimmunity in NBZ/NZW mice. *Arthritis Rheum* 1979; 22:1162.

Rozman TL and Brooks WL: Neural modulation of immune function. *J Neuroimmunol* 1985; 10:59.

Sandrini M, Guarini S, and Bertolini A: Influence of the intravenous administration of ACTH (1–24) on the characteristics of brain, heart and spleen adrenoreceptors of hemorrhage-shocked rats. *Pharmacol Res Commun* 1988; 20:739.

Sawyer WH: Neurohypophyseal hormones. *Pharmacol Rev* 1961; 13:225.

Seaman WE and Gindhart TD: Effect of estrogen on natural killer cells. *Arthritis Rheum* 1979a; 22:1234.

Seaman WE, Merigan TC, and Talal N: Natural killing in estrogen treated mice responds poorly to poly I:C despite normal stimulation of circulating interferon. *J Immunol* 1979b; 123:2903.

Shepard TH, Landing BH, and Mason DC: Familial Addison's disease: case report of two sisters with corticoid deficiency associated with hypoaldosteronism. *Am J Dis Child* 1959; 97:154.

Silverman DHS, Krueger JM, and Karnovsky ML: Specific binding sites for muramyl peptides on murine macrophages. *J Immunol* 1986; 136:2195.

Simard M, Pekary AE, Smith VP, and Hershman JM: Thyroid hormones modulate thyrotropin-releasing hormone biosynthesis in tissue outside the hypothalamic-pituitary axis of male rats. *Endocrinology* 1989; 125:524.

Singh I, Moser HW, Moser AB, and Kishimoro Y: Adrenoleukodystrophy: impaired oxidation of very long fatty acids in white blood cells, cultured skin fibroblasts and aminocytes. *Pediatr Res* 1984; 18:286.

Smith EM and Blalock JE: Human leukocyte production of corticotropin and endorphin-like substances: association with leukocyte interferon. *Proc Natl Acad Sci USA* 1981; 78:7530.

Smith EM, Phan M, Kruger TE, Coopenhaver DH, and Blalock JE: Human lymphocyte production of immunoreactive thyrotropin. *Proc Natl Acad Sci USA* 1983; 80:6010.

Smith EM, Morrill AC, Meyer WJ III, and Blalock JE: Corticotropin-releasing factor induction of leukocyte-derived immunoreactive ACTH and endorphins. *Nature* 1986; 321:881.

Smith EM, Brosnan P, Meyer WJ, Blalock JE: A corticotropin (ACTH) receptor on human mononuclear lymphocytes: correlation with adrenal ACTH receptor activity. *N Engl J Med* 1987; 317:1266.

Smith EM and Ebaugh MJ: Human lymphocyte production of immunoreactive luteinizing hormone. *Ann NY Acad Sci* 1990; 594:492.

Smith EM and Johnson EW: A molecular basis for bidirectional communication between the neuroendocrine and immune systems. In *Advances in Immunopharmacology IV* Hadden IW et al., Eds. Pergamon Press, Oxford, pp. 47–54.

Smith EM, Galin FS, LeBouf RD, et al. Nucleotide and amino acid sequence of lymphocyte-derived corticotropin: endotoxin induction of a truncated peptide. *Proc Natl Acad Sci USA* 1990; 87:1057.

Smith EM and Johnson EW: A molecular basis for bidirectional communication between the neuroendocrine and immune systems. *Adv Immunopharmacol* 1988; 4:47.

Smith EM, Meyer WJ, and Blalock JE: Virus-induced corticosterone in hypophysectomized mice: a possible lymphoid adrenal axis. *Science* 1982; 218:1311.

Steplewski Z, and Vogel WH: Changes in brain serotonin levels affect leukocytes, lymphocytes, T-cell subpopulations and natural killer cell activity in rats. *Neurosci Lett* 1985; 62:277.

Sternberg EM, Wedner HJ, Leung MK and Parker CW: Effect of serotonin (5-HT) and other monoamines on murine macrophages: modulation of interferon-γ induced phagocytosis. *J Immunol* 1987; 138:4360.

Stolc V: Inhibitory effect of pituitary factor on phagocytosis and iodine metabolism in human leukocytes. *Endocrinology* 1972a; 91:835.

Stolc V: Regulation of iodine metabolism in human leukocytes by adenosine 3:5'-monophosphate. *Biochem Biophys Res Commun* 1972b; 264:285–288.

Talal N: Sex steroid hormones and systemic lupus erythematosis. *Arthritis Rheum* 1981; 24:1054.

Tepperman J: *Metabolic and Endocrine Physiology*. Year Book Medical Publishers, Chicago, 1980, p. 73.

Thibonnier M and Roberts JM: Characterization of human platelet vasopressin receptors. *J Clin Invest* 1985; 76:1857.

Thibonnier M, Snajdar RM, and Rapp JP: Characterization of vasopressin receptors of rat urinary bladder and spleen. *Am J Physiol* 1986; 251:H115.

Torres BA and Johnson HM: Arginine vasopressin (AVP) replacement of helper cell requirement in IFN-gamma production: evidence for a novel AVP receptor on mouse lymphocytes. *J Immunol* 1988; 140(7):2179.

Tramontano D, Chin WW, Moses AC, et al. Thyrotropin and dibutyryl cAMP increase levels of cMYc and c for mRNAs in cultured rat thyroid cells. *J Biol Chem* 1986; 261:3919.

Vittet D, Rondot A, Cantau B, Landry JM, and Chevillard C: Nature and properties of human platelet vasopressin receptors. *Biochem J* 1985; 233:631.

Walker RF and Codd EE: Neuroimmunomodulatory interactions of norepinephrine and serotonin. *J Neuroimmunol* 1985; 10:41.

Webster EL and De Souza EB: Corticotropin-releasing receptors in mouse spleen: identification, autoradiographic localization, and regulation by divalent cations and guanine nucleotides. *Endocrinology* 1988; 122:609.

Weigent DA, Baxter JB, Wear WE, et al. Production of immunoreactive growth hormone by mononuclear leukocytes. *FASEB J* 1988; 2:2812.

Whitfield JF, Perris AD, Youdale T: The calcium mediated promotion of mitotic activity in rat thymocyte populations by growth hormone, neurohormones, parathyroid hormone and prolactin. *J Cell Physiol* 1969; 73:203.

Chapter

30

Neuropeptide Signals and Receptors in the Thymus

Vincent Geenen, Françoise Robert,
Jean-Jacques Legros, and Paul Franchimont
Department of Endocrinology,
Laboratory of Radioimmunology,
Neuroendocrin Unit, CHU-B23-Immunology Unit,
University of Liége — Sart Tilman,
B-4000 Liége, Belgium

INTRODUCTION

T-cell differentiation primarily occurs within the thymus and requires close interactions between developing thymocytes and thymic stromal cells. These interactions control the maturation program of T-cells, which includes the rearrangement of the genes coding for the antigen receptor (TCR) and the sequential expression of cell surface markers. At the end of the process, immunocompetent cells bearing the $CD4^+$, 8^- and $CD4^-$, 8^+ phenotypes, together with CD3 and functional TCRs, leave the thymus for the secondary peripheral immune organs. In addition, two important phenomena take place within the thymus: the tolerance-to-self major histocompatibility complex (MHC) molecules are induced by bone marrow-derived interdigitating cells, while the imprinting of MHC restrictions — which means that one T-cell will respond to one foreign antigen only if this is presented in association with one MHC molecule — is probably due to the intervention of the thymic reticular epithelium (Marrack et al., 1988; Fowlkes and Pardoll, 1989). A considerable insight into fundamental molecular mechanisms such as TCR gene rearrangement was gained these last years, but important questions remain to be answered like the molecular nature of the signals inducing TCR

TABLE I.
Neuropeptides Detected in the Thymus from Different Species

Neuropeptides	Species	References
Somatostatin	Chicken, rat	Sundler et al., 1979
		Geppetti et al., 1987
		Fuller and Verity, 1989
Neurotensin	Chicken	Sundler et al., 1979
	Human, rat, mouse, ovine	Geenen et al., 1986, 1987, 1988a
Neurohypophyseal-related peptides		Moll et al., 1988
		Markwick et al., 1986
		Ervin et al., 1988
Substance P	Rat, guinea pig	Geppetti et al., 1987
Neurokinin A	Rat, guinea pig	Geppetti et al., 1988a
Calcitonin gene-related peptide	Rat	Geppetti et al., 1988b

gene rearrangement and expression, the clonal deletion of thymocytes with high reactivity to self antigens, or the positive selection of MHC-restricted thymocytes.

For a long time, various types of peptides synthesized within the thymus were suspected to play an important role in the control of T-cell differentiation. The best characterized thymic peptides are thymulin (Bach and Dardenne, 1973; Dardenne et al., 1977), thymopoietin (Goldstein, 1974), and thymosin-α_1 (Goldstein et al., 1981). There is now strong evidence that neuropeptides can also be detected within the thymus, and the purpose of this chapter is to consider their potential role in the process of T-cell differentiation.

THYMIC NEUROPEPTIDES (TABLE I)

Peptide hormone-producing cells have been histologically and ultrastructurally characterized in the chicken thymus (Hakanson et al., 1974). Two separate populations of these cells were found to display neurotensin (NT) and somatostatin (SRIF) immunoreactivities (Sundler et al., 1978). Thymic immunoreactive (ir)-SRIF had identical characteristics with the synthetic peptide in immunochemical and chromatographical analyses, while ir-NT appeared to be of a larger molecular size. Ir-NT was not detected in rat, bovine, or rabbit thymic extracts. Immunostained thymic cells were mainly located in the medullary area. Ir-SRIF has also been evidenced in the rat thymus, and high-performance liquid chromatography (HPLC) analysis revealed that 70% of the total immunoreactivity eluted as synthetic SRIF (Geppetti et al., 1987). Very recently, SRIF gene expression was demonstrated in the rat thymus (Fuller and Verity, 1989) and shown to be partially regulated by adrenal function. Ir-SRIF has also been described in a human thymic tumor extract (Penman et al., 1980).

Ir-neurohypophyseal peptides have been detected in human and rat thymuses (Geenen et al., 1986; Markwick et al., 1986). In human thymic samples, ir-oxytocin (OT) was extracted and behaved immunochemically and chromatographically as synthetic OT. The biological activity of thymic OT on uterine contractility was also analogous to standard OT. The precursor-associated component, neurophysin (NP), was also characterized in the human thymus. This finding suggested a local synthesis, which was further supported by dot-blot positive hybridization of thymic messenger (m) RNAs with vasopressin (VP) and OT-cDNAs (Geenen et al., 1987). Complete characterization of thymic mRNA remains to be further defined, and will probably require specific amplification since preliminary assays failed to reveal positive signals on Northern blots (Schmale, personal communication) or detect in an adult thymus an OT mRNA of smaller size than the hypothalamic one (Ivell et al., 1988). Ir-neurohypophyseal peptides were detected by immunocytochemistry in two thymic cell populations, one located in the subcapsular cortex and the other in the medulla (Geenen et al., 1987, 1988a). The epithelial nature of the positive cells was demonstrated by their reactivity with an anti-cytokeratin monoclonal antibody (mAb) (Moll et al., 1988). Ir-VP-containing cells were characterized in the same areas through the use of a specific mAb (B312) (Robert et al., 1985), but their immunostaining required an amplification procedure by post-osmification of the product from the peroxidase reaction. Ir-VP has been detected and characterized by HPLC in the murine and rat thymus (Markwick et al., 1986). In the human thymus, ir-VP concentrations were 3 to 50 times lower than ir-OT concentrations (Geenen et al., 1989). Ir-vasotocin (VT), VP, and OT were detected in ovine fetal and neonatal thymic glands; thymic fetal levels of ir-VT were eight to ten times higher than neonatal levels, suggesting a role for VT in the development of thymic function (Ervin et al., 1988).

A specialized epithelial cell derived from the subcapsular cortex, the "thymic nurse cell", was immunostained with antibodies against neurohypophyseal peptides, neuron-specific enolase, and A2B5, a complex ganglioside expressed on the surface of neural crest-derived cells, neuroendocrine cell types, and glial precursors (Geenen et al., 1988a).

Recently, we had the opportunity to test different mAbs raised against synthetic OT (013, 022, 033) and kindly provided by Professor J. Urbain (University of Liége, Rhode St Genèse, Belgium). The three mAbs stained hypothalamic and extrahypothalamic central structures known to contain OT. The distribution of immunostained cell bodies and neurites was comparable to that observed with rabbit polyclonal antisera, with one remarkable exception: the suprachiasmatic nucleus contained cell bodies and terminals labeled with mAbs 022 and 033, but not with mAb 013 or with polyclonal antiserum. In the human thymus, mAb 033 and polyclonal antiserum identified the same cells in the subcapsular cortex and in the medulla, while immunostaining with mAb 013 was negative (Robert et al., manuscript in preparation).

Altogether, these data demonstrate the existence of an intrathymic synthesis of neuropeptides closely related to authentic OT and VP. But, as in other peripheral sites where they have been detected, some molecular differences with the hypothalamic peptides appear and require further investigations (Clements and Funder, 1986; Pickering et al., 1988).

Geppetti et al. ((1987, 1988a) have described the presence of ir-substance P (SP) and other tachykinins (TKs) in rat and guinea pig thymus, while the thymic levels were very low or undetectable in hamster and mouse. Pretreatment with capsaicin markedly reduced, but did not abolish the thymic TK concentrations, suggesting the association of these immunoreactivities with the sensory nervous structures of the organ. Vasoactive intestinal peptide (VIP) has also been immunocytochemically detected in varicosities of peptidergic fibers innervating the rat thymus (Felten et al., 1985). And last, the presence of calcitonin gene-related peptide (CGRP) has been reported in rat thymus (Geppetti et al., 1988b). Ir-CGRP thymic concentrations were not affected by capsaicin, suggesting that CGRP is not associated with sensory innervation of the thymus.

THYMIC NEUROPEPTIDE RECEPTORS (TABLE II)

Specific OT receptors of the uterine type have been evidenced in rat thymus through the use of a highly specific radioiodinated ligand (Elands et al., 1988); OT receptors are also expressed by rat thymocytes and their density is not modified by dexamethasone treatment (Elands, personal communication). ^{3}H-VP binding sites were also found on a thymic lymphoma cell line (RL12-NP) obtained after irradiation of C57Bl/Ka mice (Lieberman et al., 1979). Competition studies with VP antagonists or agonists indicated that VP

TABLE II.
Neuropeptide Receptors Detected in the Thymus

Receptors	Species	References
Substance P	Rat	Shigematsu et al., 1986
Oxytocin	Rat	Elands et al., 1988
LHRH	Rat	Marchetti et al., 1989a

binding sites could be related to the V_{1b} subtype as defined at the antehypophyseal level (Geenen et al., 1988b).

Specific SP binding sites were characterized in rat thymus and spleen; by quantitative autoradiography, they were localized in vascular smooth muscle and subendothelial layers of the thymic vasculature in the medulla and in the marginal sinus of the spleen white pulp (Shigematsu et al., 1986).

Recently, LHRH binding sites were described in rat thymic membranes, with a lower affinity (Kd = $8.4 \times 10^8\ M^{-1}$) than the ovarian binding site (Kd = $2.8 \times 10^9\ M^{-1}$). Their cellular distribution was not reported, but their expression by thymocytes is plausible since LHRH possessed some mitogenic activity upon these cells (Marchetti et al., 1989a, 1989b).

PHYSIOLOGICAL ACTIONS OF THYMIC NEUROPEPTIDES

The thymic contribution to the circulating levels of neuropeptides in the peripheral plasma is still undefined and is probably negligible in normal conditions. However, some thymic epithelial carcinomas may derive from neuroendocrine-like cells and are sometimes associated with a paraneoplasic syndrome like water retention by inappropriate VP secretion (Rosai et al., 1976).

Local paracrine effects on T-cell growth and differentiation are most plausible, and it has previously been reported that OT and VP could increase the mitotic index and DNA synthesis of rat thymocytes (Whitfield et al., 1969, 1970). Similar actions have been reported for neurohypophyseal peptides in rat thymic organotypic cultures (Ficek, 1983). Glucose oxidation of rat thymocytes is stimulated by OT (Goren et al., 1984), and neurohypophyseal peptides can replace interleukin-2 to induce the production of γ-interferon by mouse splenocytes, an action which seems to be mediated by a novel V_1 subtype (Johnson and Torres, 1985; Torres and Johnson, 1988).

No specific function has been attributed to SP in T-cell differentiation. The demonstration of SP receptors associated with blood vessel structures in thymic medulla support their possible intervention in the control of blood flow and vascular permeability in this organ. If further demonstrated, a local synthesis of SP within the thymus, together with the previous reports on SP receptor expression by immunocompetent cells (Payan et al., 1984; Hartung et al., 1986), would support an active role for SP in the process of T-cell differentiation and early activation.

Immunomodulatory properties have also been described for SRIF, NT, and VIP, but intrathymic actions upon T-cell differentiation have not been described until now.

CONCLUSIONS AND FRONTIERS

There is now clear evidence that an active synthesis of various neuropeptides occurs within the thymus. As outlined above, some interspecies differences may exist in the thymic neuropeptide repertoire, and the physiological reason of this specificity is still unclear. The regulation of thymic neuropeptide synthesis is still largely undefined: the adrenal activity and glucocorticoids are certainly important factors, but the role of thymic autonomous innervation remains to be further investigated. Finally, the intervention of thymic neuropeptides in the control of T-cell differentiation deserves further attention. Neuropeptide signals and their cognate receptors, coupled by G-proteins to intracellular pathways of activation like inositol-phospholipids mobilization, could contribute to the positive selection of immature T-cells. A trophic function for neuropeptides in the immune system is an attractive hypothesis, and a neuronotrophic role was recently demonstrated for CGRP (Denis-Donini, 1989). Parallel pathways of cell differentiation in the nervous and immune systems are further suggested by the finding of nerve growth factor receptor expression in chicken and rat primary lymphoid organs (Ernfors et al., 1988) as well as the expression of neural cell adhesion molecule (N-CAM) by murine developing T-cells (Brunet et al., 1989). Obviously, a deeper understanding of the molecular mechanisms involved in cellular development may be expected from the comparison of nervous and immune differentiation pathways.

ACKNOWLEDGMENTS

Vincent Geenen is Research Associate of the National Foundation for Scientific Research of Belgium which supports this work. A substantial part of the program has been supported by grants from the European Science Foundation (Grant No. 87/41) and a cooperation agreement between INSERM and the Communauté Française de Belgique (CGRI).

REFERENCES

Bach JF and Dardenne M: Studies of thymic products. II. Demonstration and characterization of a circulating thymic hormone. *Immunology* 1973; 25:353.

Brunet J-F, Hirsch M-R, Naquet P, Überla K, Diamantstein T, Lipinski M, and Goridis C: Developmentally regulated expression of the neural cell adhesion molecule (NCAM) by mouse thymocytes. *Eur J Immunol* 1989; 19:837.

Clements JA and Funder JW: Arginine vasopressin (AVP) and AVP-like immunoreactivity in peripheral tissues. *Endocr Rev* 1986; 7:449.

Dardenne M, Pléau JM, Man NK, and Bach JF: Structural study of circulating thymic factor: a peptide isolated from pig serum. I. Isolation and purification. *J Biol Chem* 1977; 252:8040.

Denis-Donini S: Expression of dopaminergic phenotypes in the mouse olfactory bulb induced by the calcitonin gene-related peptide. *Nature* 1989; 339:701.

Elands J, Resink A, and De Kloet ER: Oxytocin receptors in the rat thymic gland. *Eur J Pharmacol* 1988; 151:345.

Ernfors P, Hallböök F, Ebendal T, Shooter EM, Radeke MJ, Mislo TP, and Persson H: Developmental and regional expression of β-nerve growth factor receptor mRNA in the chick and rat. *Neuron* 1988; 1:983.

Ervin MG, Polk DH, Humme JA, Ross MG, and Leake RD: Immunoreactive vaso-tocin, vasopressin and oxytocin in ovine fetal and neonatal thymus glands. *Clin Res* 1988; 36:A217.

Felten DL, Felten SY, Carlson SL, Olschowka JA, and Livnat S: Noradrenergic and peptidergic innervation of lymphoid tissue. *J Immunol* 1985; 135:755s.

Ficek W: Physiological dependency between the hypothalamus and the thymus of Wistar rats. IV. Organotypic culture of the thymus in the presence of hypophyseal hormones, vasopressin and oxytocin. *Gegenbaurs Morphol Jahrb* 1983; 129:445.

Fowlkes BJ and Pardoll DM: Molecular and cellular events of T cell development. *Adv Immunol* 1989; 44:207.

Fuller PJ and Verity K: Somatostatin gene expression in the thymus gland. *J Immunol* 1989; 143:1015.

Geenen V, Legros JJ, Franchimont P, Baudrihaye M, Defresne M-P, and Boniver J: The neuroendocrine thymus: Coexistence of oxytocin and neurophysin in the human thymus. *Science* 1986; 232:508.

Geenen V, Legros JJ, Franchimont P, Defresne M-P, Boniver J, Ivell R, and Richter D: The thymus as a neuroendocrine organ. Synthesis of vasopressin and oxytocin in human thymic epithelium. *Ann NY Acad Sci* 1987; 495:56.

Geenen V, Defresne M-P, Robert F, Legros JJ, Franchimont P, and Boniver J: The neurohormonal thymic microenvironment: immunocytochemical evidence that thymic nurse cells are neuroendocrine cells. *Neuroendocrinology* 1988a; 47:365.

Geenen V, Robert F, Fatemi M, Defresne M-P, Boniver J, Legros JJ, and Franchimont P: Vasopressin and oxytocin: thymic signals and receptors in T cell ontogeny. In *Recent Progress in Posterior Pituitary Hormones* Yoshida S and Share L, Eds. Elsevier 1988b, pp. 303–310.

Geenen V, Robert F, Defresne M-P, Boniver J, Legros JJ, and Franchimont P: Neuroendocrinology of the thymus. *Horm Res* 1989; 31:81.

Geppetti P, Maggi CA, Zecchi-Orlandini S, Santicioli P, Meli A, Frilli S, Spillantini, MG, and Amenta F: Substance P-like immunoreactivity in capsaicin-sensitive struc-tures of the rat thymus. *Regul Peptides* 1987; 18:321.

Geppetti P, Theodorsson-Norheim E, Ballerini G, Alessandri M, Maggi CA, Santicioli P, Amenta F, and Fanciullacci M: Capsaicin-sensitive tachykinin-like immuno-reactivity in the thymus of rats and guinea-pigs. *J Neuroimmunol* 1988a; 19:3.

Geppetti P, Frilli S, Renzi D, Santicioli P, Maggi CA, Theodorsson E, and Fanciullacci M: Distribution of calcitonin gene-related peptide-like immunoreactivity in various rat tissues: correlation with substance P and other tachykinins and sensitivity to capsaicin. *Regul Peptides* 1988b; 23:289.

Goldstein AL, Low TLK, Thurman GB, Zatz MM, Hall N, Chen J, Hu S-K, Naylor PB, and McClure JE: Current status of thymosin and other hormones of the thymus gland. *Recent Prog Horm Res* 1981; 37:369.

Goldstein G: Isolation of bovine thymin: a polypeptide hormone of the thymus. *Nature* 1974; 247:11.

Goren HJ, Okabe T, Lederis K, and Hollenberg MD: Oxytocin stimulates glucose oxidation in rat thymocytes. *Proc West Pharmacol Soc* 1984; 27:461.

Hakanson R, Larsson LI, and Sundler F: Peptide and amine-producing endocrine-like cells in the chicken thymus. A chemical, histochemical and electron microscopic study. *Histochemistry* 1974; 39:25.

Hartung HP, Wolters K, and Toyka KV: Substance P: binding properties and studies on cellular responses in guinea pig macrophages. *J Immunol* 1986; 136:3856.

Johnson HM and Torres BA: Regulation of lymphokine production by arginine vasopressin and oxytocin: modulation of lymphocyte function by neurohypophyseal hormones. *J Immunol* 1985; 135:773s.

Lieberman M, Declève A, Ricciardi-Castagnoli P, Boniver J, Finn, OJ, and Kaplan HS: Establishment, characterization and virus expression of cell lines derived from radiation- and virus-induced lymphomas of C57Bl/Ka mice. *Int J Cancer* 1979; 24:168.

Marchetti B, Guarcello V, Morale MC, Bartoloni G, Farinella Z, Cordaro S, and Scapagnini U: Luteinizing hormone-releasing hormone-binding sites in the rat thymus: characteristics and biological function. *Endocrinology* 1989a; 125:1025.

Marchetti B, Guarcello V, Morale MC, Bartoloni G, Raiti F, Palumbo G Jr, Farinella Z, Cordaro S, and Scapagnini U: Luteinizing hormone-releasing hormone (LHRH) agonist restoration of age-associated decline of thymus weight, thymic LHRH receptors, and thymocyte proliferative capacity *Endocrinology* 1989b; 125:1037.

Markwick AJ, Lolait SJ, and Funder JW: Immunoreactive arginine vasopressin in the rat thymus. *Endocrinology* 1986; 119:1690.

Marrack P, Lo D, Brinster R, Palmiter R, Burkly L, Flavell RH, and Kappler J: The effect of thymus environment on T cell development and tolerance. *Cell* 1988; 53:627.

Moll UM, Lane BL, Robert F, Geenen V, and Legros JJ: The neuroendocrine thymus. Abundant occurrence of oxytocin-, vasopressin-, and neurophysin-like peptides in epithelial cells. *Histochemistry* 1988; 89:385.

Payan DG, Brewster DR, Missirian BA, Goetzl EJ: Substance P recognition by a subset of human T lymphocytes. *J Clin Invest* 1984; 74:1532.

Penman E, Wass JAH, Besser GM, and Rees LH: Somatostatin secretion by lung and thymic tumours. *Clin Endocrinol* 1980; 13:613.

Pickering BT, Birkett SD, Guldenaar SEF, Humphrys J, Nichilson HD, Worley RTS, and Yeung WSB: Biosynthesis of neurohypophyseal hormones: the questions remaining. In *Progress in Endocrinology 1988* Imura H et al, Eds. Elsevier 1988, pp. 1177–1182.

Robert F, Léon-Henri BP, Chapleur-Chateau MM, Girr MN, and Burlet AJ: Comparison of three immunoassays in the screening and characterization of monoclonal antibodies against arg-vasopressin. *J Neuroimmunol* 1985; 9:205.

Rosai J, Levine GD, Weber WR, and Higa E: Carcinoid tumors and goat cell carcinomas of the thymus. *Pathol A* 1976; 11:201.

Shigematsu K, Saavedra JM, and Kurihara M: Specific substance P binding sites in rat thymus and spleen: in vitro autoradiographic study. *Regul Peptides* 1986; 16:147.

Sundler F, Carraway RE, Hakanson R, Alumets J, and Dubois MP: Immunoreactive neurotensin and somatostatin in the chicken thymus. A chemical and histochemical study. *Cell Tissue Res* 1978; 194:367.

Torres BA and Johnson HM: Arginine vasopressin (AVP) replacement of helper cell requirement in IFN-gamma production. Evidence for a novel AVP receptor on mouse lymphocytes. *J Immunol* 1988; 140:2179.

Whitfield JF, Perris AD, and Youdale T: The calcium mediated promotion of mitotic activity in rat thymocyte populations by growth hormone, neurohormones, parathyroid hormone and prolactin. *J Cell Physiol* 1969; 73:203.

Whitfield JF, MacManus JP, and Gillan DJ: The possible mediation by cyclic AMP of the stimulation of thymocyte proliferation by vasopressin and the inhibition of this mitogenic activity by thyrocalcitonin. *J Cell Physiol* 1970; 76:65.

Part III
Animal Models of Stress and Immunity

Stress, Immunity, and Cancer

W.H. Vogel and D.B. Bower
Department of Pharmacology
Jefferson Medical College
Thomas Jefferson University
Philadelphia, Pennsylvania

INTRODUCTION

This chapter will deal with some basic concepts of the stress response and the immune system, followed by a review of selected papers which explore the interaction between stress and immunity and how this interaction affects tumor formation and growth.

THE STRESS RESPONSE

Stress is defined as a perturbation of the normal homeostasis of the body. Common indices of stress include changes in (1) biochemical parameters such as serum norepinephrine, epinephrine, and adrenal steroids, (2) physiological parameters such as heart rate and blood pressure, and (3) behavioral effects such as anxiety, fear, and tension. It is generally assumed that certain challenges or life events called stressors cause stress in animals and humans and, if stress becomes very intense or chronic, lead to stress-related diseases (Cannon, 1914; Selye, 1936). However, this phenomenon has been shown to be more complex than that. The same "stressful" event affects individuals differently and their stress responses can range from extreme to mild to absent; for example, public speaking is dreaded by some people, but enjoyed by others. Thus, attention is now focused more on the individual and his or her response to external or internal stimuli. The following sequence of events seems to describe best the origin and extent of the stress response and its ensuing health consequences (Lazarus and De Longis, 1983; Rutter, 1986; Kobasa et al., 1981; Tapp and Natelson, 1988; Vogel, 1985).

Events outside the body such as the death of a loved one or loss of a job, or inside the body such as pain, are perceived by the brain and evaluated as to their importance and consequences to the organism. This evaluation is based on several factors: a genetically determined trait of low or high stress response, previous experience (encountering the same situation for the first or tenth time), and the context of the situation (seeing a foreign soldier during war or peace). If this event is deemed to be of no importance or consequence, then the existing homeostasis of the organism will remain undisturbed, no stress response will occur, the event is considered nonstressful, and no stress-related health consequences will ensue. If the event is interpreted as important and of consequence but can be dealt with easily, no stress will be experienced and no stress-related disease will occur; again, the event remains just an "event". However, if coping with this event is perceived as difficult or if no coping strategies can be marshalled, certain brain centers are activated which affect and change the homeostasis of other brain centers and, in turn, that of the body. In this case, stress is experienced and the presence of a stress response indicates that the event is a stressor. Depending on the individual, the stress response can manifest itself in different organ systems (e.g., tension, palpitations, or stomach upset) and to different degrees (e.g., mild, moderate or disabling stress).

Stress is often considered bad and has been linked to a variety of stress-related diseases. However, stress is not necessarily bad all the time. News of winning the lottery can markedly affect our homeostasis; epinephrine levels skyrocket, but the stress response is experienced as joy. Stress can also be helpful; the stress of pending examinations helps one to study and pass the tests. Conversely, lack of stress can be bad; no punishment or stress fosters bad habits. Stress is usually bad for the organism if the experience is unpleasant and intense or chronic; in these cases, pathology is likely to follow. However, disease only develops in some, not all subjects; some individuals are very susceptible while others are resistant to the pathological effects of stress. Such health consequences can include hypertension, cardiac arrhythmias, headaches, ulcers, depression, alcoholism, or other stress-related diseases. Usually, stressed individuals will develop only one or a few of these health problems. Thus, an organ vulnerability seems to exist which determines the organ to be affected or the health problems to be caused. Stress-induced tachycardia can seriously compromise an infarcted heart and lead to a fatal heart attack, while healthy hearts do not suffer significant health consequences. Again, organ vulnerability seems to depend on genetic vulnerabilities and environmental factors.

In conclusion, stress is in the mind of the beholder. We create our own stress, make our own stressful events, and cause our own diseases. These processes are based on specific genetic vulnerabilities, individual experiences, and environmental circumstances. This explains the well-known observations that some individuals are quite stress resistant while others are stress susceptible, that stress-susceptible individuals will experience different stress reactions, and that the nature and extent of stress-related diseases vary greatly among individuals.

THE IMMUNE SYSTEM

The function of the immune system is the identification and destruction of "non-self" materials. These "non-self" materials can be foreign cells such as microorganisms or converted "self" cells such as tumor cells. Our knowledge of the immune system has expanded tremendously over the last decade, revealing a system consisting of a large variety of different humoral and cellular components with many interactions and control sites.

Immunological effector cells can be divided into phagocytic and lymphocytic cells. The phagocytes include eosinophils, neutrophils, basophils, and macrophages, which circulate as monocytes, then migrate out of the vascular space to become tissue macrophages. Lymphocytic cells are classified according to their site of maturation. Lymphocytes which mature in the thymus gland are referred to as T-lymphocytes; those which mature in other tissues are classified as B-lymphocytes. Several subclasses of T-lymphocytes have been identified: T-helper, T-suppressor, T-cytotoxic, and T-contrasuppressor cells. Another class of lymphocytes are natural killer (NK) cells which "may be important in immunological surveillance against neoplasia" (Ghoneum et al., 1987).

In addition, a large number of humoral or soluble chemicals participate in the immune response. Antibodies are glycoproteins which identify "non-self" material; the cascade system of proteases of the complement system destroys such material. Tumor necrosis factor is secreted by macrophages, causing hemorrhagic necrosis of neoplastic tissue (Creekmore and Longo, 1988). A multitude of biological response modifiers regulate and coordinate the different parts of the immune system. They include monokines, derived from circulating monocytes or tissue macrophages, and lymphokines, derived from lymphocytes. An example of the monokines is interleukin-1 (IL-1), which causes activated T-lymphocytes to divide. Stimulation of lymphocytes by antigen and mitogen results in the production of lymphokines such as interleukin-2 (IL-2), which causes activated T-cells to proliferate and induces cytotoxic T-cell reactivity. Thus, the immune system consists of a multitude of individual components which interact with and control each other to produce their effects. Until recently, it was thought that this system was self-controlling.

COMMUNICATION BETWEEN THE CENTRAL NERVOUS AND IMMUNE SYSTEMS

All physiological systems are under direct or indirect control by the central nervous system; therefore, it is not surprising that recent research has shown that the brain can affect and modulate the immune system and that the immune system can communicate information about its functional status to the brain.

The anatomic integrity of the brain has been shown to be critical in the normal functioning of the peripheral immune response. Electrolytic lesions in the anterior hypothalamus of guinea pigs (Stein et al., 1976) significantly decreased the severity of and mortality due to anaphylaxis after immunogenic challenge with ovalbumin. Similarly, hypophysectomy reduced the response of peripheral blood lymphocytes to phytohemagglutin challenge (Keller et al., 1988). Specific central neurotransmitters have been shown to affect the function of the immune system, and changes in the levels of these neurotransmitters cause marked changes in the immune system. Central (but not peripheral) chemical sympathectomy induced by treatment by 6-hydroxydopamine decreased the number of plaque forming cells found in the spleens of treated mice after immunologic challenge with sheep red blood cells (Cross et al., 1986) and markedly impaired the humoral antibody response to the T-cell dependent antigen trinitrophenyl-keyhole limpet hemocyanin (Cross and Roszman, 1988). The effect on the peripheral immune response is rather selective since the response to the T-cell-independent antigen trinitrophenyl-lipopolysaccharide was not affected under these conditions. In a similar study, Steplewski and Vogel (1985) demonstrated the involvement of 5-hydroxytryptamine (5-HT). Depletion of rat brain 5-HT by intracerebral ventricular injection of 5,6-dihydroxytryptamine significantly decreased splenic NK cell activity.

Changes in neuronal activity can be transferred to the immune system either by direct innervation or hormones; both systems seem to be involved. It has been shown that nerves from the central nervous system innervate lymph nodes and other structures of the immune system; this would assure an extremely rapid response. The split-second release of catecholamines from the adrenal medulla and sympathetic nerve terminals after nerve activation can affect oxidant production by human neutrophils (Tecoma et al., 1986), phagocytic activity of neutrophils (Henricks et al., 1986), or mitogen responsiveness of monocytes (Crary et al., 1983). Hormones released from the brain can affect various immune structures and functioning; ACTH, manufactured by the brain and released from the pituitary gland, stimulates the adrenal cortex to release cortical steroids which cause well-known effects on the immune system. Peripheral increases in endorphin levels can stimulate or depress selective parts of the immune system (Shavit et al., 1985; Ghoneum et al., 1987; Deitch et al., 1988; Morley et al., 1987). The effects of hormones on the immune system are slower in onset but usually of longer duration.

In turn, a change in the status of the immune system can affect and alter neuronal activity. An immunogenic stimulus, the intraperitoneal injection of sheep red blood cells into rats, was found to decrease norepinephrine content and turnover in hypothalamic noradrenergic neurons (Besedovsky et al., 1983). Administration of Newcastle disease virus to mice increased both cerebral tryptophan levels and cerebral biogenic amine metabolism (Smith and Blalock, 1981). IL-1 (Dinarello and Mier, 1987) and interferon-α (Creekmore and Longo, 1988) are pyrogens; systemic IL-1 stimulates hypothalamic norepinephrine metabolism (Dunn, 1988b) and alters the secretion of a variety of adenohypopheseal hormones (Bernton et al., 1987) such as corticotropin releasing factor (Sapolsky et al., 1987). Interferon-α has also been shown to bind to opiate receptors (Dafny, 1984). At present, it is not clear how these molecules penetrate into the brain since they would have to pass the blood-brain barrier. These peripheral messengers are either capable of crossing this barrier or enter at sites with no barrier such as part of the hypothalamus or area postrema. A recent review outlines the interactions between the nervous system and immune system in more detail (Dunn, 1988a).

STRESS AND IMMUNITY

During stress, a large number of chemical changes occur in the brain and periphery. Increases or decreases in many brain neurotransmitters occur, especially in the hypothalamus, where norepinephrine drops markedly (De Turck and Vogel, 1982). In the periphery, catecholamines are released from sympathetic nerve endings and the adrenal medulla within seconds and reach peak values after a few minutes; these increases can be 10 to 20 times the resting levels. Corticosteroids are released somewhat later (Livezey et al., 1985) and increases are less dramatic, rising two- to fourfold. In addition, many other chemicals change during stress, including endorphins and amino acids. Thus, stress can be expected to affect the immune system and the responses can be expected to be many-fold.

Changes in the absolute number of immune cells during or after stress have been demonstrated. During the very first minutes of an immobilization stress response, the number of circulating leukocytes in general and lymphocytes in particular increases markedly in rats (Bower and Vogel, 1989); after 15 min of stress, cell numbers normalize. This increase was found with either restraint or footshock. After 11 d of restraint stress, total lymphocytes, T-helper, and T-suppressor cells decreased markedly (Steplewski et al., 1985). Interestingly, after a 12-d recovery period, lymphocyte number rebounded and the number of circulating cells actually increased above baseline levels (Table I). Similarly, total lymphocytes, T-lymphocytes, T-helper, and T-suppressor cells in rats decreased at the end of a 30-m acute uncontrollable

TABLE I.
Effects of Acute and Chronic Immobilization Stress on Leukocytes, Lymphocytes, and Neutrophils in Rats

	Acute Stress (N = 6)		
Baseline	5 Min Stress	30 Min Stress	30 Min Recovery
Leukocytes (cells per mm³ × 10⁻³)			
12 ± 1	19 ± 0.5^a	17 ± 4	12 ± 3
Lymphocytes (% of total leukocytes)			
66 ± 8	73 ± 7	72 ± 11	54 ± 12
Neutrophils (% of total leukocytes)			
31 ± 2	24 ± 7	25 ± 19	43 ± 10

Chronic Stress (3 h/d × 11 d)		
Unstressed (N=11)	11 D Stress (N=6)	11 D Stress Plus 12 D Recovery (N=6)
Leukocytes (cells per mm³ × 10⁻³)		
10 ± 1	5.1 ± 0.5^b	11 ± 1
Lymphocytes (% of total leukocytes)		
66 ± 3	29 ± 3^b	80 ± 3^b
Neutrophils (% of total leukocytes)		
31 ± 2	68 ± 4^b	15 ± 2^b

Note: Values are expressed as means $\pm$ SEM.
[a] Indicates a significant difference ($p < 0.05$) vs. baseline.
[b] Indicates a significant difference ($p < 0.05$) vs. unstressed controls.

footshock session. This phenomenon occurred only in animals which had an intact pituitary gland, implicating a hormonal control mechanism (Keller et al., 1988).

Stress can also significantly affect the activity of the immune system. Usually, stress suppressed splenic NK cell activity (Morley et al., 1987; Steplewski et al., 1985; Shavit et al., 1984). This suppression could be reversed by the administration of naltrexone, an opiate antagonist, implicating endorphins in this action (Shavit et al., 1984). The peak number of splenic lymphocytes forming antibodies to sheep erythrocytes from stressed mice was half the number observed in controls (Esterline and Rabin, 1987). Delayed-type hypersensitivity to sheep red blood cells, phagocytosis by macrophages, and NK cell activity were reduced in stressed mice (Okimura et al., 1986). Mitogen-induced proliferation of splenic lymphocytes from rats was markedly reduced by footshock (Odio et al., 1986); however, the stress-induced decrease in mitogenic response depended on the mitogen used (Dunn, 1988a). The phagocytic activity of polymorphonuclear leukocytes obtained from stressed calves was significantly reduced (Henricks et al., 1986). Macrophages from stressed mice showed depressed functional activity (Shulze et al., 1979). Antibody formation, in particular IgG and IgM production, was reduced in footshocked rats (Keller et al., 1984). Separation stress in infant monkeys suppressed mitogen-induced lymphocyte proliferation; following reunion with the mother, normal activity was restored (Laudenslager et al., 1982). Chronic exercise stress also reduced the number of lymphocytes and their mitogen response (Hoffman-Goetz et al., 1986). Some of these changes seem to be more pronounced in older animals since 12-month-old rats, compared to 3-month-old rats, showed considerably more depression of NK cell activity (Ghoneum et al., 1987).

Human studies provide similar data in that stress is generally detrimental to the immune system. Kiecolt-Glaser et al. (1987) found that subjects under the chronic stress of caring for patients with Alzheimer's disease showed decreased percentages of total T-lymphocytes, T-helper cells, T-suppressor cells, and a reduction in the T-helper: T-suppressor cell ratio. Willis et al. (1987) reported decreased lymphocyte numbers in subjects undergoing a "major life crisis." Before surgery, NK cell activity was increased in patients but reduced after onset of anesthesia; post-operatively, NK cell activity was depressed (Tonnesen et al., 1987). The quantity of interferon produced by concanavalin A stimulated leukocytes obtained from 40 medical students during examination stress was significantly depressed. NK cell activity is reduced more in individuals reporting high levels of stressful experiences than in individuals with low levels (Dorian and Garfinkel, 1987; Kiecolt-Glaser et al., 1984). The reduction in NK cell activity in the medical student study was found to be larger in students reporting more stressful events in their lives (Glaser et al., 1986; Kiecolt-Glaser et al., 1984).

The effects of stressful events on immune function can be markedly influenced by the coping strategies available to an individual. Laudenslager et al. (1983), using tritiated thymidine incorporation in response to mitogen, measured the proliferation of lymphocytes from rats which could control (cope with) or could not control (not cope with) an electric shock. Proliferation was suppressed in rats with no control but remained normal in those animals which could control the shock. In humans, report of life stresses are often a function of "coping" strategies; the same event will be viewed as a mild stressor by a "good" coper and as a severe stressor by a "poor" coper. Since the degree of depression of immunity is related to the self-rated indemnity of the life event, coping strategies could be a major factor in the effects of challenges on the immune system.

Thus, it is evident that stress affects the immune system. At present, the exact mechanisms are still unclear and the results reported, which are sometimes contradictory, will depend on many factors such as the species or strain used, the nature, intensity and length of stress experienced; the coping mechanisms available to subjects tested, and the part of the immune system studied.

STRESS AND NEOPLASIA

While stress has been linked to a number of diseases, only the interaction between stress and neoplasia will be examined here. Although cancer as a stress-related disease is a rather novel concept, there is no doubt that stress can affect tumor growth and development. This notion is supported by several studies in animals and humans. The existence of different results with seemingly similar experimental designs indicates our ignorance of the complexity of processes involved in tumor formation, recognition, and destruction.

Riley (1975) showed that the incidence of virally induced mammary tumors in mice was significantly elevated when the animals were housed under conditions considered to be stressful. Depending on housing conditions, Steplewski et al. (1987) found marked variations in tumor formation and growth using 7,12-dimethylbenz[a]anthracene (DMBA) or mammary tumor cell injections. Animals which were group housed had somewhat larger tumors than those which were individually housed, and changing from group housing before tumor induction to individual housing afterwards dramatically increased tumor size; the latter housing conditions are considered most stressful to the animals. In this study, a sex difference was also noted; tumor cells grew slower under all three housing conditions in female as compared to male rats (Table II). This is similar to studies where mice raised under stressful conditions of social change showed the least tumor growth resistance (Sklar and Anisman, 1979). Mice receiving p815 mastocytoma and inescapable shock showed tumors earlier and died sooner than control animals. Tumor rejection of rats receiving Walker 256 sarcoma and inescapable shock was lower than that seen in unstressed controls (Visintainer et al., 1982). Tumor cell killing by macrophages isolated from mice which had been subjected to at least 18 h of restraint was significantly reduced (Pavlidis and Chirigos,

TABLE II.
Effect of Housing Conditions on the Growth of DMBA- and Adenocarcinoma Cell-Induced Tumors

| | Tumor Weight (g) | | |
| | DMBA-Induced | Tumor Cell-Induced | |
Housing	Female	Female	Male
Group	4.7 ± 5.6 (17)	5.5 ± 3.7 (6)	6.1 ± 2.8 (6)
Individual	0.7 ± 1.3 (8)[a]	3.3 ± 3.1 (6)	4.3 ± 3.2 (7)
Group, then individual	13.9 ± 12.8 (10)[a,b]	9.9 ± 3.6 (7)[a,b]	12.5 ± 2.1 (13)[a,b,c]

Note: Values are expressed as means ± SEM; number in parentheses represents number of animals.
[a] Indicates a significant difference ($p < 0.05$) from group housing.
[b] Indicates a significant difference ($p < 0.05$) from individual housing.
[c] Indicates a significant difference ($p < 0.05$) between males and females.

1980). However, more interesting are reports that stress can be beneficial to the animals and suppress tumor formation or growth. DMBA-induced tumors were found to grow slower in animals exposed to immobilization, electric shock, or overcrowding-noise stress situations (Bhattacharya and Pradhan, 1979; Pradhan and Ray, 1974; Ray and Pradhan, 1979; Amkraut and Solomon, 1972). The number and growth of DMBA-induced tumors in rats was significantly reduced by chronic restraint (Newberry et al., 1976; Goldman and Vogel, 1985). Following administration of mammary adenocarcinoma cells to rats, chronic restraint stress increased tumor burden during the stress period but significantly reduced tumor burden during the recovery period after stress (Steplewski et al., 1985). Exposing animals to footshock prior to virus inoculation decreased tumor size, but tumor size was increased when stress was experienced after innoculation (Amkraut and Solomon, 1972). Chronic cold or intermittent cold stress caused different effects on L1210 tumor-bearing mice; chronic cold stress decreased total tumor cell count while intermittent cold stress increased the number of these cells (Lahiri and Roy, 1987). Similarly, daily (Burchfield et al., 1978) or chronic (Baker, 1977) exposure to cold stress reduced the growth or incidence of chemically induced tumors in rats. The differential effects of stress on tumor growth or formation are probably the result of different stressors and time points at which the effects are assessed.

Among the many factors which play a role in the interaction between experimentally induced tumors and stress is the controllability or coping strategy of the organism (Sklar and Anisman, 1979; Visintainer et al., 1982). If rats could control an aversive, stressful event (by terminating an electric footshock), they more easily rejected implanted tumors or reduced tumor growth compared to rats which could not control or could not cope with this event (could not terminate the shock; in both instances, animals were yoked and received the same number of identical shocks).

In humans, anecdotal reports over the centuries have shown that stress can be beneficial or detrimental to cancer formation and development (Le Shan, 1959). Exact data are often difficult to obtain or existing data are difficult to interpret. Nevertheless, certain personalities, prone to stress, are more likely to show tumors (Lehrer, 1980; Jacobs and Charles, 1980; Kissen et al., 1969). Vulnerability to breast cancer increased with the perceived stressful lack of social support (Levy et al., 1987), and stress-relieving social support has been claimed to act as a buffer for adult cancer patients (Revenson et al., 1983). This is in agreement with a study of the effect of stress on the rate of breast cancer recurrence (Ramirez et al., 1989); severely threatening life events and difficulties were associated with the first recurrence of this disease. However, other reports do not show such a correlation. No difference was found in the number of stressful life events by patients with benign and malignant tumors, and controls without disease actually reported significantly higher levels of stress exposure (Priestman et al., 1985); the latter could be interpreted that stress was beneficial and prevented cancer formation. No correlation was found between survival of cancer patients and several psychological factors, including marital stress (Cassileth et al., 1985). Thus, the human picture is even more complex and diffuse than that seen in animals.

Although the exact nature of the stress-cancer interaction is unknown, factors similar to those seen in stress and immune function will play a role. Stress-induced reductions in the concentrations of brain norepinephrine and serotonin should change the peripheral immune response and tumor surveillance leading to altered tumor formation and growth. However, no major changes in these neurotransmitters are found during successful coping with adverse conditions (Swenson and Vogel, 1983); this correlates with findings that tumor rejection or growth is slowed in coping as compared to noncoping animals. During depression, norepinephrine and serotonin are believed to be reduced, leading to a weakening of the immune system, and increased cancer occurred in some of those patients (Shekelle et al., 1981). A correlation was also found between striatal dopamine-stimulated adenylate cyclase activity and susceptibility of rats to DMBA-induced mammary tumor development (Goldman and Vogel, 1984). Steroids, endorphins, and catecholamines, the levels of all of which are elevated during stress, must affect the immune system in such a way as to increase or decrease tumor surveillance (Shulze et al., 1979; Peters and Kelly, 1977). Estradiol and prolactin might be involved; increased levels of estradiol and decreased levels of prolactin have been correlated with tumor growth in DMBA-treated rats (Smithline et al., 1975; Goldman and Vogel, 1985). Stress might act on an even more basic level to affect tumor formation and growth. Rats exposed to carcinogens and stress displayed reduced levels of the enzyme methyl transferase, a DNA repair enzyme (Glaser et al., 1985). DNA repair in X-irradiated lymphocytes from severely distressed psychiatric patients was significantly reduced compared to controls (Kiecolt-Glaser et al., 1985).

CONCLUSIONS

Stress is a highly personalized experience determined by genetic and environmental factors. Individuals view the world and its challenges with their own perceptions and interpretations. They determine which events are stressful and which health consequences will ensue. The latter is again determined by a genetic organ vulnerability and specific environmental factors. If the immune system is susceptible to stress, increased or decreased resistance to infections, survival of transplanted organs, or tumor formation or growth can be expected. Thus, stress must not be viewed as only "bad" and must not necessarily be reduced or abolished at any expense in order to remain healthy. Stress can be both "good" and "bad", depending on its nature and intensity in a particular individual.

The fact that stress can modulate tumor formation, growth, and metastasis gives us another approach to the understanding of the formation and growth of tumors by studying the chemical changes which occur during stress and which either enhance or inhibit this pathological process.

REFERENCES

Amkraut A and Solomon GF: Stress and murine sarcoma virus (Moloney)-induced tumors. *Cancer Res* 1972; 32:1428.

Baker DG: Influence of a chronic environmental stress on the incidence of methylcholanthrene-induced tumors. *Cancer Res* 1977; 37:3939.

Bernton EW, Beach JE, Holaday JW, Smallridge RC, and Fein HG: Release of multiple hormones by a direct action of interleukin-1 on pituitary cells. *Science* 1987; 238:519.

Besedovsky H, Del Rey A, Sorkin E, Da Prada M, Burri R, and Honneger C: The immune response evokes changes in brain noradrenergic neurons. *Science* 1983; 221:564.

Bhattacharya AK and Pradhan SN: Effects of stress on DMBA-induced tumor growth, plasma corticosterone, and brain biogenic amines in rats. *Res Commun Chem Pathol Pharmacol* 1979; 23:107.

Bower DB and Vogel WH: Effects of acute stress on circulating white blood cells in rats. Manuscript in preparation (1989).

Burchfield SR, Woods SC, and Elich MS: Effects of cold stress on tumor growth. *Physiol Behav* 1978; 21:537.

Cannon WB: The emergency function of the adrenal medulla in pain and major emotions. *Am J Physiol* 1914; 33:356.

Cassileth BR, Lusk EJ, Miller DS, Brown LL, and Miller C: Psychosocial correlates of survival in advanced malignant disease? *N Engl J Med* 1985; 312(24):1551.

Crary B, Hauser SL, Borysenko M, Kutz I, Hoban C, Ault KA, Weiner HL and Benson H: Decrease in mitogen responsiveness of mononuclear cells from peripheral blood after epinephrine administration in humans. *J Immunol* 1983; 130(2):694.

Creekmore SP and Longo DL: Biologic response modifiers: interferons, interleukins, and other cytokines. *Res Staff Physician* 1988; 34(8):23.

Cross RJ and Roszman TL: Central catecholamine depletion impairs in vivo immunity but not in vitro lymphocyte activation. *J Neuroimmunol* 1988; 19:33.

Cross RJ, Jackson JC, Brooks WH, Sparks DL, and Markesbery WR: Neuroimmunomodulation: impairment of humoral immune responsiveness by 6-hydroxydopamine treatment. *Immunology* 1986; 57:145.

Dafny N: Interferon: a candidate as the endogenous substance preventing tolerance and dependence to brain opioids. *Prog Neuropsychopharmacol Biol Psychiatry* 1984; 8:351.

De Turck KH and Vogel WH: Effects of acute ethanol on plasma and brain catecholamine levels in stressed and unstressed rats: evidence for an ethanol-stress interaction. *J Pharmacol Exp Ther* 1982; 223:348.

Deitch EA, Xu D, and Bridges RM: Opioids modulate human neutrophil and lymphocyte function: thermal injury alters plasma β-endorphin levels. *Surgery* 1988; 104(1):41.

Dinarello CA and Mier JW: Lymphokines. *N Eng J Med* 1987; 317(13):940.

Dorian B and Garfinkel PE: Stress, immunity and illness — a review. *Psychol Med* 1987; 17:393.

Dunn AJ: Nervous system-immune system interactions: an overview. *J Recept Res* 81988a; (1–4):589.

Dunn AJ: Systemic interleukin-1 administration stimulates hypothalamic norepinephrine metabolism paralleling the increased plasma corticosterone. *Life Sci* 1988b; 43:429.

Esterline B and Rabin BS: Stress-induced alteration of T-lymphocyte subsets and humoral immunity in mice. *Behav Neurosci* 1987; 101(1):115.

Ghoneum M, Gill G, Assanah P, and Stevens W: Susceptibility of natural killer cell activity of old rats to stress. *Immunology* 1987; 60:461.

Glaser R, Kiecolt-Glaser JK, Stout JC, Tarr KL, Speicher CE, and Holliday JE: Stress-related impairment in cellular immunity. *Psychol Res* 1985; 16:233.

Glaser R, Rice J, Speicher CE, Stout JC, and Kiecolt-Glaser JK: Stress depresses interferon production by leukocytes concomitant with a decrease in natural killer cell activity. *Behav Neurosic* 1986; 100(5):675.

Goldman PR and Vogel WH: Striatal dopamine-stimulated adenylate cyclase activity reflects susceptibility of rats to 7,12-dimethylbenz[*a*]-anthracene induced mammary tumor development. *Carcinogenesis* 1984; 5:971.

Goldman PR and Vogel WH: Plasma estradiol and prolactin levels and their response to stress in two strains of rats with different sensitivites to 7,12-dimethylbenz[*a*]anthracene-induced tumors. *Cancer Lett* 1985; 25:277.

Henricks PAJ, Binkhorst GJ, and Nijkamp FP: Stress influences phagocytic cell function in calves. *Agents Actions* 1986; 19(5/6):355.

Hoffman-Goetz L, Keir R, Thorne R, Houston ME, and Young C: Chronic exercise stress in mice depresses splenic T lymphocyte mitogenesis in vitro. *Clin Exp Immunol* 1986; 66:551.

Jacobs TJ and Charles E: Life events and the occurrence of cancer in children. *Psychosom Med* 1980; 42:11.

Keller SE, Schleifer SJ, Camerino MA, Falini JA, Halperin J, and Stein M: Stress-induced suppression of antibody production and PFCs in the rat. *Psychosom Med* 1984; 46(3):286.

Keller SE, Schleifer SJ, Liotta AS, Bond RN, Farhoody N, and Stein M: Stress-induced alterations of immunity in hypophysectomized rats. *Proc Natl Acad Sci USA* 1988; 85:9297.

Kiecolt-Glaser JK, Garner W, Speicher C, Penn GM, Holliday J, and Glaser R: Psychosocial modifiers of immunocompetence in medical students. *Psychosom Med* 1984; 46(1):7.

Kiecolt-Glaser JK, Glaser R, Shuttleworth EC, Dyer CS, Ogrocki P, and Speicher CE: Chronic stress and immunity in family caregivers of Alzheimer's disease victims. *Psychosom Med* 1987; 49:523.

Kiecolt-Glaser JK, Stephens RE, Lipetz PD, Speicher CE, and Glaser R: Distress and DNA repair in human lymphocytes. *J Behav Med* 1985; 8:311.

Kissen DM, Brown RIF, and Kissen M: A further report on personality and psychosocial factors in lung cancer. *Ann NY Acad Sci* 1969; 164:535.

Kobasa SC, Maddi WR, and Courington S: Personality and constitution as mediators in the stress-illness relationship. *J Health Serv Behav* 1981; 22:368.

Lahiri T and Roy D: Effects of chronic and intermittent cold stress on physiological and tumour response in mice. *Ind J Exp Biol* 1987; 25:285.

Laudenslager ML, Reite M, and Harbeck RJ: Suppressed immune response in infant monkeys associated with maternal separation. *Behav Neural Biol* 1982; 36:40.

Laudenslager ML, Ryan SM, Drugan RC, Hyson RL, and Maier SF: Coping and immunosuppression: inescapable but not escapable shock suppresses lymphocyte proliferation. *Science* 1983; 221:568.

Lazarus RS and De Longis A: Psychological stress and coping in aging. *Am Psychol* 1983; (March):245.

Le Shan L: Psychological states as factors in the development of malignant disease: a critical review. *J Natl Cancer Inst* 1959; 22:1.

Lehrer S: Life change and gastric cancer. *Psychosom Med* 1980; 42:499.

Levy S, Herberman R, Lippman M, and d'Angelo T: Correlation of stress factors with sustained depression of natural killer cell activity and predicted prognosis in patients with breast cancer. *J Clin Oncol* 1987; 5(3):348.

Livezey GT, Miller JM, and Vogel WH: Plasma norepinephrine, epinephrine and corticosterone stress responses to restraint in individual male and famale rats, and their correlations. *Neurosci Lett* 1985; 62:51.

Morley JE, Kay NE, Solomon GF, and Plotnikoff NP: Neuropeptides: conductors of the immune orchestra. *Life Sci* 1987; 41:527.

Newberry BH, Gildow J, Wogan J, and Reese RL: Inhibition of Huggins tumors by forced restraint. *Psychosom Med* 1976; 38(3):155.

Odio M, Goliszek A, Brodish A, and Ricardo MJ: Impairment of immune function after cessation of long-term chronic stress. *Immunol Lett* 1986; 13:25.

Okimura T, Ogawa M, and Yamauchi T: Stress and immune responses. III. Effect of restraint stress on delayed type hypersensitivity (DTH) response, natural killer (NK) activity and phagocytosis in mice. *Jpn J Pharmacol* 1986; 41:229.

Pavlidis N and Chirigos M: Stress-induced impairment of macrophage tumoricidal function. *Psychcom Med* 1980; 42:47.

Peters LJ and Kelly H: The influence of stress and stress hormones on the transplantability of a non-immunogenic syngeneic murine tumor. *Cancer* 1977; 39:1482.

Pradhan SN and Ray P: Effects of stress on growth of transplanted and 7,12-dimethylbenz[*a*]anthracene-induced tumors and their modification by psychotropic drugs. *J Natl Cancer Inst* 1974; 53:1241.

Priestman TJ, Priestman SG, and Bradshaw C: Stress and breast cancer. *Br J Cancer* 1985; 51:493.

Ramirez AJ, Craig TKJ, Watson JP, Fentiman IS, North WRS, and Rubens RD: Stress and relapse of breast cancer. *Br Med J* 1989; 298(6669):291.

Ray P and Pradhan SN: Growth of transplanted and induced tumors in rats under a schedule of punished behavior. *J Natl Cancer Inst* 1979; 52:575.

Revenson TA, Wollman CA, and Felton BJ: Social supports as stress buffers for adult cancer patients. *Psychosom Med* 1983; 45(4):321.

Riley V: Mouse mammary tumors: alteration of incidence as apparent function of stress. *Science* 1975; 189:465.

Rossi V, Breviario F, Ghezzi P, Dejana E, and Mantovani A: Prostacyclin synthesis induced in vascular cells by interleukin-1. *Science* 1985; 229:174.

Rutter M: Meyerian psychobiology, personality development and the role of life experiences. *Am J Psychiatry* 1986; 143:1077.

Sapolsky R, Rivier C, Yamamoto G, Plotsky P, and Vale W: Interleukin-1 stimulates the secretion of hypothalamic corticotropin-releasing factor. *Science* 1987; 238:522.

Selye H: A syndrome produced by diverse nocuous agents. *Nature (London)* 1936; 138:32.

Shavit Y, Lewis JW, Terman GW, Gale RP, and Liebeskind JC: Endogenous opioids may mediate the effects of stress on tumor growth and immune function. *Science* 1984; 223:188.

Shavit Y, Terman GW, Martin FC, Lewis JW, Liebeskind JC, and Gale RP: Stress, opioid peptides, the immune system, and cancer. *J Immunol* 1985; 135(2):834s.

Shekelle RB, Raynor WJ, Ostfeld AM, Garron DC, Bieliauskas L, Liu SC, Maliza C, and Paul O: Psychological depression and 17 year risk of death from cancer. *Psychosom Med* 1981; 43:117.

Shulze R, Chirigos MA, Stoychkov JN, and Pavlidis NA: Factors affecting macrophage cytotoxic activity with particular emphasis on corticosteroids and acute stress. *J Reticuloendothel Soc* 1979; 26(1):83.

Sklar L and Anisman H: Stress and coping factors influence tumor growth. *Science* 1979; 205:513.

Smith EM and Blalock JE: Human lymphocyte production of ACTH and endorphin-like substances: association with leukocyte interferon. *Proc Natl Acad Sci USA* 1981; 78:7530.

Smithline F, Sherman L, and Kolodny HD: Prolactin and breast carcinoma. *N Engl J Med* 1975; 292:784.

Stein M, Keller SE, and Schleifer SJ: Stress and immunomodulation: the role of depression and neuroendocrine function. *J Immunol* 1985; 135(2):827s.

Stein M, Schiavi RC, and Camerino M: Influence of brain and behavior on the immune system. *Science* 1976; 191:435.

Steplewski Z, Goldman PR, and Vogel WH: Effect of housing stress on the formation and development of tumors in rats. *Cancer Lett* 1987; 34:257.

Steplewski Z and Vogel WH: Changes in brain serotonin levels affect leukocytes, lymphocytes, T-cell subpopulations and natural killer cell activity. *Neurosci Lett* 1985; 62:277.

Steplewski Z, Vogel WH, Ehya H, Poropatich C, and Smith JM: Effects of restraint stress on inoculated tumor growth and immune response in rats. *Cancer Res* 1985; 45:5128.

Swenson RM and Vogel WH: Plasma catecholamine and corticosterone as well as brain catecholamine changes during coping in rats exposed to stressful footshock. *Biochem Pharmacol Behav* 1983; 18:689.

Tapp WN and Natelson BH: Consequences of stress: a multiplicative function of health status. *FASEB J* 1988; 2:2268.

Tecoma ES, Motulsky HJ, Traynor AE, Omann GM, Muller H, and Sklar LA: Transient catecholamine modulation of neutrophil activation: kinetic and intracellular aspects of isoproterenol action. *J Leukocyte Biol* 1986; 40:629.

Tonnesen E, Brinklov MM, Christensen NJ, Olesen AS, and Madsen T: Natural killer cell activity and lymphocyte function during and after coronary artery bypass grafting in relation to the endocrine stress response. *Anesthesiology* 1987; 67:526.

Visintainer MA, Volpicelli JR, and Seligman MEP: Tumor rejection in rats after inescapable or escapable shock. *Science* 1982; 216:437.

Vogel WH: Coping, stress, stressors and health consequences. *Neuropsychobiology* 1985; 13:129.

Willis L, Thomas P, Garry PJ, and Goodwin JS: A prospective study of response to stressful life events in initially healthy elders. *J Gerontol* 1987; 42(6):627.

Stress-Induced Alterations of Immunity in Rodents

Donald T. Lysle
Department of Psychology
University of North Carolina
Chapel Hill, North Carolina

Joan E. Cunnick
Department of Microbiology, Immunology,
and Preventative Medicine
Iowa State University
Ames, Iowa

Bruce S. Rabin
Department of Pathology
University of Pittsburgh
Pittsburgh, Pennsylvania

INTRODUCTION

There is evidence that activation of nervous system pathways by the presentation of a stressor can induce alterations of immune function in rodents (e.g., Ackerman et al., 1987; Alito et al., 1985; Besedovsky et al., 1979; Braun et al., 1986; Felten et al., 1985; Felten and Olschowka, 1987; Kasahara, et al., 1977; Keller et al., 1981; Shavit et al., 1984). However, there is little or no consensus among researchers about which is the most appropriate environmental stimulation to use in this type of research. In addition, some question arises as to whether alterations of *in vitro* immune function indicates a change in disease susceptibility. The status of these effects is further complicated by reports which indicate that the effect of environmental manipulations on immune function is not consistent across different species and strains of rodents (e.g., Irwin and Livnat, 1987; Rabin et al., 1987).

The purpose of this chapter is to present some of our research with rodents examining the effect of stress on immune function and communicate how our findings address these issues. We would also like to convey some of our concerns about this area of research which extend beyond the rodent model.

ISSUES CONCERNING THE SELECTION OF A STRESSOR

The term "stress" is commonly used in many different ways. For example, a stressor can be defined as any environmental event that is not preferred, or one that induces a specific set of behavioral or physiological responses such as an increase in glucocorticoids. For the most part, animal studies have viewed any severe environmental stimulation as a stressor.

Several types of environmental stimulation have been used as stressors in animals, but there has been little agreement about the type of stressor that should be employed in the investigation of the effect of stress on immune function. Furthermore, even when a particular type of stressor is used, there is often wide variability across laboratories in the selection of parameters for that stressor. One focus of our research has been to determine whether different types of stressors influence immune function in a similar manner. In addition, our investigations have been directed at determining whether the particular parameters of the stressor (i.e., frequency of stressor presentations within and across days) can influence the direction or level of immune alteration. These studies have included assessments of different compartments of the immune system.

Our initial study employed Lewis rats and electric footshock as the stressor (Lysle et al., 1987). In this study, rats were presented with 4, 8, or 16 signaled shocks on a 4-min variable-time schedule for 1, 3, or 5 successive daily sessions. The shock was 5.0 s in duration and was always preceded by a 15-s clicker signal. Immediately following the last shock experience, the subjects were sacrificed and a sample of peripheral blood and spleen was removed. Lymphocytes from both tissues were evaluated for their responsiveness to the nonspecific mitogen concanavalin A (ConA).

The results for the groups that received 16 shocks per session are shown in Table I. Following a single shock session, the spleen and peripheral blood lymphocytes showed only 6 and 12% of the normal response to ConA, respectively. However, the suppression of responsiveness of the spleen lymphocytes completely diminished with the increase in the number of shock sessions. In contrast, the peripheral blood lymphocytes showed no attenuation

TABLE I.
Shock-Induced Immune Modulation

Number of Shock Sessions	Mitogen Response (ConA)*	
	Spleen	Blood
1	6 ± 2.1	12 ± 3.0
3	35 ± 16.9	4 ± 2.2
5	101 ± 3.7	5 ± 1.2

* Values are expressed as a mean percentage of the response of unshocked, homecage control subjects, ± SEM.

of suppressed mitogenic responsiveness with the increase in the number of shock sessions. Similar effects were obtained for the groups that received 8 shocks per session, whereas those groups which received 4 shocks per session showed little change from nonshocked controls. These results show that presentation of a stressor can have a dramatic effect on immune function, but the magnitude of the effect is dependent upon the compartment of the immune system assayed, as well as the frequency of the stressor presentations both within and across days.

Although these results indicate that different compartments of the immune system are differentially sensitive to variation in the stressor, they are limited in that the assessments are confined to the use of electric shock as the stressor. Therefore, we investigated whether similar effects would occur with the chemical stressor, 2-deoxy-D-glucose (2-DG) (Lysle et al., 1988). The injection of 2-DG, an antimetabolic glucose analog, produces an acute intracellular glucoprivation. Acute glucoprivation is a metabolic condition which shows the physiological hallmarks of a physical stressor (Brown, 1962; Himsworth, 1968; Ritter and Neville, 1976; Smith and Epstein, 1969; Smith and Root, 1969). However, glucoprivation is an interoceptive condition and thus induces behavioral responses that are different from the behavioral responses induced by exteroceptive stressors such as footshock. For example, footshock characteristically produces an increase in locomotor activity and escape responses, whereas glucoprivation is accompanied by a decrease in motor activity (Smith and Epstein, 1969). Thus, although the neural and endocrine patterns indicate that 2-DG administration is stressful, the behavioral consequences indicate that it is distinctly different from electric shock.

In this study, different groups of rats received either 1, 3, or 5 injections of 2-DG or the phosphate-buffered saline vehicle. The subjects were sacrificed 1 h after their last injection. Blood and spleen lymphocytes were subjected to a mitogen stimulation assay. The results showed that a single injection of 2-DG decreased reactivity in both blood and spleen lymphocytes, as determined by mitogenic stimulation to ConA and phytohemagglutinin (PHA). The suppressed reactivity for the spleen lymphocytes attenuated with repeated injections, but the blood lymphocytes did not show any attenuation. Thus, the results of this investigation demonstrate a pattern of immunologic alteration identical to that obtained with electric shock.

Our study using 2-DG as the stressor was extended to include an evaluation of lymphocytes from the mesenteric lymph nodes and thymus. The results for the mesenteric lymph nodes did not show any significant change in mitogenic responsiveness due to 1, 3, or 5 injections of 2-DG. However, lymphocytes from the thymus showed functional changes dependent on the number of injections of 2-DG that were opposite to that of the spleen lymphocytes. A single injection of 2-DG was not sufficient to induce suppression of thymus-derived lymphocyte responsiveness, but suppression of mitogenic responsiveness was observed following five administrations of 2-DG.

Collectively, these studies show that different types of stressors can have similar effects on immune function provided that there is a similar amount of exposure to the stressor. These studies also indicate that the restriction of immunologic assessments to certain compartments of the immune system and a particular stressor parameter can lead to incomplete conclusions. For example, in the above work, assessment of only the peripheral blood lymphocytes would have led to the conclusion that presentation of electric shock or 2-DG induces a suppression of lymphocyte function which is maintained with additional exposure. In contrast, the assessment of only splenic lymphocytes would have led to different conclusions; namely, that presentation of stressor induces an alteration of lymphocyte function following a single session, but additional sessions induce little or no alteration in immune function. Neither of these conclusions alone provides an accurate account of the effect of presentations of a stressor on the immune system. Thus, it is important to systematically evaluate several immune compartments across different parameters of a stressor.

The above findings suggest that either different pathways exist by which the nervous system interacts with the compartments of the immune system or that there are qualitative differences among populations of lymphocytes in the various compartments. However, this suggestion may be an oversimplification in that our subsequent work using splenic lymphocytes showed that the factor which induces the functional suppression of natural killer (NK) cell activity and the factor which induces the suppression of mitogenic responsiveness in T-lymphocytes are not identical (Cunnick et al., 1988). In that work, we measured the activity of splenic NK cells in rats exposed to 1 or 5 sessions of electric shock. The results showed that in contrast to mitogenic responsiveness of T-lymphocytes, both single and multiple sessions of electric shock induced a suppression of splenic NK activity.

Shavit and colleagues (1984) provide evidence that opioid activity is responsible for the stress-induced alterations of NK cells. To assess opioid involvement, we pretreated rats with the opiate antagonist naltrexone or saline prior to exposing them to electric shock. The results showed that naltrexone inhibited the functional alteration of splenic-derived NK cells, but had no effect on the shock-induced suppression of mitogenic responsiveness of splenic lymphocytes (Cunnick et al., 1988). These findings suggest that NK cells and lymphocytes within the spleen are altered through different mechanisms or pathways. Thus, not only are immune compartments differentially affected by exposure to the same stressor, but different cell populations within those compartments can be affected by different stress-related factors.

The investigations of stress-induced alterations in animals have almost exclusively used physically aversive stimulation as the stressor. One of our interests was whether the psychological aspects of a stressful experience would induce an alteration of immune function independently of physically aversive stimulation. The human literature suggests that psychological stress can alter immune function, but those studies are confounded by possible physical factors, as well as changes in dietary and health-related habits. Therefore, we cannot conclude from those studies that psychological stress itself impairs immune function.

The studies reported above provided the necessary parametric data to enable us to conduct a series of three experiments designed to study the immunomodulatory effects of a pure psychological stressor, i.e., a conditioned aversive stimulus (Lysle et al., 1988). A conditioned aversive stimulus (CS) is an environmental event that is not inherently aversive, but acquires that property by predicting an event (like shock) that is inherently aversive. Our first experiment assessed whether aversive conditioning would enable the CS by itself to suppress the responsiveness of lymphocytes to mitogen stimulation. To control for different factors ancillary to the conditioning process (e.g., shock effects and handling of the subjects), our first experiment employed five groups of rats (see Table II). Two groups (designated A+ and B+) were given two consecutive days of conditioning during which there were ten

TABLE II.
Conditioned Immune Modulation

Group Designation	Training Days 1 and 2*	Test Session Day 8	CONA (mean cpm ± SEM)
A +	Stimulus A/shock	Stimulus A	50,477 ± 12,147
B +	Stimulus B/shock	Stimulus A	126,055 ± 9,475
A + /B −	Stimulus A/shock and Stimulus B/no shock	Stimulus A	64,549 ± 9,468
A − /B +	Stimulus A/no shock and Stimulus B/shock	Stimulus A	117,222 ± 9,160
X	Apparatus only	Apparatus only	112,806 ± 2,603

* For all groups, stimulus A and B was a clicker or light stimulus balanced within groups.

daily presentations, on a 4-min variable-time (VT) schedule, of either a 15-s A or a 15-s B stimulus (A and B are the designations used for a light- or clicker-conditioned stimulus, balanced within groups) that coterminated with a 5-s, 1.6-mA footshock. Then, after a 6-d recovery period in their home cages, both groups were given a single test session involving ten presentations, on a 4-min VT schedule, of just the A stimulus, which was a conditioned aversive stimulus for group A+ and a novel stimulus for group B+. Because a novel stimulus can elicit fear and possibly generate stress, two other groups were given differential conditioning to A and B, so as to familiarize the subjects with both stimuli. On each of their two conditioning days, one group (A+/B−) received ten presentations of A paired with the shock, as above, and ten presentations of stimulus B unpaired with the shock; the other group (A−/B+) received just the reverse. For those groups, the A and B trials occurred randomly on a 2-min VT schedule. On the test day, following the 6-d recovery period, both groups also received ten presentations, on a 4-min VT schedule, of just the A stimulus, which was a conditioned stimulus for group A+/B− and a nonconditioned, familiar stimulus for group A−/B+. To control for any stressful effects stemming from handling and transportation of the subjects, the fifth group was given the same treatment as the other four groups except that its exposure to the apparatus during the conditioning and test sessions did not include presentations of A, B, or the shock.

Immediately after the test session, the subjects were sacrificed and their spleens removed for a mitogen-stimulation assay using both ConA and PHA. The results for all concentrations of ConA and PHA were similar. Table 2 shows the results for the optimal concentration of ConA expressed as counts per minute of ^{3}H-thymidine incorporation by actively dividing lymphocytes. The results show that there was a comparably pronounced suppression of the reactivity of splenic lymphocytes for the A+ and A+/B− groups relative to the other three groups, which did not differ. These results demonstrate that a conditioned or psychological stressor can induce a decrease in mitogenic responsiveness which is independent of the effect of the shock experience, handling, and exposure to the stimuli used in conditioning.

We conducted two experiments evaluating whether the suppression of lymphocyte reactivity induced by the conditioned stimulus would be attenuated by operations known to degrade that stimulus as a signal for electric shock, viz., extinction and preexposure (Lysle et al., 1988). In one experiment, two experimental groups were given the same conditioning, recovery, and test treatments as group A+ above, except that conditioning to A was limited to one session and six additional days intervened between conditioning and the test session. On those additional days, one group was given extinction training, involving ten daily presentations of A without the shock on a 4-min VT schedule. The other group was left undisturbed in the home cages.

Two control groups received exactly the same treatments as the experimental groups, except that on the test day, the controls were exposed to the conditioning chambers without any presentations of A. Our use of both controls was to assess whether extinction training resulted in a change in the baseline mitogenic response.

The second experiment duplicated the first, with the exception that the six additional days occurred prior to, rather than after, the conditioning session and involved exposure to the conditioning chambers with or without ten daily presentations of A. Such preexposure to a conditioned stimulus is known to produce "latent inhibition" and to retard subsequent conditioning of that stimulus (Lubow, 1973). As before, all subjects were sacrificed immediately after the test session and their spleens removed for mitogen-stimulation assays involving both ConA and PHA.

The results of those assays showed that test presentations of a conditioned aversive stimulus induced a pronounced suppression of lymphocyte reactivity, and that suppression was significantly attenuated for the experimental subjects that had received preexposure or extinction training. The lymphocyte reactivity for those subjects was still reliably suppressed relative to the baseline performance of the controls, which did not differ. That outcome speaks to the robustness of our conditioning effects because it indicates that psychological stress in the form of conditioned fear can still suppress immune activity in spite of manipulations specifically designed to attenuate it.

In summary, research using rodents as subjects has provided us with the opportunity to evaluate the immunologic consequence of both physical and psychological forms of stress. To date, the stressors that we have tested induced similar immune alterations, when the parameters of the stressors are similar. Furthermore, research with rodent subjects has indicated that a complete understanding of the relationship between stress and immune function requires the assessment of multiple immune compartments.

ISSUES CONCERNING ENVIRONMENTAL MANIPULATION IN OTHER RODENT SPECIES

Although rodents are related phylogenetically, there is evidence suggesting that the effect of stress on immune function will not be the same for different species and strains. For example, Irwin and Livnat (1987) exposed three different strains of mice to acute inescapable footshock. Two strains, CD-1 and C57BL/6J, showed a decrease in NK cell activity and one strain, DBA/2J, showed no effect. These results suggest that genetic factors can participate in the immunologic alteration induced by a stressor. However, the locus of the genetic influence is not known, and the different effects for the strains may well be related to an interaction between genetic and environmental variables.

The interaction of genetic and environmental variables is evident in studies investigating the effect of different housing conditions on immune function in mice. For example, we evaluated the immune alterations induced by housing mice 1 or 5 per cage (Rabin et al., 1987). Those studies used five different strains of mice. The strains were originally selected on the basis of their histocompatibility. That is, they either shared or did not share the H_2K and/ or the H_2D locus with the C_3H/HeJ mouse.

The immune response of individually housed, male C_3H/HeJ mice showed greater T-cell function as measured by mitogenic responsiveness, interleukin-2 (IL-2) production, and plaque-forming cell response to sheep erythrocytes in comparison to the group-housed mice. Another mouse strain, $C_3H·SW/SN$, which shares neither the H_2D or H_2K loci with the C_3H strain, also showed greater immunologic response to sheep erythrocytes when housed individually. In contrast, two other strains of mice, B10.Br/SgSN and C_3H-H-2^{02}/SFSN, which partially shared alleles at the major histocompatibility locus, failed to show any difference in their response to sheep erythrocytes based on housing. These results indicate that different strains of mice do not show similar alterations of immune function based on housing conditions, and that these strain differences are not related to the major histocompatibility complex.

The sex of the rodent can also influence the immune alterations induced by differential housing. In contrast to the male C_3H/HeJ mice, female C_3H/HeJ mice housed 1 or 5 per cage did not show a difference in their immunologic reactivity as assessed by mitogenic responsiveness, IL-2 production, and production of plaque-forming cells. In contrast, our investigation of the CD-1 mouse strain showed that both males and females which were individually housed exhibited greater mitogenic responsiveness and a greater PFC response to sheep erythrocytes in comparison to group-housed mice (Rabin et al., 1987). These data indicate that sex differences can interact with housing conditions to lead to immune alteration, but that the interaction is dependent upon the strain of mouse.

The interaction of strain and sex with housing conditions indicates the complexity in selecting a rodent subject for the investigation of stress-induced immune alterations. Studies using rodents have produced some very interesting and provocative data, but the evaluation of environmentally induced alterations of immune function must be considered in the context of the species, the strain, and the sex of animals.

ISSUES CONCERNING IMMUNOLOGIC TESTING

Although there is strong evidence demonstrating that presentations of a stressor can alter immune function, there is little evidence that alteration of *in vitro* immune function indicates a change in susceptibility or resistance to immunologically mediated disease (infection, malignancy, and autoimmunity). Statistical procedures can be used to identify stress-induced alterations of *in vitro* immune responses, with the implied assumption that those effects indicate a change in susceptibility to disease. However, there is little evidence to support this relationship. Furthermore, there is evidence which suggests that *in vitro* test values alone are poor predictors of alterations in disease susceptibility.

The normal concentration of immunoglobulin in humans provides an excellent example of the difficulty in relating immunologic changes with altered disease susceptibility. In humans, serum IgG has a normal concentration of approximately 1200 mg/dl. Two standard deviations below the mean is approximately 700 mg/dl. Therefore, it could safely be assumed that an individual with 300 mg/dl of serum IgG would be at high risk for developing infections with pyogenic bacteria. However, most such individuals are entirely healthy and free of infection. In fact, other investigations have indicated that 150 mg/dl of IgG is entirely adequate to prevent pyogenic infection. Thus, the physiologic normal range may not be related to the statistical normal range.

The interpretation of alterations in immune parameters is further complicated when one considers IgA deficiency. Approximately 1 in 500 individuals lack IgA and have no immunologically related disease problems. In contrast, other individuals with an IgA deficiency have problems with either upper respiratory, gastrointestinal, allergic, or autoimmune diseases. One account of this inconsistency is that the latter individuals have additional immunologic abnormalities which were not assayed. Thus, without knowing all of the immunologic abnormalities, one may wrongly associate an immune test result that is outside of the normal range with altered disease susceptibility.

The relationship of *in vitro* immune measures to disease susceptibility is also obscured by our limited knowledge of the relationship between different immunologic functions. For example, a decrease in the number of T-helper lymphocytes should increase susceptibility to pathogens which are held in check via T-cell-dependent pathways. However, it is not known how substantial a reduction in T-helper activity is required before cells dependent on that activity are unable to respond at a normal level. Relatedly, it is also not known whether the alteration of a single immune parameter is sufficient to increase the risk of disease susceptibility, or whether several alterations must occur simultaneously to produce a marked effect on the quality of health. Thus, we must determine the hierarchical relationship of the different immune mechanisms, as well as determine whether multiple immunologic alterations act additively or synergistically to increase susceptibility to infectious diseases, malignancy, or autoimmunity.

The complexity of making such a determination is magnified when one considers the methodology for the *in vitro* measurement of cellular components of the immune system. Not only are there no clear indications as to the amount of functional activity required to provide adequate resistance to infectious disease, but the optimum way of measuring *in vitro* cellular immune reactivity has not been determined. For example, the use of lymphocyte transformation to nonspecific mitogens as a test of lymphocyte function can be performed with whole blood cultures or separated lymphocytes. The cells can be cultured in autologous plasma, normal plasma of the same species, serum from a different species, or serum free medium. The assay conditions can be dramatically different across laboratories with regard to the type and concentration of mitogen, the duration of incubation, the duration of the radioactive pulse, the method of cell harvest, and the determination of radioactivity in cultured cells. To help overcome these problems, it is necessary for researchers in this field to study changes in several immune measures, to use disease models to observe changes in disease susceptibility, and to precisely report procedures and attempt to standardize all immunológic procedures.

STRESS AND DISEASE

Although there is substantial evidence that stress can alter immune function, there is very little evidence demonstrating a relationship between stress and disease pathogenesis. Recently, Moynihan and colleagues, at the University of Rochester, compared the survival rates of MRL-1pr/1pr mice that received electric shock with apparatus and home cage control animals (Moynihan et al., 1989). MRL-1pr/1pr mice develop autoimmunity that is characterized by the production of autoantibodies to a wide spectrum of self-antigens. These animals die beginning at approximately 20 weeks of age from complications related to their autoimmune status. The results indicated that electric footshock significantly prolonged the survival of these mice relative to the apparatus and home cage control.

We also have initiated a study investigating the ability of stress to alter the incidence and severity of a disease state. Our investigation employed an animal model of rheumatoid arthritis, adjuvant-induced arthritis. Arthritis can be induced in rats by the injection of complete Freunds adjuvant containing *Mycobacterium tuberculosis*. In approximately 14 to 16 d, 70 to 80% of normal rats begin to develop arthritis in one or more paws. The severity of the disease can be scored, based on swelling, redness, and deformity of the ankles using a 14-point scale. A score of 14 indicates very severe disease in all four paws and zero equals no change. The investigation of this disease is particularly relevant to our investigation of stressor-induced alteration of peripheral blood lymphocytes, as the disease is induced by circulating lymphocytes.

The results of a series of experiments conducted at the University of North Carolina, by Linda J. Luecken and Donald T. Lysle, showed that presentations of a CS on days 12, 14, and 16 following injection with adjuvant containing *Mycobacterium tuberculosis,* produced a pronounced suppression in the development of arthritis as measured by the clinical disease severity rating scale. In contrast, presentation of the CS on day 0, 2, and 4 following injection did not have any effect on the development of arthritis. These results demonstrate that a CS can alter the development of adjuvant-induced arthritis, but that the effect is dependent upon the timing of the antigen exposure and the presentation of the CS.

One of the paradoxical findings in the human literature is that a stressor decreases immunocompetence, but has been reported to increase the development of autoimmune disease. Our research provides some insight into that paradox, for it demonstrates that the temporal relationships of the stressor, the antigen exposure, and the disease onset, are important to the development of the disease and its symptoms.

SUMMARY

The aim of the research that has been described was to investigate the relationship between stressful stimulation and immune function in rodents. Although we have provided evidence that the relationship is ubiquitous, we are only beginning to understand the factors which control it. Our work has shown that the effect of stress on immune function is dependent on the amount of stressor presentation, as well as the compartment of the immune system used in the evaluation. Furthermore, it has indicated that psychological stress in the form of a conditioned aversive stimulus can induce alterations of immune function independent of physically aversive stimulation. To be cautious, we have identified that the species and strain of rodent used in the evaluation can influence the relationship.

We have also raised some issues about the meaningfulness of some of the immunologic procedures used in this area of research. There is very little evidence that procedures such as mitogen stimulation, antibody titers, and NK cell activity accurately predict resistance or susceptibility to disease. Our research, along with that of others, has demonstrated that stressful stimulation can have an effect on the pathogenesis of disease, but the relationship of those disease states to immune function is uncertain.

What is certain is that this area of research will remain a rich source of empirical inquiry, as well as a practical concern. Rodent models will assume an increasingly important role in the investigation of the relationship between stress and disease, for these models can be used to determine the importance of the different immune compartments in health and disease.

ACKNOWLEDGMENTS

This research was supported in part by Grants from the National Institutes of Mental Health (MH43411 and MH46284). A major part of the data reported in this chapter was collected while JEC and DTL were postdoctoral fellows at the University of Pittsburgh.

REFERENCES

Ackerman KD, Felten SY, and Bellinger DL: Noradrenergic sympathetic innervation of spleen and lymph nodes in relation to specific cellular compartments. *Prog Immunol* 1987; 6:588.

Alito AE, Carlomagno MA, Cardinali DP, and Braun M: Effect of regional sympathetic denervation on local immune reactions. *Fed Proc* 1985; 44:564.

Besedovsky HO, del Rey AE, Sorkin E, Da Prada M, and Keller HH: Immunoregulation mediated by the sympathetic nervous system. *Cell Immunol* 1979; 48:346.

Braun M, Alito A, Baler R, Romeo H, and Cardinali D: Effect of the autonomic nervous system on immune responses. In *Proc 6th Int Congr Immunology* (1986), p. 479.

Brown J: Effects of 2-deoxyglucose on carbohydrate metabolism: review of the literature and studies in the rat. *Metabolism* 1962; 11:1098.

Cunnick JE, Lysle DT, Armfield A, and Rabin BS: Shock-induced modulation of lymphocyte responsiveness and natural killer activity: differential mechanisms of induction. *Brain Behav Immun* 1988; 2:102.

Felten DL, Felten SY, Carlson SL, Olschowka JA, and Livnat S: Noradrenergic and peptidergic innervation of lymphoid tissue. *J Immunol* 1985; 135:755s.

Felten SY and Olschowka JA: Noradrenergic sympathetic innervation of the spleen. II. Tyrosine hydroxylase (TH)-positive nerve terminals form synaptic-like contacts on lymphocytes in the splenic white pulp. *J Neurosci Res* 1987; 18:37.

Himsworth RL: Compensatory reactions to a lack of metabolizable glucose. *J Physiol* 1968; 198:451.

Irwin J and Livnat S: Behavioral influences on the immune system: stress and conditioning. *Prog Neuropsychopharmacol Biol Psychiatry* 1987; 11:137.

Keller ES, Weiss JM, Schleifer SJ, Miller NE, and Stein LM: Suppression of immunity by stress: effect of a graded series of stressors on lymphocyte stimulation in the rat. *Science* 1981; 213:1397.

Lysle DT, Cunnick JE, Wu R, Caggiula AR, Wood PG and Rabin BS: 2-Deoxy-D-glucose modulation of T-lymphocyte reactivity: differential effects on lymphoid compartments. *Brain Behav Immun* 1988; 2:212.

Lysle DT, Cunnick JE, Fowler H, and Rabin BS: Pavlovian conditioning of shock-induced suppression of lymphocyte reactivity: acquisition, extinction, and preexposure effects. *Life Sci* 1988; 42:2185.

Lysle DT, Lyte M, Fowler H, and Rabin BS: Shock-induced modulation of lymphocyte reactivity: suppression, habituation, and recovery. *Life Sci* 1987; 41:1805.

Lubow RE: Latent inhibition. *Psychol Bull* 1973; 79:398.

Moynihan J, Schmidt S, Schachtman T, Grota L, Cohen N, and Ader R: Inescapable footshock stress prolongs survival of autoimmune MRL-1pr/1pr mice. Paper presented at 7th Int Congr Immunology. (1989).

Rabin BS, Lyte M, and Hamill E: The influence of mouse strain and housing on the immune response. *J Neuroimmunol* 1987; 17:11.

Ritter RC and Neville M: Hypothalamic noradrenaline turnover is increased during glucoprivic feeding. *Fed Proc* 1976; 35:642.

Shavit Y, Lewis JW, Terman GW, Gale RP, and Liebeskind JC: Opioid peptides mediate the suppressive effect of stress on natural killer cell cytoxicity. *Science* 1984; 223:188.

Smith GP and Epstein AN: Increased feeding in response to decreased glucose utilization in the rat and monkey. *Am J Physiol* 1969; 217:1082.

Smith GP and Root AW: Effects of feeding on hormonal responses to 2-deoxy-D-glucose with conscious monkeys. *Endocrinology* 1969; 85:963.

Chapter 33

Chronic Stress and the Immune Response

Will J. Kort and Ineke M. Weijma
*Laboratory for Experimental Surgery,
Erasmus University, Medical Faculty,
3000 DR Rotterdam, The Netherlands*

THE DEFINITIONS

Stress is a term that knows many definitions, but in the context of research on the pathophysiological effects, stress is mostly defined as "the reactions of the body to forces of a deleterious nature, infections and various abnormal states that tend to disturb its normal physiological equilibrium (homeostasis)" (Burgess, 1987; Sklar and Anisman, 1981; Stott, 1981; Riley, 1981). The stimulus that causes such a disruption is sometimes called "the stressor", but is very often called "stress" too. This implies that not only the reactions of the body are named "stress", but that stress is also defined as "the physical or psychological stimulus which when impinging upon an individual produced strain or disequilibrium". Although this may sound confusing, actually it does not appear to be a problem when the word stress is used for both concepts. In the present article, we have used the word stress in its second defined meaning, which implies that "we exposed our animals to stress", and that "the animals underwent stress".

The term stress may then be clear, but to fully understand the physiological consequences of stress, the type of stress has to be specified in substantial detail. Contradictory results were found, depending upon the nature of the stress stimuli. In order to obtain a certain classification of stress, stress was divided into a number of categories according to the nature and the severity of the stress. As such, acute and chronic stress were distinguished, which were further divided into a number of subcategories, e.g., unavoidable vs. avoidable, severe vs. mild, and physical vs. physiological. Furthermore, it seems logical that many types of physical stress will have direct metabolic consequences (e.g., cold exposure), which implies that such a type of stress is very specific in the nature of its effect on the individual's physiology, and therefore such a stress cannot be compared with any other type of stress.

INTRODUCTION TO STRESS

Much of the knowledge on stress was developed from animal experiments and it was, for instance, the pioneering animal studies of Rasmussen (1969), and of Solomon (1969), which produced evidence for the relationship between stress and decreased immunocompetence. These findings led others to investigate the role of stress-induced depression of immunity and cancer (Lahiri and Banerjee, 1986; Nieburgs et al., 1979; Shavit et al., 1985; Solomon and Amkraut, 1979; Tanemura et al., 1982). Also, there was evidence that such a relationship could be possible in man (Bartrop et al., 1977; Cox and MacKay, 1982; Goodkin et al., 1986; Grossart-Maticek et al., 1982; Levy et al., 1987; Richardson and Keeling, 1981; Yoshihara et al., 1986).

A role of stress in carcinogenesis in man has been suspected since long ago. Galen, in the second century, believed that melancholic women were more likely to develop cancer than those who were more confident and vital. The supposition that persons with a certain personality structure are more prone to stress and, as a result of this, to illness is still a concept that gets much attention (Bahnson, 1980; Bahnson, 1981; Cooper, 1984; Cox and MacKay, 1982; Grossart-Maticek et al., 1982). In this concept, the term "cancer-prone personality" was introduced, a term given for individuals with an inhibited lifestyle, melancholic and easily giving up, and the propensity to withdraw from unacceptable realities.

Also on the basis of epidemiologic studies in man, cancer and stress were associated. Substantial evidence was provided that environmental factors could contribute to cancer occurrence (Doll and Peto, 1981; Wynder and Gori, 1977; Wynder and Hirayama, 1977). Furthermore, in the context of environmental factors and cancer, stress was mentioned as an important risk to cancer (Doll and Peto, 1981; Higginson, 1980; Nieburgs et al., 1979; Phillips, 1975). Although stress-induced immunosuppression (by increased levels of adrenal hormones) seemed to most investigators the most plausible explanation for the stress-induced enhancement of cancer incidence (Cox and MacKay, 1982; Curti et al., 1982; Grossart-Maticek et al., 1982; Levy et al., 1987; Riley, 1981; Sklar and Anisman, 1981; Steplewski and Vogel, 1986), other explanations were forwarded as well, e.g., activation of the pituitary-adrenal and pituitary-thyroid axis (Armario et al., 1984) or release of opioid peptides (Shavit et al., 1985; Young and Akil, 1985).

STRESS INDUCTION IN ANIMAL MODELS

In experimental animals, many ways are available to induce stress. One of the most commonly used devices to induce stress is the shuttle box. This apparatus can be used to induce avoidable and unavoidable pain stress, mostly in acute or repeated stress experiments. Furthermore, stress is induced by swimming, restraint, isolation, overcrowding, light flashes, offensive noises, etc. Some of these forms of stress can also be used repeatedly, in such a way inducing chronic stress. For a more comprehensive treatise on the different methods of stress, we refer to the review articles on that subject by Borysenko and Borysenko (1982), Sklar and Anisman (1981), and Riley (1979).

Preferences for a particular method of stress are mostly personal considerations of a certain research group, although a number of general considerations should also be taken into account. In the first place, for ethical reasons, very harsh types of stress, such as long periods of cold swim stress, should not be allowed in any study. Moreover, neither type of extensive stress can be translated to "normal" stress situations in clinical practice, and should as such be banned in studies in experimental animals. Types of mild stress, such as proposed by Riley (1981), using a turntable device, will give a better reproducibility and liability of results and are not harmful procedures to the animals. Furthermore, it is important to realize that a certain basal level of stress is unavoidable; stress induced by handling, background noises, etc. will affect some stress parameters, such as corticosteroid levels (Riley, 1981; Gärtner et al., 1980). This means that baseline levels of stress should be kept as low as possible by minimizing the factors involved. If this is not possible, one should at least care to control the conditions in the animal rooms, and avoid subjecting certain animals to more background noises (e.g., from air conditioning) or not equally exposing them to light and temperature changes. It was also our experience that the social structure (pecking order) in a certain cage may influence baseline levels of stress. In long-term experiments, one can avoid such fluctuations in stress by randomizing the animals again after some time (Kort et al., 1986a).

In contrast to acute stress, it is difficult to expose animals to chronic stress effectively. Prolonged means of stress hostile and adverse to the animal will irrevocably lead to adaptation, whereas less hostile stress leads to habituation. To illustrate this problem, in an experiment on chronic noise stress, either loss of hearing occurred with severe stress or with mild noise stress, habituation (Borg and Moller, 1978). To overcome this problem, we preferred for our studies on stress and cancer (Kort et al., 1982, 1986a, 1986b; Kort and Weijma, 1982) a way of unavoidable physiological stress, light-dark (L/D) shift stress. Reversing the L/D cycle of man and animal interferes with the individual's sleep-wakefulness pattern and as such with eating and drinking behavior as well (Glantz, 1967). Hormone levels and those of other metabolites following a circadian rhythm have to be reset. Hence, rats undergoing repeated L/D shifting are exposed to changes of homeostasis, and with each shift homeostasis will necessarily be altered again. Because adaptation to light and dark comes about endogenously, this will not lead to habituation of the biological system. In experiments in which L/D shifts were studied, it was found that reestablishment of the eating and drinking pattern took place after 7 to 9 d (Zucker, 1971), which means that weekly shifting permanently leads to adaptation to the new L/D regimen.

Another attractive aspect of the method of L/D shift stress is its simplicity. Where other possible methods of chronic stress give many logistic problems when carried out for long periods of time, such as is the case with repeated bleeding, isolation stress, etc., L/D shift is carried out by simply altering the timer controlling light and dark in the animal room. Only one problem had to be coped with, handling of the animals during daytime when they are in the dark phase. This was overcome by doing all necessary handling by infrared lighting.

Control animals were housed in an animal room identical to the L/D shift room in terms of background noise, light intensity, and number of hours of light and dark.

MEASUREMENT OF STRESS

Most often, stress is measured by determining adrenal hormone levels. Stress and increased corticosteroid levels are very closely related, and sometimes stress is not called stress until increased corticosterone levels are detected. However, although this may be true for acute stress, it certainly is not for chronic stress; in chronic stress, decreased levels of corticosterone were found more often. Apart from other parameters that are directly or indirectly associated with adrenal activity, such as immunity, and hormones other than corticosteroids and adrenalin, it seems to be particularly sensible to use those parameters that are directly related to the stress type involved. This means that in stress experiments on water deprivation, renal function should be measured, and in our experiments, with a stress type that deregulates eating and drinking behavior, body weights or blood glucose values should be determined.

CHRONIC STRESS AND THE IMMUNE RESPONSE

When compared to acute stress, chronic stress seems to have opposing effects on many parameters of stress, but the effect on the immune system is uniformly found to be the same in both types of stress, e.g., suppressed

TABLE I.
Determinations After 7 and 52 Weekly L/D Shifts

	Stress Mean ± SEM (n)	Controls
7 Weeks		
Peripheral Lymphocytes (× 10⁶/ml)	5.4 ± 0.2 (20)	9.3 ± 0.7 (20)*
ConA Stimulation (counts/min/culture)	13,106 ± 2,964 (10)	43,439 ± 5,130 (10)*
PLNA (mg)	29.2 ± 1.4 (10)	37.0 ± 1.8 (10)*
52 Weeks		
Peripheral Lymphocytes (× 10⁶/ml)	4.3 ± 0.2 (10)	5.3 ± 0.7 (10)**
ConA Stimulation (counts/min/culture)	25,822 ± 5,427 (10)	59,945 ± 13,375 (10)*
PLNA (mg)	22.5 ± 1.1 (10)	25.2 ± 1.5 (10)

Note: PLNA = popliteal lymph node assay.
* Statistically significantly different ($p < 0.01$).
** Statistically significantly different ($p < 0.05$).

(Armario et al., 1984; Borg, 1978; Dorian and Garfunkel, 1987; Godkin et al., 1986; Lahiri and Banerjee, 1986; Stott, 1981; Steplewski and Vogel, 1986). The latter finding was confirmed in our studies (Kort et al., 1982; Kort and Weijma, 1982). In these studies, we used the method of L/D shift to test alterations in a number of immune and endocrine parameters.

For this purpose, we measured plasma corticosterone, corticosterone synthesis capacity *in vitro,* blood glucose, peripheral blood leucocyte, and concanavalin A stimulation of peripheral blood (ConA) and popliteal lymph node assay (PLNA), the latter two expressing the cellular immune response. Moreover, the spleen and adrenal glands were weighed at autopsy.

Cellular immune response measured after seven weekly L/D shifts (the number of shifts given to the animals in which transplantable tumors were inoculated) and after 1 year of stress showed (Table I) that the cellular immune response was significantly inhibited in those animals receiving L/D shift stress. Also, the number of peripheral lymphocytes was substantially decreased in the rats under stress.

After 35 weeks of L/D shift stress, and with other parameters, the results showed (Table II) that serum corticosterone was not affected, and the corticosterone *in vitro* assay even showed slightly decreased values. These results confirm the findings of many other investigators that chronic stress, in contrast to acute stress, does not augment corticosterone values (Armario et al., 1984; Monjan and Collector, 1977; Sklar and Anisman, 1981; Stott, 1981).

However, other parameters did show statistically significant differences, e.g., blood glucose values were statistically significantly decreased in the L/D-shifted rats. At autopsy, when adrenal glands and spleens were weighed, the adrenal gland weights of L/D-shifted rats showed a statistically significant decrease, but spleen weights were the same in both experimental groups (Table II). Also, body weights showed a retardation in the L/D-shifted rats.

We concluded from these results that L/D shift is an effective way to induce chronic stress with direct consequences of immunological alterations, implying that diseases associated with changes in the immune capacity may be altered in incidence or severity. With regard to the hormonal alterations measured (corticosterone and insulin), differences between L/D shift-stressed animals and controls were small and do not seem to be significant.

STRESS AND SPONTANEOUS TUMOR INCIDENCE

Due to the many logistic problems that one encounters when the effect of chronic stress is studied in models of spontaneous tumors, these models have not been used very often. Still, this particular experimental design may be the best approach for those wanting to study a possible connection between psychological stress and cancer in humans. The BN rat strain shows a spontaneous tumor incidence with large variations according to tumor site, and one may expect to find a total tumor incidence of 70 to 80% (Burek, 1978). When spontaneous tumor incidence is taken as a model, not only can tumor incidence be established, but also growth pattern and the age of the rat at the time of tumor incidence.

All these arguments were enough reason for us to study a possible association between chronic stress and cancer in the model of spontaneous tumor incidence in the BN female rat (Kort et al., 1986a). For this purpose, 100

TABLE II.
Determination After 35 Weekly L/D Shifts

	Stress Mean ± SEM (n)	Controls
Serum Corticosterone (μg/100 ml)	39.0 ± 3.3 (9)	38.0 ± 3.4 (10)
Corticosterone *in vitro* (μg/100 mg adrenal gland/h)	17.5 ± 0.9 (21)	19.5 ± 1.2 (19)
Plasma Insulin (mmol/l)	21.6 ± 2.8 (10)	17.3 ± 9.0 (10)
Blood Glucose (mmol/l)	4.9 ± 0.1 (39)	5.5 ± 0.2 (40)*
Adrenal Glands L + R (mg)	45.3 ± 0.6 (39)	51.5 ± 0.8 (40)*
Spleen (mg)	337.6 ± 5.3 (39)	344.5 ± 6.6 (40)
Body Weight (g)	177.3 ± 1.4 (39)	183.7 ± 1.6 (40)*

* Statistically significantly different (blood glucose, $p < 0.05$; adrenal gland weight, $p < 0.001$; body weight, $p < 0.01$)

TABLE III.
Incidence of Spontaneous Tumor and Mean Age

Tumors	Mean Age ± SEM (weeks) and Tumor Incidence			
	Stress	n	Controls	n
Tumor (general)	138.5 ± 2.2	74	140.5 ± 2.5	85
Mammary Gland	132.2 ± 5.0	15	120.8 ± 6.9	19
Adrenal Cortex	138.7 ± 5.3	11	135.6 ± 4.0	14
Adrenal Medulla	142.0 ± 5.4	6	137.1 ± 7.2	8
Pituitary Gland	138.4 ± 2.7	32	142.4 ± 2.1	29
Pancreas Islets	148.4 ± 0.9	25	147.1 ± 1.2	21
Cervix/Uterus	121.9 ± 8.7	9	136.1 ± 5.0	17
Lymphoreticular System	128.2 ± 4.8	13	117.1 ± 7.0	11

Note: No statistically significant differences; n = number of animals.

TABLE IV.
Incidence of Nontumor Processes and Mean Age

Nontumor Process	Mean Age ± SEM (weeks) and Nontumor Incidence			
	Stress	n	Controls	n
Uterine Infection	130.0 ± 14.4	8	140.6 ± 4.1	10
Hydronephrosis	135.4 ± 2.5	52	136.8 ± 2.8	49
Biliary Cysts	137.5 ± 3.6	35	137.1 ± 2.7	49
Pancreatic Atrophy	144.0 ± 3.6	14	134.4 ± 4.5	22
Mammary Hyperplasia	136.4 ± 2.6	49	139.8 ± 1.9	53
Cardiac Ischemia	137.1 ± 3.8	14	135.8 ± 3.0	22

Note: No statistical significant differences; n = number of animals.

BN female rats underwent L/D shift stress during their whole lifespan (from weaning to maximally 150 weeks). A control group received a standard lighting regimen (7 a.m.—7 p.m., light; 7 p.m.—7 a.m., dark).

The survival curves of both groups were almost identical. There were no significant differences in the tumor incidence rates of the most frequently encountered tumors (Table III), nor in the mean age of the animals at tumor occurrence. Furthermore, the incidence of nontumor processes, for which at least uterine infection might have had some relation with impaired immunity, did not show any difference as well (Table IV). Body weights of animals undergoing stress were statistically significantly different from the control group from week 20 onwards, reaching a maximum difference of 15 g at termination (mean ± SEM: 222 ± 2.8 vs. 237 ± 3.0 g for L/D shift and controls, respectively). These results confirm the particular findings in our previous experiments. Again, differences in the adrenal gland weights were not statistically significant (mean ± SEM: 74 ± 1.8 vs. 78 ± 2.6 g for L/D shift and controls, respectively).

An important disadvantage of models of spontaneous tumors in the rat is the fact that only a very limited number of tumors that arise do metastasize (Table V). This implies that this particular aspect of carcinogenesis can hardly be studied in spontaneous tumor models, and can be studied more accurately in transplantable tumor models with metastatic capacities. The only tumor in this rat strain with a high metastatic rate is the adrenal cortical carcinoma, which was found in five of nine and three of nine animals in the L/D-shifted and control groups, respectively. No statistically significant differences in metastasis were seen.

We concluded that chronic stress does seem to impede tumor incidence or longevity in rats. On the contrary, in light of the results of the total tumor incidence, one may even draw the conclusion that stress has a slightly inhibiting effect on cancer, a conclusion that is confirmed by other investigators using different types of chronic stress and other models (Lahiri and Banerjee, 1986; Nieburgs et al., 1979; Sklar and Anisman, 1979), and also by us with the results of L/D shift stress in transplantable tumor models (Kort et al., 1986b).

STRESS AND TRANSPLANTABLE TUMOR GROWTH

As a next step in our effort to determine a possible relationship between stress and cancer, L/D shift stress was given to rats into which transplantable tumors were inoculated (Kort et al., 1986b). For this, 6-week-old BN female rats underwent L/D shift stress from 7 weeks prior to tumor inoculation until the animals were sacrificed. The rats received one of the following types of

TABLE V.
Number of Tumors Found with Distant Metastases

	Total No. Tumors/ No. Tumors with Metastases	
	Stress	Control
Adrenal Gland (cortical carcinoma)	9/5	9/3
Adrenal Gland (medullary pheochromacytoma)	6/0	8/1
Pancreas (Langerhans islet carcinoma)	2/1	1/0
Bone (osteosarcoma)	1/1	—

Note: No statistically significant differences. The tumors were metastasized to lungs (cortical carcinoma, medullary pheochromacytoma), liver (cortical carcinoma), brains (cortical carcinoma), and pleura (Langerhans islet carcinoma).

TABLE VI.
Characteristics of Transplantable Tumor Models[a]

	BN175	BN248	BN569	BN1312	WR1618
Weeks before take[b]	<1	1	2	1	1
Growth rate[c]	4	7	14	1–2	13
Immunogenicity	Neg	Neg	Neg	Neg	Pos
Morphology[d]	Mes	Mes	Epi	Mes	Epi
Strain	BN	BN	BN	BN	WR
Metastasizing	Pos	Neg	Neg	Neg	Neg
Hormone response	Pos	Neg	Neg	Pos	Neg
Original	Soft	Cervix,	Ureter	Lympho-	Skin
anatomical site[e]	tissue	uterus		ret.	
	pancreas			system	

[a] Rats on standard housing conditions.
[b] Number of weeks before detectable tumor growth.
[c] Number of days between tumor size 10 mm and 20 mm, except for tumor BN1312, for which was taken the number of days between 5×10^5 and 1×10^6 tumor cells in the spleen.
[d] Mes = mesenchymal tumor; epi = epithelial tumor.
[e] BN175 grew more rapidly in female rats; BN1312 grew more rapidly in ovariectomized and in adrenalectomized rats. BN248, BN569, and WR1618 did not show any difference in tumor growth, either inoculated in male or in female rats.

tumor inoculae: leiomyosarcoma, squamous cell carcinoma, basal cell carcinoma, fibrosarcoma, or a myeloid leukemia. The biological characteristics of these tumors with regard to hormonal responsiveness, metastatic behavior, etc. are summarized in Table VI.

The fibrosarcoma (BN175) and the myeloid leukemia (BN1312) showed a retardation of tumor growth in those rats receiving L/D shift stress, compared with the control rats (Table VII). No significant differences in tumor growth by L/D shift stress were observed in the other tumor models, despite the fact that among these tumors one, the WR1618, was immunogenic.

Both "stress-responsive" tumors were distinguished from the other ones by the fact that these two tumors had proved to be "hormone responsive" (hormone responsiveness was established in parallel experiments, by determining differences in tumor growth between control rats and rats that were either adrenalectomized or ovariectomized). Hence, it seems logical to consider that this fact in particular may have contributed to the different growth characteristics of the myeloid leukemia and the fibrosarcoma.

The metastatic behavior of tumor BN175, the one tumor that metastasizes spontaneously when inoculated subcutaneously, was not statistically different in either L/D shift-stressed rats or controls. Nevertheless, the mean score (rating, 0 to 5) of the number of metastatic nodules in the L/D-shifted rats was less than that of the controls (mean ± SEM [n]: 2.7 ± 0.3 [10] vs. 3.7 ± 0.4 [10] for L/D shift stress and controls, respectively). This indicates that it is certainly out of the question that mild stress enhances tumor metastasis. However, in a study of acute stress and tumor metastasis, Tanemura et al. (1982) found an increase in the number of metastases, whereas Zimel et al. (1977), with a model of chronic stress, confirmed our results.

The results of our experiments on mild chronic stress, both in spontaneous and transplantable tumor models in the rat, strengthen our belief that chronic stress does not lead to enhanced tumor growth or incidence, although it still may be detrimental to other illnesses, particularly those mediated by an impaired immune capacity.

DISCUSSION

Chronic stress, unlike acute stress, does not lead to enhanced tumor incidence or growth. One may criticize this statement on the basis of our results and may argue, for instance, that the type of stress given was too weak to induce measurable stress effects. However, in the first place, our findings are in line with those of other investigators on chronic stress and cancer (Lahiri and Banerjee, 1986; Nieburgs et al., 1979; Sklar and Anisman, 1979), and it seems, therefore, that the found enhancement of cancer is restricted to acute stress or repeated stress (Bahnson, 1980, 1981; Riley, 1981; Shavit et al., 1985; Sklar and Anisman, 1981). Second, it is our opinion that one should not exaggerate stress conditions in animal studies, as we believe that such conditions are not comparable to any stress situation in humans. Third, the model of L/D shift stress has its human equal. Shift work is considered a stressful situation, with many social and medical implications (Åkerstedt, 1977; Curti et al., 1982; Koller, 1983; Smith and Colligan, 1982; Winget et al., 1978). It will be clear that exclusively physiological conse-

TABLE VII.
Growth Rate After L/D Shift Stress

Tumors	Stress tgα ± SEM	Controls
BN175	17.7 ± 1.4 (10)	21.4 ± 1.1 (10)*
BN248	10.8 ± 0.7 (9)	11.5 ± 0.6 (8)
BN569	4.5 ± 0.3 (9)	4.8 ± 0.6 (7)
BN1312	1854.5 ± 75.4 (10)	2220.7 ± 50.3 (10)
WR1618	5.3 ± 0.5 (9)	5.6 ± 0.5 (6)*

Note: Growth of tumors BN248, BN569, and WR1618 is given as the mean of the individual tgα values (tgα is the regression coefficient of the linear regression plotted from the individual's weekly tumor sizes), BN1312 is given as the mean spleen weight at day of termination, and BN175 is given as mean tumor size (mean of length and width) at day 7.

* Statistically significantly different ($p < 0.05$).

quences of shift stress can be mimicked in animal models, and not the psychological disturbances, but it is our opinion that mimicking psychological stress in an animal model is not possible.

It is as yet unclear which forms of stress in humans have to be considered acute stress, and which as chronic ones. Hospitalization, surgery, or bereavement could be acute stress, whereas persons with certain psychological characteristics might be considered to suffer from chronic stress. Therefore, the often-observed negative effect of surgery on cancer patients could have been the result of acute stress, caused by anesthesia, tissue damage, blood loss, blood transfusions, etc. (Lundy, 1980; Tanemura et al., 1982; Yoshihara et al., 1986).

Although mild chronic stress may be relatively insignificant with respect to cancer risk, its importance to other diseases will have to be considered carefully. After all, it seems that chronic stress does increase the susceptibility to coronary heart disease and bacterial or virus diseases (Alfredson et al., 1982; Koller, 1983; Smith and Colligan, 1982).

Consequences of (Unwanted) Stress in Animal Experiments

Results of animal experiments uniformly show large variations. This fact has been ascribed to biological variations, but environmental conditions, i.e., the conditions of the animal in the animal room, pre- and post-operatively, will be of importance too. Many investigators will confirm that although conditions are optimized as much as possible using SPF (specified pathogen-free) animals, inbred strains of animals, controlled lighting and air conditioning in animal houses, etc. — large variations in results still will occur.

One such variation we made a subject of study (Kort et al., 1976, 1979). In studies of allogenic kidney transplantation in rats, large variations were found in the untreated control groups. Despite the fact that no immunosuppressive treatment was given, 10% of the animals lived much longer than the "normal" rejection time of 10 to 12 d. As we could not think of explanations for the found variation other than differences in post-operative stress, we willingly varied stress post-operatively in order to investigate the effect of stress on kidney graft survival. The results showed that kidney graft survival was significantly enhanced when 1 d of restraint stress was given. This meant that only a relatively slight variation in the post-operative stress was able to induce immunosuppressive alterations that prolonged kidney graft survival. These results once again show the importance of controlling baseline levels of stress — not only in experiments on stress, as was earlier emphasized by Riley (1981), but also in experiments in which alterations of the immune system may have important consequences on the results.

REFERENCES

Åkerstedt T: Inversion of sleep wakefulness pattern: effects on circadian variations in psychophysiological activation. *Ergonomics* 1977; 20:459.

Alfredsson L, Karasek R, and Theorell T: Myocardial infarction risk and psychosocial work environment: an analysis of the male Swedish working force. *Swed Soc Sci Med* 1982; 16:463.

Armario A, Castellanos JM, and Balasch J: Effect of acute and chronic psychogenic stress on corticoadrenal and pituitary-thyroid hormones in male rats. *Horm Res* 1984; 20:241.

Bahnson CB: Stress and cancer: the state of the art. I. *Psychosomatics* 1980; 21:975.

Bahnson CB: Stress and cancer: the state of the art. II. *Psychosomatics* 1981; 22:207.

Bartrop RW, Lazarus L, Luckhurst E, and Kiloh LG: Depressed lymphocyte function after bereavement. *Lancet* 1977; 1:834.

Borg E and Moller AR: Noise and blood pressure: effect of lifelong exposure in the rat. *Acta Physiol Scand* 1978; 103:340.

Borysenko M and Borysenko J: Stress, behavior, and immunity: animal models and mediating mechanisms. *Gen Hosp Psychiatry* 1982; 4:59.

Burchfield SR, Woods SC, and Elich MS: Pituitary adrenocortical response to chronic intermittant stress. *Physiol Behav* 1980; 24:297.

Burek JD: *Pathology of Aging Rats* CRC Press, Boca Raton, FL (1979).

Burgess C: Stress and cancer. *Cancer Surv* 1987; 6:403.

Chang S-S and Rasmussen AF: Stress-induced suppression of interferon production in virus-infected mice. *Nature* 1965; 205:623.

Cooper CL: The social-psychological precursors to cancer. *J Hum Stress* 1984; 10:4.

Cox T and MacKay C: Psychosocial factors and psychophysiological mechanisms in the aetiology and development of cancers. *Soc Sci Med* 1982; 16:381.

Curti R, Radice L, Cesane GC, Zanettini R, and Grieco A: Work stress and immune system: lymphocyte reactions during rotating shift work. Preliminary results. *Med Lav* 1982; 6:564.

Doll R and Peto R: The causes of cancer: quantitative estimates of avoidable risks of cancer in the United States today. *JNCI* 1981; 66:1191.

Dorian B and Garfinkel PE: Stress, immunity and illness — a review. *Psychol Med* 1987; 17:393.

Gärtner K, Büttner D, Döhler K, Friedel R, Lindena J, and Trautschold I: Stress response of rats to handling and experimental procedures. *Lab Anim* 1980; 14:267.

Glantz RM: Circadian rhythms in the albino rat: effect of illumination on urine excretion, water intake, and the formation of antidiuretic hormone. *Physiol Behav* 1967; 2:49.

Goodkin K, Antoni MH, and Blaney PH: Stress and hopelessness in the promotion of cervical intraepithelial neoplasia to invasive squamous cell carcinoma of the cervix. *J Psychosom Res* 1986; 30:67.

Grossart-Maticek R, Kanazir DT, Schmidt P, and Vetter H: Psychosomatic factors and psychophysiological mechanisms in the aetiology and development of cancers. *Psychother Psychosom* 1982; 38:284.

Higginson J: Importance of environmental and occupational factors in cancer. *J Toxicol Environ Health* 1980; 6:941.

Koller M: Health risks related to shift work. An example of time-contingent effects of long-term stress. *Int Arch Occup Environ Health* 1983; 53:59.

Kort WJ, van Dongen JJ, and Westbroek DL: The effect of stress on the survival of grafted organs. *Microchirugie* 1976; 1:21.

Kort WJ, Weijma IM, and Westbroek DL: Effect of stress and dietary fatty acids on allograft survival in the rat. *Eur Surg Res* 1979; 11:434.

Kort WJ and Weijma IM: Effect of chronic light-dark shift stress on the immune response of the rat. *Physiol Behav* 1982; 29:1083.

Kort WJ, Weijma IM, Bijma AM, and Westbroek DL: Effect of chronic stress, dietary linoleic acid on immune response and tumor growth in rats. *Langenbecks Arch Chir* 1982; 357:194.

Kort WJ, Zondervan PE, Hulsman LO, Weijma IM and Westbroek DL: Light-dark shift stress, with special reference to spontaneous tumor incidence in female BN rats. *JNCI* 1986a; 76:439.

Kort WJ, Weijma IM, Zondervan PE, and Westbroek DL: The effect of chronic stress on tumor growth: an experimental study in the rat. *J Exp Clin Cancer Res* 1986b; 5:233.

Lahiri T and Banerjee M: Differential responses of carcinogen-induced fibrosarcoma of mice to altered regimes of cold exposure. *Neoplasma* 1986; 33:307.

Levy S, Herberman R, Lippman M, and d'Angelo T: Correlation of stress factors with sustained depression of natural killer cell activity and predicted prognosis in patients with breast cancer. *J Clin Oncol* 1987; 5:348.

Lundy J: Anesthesia and surgery: a double-edged sword for the cancer patient. *J Surg Oncol* 1980; 14:61.

Monjan AA and Collector MI: Stress-induced modulation of the immune response. *Science* 1977; 196:307.

Nieburgs HE, Weiss J, Navarette M, Strax P, Teirstein A, Grillione G, and Siedlechi B: The role of stress in human and experimental oncogenesis. *Cancer Detect Prev* 1979; 2:307.

Phillips RL: Role of life-style and dietary habits in risks of cancer among Seventh Day Adventists. *Cancer Res* 1975; 35:3513.

Rasmussen AF: Emotions and immunity. *Ann NY Acad Sci* 1969; 164:458.

Richardson J and Keeling M: The mechanism of stress and immunosuppression. *Med Hypoth* 1981; 7:765.

Riley V: Cancer and stress: overview and critique. *Cancer Detect Prev* 1979; 2:163.

Riley V: Psychoneuroendocrine influences on immunocompetence and neoplasia. *Science* 1981; 212:1100.

Shavit Y, Terman GW, Martin FC, Lewis JW, Liebeskind JC and Gale RP: Stress, opioid peptides, and the immune system, and cancer. *J Immunol* 1985; 135:834a.

Sklar LS and Anisman H: Stress and cancer. *Psychol Bull* 1981; 89:369.

Smith MJ and Colligan MJ: Health and safety consequences of shift work in the food processing industry. *Ergonomics* 1982; 25:133.

Solomon GF: Stress and antibody response in rats. *Int Arch Allergy Appl Immunol* 1969; 35:97.

Solomon GF and Amkraut AA: Neuroendocrine aspects of the immune response and their implications for stress effects on tumor immunity. *Cancer Detect Prev* 1979; 2:197.

Steplewski Z and Vogel WH: Total leukocytes, T cell subpopulation and natural killer (NK) cell activity in rats exposed to restraint stress. *Life Sci* 1986; 38:2419.

Stott GH: What is animal stress and how is it measured? *J Anim Sci* 1981; 52:150.

Tanemura H, Sakata K, Kunieda T, Saji S, Yamamoto S, and Takekoshi T: Influences of operative stress on cell-mediated immunity and on tumor metastasis and their prevention by nonspecific immunotherapy: experimental studies in rats. *J Surg Oncol* 1982; 21:189.

Winget C, Hughes L, and Ladou J: Physiological effects of rotational work shifting: a review. *JOM* 1978; 20:204.

Wynder EL and Gori GB: Guest editorial. Contribution of the environment to cancer incidence: an epidemiologic exercise. *J Natl Cancer Inst* 1977; 58:825.

Wynder EL and Hirayama T: A comparative epidemiologic study of the United States and Japan with special reference to cancer. *Prev Med* 1977; 6:567.

Yoshihara H, Tanaka N, and Orita K: Suppression of natural killer cell activity by surgical stress in cancer patients and the underlying mechanisms. *Acta Med Okayama* 1986; 40:113.

Young E and Akil H: Changes in releasability of ACTH and beta-endorphin with chronic stress. *Neuropeptides* 1985; 5:545.

Zimel H, Zimel A, Petrescu R, Ghinea E, and Tasca C: Influence of stress and of endocrine imbalance on the experimental metastasis. *Neoplasia* 1977; 24:151.

Zucker I: Light-dark rhythms in rat eating and drinking behavior. *Physiol Behav* 1971; 6:115.

Index

INDEX

A